Core Curriculum for Nephrology Nursing

Sixth Edition

Editor: Caroline S. Counts, MSN, RN, CNN

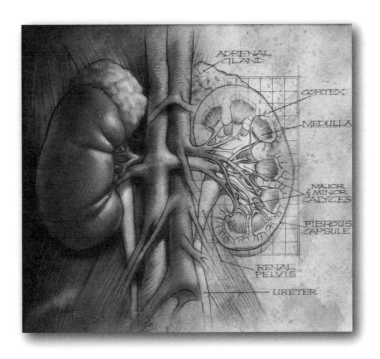

MODULE 3

Treatment Options for Patients with Chronic Kidney Failure

ANNA American Nephrology Nurses' Association
www.annanurse.org

Core Curriculum for Nephrology Nursing, 6th Edition

Editor and Project Director
Caroline S. Counts, MSN, RN, CNN

MODULE 3 • Treatment Options for Patients with Chronic Kidney Failure

Publication Management
Anthony J. Jannetti, Inc.
East Holly Avenue/Box 56
Pitman, New Jersey 08071-0056

Managing Editor: Claudia Cuddy
Editorial Coordinator: Joseph Tonzelli
Layout Design and Production: Claudia Cuddy
Layout Assistants: Kaytlyn Mroz, Katerina DeFelice, Casey Shea, Courtney Klauber
Design Consultants: Darin Peters, Jack M. Bryant
Proofreaders: Joseph Tonzelli, Evelyn Haney, Alex Grover, Nicole Ward
Cover Design: Darin Peters
Cover Illustration: Scott M. Holladay © 2006
Photography: Kim Counts and Marty Morganello (*unless otherwise credited*)

ANNA National Office Staff
Executive Director: Michael Cunningham
Director of Membership Services: Lou Ann Leary
Membership/Marketing Services Coordinator: Lauren McKeown
Manager, Chapter Services: Janet Betts
Education Services Coordinator: Kristen Kellenyi
Executive Assistant & Marketing Manager, Advertising: Susan Iannelli
Co-Directors of Education Services: Hazel A. Dennison and Sally Russell
Program Manager, Special Projects: Celess Tyrell
Director, Jannetti Publications, Inc.: Kenneth J. Thomas
Managing Editor, *Nephrology Nursing Journal*: Carol Ford
Editorial Coordinator, *Nephrology Nursing Journal*: Joseph Tonzelli
Subscription Manager, *Nephrology Nursing Journal*: Rob McIlvaine
Managing Editor, *ANNA Update, ANNA E-News,* & Web Editor: Kathleen Thomas
Director of Creative Design & Production: Jack M. Bryant
Layout and Design Specialist: Darin Peters
Creative Designer: Bob Taylor
Director of Public Relations and Association Marketing Services: Janet D'Alesandro
Public Relations Specialist: Rosaria Mineo
Vice President, Fulfillment and Information Services: Rae Ann Cummings
Director, Internet Services: Todd Lockhart
Director of Corporate Marketing: Tom Greene
Exhibit Coordinator: Miriam Martin
Conference Manager: Jeri Hendrie
Comptroller: Patti Fortney

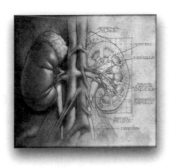

Foreword

The American Nephrology Nurses' Association has had a long-standing commitment to providing the tools and resources needed for individuals to be successful in their professional nephrology roles. With that commitment, we proudly present the sixth edition of the *Core Curriculum for Nephrology Nursing*.

This edition has a new concept and look that we hope you find valuable. Offered in six separate modules, each one will focus on a different component of our specialty and provide essential, updated, high-quality information. Since our last publication of the *Core Curriculum* in 2008, our practice has evolved, and our publication has been transformed to keep pace with those changes.

Under the expert guidance of Editor and Project Director Caroline S. Counts, MSN, RN, CNN (who was also the editor for the 2008 *Core Curriculum*!), this sixth edition continues to build on our fundamental principles and standards of practice. From the basics of each modality to our roles in advocacy, patient engagement, evidence-based practice, and more, you will find crucial information to facilitate the important work you do on a daily basis.

The ANNA Board of Directors and I extend our sincerest gratitude to Caroline and commend her for the stellar work that she and all of the section editors, authors, and reviewers have put forth in developing this new edition of the *Core Curriculum for Nephrology Nursing*. These individuals have spent many hours working to provide you with this important nephrology nursing publication. We hope you enjoy this exemplary professional resource.

Sharon Longton, BSN, RN, CNN, CCTC
ANNA President, 2014-2015

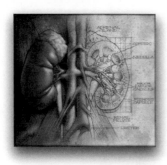

What's new in the sixth edition?

The 2015 edition of the *Core Curriculum for Nephrology Nursing* reflects several changes in format and content. These changes have been made to make life easier for the reader and to improve the scientific value of the *Core*.

1. The *Core Curriculum* is divided into six separate modules that can be purchased as a set or as individual texts. Keep in mind there is likely additional relevant information in more than one module. For example, in Module 2 there is a specific chapter for nutrition, but the topic of nutrition is also addressed in several chapters in other modules.

2. The *Core* is available in both print and electronic formats. The electronic format contains links to other websites with additional helpful information that can be reached with a simple click. With this useful feature comes a potential issue: when an organization changes its website and reroutes its links, the URLs that are provided may not connect. When at the organization's website, use their search feature to easily find your topic. The links in the *Core* were updated as of March 2015.

3. As with the last edition of the *Core*, the pictures on chapter covers depict actual nephrology staff members and patients with kidney disease. Their willingness to participate is greatly appreciated.

4. Self-assessment questions are included at the end of each module for self-testing. Completion of these exercises is not required to obtain CNE. CNE credit can be obtained by accessing the Evaluation Forms on the ANNA website.

5. References are cited in the text and listed at the end of each chapter.

6. We've provided examples of references in APA format at the beginning of each chapter, as well as on the last page of this front matter, to help the readers know how to properly format references if they use citations from the *Core*. The guesswork has been eliminated!

7. The information contained in the *Core* has been expanded, and new topics have been included. For example, there is information on leadership and management, material on caring for Veterans, more emphasis on patient and staff safety, and more.

8. Many individuals assisted in making the *Core* come to fruition; they brought with them their own experience, knowledge, and literature search. As a result, a topic can be addressed from different perspectives, which in turn gives the reader a more global view of nephrology nursing.

9. This edition employs usage of the latest terminology in nephrology patterned after the National Kidney Foundation.

10. The *Core Curriculum for Nephrology Nursing*, 6th edition contains 233 figures, 234 tables, and 29 appendices. These add valuable tools in delivering the contents of the text.

Thanks to B. Braun Medical Inc. for its grant in support of ANNA's *Core Curriculum*.

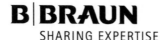

SHARING EXPERTISE

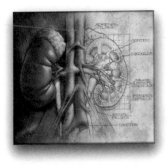

Preface

The sixth edition of the *Core Curriculum for Nephrology Nursing* has been written and published due to the efforts of many individuals. Thank you to the editors, authors, reviewers, and everyone who helped pull the *Core* together to make it the publication it became. A special thank you to Claudia Cuddy and Joe Tonzelli, who were involved from the beginning to the end — I could not have done my job without them!

The overall achievement is the result of the unselfish contributions of each and every individual team member. At times it was a daunting, challenging task, but the work is done, and all members of the "Core-team" should feel proud of the end product.

Now, the work is turned over to you — the reader and learner. I hope you learn at least half as much as I did as pieces of the *Core* were submitted, edited, and refined. Considering the changes that have taken place since the first edition of the *Core* in 1987 (322 pages!), one could say it is a whole new world! Even since the fifth edition in 2008, many changes in nephrology have transpired. This, the 2015 edition, is filled with the latest information regarding kidney disease, its treatment, and the nursing care involved.

But, buyer, beware! Evolution continues, and what is said today can be better said tomorrow. Information continues to change and did so even as the chapters were being written; yet, change reflects progress. Our collective challenge is to learn from the *Core*, be flexible, keep an open mind, and question what could be different or how nephrology nursing practice could be improved.

Nephrology nursing will always be stimulating, learning will never end, and progress will continue! So, the *Core* not only represents what we know now, but also serves as a springboard for what the learner can become and what nephrology nursing can be. A Chinese proverb says this: "Learning is like rowing upstream; not to advance is to drop back."

A final thank-you to the Core-team and a very special note of appreciation to those I love the most. (Those I love the most have also grown since the last edition!) For their love, support, and encouragement, I especially thank my husband, Henry, who thought I had retired; my son and daughter-in law, Chris and Christina, and our two amazing grandchildren, Cate and Olin; and my son-in-law, Marty Morganello, and our daughter, Kim, who provided many of the photographs used in this version of the *Core*. It has been a family project!

Last, but certainly not least, I thank the readers and learners. It is your charge to use the *Core* to grow your minds. Minds can grow as long as we live — don't drop back!

Caroline S. Counts
Editor, Sixth Edition

Module 3

The contents in Module 3 took me on a trip down memory lane. I began my career in nephrology nursing on August 23, 1970. I still remember my reaction when I walked into the unit on that day: "What have I done? I will never learn all of this equipment!" Patients were dialyzing on what looked like washing machines. The dialysate fluid was made in a single batch that lasted for the 6-hour treatment. The water came straight from the spigot on the wall – there was no water treatment. Patients had external shunts, the only type of vascular access available. Achieving ultrafiltration was a hit-and-a-miss by the turn-of-a-screw clamp on the venous bloodline. My saving grace was the thought, "I am a registered nurse. If people with no medical background can do these treatments at home, I can learn." Home dialysis was the only option in our area; there were no outpatient dialysis units. And, for cost savings, all home patients reprocessed their dialyzers.

Peritoneal dialysis was just as antiquated. It involved glass bottles hanging over the patient's bed. Run the fluid in 20 minutes, wait 20 minutes, run the fluid out in 20 minutes – and so it went for 24 to 48 hours while the patient was in the hospital. Transplant was always the treatment of choice, but the immunosuppression was brutal. The reverse isolation and hospital stay were long and arduous.

I remember one patient quipping in those days that she could not wait for a "wearable kidney." I chuckled. I don't chuckle anymore, but wait with great enthusiasm. The progress in technology is almost miraculous; the "almost" could probably be deleted. Orientation to the specialty consisted of one article and handwritten notes on the steps to take to initiate and terminate dialysis. Progress has been made in that realm as well. It really is a whole new world!

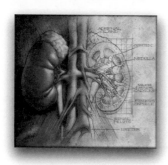

Chapter Editors and Authors

Lisa Ales, MSN, NP-C, FNP-BC, CNN
Clinical Educator, Renal
Baxter Healthcare Corporation
Deerfield, IL
Author: Module 3, Chapter 4

Kim Alleman, MS, APRN, FNP-BC, CNN-NP
Nurse Practitioner
Hartford Hospital Transplant Program
Hartford, CT
Editor: Module 6

Billie Axley, MSN, RN, CNN
Director, Innovations Group
FMS Medical Office
Franklin, TN
Author: Module 4, Chapter 3

Donna Bednarski, MSN, RN, ANP-BC, CNN, CNP
Nurse Practitioner, Dialysis Access Center
Harper University Hospital
Detroit, MI
Editor & Author: Module 1, Chapter 3
Editor & Author: Module 2, Chapter 3
Author: Module 6, Chapter 3

Brandy Begin, BSN, RN, CNN
Pediatric Dialysis Coordinator
Lucile Packard Children's Hospital at Stanford
Palo Alto, CA
Author: Module 5, Chapter 1

Deborah Brommage, MS, RDN, CSR, CDN
Program Director
National Kidney Foundation
New York, NY
Editor & Author: Module 2, Chapter 4
Editor: Module 4, Chapter 3

Deborah H. Brooks, MSN, ANP-BC, CNN, CNN-NP
Nurse Practitioner
Medical University of South Carolina
Charleston, SC
Author: Module 6, Chapter 1

Colleen M. Brown, MSN, APRN, ANP-BC
Transplant Nurse Practitioner
Hartford Hospital
Hartford, CT
Author: Module 6, Chapter 3

Loretta Jackson Brown, PhD, RN, CNN
Health Communication Specialist
Centers for Disease Control and Prevention
Atlanta, GA
Author: Module 2, Chapter 3

Molly Cahill, MSN, RN, APRN, BC, ANP-C, CNN
Nurse Practitioner
KC Kidney Consultants
Kansas City, MO
Author: Module 2, Chapter 3

Sally F. Campoy, DNP, ANP-BC, CNN-NP
Nurse Practitioner, Renal Section
Department of Veterans Affairs
Eastern Colorado Health System
Denver VA Medical Center, Denver, CO
Author: Module 6, Chapter 2

Laurie Carlson, MSN, RN
Transplant Coordinator
University of California –
   San Francisco Medical Center
San Francisco, CA
Author: Module 3, Chapter 1

Deb Castner, MSN, APRN, ACNP, CNN
Nurse Practitioner
Jersey Coast Nephrology & Hypertension
   Associates
Brick, NJ
Author: Module 2, Chapter 3
Author: Module 3, Chapter 2

Louise Clement, MS, RDN, CSR, LD
Renal Dietitian
Fresenius Medical Care
Lubbock, TX
Author: Module 2, Chapter 4

Jean Colaneri, ACNP-BC, CNN
Clinical Nurse Specialist and Nurse
   Practitioner, Dialysis Apheresis
Albany Medical Center Hospital, Albany, NY
Editor & Author: Module 3, Chapter 1

Ann Beemer Cotton, MS, RDN, CNSC
Clinical Dietitian Specialist in Critical Care
IV Health/Methodist Campus
Indianapolis, IN
Author: Module 2, Chapter 4
Author: Module 4, Chapter 2

Caroline S. Counts, MSN, RN, CNN
Research Coordinator, Retired
Division of Nephrology
Medical Unversity of South Carolina
Charleston, SC
Editor: Core Curriculum for Nephrology Nursing
Author: Module 1, Chapter 2
Author: Module 2, Chapter 6
Author: Module 3, Chapter 3

Helen Currier, BSN, RN, CNN, CENP
Director, Renal Services, Dialysis/Pheresis,
   Vascular Access/Wound, Ostomy,
   Continence, & Palliative Care Services
Texas Children's Hospital, Houston, TX
Author: Module 6, Chapter 5

Kim Deaver, MSN, RN, CNN
Program Manager
University of Virginia
Charlottesville, VA
Editor & Author: Module 3, Chapter 3

Anne Diroll, MA, BSN, BS, RN, CNN
Consultant
Volume Management
Rocklin, CA
Author: Module 5, Chapter 1

Daniel Diroll, MA, BSN, BS, RN
Education Coordinator
Fresenius Medical Care North America
Rocklin, CA
Author: Module 2, Chapter 3

Sheila J. Doss-McQuitty, MBA, BSN, RN, CNN, CCRA
Director, Clinical Programs and Research
Satellite Healthcare, Inc., San Jose, CA
Author: Module 2, Chapter 1

Paula Dutka, MSN, RN, CNN
Director, Education and Research
Nephrology Network
Winthrop University Hospital, Mineola, NY
Author: Module 2, Chapter 1

Andrea Easom, MA, MNSc, APRN, FNP-BC, CNN-NP
Instructor, College of Medicine
Nephrology Division
University of Arkansas for Medical Sciences
Little Rock, AR
Author: Module 6, Chapter 2

Rowena W. Elliott, PhD, RN, CNN, CNE, AGNP-C, FAAN
Associate Professor and Chairperson
Department of Advanced Practice
College of Nursing
University of Southern Mississippi
Hattiesburg, MS
Editor & Author: Module 5, Chapter 2

Susan Fallone, MS, RN, CNN
Clinical Nurse Specialist, Retired
Adult and Pediatric Dialysis
Albany Medical Center, Albany, NY
Author: Module 4, Chapter 2

Jessica J. Geer, MSN, C-PNP, CNN-NP
Pediatric Nurse Practitioner
Texas Children's Hospital, Houston, TX
Instructor, Renal Services, Dept. of Pediatrics
Baylor College of Medicine, Houston, TX
Author: Module 6, Chapter 5

Silvia German, RN, CNN
Clinical Writer, CE Coordinator
Manager, DaVita HealthCare Partners Inc.
Denver, CO
Author: Module 2, Chapter 6

Elaine Go, MSN, NP, CNN-NP
Nurse Practitioner
St. Joseph Hospital Renal Center
Orange, CA
Author: Module 6, Chapter 3

Norma Gomez, MSN, MBA, RN, CNN
Nephrology Nurse Consultant
Russellville, TN
Editor & Author: Module 1, Chapter 4

Janelle Gonyea, RDN, LD
Clinical Dietitian
Mayo Clinic
Rochester, MN
Author: Module 2, Chapter 4

Karen Greco, PhD, RN, ANP-BC, FAAN
Nurse Practitioner
Independent Contractor/Consultant
West Linn, OR
Author: Module 2, Chapter 1

Bonnie Bacon Greenspan, MBA, BSN, RN
Consultant, BBG Consulting, LLC
Alexandria, VA
Author: Module 1, Chapter 1

Cheryl L. Groenhoff, MSN, MBA, RN, CNN
Clinical Educator, Baxter Healthcare
Plantation, FL
Author: Module 2, Chapter 3
Author: Module 3, Chapter 4

Debra J. Hain, PhD, ARNP, ANP-BC, GNP-BC, FAANP
Assistant Professor/Lead AGNP Faculty
Florida Atlantic University
Christine E. Lynn College of Nursing
Boca Raton, FL
Nurse Practitioner, Cleveland Clinic Florida
Department of Nephrology, Weston, FL
Editor & Author: Module 2, Chapter 2

Lisa Hall, MSSW, LICSW
Patient Services Director
Northwest Renal Network (ESRD Network 16)
Seattle, WA
Author: Module 2, Chapter 3

Mary S. Haras, PhD, MS, MBA, APN, NP-C, CNN
Assistant Professor and Interim Associate Dean of Graduate Nursing
Saint Xavier University School of Nursing
Chicago, IL
Author: Module 2, Chapter 2

Carol Motes Headley, DNSc, ACNP-BC, RN, CNN
Nephrology Nurse Practitioner
Veterans Affairs Medical Center
Memphis, TN
Editor & Author: Module 2, Chapter 1

Mary Kay Hensley, MS, RDN, CSR
Chair/Immediate Past Chair
Renal Dietitians Dietetic Practice Group
Renal Dietitian, Retired
DaVita HealthCare Partners Inc.
Gary, IN
Author: Module 2, Chapter 4

Kerri Holloway, RN, CNN
Clinical Quality Manager
Corporate Infection Control Specialist
Fresenius Medical Services, Waltham, MA
Author: Module 2, Chapter 6

Alicia M. Horkan, MSN, RN, CNN
Assistant Director, Dialysis Services
Dialysis Center at Colquitt Regional Medical Center
Moultrie, GA
Author: Module 1, Chapter 2

Katherine Houle, MSN, APRN, CFNP, CNN-NP
Nephrology Nurse Practitioner
Marquette General Hospital
Marquette, MI
Editor: Module 6
Author: Module 6, Chapter 3

Liz Howard, RN, CNN
Director
DaVita HealthCare Partners Inc.
Oldsmar, FL
Author: Module 2, Chapter 6

Darlene Jalbert, BSN, RN, CNN
HHD Education Manager
DaVita University School of Clinical Education Wisdom Team
DaVita HealthCare Partners Inc., Denver, CO
Author: Module 3, Chapter 2

Judy Kauffman, MSN, RN, CNN
Manager, Acute Dialysis and Apheresis Unit
University of Virginia Health Systems
Charlottesville, VA
Author: Module 3, Chapter 2

Tamara Kear, PhD, RN, CNS, CNN
Assistant Professor of Nursing
Villanova University, Villanova, PA
Nephrology Nurse, Fresenius Medical Care
Philadelphia, PA
Editor & Author: Module 1, Chapter 2

Lois Kelley, MSW, LSW, ACSW, NSW-C
Master Social Worker
DaVita HealthCare Partners Inc.
Harrisonburg Dialysis
Harrisonburg, VA
Author: Module 2, Chapter 3

Pamela S. Kent, MS, RDN, CSR, LD
Patient Education Coordinator
Centers for Dialysis Care
Cleveland, OH
Author: Module 2, Chapter 4

Carol L. Kinzner, MSN, ARNP, GNP-BC, CNN-NP
Nurse Practitioner
Pacific Nephrology Associates
Tacoma, WA
Author: Module 6, Chapter 3

Kim Lambertson, MSN, RN, CNN
Clinical Educator
Baxter Healthcare
Deerfield, IL
Author: Module 3, Chapter 4

Sharon Longton, BSN, RN, CNN, CCTC
Transplant Coordinator/Educator
Harper University Hospital
Detroit, MI
Author: Module 2, Chapter 3

Maria Luongo, MSN, RN
CAPD Nurse Manager
Massachusetts General Hospital
Boston, MA
Author: Module 3, Chapter 5

Suzanne M. Mahon, DNSc, RN, AOCN, APNG
Professor, Internal Medicine
Division of Hematology/Oncology
Professor, Adult Nursing, School of Nursing
St. Louis University, St. Louis, MO
Author: Module 2, Chapter 1

Nancy McAfee, MN, RN, CNN
CNS – Pediatric Dialysis and Vascular Access
Seattle Children's Hospital
Seattle, WA
Editor & Author: Module 5, Chapter 1

Maureen P. McCarthy, MPH, RDN, CSR, LD
Assistant Professor/Transplant Dietitian
Oregon Health & Science University
Portland, OR
Author: Module 2, Chapter 4

M. Sue McManus, PhD, APRN, FNP-BC, CNN
Nephrology Nurse Practitioner
Kidney Transplant Nurse Practitioner
Richard L. Roudebush VA Medical Center
Indianapolis, IN
Author: Module 1, Chapter 2

Lisa Micklos, BSN, RN
Clinical Educator
NxStage Medical, Inc.
Los Angeles, CA
Author: Module 1, Chapter 2

Michele Mills, MS, RN, CPNP
Pediatric Nurse Practitioner
Pediatric Nephrology
University of Michigan
C.S. Mott Children's Hospital, Ann Arbor, MI
Author: Module 5, Chapter 1

Geraldine F. Morrison, BSHSA, RN
Clinical Director, Home Programs & CKD
Northwest Kidney Center
Seattle, WA
Author: Module 3, Chapter 5

Theresa Mottes, RN, CDN
Pediatric Research Nurse
Cincinnati Children's Hospital & Medical Center
Center for Acute Care Nephrology
Cincinnati, OH
Author: Module 5, Chapter 1

Linda L. Myers, BS, RN, CNN, HP
RN Administrative Coordinator, Retired
Home Dialysis Therapies
University of Virginia Health System
Charlottesville, VA
Author: Module 4, Chapter 5

Clara Neyhart, BSN, RN, CNN
Nephrology Nurse Clinician
UNC Chapel Hill
Chapel Hill, NC
Editor & Author: Module 3, Chapter 1

Mary Alice Norton, BSN, FNP-C
Senior Heart Failure/LVAD/Transplant
  Coordinator
Albany Medical Center Hospital
Albany, NY
Author: Module 4, Chapter 6

Jessie M. Pavlinac, MS, RDN, CSR, LD
Director, Clinical Nutrition
Oregon Health and Science University
Portland, OR
Author: Module 2, Chapter 4

Glenda M. Payne, MS, RN, CNN
Director of Clinical Services
Nephrology Clinical Solutions
Duncanville, TX
Editor & Author: Module 1, Chapter 1
Author: Module 3, Chapter 2
Author: Module 4, Chapter 4

Eileen J. Peacock, MSN, RN, CNN,
  CIC, CPHQ, CLNC
Infection Control and Surveillance
  Management Specialist
DaVita HealthCare Partners Inc.
Maple Glen, PA
Editor & Author: Module 2, Chapter 6

Mary Perrecone, MS, RN, CNN, CCRN
Clinical Manager
Fresenius Medical Care
Charleston, SC
Author: Module 4, Chapter 1

Susan A. Pfettscher, PhD, RN
California State University Bakersfield
  Department of Nursing, Retired
Satellite Health Care, San Jose, CA, Retired
Bakersfield, CA
Author: Module 1, Chapter 1

Nancy B. Pierce, BSN, RN, CNN
Dialysis Director
St. Peter's Hospital
Helena, MT
Author: Module 1, Chapter 1

Leonor P. Ponferrada, BSN, RN, CNN
Education Coordinator
University of Missouri School of Medicine –
  Columbia
Columbia, MO
Author: Module 3, Chapter 4

Lillian A. Pryor, MSN, RN, CNN
Clinical Manager
FMC Loganville, LLC
Loganville, GA
Author: Module 1, Chapter 1

Timothy Ray, DNP, CNP, CNN-NP
Nurse Practitioner
Cleveland Kidney & Hypertension Consultants
Euclid, OH
Author: Module 6, Chapter 4

Cindy Richards, BSN, RN, CNN
Transplant Coordinator
Children's of Alabama
Birmingham, AL
Author: Module 5, Chapter 1

Karen C. Robbins, MS, RN, CNN
Nephrology Nurse Consultant
Associate Editor, *Nephrology Nursing Journal*
Past President, American Nephrology Nurses'
  Association
West Hartford, CT
Editor: Module 3, Chapter 2

Regina Rohe, BS, RN, HP(ASCP)
Regional Vice President, Inpatient Services
Fresenius Medical Care, North America
San Francisco, CA
Author: Module 4, Chapter 8

Francine D. Salinitri, PharmD
Associate (Clinical) Professor of
  Pharmacy Practice
Wayne State University, Applebaum College of
  Pharmacy and Health Sciences, Detroit, MI
Clinical Pharmacy Specialist, Nephrology
Oakwood Hospital and Medical Center
Dearborn, MI
Author: Module 2, Chapter 5

Karen E. Schardin, BSN, RN, CNN
Clinical Director, National Accounts
NxStage Medical, Inc.
Lawrence, MA
Editor & Author: Module 3, Chapter 5

Mary Schira, PhD, RN, ACNP-BC
Associate Professor
Univ. of Texas at Arlington – College of Nursing
Arlington, TX
Author: Module 6, Chapter 1

Deidra Schmidt, PharmD
Clinical Pharmacy Specialist
Pediatric Renal Transplantation
Children's of Alabama
Birmingham, AL
Author: Module 5, Chapter 1

Joan E. Speranza-Reid, BSHM, RN, CNN
Clinic Manager
ARA/Miami Regional Dialysis Center
North Miami Beach, FL
Author: Module 3, Chapter 2

Jean Stover, RDN, CSR, LDN
Renal Dietitian
DaVita HealthCare Partners Inc.
Philadelphia, PA
Author: Module 2, Chapter 4

Charlotte Szromba, MSN, APRN, CNNe
Nurse Consultant, Retired
Department Editor, Nephrology Nursing
  Journal
Naperville, IL
Author: Module 2, Chapter 1

Kirsten L. Thompson, MPH, RDN, CSR
Clinical Dietitian
Seattle Children's Hospital, Seattle, WA
Author: Module 5, Chapter 1

Lucy B. Todd, MSN, ACNP-BC, CNN
Medical Science Liaison
Baxter Healthcare
Asheville, NC
Editor & Author: Module 3, Chapter 4

Susan C. Vogel, MHA, RN, CNN
Clinical Manager, National Accounts
NxStage Medical, Inc.
Los Angeles, CA
Author: Module 3, Chapter 5

Joni Walton, PhD, RN, ACNS-BC, NPc
Family Nurse Practitioner
Marias HealthCare
Shelby, MT
Author: Module 2, Chapter 1

Gail S. Wick, MHSA, BSN, RN, CNNe
Consultant
Atlanta, GA
Author: Module 1, Chapter 2

Helen F. Williams, MSN, BSN, RN, CNN
Special Projects – Acute Dialysis Team
Fresenius Medical Care
Denver, CO
Editor: Module 4
Editor & Author: Module 4, Chapter 7

Elizabeth Wilpula, PharmD, BCPS
Clinical Pharmacy Specialist
Nephrology/Transplant
Harper University Hospital, Detroit, MI
Editor & Author: Module 2, Chapter 5

Karen Wiseman, MSN, RN, CNN
Manager, Regulatory Affairs
Fresenius Medical Services
Waltham, MA
Author: Module 2, Chapter 6

Linda S. Wright, DrNP, RN, CNN, CCTC
Lead Kidney and Pancreas Transplant
   Coordinator
Thomas Jefferson University Hospital
Philadelphia, PA
Author: Module 1, Chapter 2

Mary M. Zorzanello, MSN, APRN
Nurse Practitioner, Section of Nephrology
Yale University School of Medicine
New Haven, CT
Author: Module 6, Chapter 3

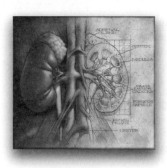

Reviewers

The Blind Review Process

The contents of the *Core Curriculum* underwent a "blind" review process by qualified individuals. One or more chapters were sent to chosen people for critical evaluation. The reviewer did not know the author's identity at the time of the review.

The work could be accepted (1) as originally submitted without revisions, (2) with minor revisons, or (3) with major revisions. The reviewers offered tremendous insight and suggestions; some even submitted additional references they thought might be useful. The results of the review were then sent back to the chapter/module editors to incorporate the suggestions and make revisions.

The reviewers will discover who the authors are now that the *Core* is published. However, while there is this published list of reviewers, no one will know who reviewed which part of the *Core*. That part of the process remains blind.

Because of the efforts of individuals listed below, value was added to the sixth edition. Their hard work is greatly appreciated.

Caroline S. Counts, Editor

Marilyn R. Bartucci, MSN, RN, ACNS-BC, CCTC
Case Manager
Kidney Foundation of Ohio
Cleveland, OH

Christina M. Beale, RN, CNN
Director, Outreach and Education
Lifeline Vascular Access
Vernon Hills, IL

Jenny Bell, BSN, RN, CNN
Clinical Transplant Coordinator
Banner Good Samaritan Transplant Center
Phoenix, AZ

M. Geraldine Biddle, RN, CNN, CPHQ
President, Nephrology Nurse Consultants
Pittsford, NY

Randee Breiterman White, MS, RN
Nurse Case Manager Nephrology
Vanderbilt University Hospital
Nashville, TN

Jerrilynn D. Burrowes, PhD, RDN, CDN
Professor and Chair
Director, Graduate Programs in Nutrition
Department of Nutrition
Long Island University (LIU) Post
Brookville, NY

Sally Burrows-Hudson, MSN, RN, CNN
Deceased 2014
Director, Nephrology Clinical Solutions
Lisle, IL

LaVonne Burrows, APRN, BC, CNN
Advanced Practice Registered Nurse
Springfield Nephrology Associates
Springfield, MO

Karen T. Burwell, BSN, RN, CNN
Acute Dialysis Nurse
DaVita HealthCare Partners Inc.
Phoenix, AZ

Laura D. Byham-Gray, PhD, RDN
Associate Professor and Director
Graduate Programs in Clinical Nutrition
Department of Nutritional Sciences
School of Health Related Professions
Rutgers University
Stratford, NJ

Theresa J. Campbell, DNP, APRN, FNP-BC
Doctor of Nursing Practice
Family Nurse Practitioner
Carolina Kidney Care
Adjunct Professor of Nursing
University of North Caroline at Pembroke
Fayetteville, NC

Monet Carnahan, BSN, RN, CDN
Renal Care Coordinator Program Manager
Fresenius Medical Care
Nashville, TN

Jacke L. Corbett, DNP, FNP-BC, CCTC
Nurse Practitioner
Kidney/Pancreas Transplant Program
University of Utah Health Care
Salt Lake City, UT

Christine Corbett, MSN, APRN, FNP-BC, CNN-NP
Nephrology Nurse Practitioner
Truman Medical Centers
Kansas City, MO

Sandra Corrigan, FNP-BC, CNN
Nurse Practitioner
California Kidney Medical Group
Thousand Oaks, CA

Maureen Craig, MSN, RN, CNN
Clinical Nurse Specialist – Nephrology
University of California Davis Medical Center
Sacramento, CA

Diane M. Derkowski, MA, RN, CNN, CCTC
Kidney Transplant Coordinator
Carolinas Medical Center
Charlotte, NC

Linda Duval, BSN, RN
Executive Director, FMQAI: ESRD Network 13
ESRD Network
Oklahoma City, OK

Damian Eker, DNP, GNP-C
ARNP, Geriatrics & Adult Health
Adult & Geriatric Health Center
Ft. Lauderdale, FL

Elizabeth Evans, DNP
Nephrology Nurse Practitioner
Renal Medicine Associates
Albuquerque, NM

Susan Fallone, MS, RN, CNN
Clinical Nurse Specialist, Retired
Adult and Pediatric Dialysis
Albany Medical Center
Albany, NY

Karen Joann Gaietto, MSN, BSN, RN, CNN
Acute Clinical Service Specialist
DaVita HealthCare Partners Inc.
Tiffin, OH

Deborah Glidden, MSN, ARNP, BC, CNN
Nurse Practitioner
Nephrology Associates of Central Florida
Orlando, FL

David Jeremiah Grubbs, RN, CDN, Paramedic, ACLS, PALS, BCLS, TNCC, NIH
Clinical Nurse Manager
Crestwood, KY

Debra J. Hain, PhD, ARNP, ANP-BC, GNP-BC, FAANP
Associate Professor/Lead Faculty AGNP Track
Florida Atlantic University
Christine E. Lynn College of Nursing
Boca Raton, FL
Nurse Practitioner, Cleveland Clinic Florida
Department of Nephrology
Weston, FL

Brenda C. Halstead, MSN, RN, AcNP, CNN
Nurse Practitioner
Mid-Atlantic Kidney Center
Richmond and Petersburg, VA

Emel Hamilton, RN, CNN
Director of Clinical Technology
Fresenius Medical Care
Waltham, MA

Mary S. Haras, PhD, MBA, APN, NP-C, CNN
Associate Dean, Graduate Nursing Programs
Saint Xavier University School of Nursing
Chicago, IL

Malinda C. Harrington, MSN, RN, FNP-BC, ANCC
Pediatric Nephrology Nurse Practitioner
Vidant Medical Center
Greenville, NC

Diana Hlebovy, BSN, RN, CHN, CNN
Nephrology Nurse Consultant
Elyria, OH

Sara K. Kennedy, BSN, RN, CNN
UAB Medicine, Kirklin Clinic
Diabetes Care Coordinator
Birmingham, AL

Nadine "Niki" Kobes, BSN, RN
Manager Staff Education/Quality
Fresenius Medical Care – Alaska JV Clinics
Anchorage, AK

Deuzimar Kulawik, MSN, RN
Director of Clinical Quality
DaVita HealthCare Partners Inc.
Westlake Village, CA

Kristin Larson, RN, ANP, GNP, CNN
Clinical Instructor
College of Nursing
Family Nurse Practitioner Program
University of North Dakota
Grand Forks, ND

Deborah Leggett, BSN, RN, CNN
Director, Acute Dialysis
Jackson Madison County General Hospital
Jackson, TN

Charla Litton, MSN, APRN, FNP-BC, CNN
Nurse Practitioner
UHG/Optum
East Texas, TX

Greg Lopez, BSN, RN, CNN
IMPAQ Business Process Manager
Fresenius Medical Care
New Orleans, LA

Terri (Theresa) Luckino, BSN, RN, CCRN
President, Acute Services
RPNT Acute Services, Inc.
Irving, TX

Alice Luehr, BA, RN, CNN
Home Therapy RN
St. Peter's Hospital
Helena, MT

Maryam W. Lyon, MSN, RN, CNN
Education Coordinator
Fresenius Medical Care
Dayton, OH

Christine Mudge, MS, RN, PNP/CNS, CNN, FAAN
Mill Valley, CA

Mary Lee Neuberger, MSN, APRN, RN, CNN
Pediatric Nephrology
University of Iowa Children's Hospital
Iowa City, IA

Jennifer Payton, MHCA, BSN, RN, CNN
Clinical Support Specialist
HealthStar CES
Goose Creek, SC

April Peters, MSN, RN, CNN
Clinical Informatics Specialist
Brookhaven Memorial Hospital Medical Center
Patchogue, NY

David J. Quan, PharmD, BCPS
Health Sciences Clinical Professor of Pharmacy
Clinical Pharmacist, Liver Transplant Services
UCSF Medical Center
San Francisco, CA

Kristi Robertson, CFNP
Nephrology Nurse Practitioner
Nephrology Associates
Columbus, MS

E. James Ryan, BSN, RN, CDN
Hemodialysis Clinical Services Coordinator
Lakeland Regional Medical Center
Lakeland, FL

June Shi, BSN, RN
Vascular Access Coordinator
Transplant Surgery
Medical University of South Carolina
Charleston, SC

Elizabeth St. John, MSN, RN, CNN
Education Coordinator, UMW Region
Fresenius Medical Care
Milwaukee, WI

Sharon Swofford, MA, RN, CNN, CCTC
Transplant Case Manager
OptumHealth
The Villages, FL

Beth Ulrich, EdD, RN, FACHE, FAAN
Senior Partner, Innovative Health Resources
Editor, *Nephrology Nursing Journal*
Pearland, TX

David F. Walz, MBA, BSN, RN, CNN
Program Director
CentraCare Kidney Program
St. Cloud, MN

Gail S. Wick, MHSA, BSN, RN, CNNe
Consultant
Atlanta, GA

Phyllis D. Wille, MS, RN, FNP-C, CNN, CNE
Nursing Faculty
Danville Area Community College
Danville, Il

Donna L. Willingham, RN, CPNP
Pediatric Nephrology Nurse Practitioner
Washington University St. Louis
St. Louis, MO

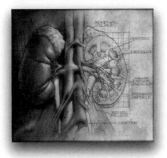

Contents at a Glance

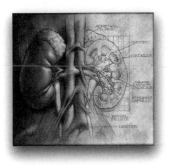

Expanded Contents

The table of contents contains chapters and sections with editors and authors for all six modules. The contents section of this specific module is highlighted in a blue background.

Module 1   Foundations for Practice in Nephrology Nursing

Module 2   Physiologic and Psychosocial Basis
for Nephrology Nursing Practice

Module 3   Treatment Options for Patients with Chronic Kidney Failure

Module 4 Acute Kidney Injury

Module Editor: Helen F. Williams

Module 5   Kidney Disease in Patient Populations Across the Life Span

Module 6   The APRN's Approaches to Care in Nephrology

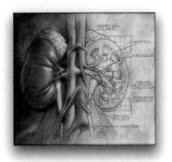

Examples of APA-formatted references

A guide for citing material from Module 3 of the *Core Curriculum for Nephrology Nursing, 6th edition.*

Module 3, Chapter 1

Example of reference for Chapter 1 in APA format. Use author of the section being cited. This example is based on Section C – Chronic Kidney Disease in Transplant Recipients.

Neyhart, C. (2015). Transplantation: Chronic kidney disease in transplant recipients. In C.S. Counts (Ed.), *Core curriculum for nephrology nursing: Module 3. Treatment options for patients with chronic kidney failure* (6th ed., pp. 1–68). Pitman, NJ: American Nephrology Nurses' Association.

Interpreted: Section author(s). (2015). Title of chapter: Title of section. In ...

For citation in text: (Neyhart, 2015) (Use the author of the section you are citing.)

Module 3, Chapter 2

Example of reference for Chapter 2 in APA format. Use author of the section being cited. This example is based on Section F – Dialyzer Reprocessing.

Jalbert, D. (2015). Hemodialysis: Dialyzer reprocessing. In C.S. Counts (Ed.), *Core curriculum for nephrology nursing: Module 3. Treatment options for patients with chronic kidney failure* (6th ed., pp. 69-166). Pitman, NJ: American Nephrology Nurses' Association.

Interpreted: Section author(s). (2015). Title of chapter: Title of section. In ...

For citation in text: (Jalbert, 2015) (Use the author of the section you are citing.)

Module 3, Chapter 3

Example of reference for Chapter 3 in APA format. Two authors for entire chapter.

Deaver, K., & Counts, C. (2015). Vascular access for hemodialysis. In C.S. Counts (Ed.), *Core curriculum for nephrology nursing: Module 3. Treatment options for patients with chronic kidney failure* (6th ed., pp. 167-226). Pitman, NJ: American Nephrology Nurses' Association.

Interpreted: Section author(s). (2015). Title of chapter: Title of section. In ...

For citation in text: (Deaver & Counts, 2015)

Module 3, Chapter 4

Example of reference for Chapter 4 in APA format. Use author of the section being cited. This example is based on Section A – Peritoneal Dialysis.

Lambertson, K. (2015). Peritoneal dialysis: Peritoneal dialysis access. In C.S. Counts (Ed.), *Core curriculum for nephrology nursing: Module 3. Treatment options for patients with chronic kidney failure* (6th ed., pp. 227-278). Pitman, NJ: American Nephrology Nurses' Association.

Interpreted: Section author(s). (2015). Title of chapter: Title of section. In ...

For citation in text: (Lambertson, 2015) (Use the author of the section you are citing.)

Module 3, Chapter 5

Example of reference for Chapter 5 in APA format. Use author of the section being cited. This example is based on Section C – Home Peritoneal Dialysis.

Luongo, M. (2015). Home dialysis: Home peritoneal dialysis. In C.S. Counts (Ed.), *Core curriculum for nephrology nursing: Module 3. Treatment options for patients with chronic kidney failure* (6th ed., pp. 279-310). Pitman, NJ: American Nephrology Nurses' Association.

Interpreted: Section author. (Date). Title of chapter: Title of section. In ...

For citation in text: (Luongo, 2015) (Use the author of the section you are citing.)

CHAPTER **1**
Transplantation

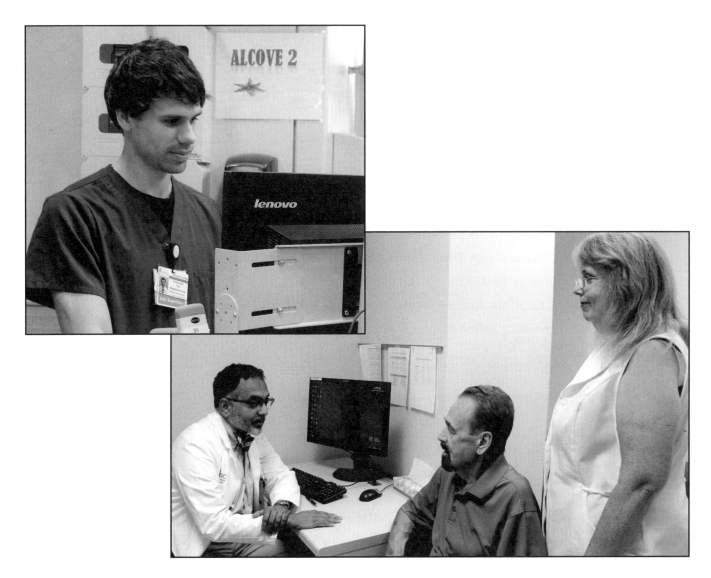

Chapter Editors
Jean Colaneri, ACNP-BC, CNN
Clara Neyhart, BSN, RN, CNN

Authors
Jean Colaneri, ACNP-BC, CNN
Clara Neyhart, BSN, RN, CNN
Laurie Carlson, MSN, RN

CHAPTER **1**
Transplantation

This offering for **2.0 contact hours with 1.0 contact hour of pharmacology content** is provided by the American Nephrology Nurses' Association (ANNA).

American Nephrology Nurses' Association is accredited as a provider of continuing nursing education by the American Nurses Credentialing Center Commission on Accreditation.

ANNA is a provider approved by the California Board of Registered Nursing, provider number CEP 00910.

This CNE offering meets the continuing nursing education requirements for certification and recertification by the Nephrology Nursing Certification Commission (NNCC).

To be awarded contact hours for this activity, read this chapter in its entirety. Then complete the CNE evaluation found at **www.annanurse.org/corecne** and submit it; or print it, complete it, and mail it in. Contact hours are not awarded until the evaluation for the activity is complete.

Example of reference for Chapter 1 in APA format. Use author of the section being cited. This example is based on Section C.

Neyhart, C. (2015). Transplantation: Chronic kidney disease in transplant recipients. In C.S. Counts (Ed.), *Core curriculum for nephrology nursing: Module 3. Treatment options for patients with chronic kidney failure* (6th ed., pp. 1–68). Pitman, NJ: American Nephrology Nurses' Association.

Interpreted: Section author(s). (2015). Title of chapter: Title of section. In ...

Cover photo by Counts/Morganello.

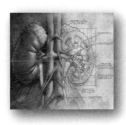

CHAPTER 1

Transplantation

Purpose

The purpose of this chapter is to discuss concepts related to kidney transplantation and simultaneous kidney and pancreas transplantation (SPK). It also addresses chronic kidney disease (CKD) and the relationship to the transplantation of livers, hearts, and lungs. In addition, the topics of HIV and hepatitis C are included.

Objectives

Upon completion of this chapter, the learner will be able to:
1. Discuss acceptance criteria for transplantation.
2. Discuss criteria for living and deceased organ donation.
3. Explain methods for modification of the immune system after transplantation.
4. List major side effects of selected immunosuppressive medications.
5. Discuss the signs and symptoms of transplant rejection.
6. Identify short-term and long-term complications of transplantation.

SECTION A
Kidney Transplantation
Jean Colaneri, Clara Neyhart

Part 1. Introduction

I. **Kidney transplantation has evolved from an experimental procedure to an accepted modality for kidney replacement therapy (KRT).** The 1950s offered the first long-term successful transplant. Since that period of time, advances in immunosuppression, understanding of the immune system, and refinement of surgical techniques have served to improve the morbidity and mortality of patients with chronic kidney disease.

II. **Overview of statistics.**

A. Kidney transplantation is the preferred treatment modality for most patients with CKD stage 4 or kidney failure (Abecassis et al., 2008; G. Danovitch, 2010a).

B. Preemptive kidney transplantation (transplant prior to dialysis) is the best option, but this only happens in about 10% of the patients with kidney failure and usually with an available living donor (Abecassis et al., 2008).

C. A patient must have a glomerular filtration rate (GFR) less than or equal to 20 cc per minute to gain waiting time points on the United Network for Organ Sharing (UNOS) List (UNOS, 2013b).

D. Overall graft survival is 89% at 1 year and 66% at 5 years. The actual half-life is less than 10 years for deceased (formerly referred to as "cadaveric") donor kidney transplants.

E. Survival statistics (UNOS, 2013a).
1. Patient survival at 1 year with a deceased donor transplant is 94.4%.
2. Patient survival at 5 years with a deceased donor transplant is 81.8%.
3. Graft survival at 1 year with a deceased donor transplant is 89.0%.
4. Graft survival at 5 years with a deceased donor transplant is 66.6%.
5. Patient survival at 1 year with a living donor transplant is 97.9%.
6. Patient survival at 5 years with a living donor transplant is 90.1%.
7. Graft survival at 1 year with a living donor transplant is 95.1%.
8. Graft survival at 5 years with a living donor transplant is 79.8%.

F. The transplant process can be viewed in four phases.
1. Pretransplant.
2. Maintenance on the waiting list.
3. Transplant.
4. Posttransplant.

III. Brief history of transplantation.

A. Surgical techniques for vascular suturing were first developed in the early 20th century by Drs. Alexis Carrel and Charles Guthrie.

B. The first successful kidney transplant was performed by Dr. Joseph Murray and Dr. Hartwell Harrison in 1954, at Peter Bent Brigham Hospital in Boston. The kidney was donated by an identical twin.

C. The importance of the immune system and immunology began to be recognized and understood, first during World War II, then even more so during the 1950s (Townsend et al., 2012).

D. The development and refinement of immunosuppressive medications and regimens have continued to advance the field.
1. Azathioprine was developed in the 1950s, and along with corticosteroids, was the mainstay of immunosuppressant therapy for decades.
2. The development of these drugs allowed non-identical transplants to be successful (Townsend et al., 2012).

E. Tissue typing became the accepted procedure to match donor and recipient in 1962 (Terasaki, 2012).

F. Later in the 1960s, the relationship between a positive crossmatch and hyperacute rejection was recognized (Terasaki, 2012).

G. In the 1970s, the use of deceased organ donors became accepted practice, and the concept of brain death was established.

H. In 1972, a landmark contribution to end-stage renal disease treatment was the passage of Public Law 92-603 (HR-1), which provided Medicare coverage for dialysis and kidney transplantation (http://www.cms.gov/medicare/End-stage-renal-disease).

I. In 1978, cyclosporine was first used in clinical trials as an immunosuppressant (Townsend et al., 2012).

J. In 1978, the use of HLA-DR matching became accepted practice.

K. In 1987, the United Network for Organ Sharing was awarded the federal government contract to govern organ sharing distribution and establish scientific registries.

L. In 1991, the Banff criteria of renal allograft pathology was developed, which allowed better tailoring of medical therapy and decreased broad use of powerful immunosuppressive medications (Solez, 2010).

M. Development of newer immunosuppressive medications, antibody reduction protocols, clearer understanding of immunology, and other research continue to advance the field.

Part 2. Organ Donation and Preservation

I. Living donor.

A. Related or biologically related: parent, sibling, child, aunt, uncle, cousin, and grandparent.

B. Unrelated or biologically unrelated: spouse, in-laws, adoptive parent, friend, significant other, and anonymous or altruistic. Donors should be willing to donate, free of coercion, fully aware of risks and benefits, medically and psychologically suitable, and competent to give consent (Delmonico & Dew, 2007).

C. Evaluation.
1. Information and explanation of process. UNOS guidelines require transplant centers to provide all living donors an independent donor advocate (IDA) to guide the potential donor through the evaluation process and provide nonbiased counsel as needed. This IDA is not involved in any way with the kidney recipient's care or evaluation (UNOS, 2013a).
   a. Information on donation process.
      (1) Orientation conference.
      (2) Review medical and psychological benefits and risks to recipient.
         (a) Explain an additional treatment option for CKD.
         (b) Procedure is elective, not life-saving.
      (3) Medical and psychological risks of evaluation process for donor.
         (a) Allergic reactions to contrast.
         (b) Discovery of reportable infections.
         (c) Discovery of serious medical conditions.
         (d) Discovery of adverse genetic findings.
         (e) Abnormal findings requiring more evaluation at donor expense (UNOS, 2013a).
      (4) Donor evaluation process.
      (5) Surgical procedure.
      (6) Postoperative recovery.
      (7) Long-term risks and benefits.

b. Discuss with someone who has donated a kidney.
c. Psychosocial assessment may include social worker, psychiatric nurse, psychologist, and/or psychiatrist.
d. Assessment of willingness to donate.
e. Assess family dynamics.
   (1) Relationship between donor and recipient.
   (2) Consideration of other family members' opinions on donation.
   (3) Assess any history of depression or psychological disorders.
      (a) Psychological disorders do not rule out donation, but the focus and concern should be the effect of stress on the donor's well-being, with a risk/benefit assessment.
      (b) Contraindications to donation would include:
         i. Ambivalence about, or significant fear of donation.
         ii. Current psychiatric disorder that may be made worse by the stress of donation.
         iii. Current substance use problems.
         iv. Concerns about coercion of the donor or pressure to donate.
         v. Inability to understand risks and benefits to the donor and recipient (Delmonico & Dew, 2007; Sharif, 2013).
f. Financial considerations.
   (1) Potential future health insurance implications.
   (2) Personal/family expenses while off work for evaluation and postoperative recovery.
   (3) Cost of further evaluation of any medical condition found during workup.
   (4) Travel to transplant center for donation and follow-up (Dew et al., 2007; UNOS, 2013a).
g. Implications of recipient graft loss or death.
2. Medical assessment varies by transplant center, but usually includes:
a. ABO typing.
   (1) ABO incompatibility does not necessarily rule out donation.
   (2) Several centers offer ABO incompatibility protocols using immunosuppression, intravenous immunoglobulin (IVIG), and plasmapheresis (or combinations thereof) (Becker et al., 2013; Montgomery et al., 2009).
b. Histocompatibility testing.
c. Age is generally between 18 and 65 years.
   (1) Each donor is considered individually in terms of medical and psychological health.
   (2) An older donor with normal kidney function and no health concerns can

donate and have an excellent prognosis for a normal life after donation.
   (3) Most centers consider the lower age limit for donation to be 18.
      (a) For some centers, the limit is 21 years of age.
      (b) The issue is whether the very young donor can fully understand the potential risks of donation over the course of a lifetime (G. Danovitch, 2010a; Ponticelli & Graziani, 2012; Townsend et al., 2012).
d. Thorough health history and physical assessment.
   (1) Rule out hypertension, although mild, controlled hypertension may be acceptable at some centers; diabetes mellitus; cardiovascular disease; pulmonary disease; kidney disease; malignancies; infections; substance abuse; obesity; current pregnancy; and other systemic diseases with implications for kidney involvement.
   (2) Review family and social history.
   (3) Review current medications, nonprescription medications, and herbal preparations (G. Danovitch, 2010a; Delmonico & Dew, 2007; Mandelbrot et al., 2007).
e. Chest x-ray.
f. EKG.
g. Hematology, chemistries, serologies, and cultures.
h. Urine studies to assess kidney function.
i. Spiral CT scan or MRI/MRA to document anatomy of kidneys, ureter, bladder (Townsend et al., 2012).
3. Living donor follow-up.
a. UNOS mandates that living donor follow-up data be collected at 6 months, 1 year, and 2 years after donation. This follow-up can be done at the transplant center or by a primary care physician. The data collection form can be referenced at http://www.unos.org/donation/index.php?topic=data_collectionhttp://www.unos.org/donation/index.php?topic=data_collection
b. After 2 years, living donors are encouraged to see their primary care physicians for annual exams and blood pressure checks and to receive routine health maintenance screenings at recommended intervals.

II. Deceased donor.

A. Changes in terminology.
1. Deceased donation encompasses donors with brain death and donation after circulatory death (not clinically brain dead, but determined to have no hope of functional recovery after brain injury).

2. Brain death also referred to as "death determined by neurologic criteria."
3. Donation after circulatory death (DCD), formerly "non-heart-beating donor" also referred to as "death determined by cardiorespiratory criteria" (O'Connor et al., 2010).
4. The Kidney Donor Profile Index (KDPI) will replace the terms "standard" (SCD) and "extended" criteria donor kidney (ECD). This is due to the fact that some ECD kidneys were of better estimated quality than some SCD kidneys, and there is a wide range of quality for ECD kidneys (UNOS, 2013b).

B. Criteria for deceased donation.
1. Heart-beating donor must have irreversible cessation of spontaneous brain function (brain death) with a known cause of brain injury. Diagnosis of brain death should be made by a physician who does not work with the transplantation team and has no conflict of interest (O'Connor et al., 2010).
   a. No seizures or posturing.
   b. No response to pain in cranial nerve distribution; spinal reflexes may be present.
   c. Apnea in response to acidosis or hypercarbia.
   d. No pupillary or corneal reflexes.
   e. No oculocephalic or vestibular reflexes.
   f. No tracheobronchial reflexes.
   g. Absent cerebral and brain stem function (O'Connor et al., 2010).
2. KDPI calculates donor clinical information and demographics into a number that quantifies the quality of the donor kidneys.
   a. This is used to decide which recipient would best benefit from a specific donor kidney.
   b. The KDPI is calculated from the Kidney Donor Risk Index (KDRI).
      (1) It estimates the relative risk of posttransplant kidney failure in an average adult recipient from a particular deceased donor.
      (2) Lower KDRI scores correlate with increased donor quality while higher KDRI values correlate with lower donor quality (UNOS, 2013b).
      (3) KDRI values are calculated based on age, height, weight, ethnicity, history of hypertension and diabetes, cause of death, serum creatinine, hepatitis C virus status, donation after circulatory death status (UNOS, 2013b).
      (4) Removed from consideration with this formula are the degree of HLA matching, cold ischemic time, and transplant procedure type (single vs. double vs. en-bloc) (Massie et al., 2011).

(5) Kidneys with high KDRI values are usually biopsied to ensure adequate numbers of glomeruli prior to transplantation.
   (a) They are also usually placed on perfusion pump to determine renal vasculature resistance.
   (b) High resistance (> 0.40) generally indicates that the donor kidneys are compromised and may not be suitable for transplantation (O'Connor et al., 2010).
3. Donation after circulatory death.
   a. Irreversible brain injury, but does not meet criteria for brain death; either a controlled or an uncontrolled situation.
      (1) Controlled situation.
         (a) Family gives informed consent prior to discontinuation of ventilator support.
         (b) Discontinuation of ventilatory support takes place in operating room. Cardiopulmonary arrest should occur within 1 hour of discontinuation of ventilatory support.
      (2) Uncontrolled situation.
         (a) Cardiopulmonary arrest occurs.
         (b) No response to cardiopulmonary resuscitation and death is declared.
         (c) Family gives informed consent.
         (d) Organs are recovered immediately to minimize warm ischemic time.
   b. As above, kidneys are usually biopsied prior to transplantation.
4. Medical criteria for deceased donors.
   a. Absence of malignancy except for some primary brain tumors or skin cancers.
   b. Absence of active systemic infections or transmissible disease.
   c. Absence of significant kidney disease or uncontrolled hypertension.
   d. Acceptable evaluation of organ function.
   e. Nucleic acid test (NAT) is drawn on donors at risk for infection: Hepatitis B and C, HIV.
      (1) Results can be determined faster than those from antibody testing.
      (2) Decreases the window for detection of infectivity.
5. Deceased donor care.
   a. Maintenance of adequate blood pressure and urine output with intravenous solution, such as crystalloid, colloid, and inotropic medications.
   b. Psychosocial support for the donor family throughout the process.
6. Other considerations.
   a. Mandatory request protocols for every hospital require the designated trained hospital representative (physician, nurse, chaplain, social worker) or Organ Procurement

Organization (OPO) coordinator to offer the option of organ and tissue donation to families of patients who meet the criteria for donation.

b. Permission is obtained from next of kin or as indicated by patient on organ donor registry.

c. Impact of multi-organ procurement.
   (1) Since different organs have different requirements for management, protocols have been developed to satisfy competing issues.
   (2) The retrieval process for multiple organs and tissues often results in multiple teams simultaneously in operating room.
   (3) May cause delays in the organ recovery process.
   (4) Preferred order of removal is heart or lungs first, liver or pancreas second, and kidneys last. The kidneys are protected against ischemia by cold flush and surface cooling during the 15 minutes needed to remove the other organs (O'Connor et al., 2010).

d. Education of healthcare professionals, especially those who work in the critical care units and emergency departments, about the need for organs and tissues is vital to promote organ donation.

e. Organ recovery.
   (1) Warm ischemia time is the period between circulatory arrest and cold storage.
      (a) Warm ischemia time is minimized using an in situ flush of cold storage solution.
      (b) After 20 minutes of warm ischemia time, delayed and nonfunction of the graft increase significantly.
   (2) Care is taken to preserve vasculature and prevent intimal tears in the renal veins and arteries, which may result in thrombosis or partial occlusion and graft loss.
   (3) Coordination of multi-organ retrieval. One surgeon leads multiple teams to ensure the optimal outcome for all organs to be procured.

f. Organ preservation. Both cold storage and pulsatile perfusion induce hypothermia to minimize ischemic injury (O'Connor et al., 2010).
   (1) Cold storage.
      (a) Kidneys are flushed with cold-storage solution, packed in sterile containers, and packed in ice.
      (b) The most common method of storage.
   (2) Hypothermic pulsatile storage.
      (a) The perfusion machine pumps solution cooled to 4° C through the renal vasculature to continuously cool, oxygenate, and allow for longer storage times than simple cold storage provides.
      (b) May reduce the incidence of delayed graft function vs. cold storage (Moers et al., 2009).
      (c) Use of pulsatile perfusion has increased in prevalence with the increase of donors with higher KDPI scores.
   (3) The goal is to transplant the kidney in less than 24 hours.
      (a) Reduces the possibility of delayed graft function.
      (b) Most centers prefer not to use the kidney after it is maintained in cold storage for over 36 hours, but exceptions are made (O'Connor et al., 2010).

g. Histocompatibility testing is done as soon as possible after donor identification.
   (1) When possible, donor lymph nodes, rich in white blood cells, are obtained for lymphocyte crossmatching with potential recipients.
   (2) Peripheral blood samples may be used when lymph node retrieval is not feasible.

III. Organ sharing and distribution.

A. United Network for Organ Sharing (UNOS).
   1. Awarded the Organ Procurement and Transplantation (OPTN) contract in 1986 with the passage of the National Organ Transplant Act of 1984 (NOTA). UNOS has received the contract every year since 1986.
   2. Established membership standards for transplant centers and organ procurement organizations (OPO).
   3. Established an equitable organ allocation system throughout country.
      a. Allocation system changes are made by UNOS every few years to reflect analyses of factors that contribute to long-term transplant success based on data collected by the Scientific Registry for Transplant Recipients (SRTR).
      b. The most recent policy revisions can be accessed on the UNOS website at http://www.unos.org
      c. Waiting patients are placed into a rank position by a central computer located in UNOS offices in Richmond, Virginia. The patient's rank within each blood group is determined by:
         (1) Time waiting: based on either a single GFR less than 20 mL/min or initiation of kidney replacement therapy. These dates may precede the actual transplant listing date, and candidates will have an advantage in increased waiting days.

(2) Histocompatibility (HLA) matching: A, B, DR.

(3) Panel-reactive antibody (PRA): level of preformed antibodies. Candidates with more preformed antibodies receive more points since it is difficult to find crossmatch negative donor kidneys.

(4) Pediatric recipients receive priority for donors younger than 35 years.

(5) Previous living donors who subsequently experience kidney failure receive priority points and will receive a transplant sooner.

4. Facilitates organ placement throughout the country.
   a. Organs are distributed locally, regionally, and nationally.
   b. Preferential local distribution when possible to decrease cold ischemia time and subsequent incidence of delayed graft function.
   c. Mandatory allocation of phenotypically identical (zero antigen mismatch) kidney to a highly sensitized patient no matter where located.
5. Monitors distribution and disposition (i.e., transplanted or discarded) of all organs in the United States.
6. Maintains scientific registries for all organs to facilitate data acquisition and management. Results are reported through the SRTR.

Part 3. Organ Transplantation

I. Definition of terminology.

A. Autograft.
   1. Transplantation of a person's own tissue from one body site to another (e.g., skin for a skin graft or a vein for a coronary artery bypass graft).
   2. Because no foreign antigens are introduced, there are no problems with rejection.

B. Isograft. Transplantation of tissues between monozygotic identical twins.

C. Allograft or homograft.
   1. Transplantation of tissues between the same species (from one person to another with different genetic makeup).
   2. Since foreign antigens are introduced into the recipient, rejection of an allograft would occur without the addition of immunosuppressive medications.

D. Xenograft.
   1. Transplantation of tissues between members of different species.
   2. Because of the extreme antigenic differences between the donor and recipient of a xenograft, the incidence of rejection is 100%.

II. Evaluation of the kidney transplant candidate.

A. All Medicare ESRD patients are entitled to be referred for transplant (CMS, 2008).

B. The patient is referred to a transplant center by the nephrologist, nurse, or social worker at the dialysis unit. Some patients are self-referred.

C. Early referral, prior to initiation of dialysis, is encouraged.

D. The purpose of the pretransplant evaluation is to determine the patient's suitability for transplant by identifying and, where possible, correcting those medical and psychosocial factors that would affect a successful outcome in the short and long term.

E. A patient's candidacy is considered on an individual basis. Broad groups of patients are no longer automatically excluded.

F. Transplant centers vary in the way that they accomplish the evaluation, but the transplant team members in this initial phase usually include:
   1. Transplant coordinator.
   2. Transplant surgeon.
   3. Transplant nephrologist/APRN/PA.
   4. Transplant social worker.
   5. Financial coordinator.
   6. Dietitian.
   7. Transplant pharmacist or pharmacologist.

III. Pretransplant patient education.

A. An informational session allows patients to consider if transplantation is the right choice for them.

B. Patient education about transplant includes an outline of center specific evaluation procedures.
   1. Medical evaluation.
   2. Psychosocial evaluation.
   3. Financial evaluation.
   4. Outcomes and setting expectations (G. Danovitch, 2010a; UNOS, 2013b).
      a. Transplant as one of the options for CKD stage 5, but not a "cure."
      b. Patient and graft survival statistics.
      c. The risks and benefits of transplantation.

5. Surgical procedure or hospitalization (G. Danovitch, 2010a; Townsend et al., 2012).
6. Postoperative care (CMS, 2008; G. Danovitch, 2010a; International Transplant Nurses Society [ITNS], http://www.itns.org).
7. Patient responsibilities and self-management.
   a. Patients must understand that one of the main determinants of successful transplantation is patient adherence to medication regimens, clinic visits, and communication of problems to the transplant team.
   b. It is imperative that the patient's role of self-management and monitoring is covered in patient education (Ponticelli & Graziani, 2012).
8. Potential complications of surgery and immunosuppression.
9. Potential long-term complications including, but not limited to, rejection, infection, malignancy, potential kidney disease recurrence, and diabetes (ITNS, 2007; Ponticelli, 2007).
10. Sources of donors.
    a. Living.
       (1) Living related.
       (2) Living unrelated.
       (3) Altruistic.
    b. Deceased.
       (1) Low KDRI. See criteria for deceased donation.
       (2) High KDRI. See criteria for deceased donation.
       (3) Donation after circulatory death.
11. Advantages and disadvantages of living vs. deceased donor kidney.
12. Small but possible risk of disease transmission (infection, cancer) despite donor testing (Ponticelli, 2007; Townsend et al., 2012).
13. Discussion regarding the illegality of buying and selling of organs (Delmonico & Dew, 2007).
14. UNOS policy and the center's policy regarding nontraditional donors; solicitation of donors, including the Internet.
15. UNOS deceased donor waiting list and organ allocation policies (UNOS, 2013b).
16. Options of multiple listing and wait time transfer.
17. Discussion of special programs throughout the country.
    a. Living donor paired exchange ("swap") (Delmonico & Dew, 2007; Sharif, 2013).
    b. ABO incompatible recipient and donor (Becker et al., 2013).
    c. Crossmatch positive recipient and donor (Montgomery et al., 2009).
    d. HIV-positive patients. See separate section on transplantation in HIV-positive patients.
    e. Older patients (> age 70) (Keith, 2013; Rodelo et al., 2013).
    f. Hepatitis C positive donors.
    g. Hepatitis B Core Antibody positive donors.
18. Rights and responsibilities of patients and transplant staff.
19. Other educational resources.
    a. UNOS (United Network for Organ Sharing).
    b. NKF (National Kidney Foundation).
    c. AKF (American Kidney Fund).
    d. AST (American Society of Transplant).
    e. ANNA (American Nephrology Nurses' Association).
    f. ITNS (International Transplant Nurses Society) (G. Danovitch, 2010a; Pham et al., 2010).
    g. NATCO (North American Transplant Coordinators Organization).

IV. Workup and selection of potential recipient.

A. Every transplant center has its own acceptance criteria for candidacy, protocol for evaluation, and absolute and relative contraindications. However, most centers are in agreement regarding major indications and contraindications for transplant.

B. Contraindications.
1. Current or recent malignancy, excluding noninvasive skin cancers.
2. Active or chronic untreated infection.
3. Severe irreversible extrarenal disease (e.g., inoperable cardiac disease, chronic lung disease, severe peripheral vascular disease) (G. Danovitch, 2010a; Pham et al., 2010).
4. Active autoimmune disease (Marinaki et al., 2013; Senglemark, 2013).
5. Morbid obesity (BMI > 35).
   a. This is a center-specific determination.
   b. There is evidence that obesity places transplant recipients at risk for surgical site infections, wound dehiscence, increased length of stay, and other complications.
   c. However, there is still controversy regarding the use of BMI as the cutoff criterion for transplant candidacy.
   d. BMI is an indirect measurement of obesity as it does not address muscle mass or body distribution of fat (such as waist circumference).
   e. The transplant surgeon will determine if the risk of a patient's obesity outweighs the anticipated benefit of transplant (Lentine, Santos et al., 2012; Teta, 2010).
6. Current substance abuse.
7. Psychiatric illness that would prevent informed consent or adherence to treatment regimen (I. Danovitch, 2010; Maldonado et al., 2012).
8. Significant history of nonadherence to treatment regimens.
9. Immunologic circumstances: ABO incompatibility and positive T-cell crossmatch are often

contraindications. However, in some circumstances, these may be addressed with desensitization protocols (G. Danovitch, 2010b; Pham et al., 2010; Townsend et al., 2012).

C. Relative contraindications and special circumstances.
  1. Housing concerns.
    a. Patients who are homeless or are otherwise unable to obtain or store medications properly, as well as having inconsistent or no mailing address, are at potential risk for posttransplant complications related to follow-up and self-maintenance.
    b. Transplant centers will generally try to assist patients in finding stable living circumstances to support home monitoring, medication storage and administration, good hygiene, access to safe food and water, and ability to communicate easily with the transplant center.
    c. However, a transplant center may consider concerns of this nature to be a contraindication to kidney transplantation.
  2. Non-United States citizenship.
    a. Many transplant centers in the United States of America will provide kidney transplant services only to citizens of the USA.
    b. This is related to financial coverage for surgery, hospitalization, medications, and follow-up care, since ESRD care is federally funded through the Medicare program.

D. History and physical examination.
  1. Age.
    a. Physiologic age is more important than chronologic age.
    b. Patients over age 70 are accepted at some centers (Keith, 2013).
    c. Older patients are at increased risk of death related to cardiovascular disease (Keith, 2013; Rodelo et al., 2013).
    d. Rejection episodes may be due to a less reactive immune system in older adults (G. Danovitch, 2010b; Keith, 2013).
    e. For pediatric patients transplant is the treatment of choice, and when possible, pre-emptive with a living donor. The goal of pediatric transplant is to improve delayed skeletal growth, promote sexual and reproductive maturity, improve cognitive development, and enhance psychosocial functioning (I. Danovitch 2010).
  2. Etiology of kidney disease.
    a. Determine native kidney disease.
      (1) Obtain renal biopsy results, if done.
      (2) Important to know the cause since some diseases can recur in the transplanted kidney, and some have comorbidities that

could influence outcome (Marinaki et al., 2013; Senglemark, 2013).
      (3) It can also affect the type of donor chosen, especially when living donation is being considered. Some kidney diseases such as polycystic kidney disease are inherited. A family member donor may be found to have kidney disease.
    b. Type of dialysis, how long, response to treatment.
    c. Determine if patient has had a previous transplant. It is important to know transplant course, treatment, and complications to assess risk in next transplant. Immunosuppression is a cumulative event, and therefore the risk is also cumulative for infection and malignancy (Alberú, 2010; Kosmadakis et al., 2013).
    d. Diabetes mellitus is associated with cardiovascular disease, cerebrovascular disease, peripheral vascular disease, infections, gastroparesis, and neuropathy (neurogenic bladder). All can increase the risk for perioperative and postoperative complications (Guerra, Ilahe, & Ciancio, 2012; Welsh et al., 2011).
    e. Autoimmune diseases need to be quiescent prior to transplant (Segelmark, 2013).
    f. Polycystic kidney disease may require nephrectomy prior to or after transplant if very enlarged or excessive bleeding from cysts or recurrent infections. Recommend cerebral imaging to rule out associated aneurysm (G. Danovitch, 2010a).
    g. Chronic pyelonephritis may also require nephrectomy to prevent infection posttransplant.
    h. Many diseases may recur in the transplanted kidney including:
      (1) Focal and segmental glomerulosclerosis (FSGS).
      (2) MPGN I and II.
      (3) IgA nephropathy.
      (4) Membranous nephropathy.
      (5) Diabetic nephropathy.
      (6) Certain types of oxalosis.
      (7) Wegener's disease.
      (8) Fabry disease.
      (9) Systemic lupus erythematosus.
      (10) Thrombotic thrombocytopenic purpura (TTP) (Canaud et al., 2012; Marinaki et al., 2013).
  3. Urinary tract.
    a. Patients with a history of recurrent infection, reflux, kidney or bladder stones, chronic urinary diversion, bladder dysfunction, neurogenic bladder, benign prostatic hypertrophy, or obstructive uropathy will

require evaluation to ensure bladder function after transplant (Karem & Giessing, 2011; Pham et al., 2010; Power et al., 2004; Townsend et al., 2012).

b. The patient must be free of active urinary tract infections due to the large amount of immunosuppression used at the time of transplant.

c. Urine output is important to assess before transplant as it may be important to assess early function of the allograft (Karam & Giessing, 2011).

d. Assessment of bladder function.

(1) The urologic tract must be evaluated for sufficient urinary storage in terms of capacity and low pressure, functional urethral control to maintain continence, and a clear passageway for complete bladder evacuation by voiding or self-catheterization (Power et al., 2004).

(2) Patients with neurogenic bladders or atonicity may be required to perform periodic self-catheterization (Karam & Giessing, 2011).

(3) Voiding cystourethrogram with postvoid films, if indicated.

(4) Urodynamic studies, if indicated.

(5) Routine urinalysis and culture, if indicated.

(6) Catheterization for post-void residual, if indicated (Karam & Giessing, 2011; Power et al., 2004).

(7) Men: Examination of prostate size and character and prostate-specific antigen (PSA) if recommended by physician.

(8) Women: Gynecologic examination may reveal related causes of urologic dysfunction, which may need to be addressed (Karam & Giessing, 2011; Power et al., 2004).

(9) Cystoscopy for patients treated with cyclophosphamide for immune-mediated kidney disease (such as antineutrophil cytoplasmic antibody-associated vasculitis or granulomatosis with polyangiitis) due to association of cyclophosphamide with urinary tract malignancy (Mahr et al., 2013).

4. Cardiovascular system.

a. Cardiac disease is the leading cause of death with functioning graft in transplant recipients. Pretransplant cardiovascular evaluation is done to decrease cardiovascular morbidity and mortality as much as possible.

b. High risk patients who are likely to be deferred pending intervention or waiting time include those with active cardiac conditions such as unstable angina or recent myocardial infarction, significant arrhythmia, severe valvular disease, and decompensated heart failure (G. Danovitch, 2010a; Lentine, Costa et al., 2012).

c. Centers differ in whether invasive or noninvasive testing is used to assess cardiovascular risk.

(1) For patients in CKD stage 4 or 5, angiography carries the risk of worsening kidney function, resulting in the need for dialysis.

(2) The decision whether or not to use invasive testing to evaluate cardiovascular risk is generally determined by a combination of stage of CKD plus number of relevant risk factors including: left ventricular hypertrophy, age > 60 years, smoking, hypertension, dyslipidemia, diabetes mellitus, prior cardiovascular disease, and > 1 year on dialysis.

d. Risk of surgery is increased by ischemic heart disease, therefore preemptive treatment, medically or surgically, is recommended (Lentine et al., 2005; Lentine, Costa et al., 2012).

e. Patients with peripheral vascular disease and/or aortoiliac disease may have compromised blood flow to the transplanted kidney or lower extremities, with higher rates of delayed graft function and graft failure.

(1) Also, patients with peripheral vascular disease have a higher rate of all cause and cardiovascular mortality.

(2) Patients with a history of claudication, lower extremity amputations, or history of cardiovascular or cerebrovascular disease warrant further investigation (Brar et al., 2013).

f. The patient must have:

(1) Adequate cardiac function.

(2) Patent iliac vasculature.

(3) Absence of severe atherosclerosis.

(4) A thorough assessment of prior cardiac and vascular events.

(5) Corrective interventions may be required prior to transplantation: coronary artery bypass surgery, stent placement, valve replacement, peripheral bypass surgery per recommendation by a cardiologist, cardiovascular surgery, and transplant surgery.

(6) Evaluation of any arrhythmias with adequate control determined by cardiologist, with explanation of operative risks to patient. In particular, pre-existing atrial fibrillation is associated with higher mortality and ischemic stroke events posttransplant (Lenihan et al., 2013).

g. Screening of asymptomatic patients with risk factors for coronary artery disease is recommended.

h. Assessment.
   (1) History and physical examination.
   (2) EKG.
   (3) Echocardiogram, if indicated.
   (4) If there are any positive findings in the history, the patient may also need stress testing, cardiac catheterization, evaluation by a cardiologist, and Doppler studies.
   (5) CT or MRA of abdominal and pelvic vessels, if indicated.
   (6) Noninvasive lower extremity arterial studies with measurement of ABI (ankle brachial index), if indicated.
   (7) Angiography, if indicated.
   (8) Evaluation by vascular surgeon, if indicated (Brar et al., 2013; Lentine, Costa et al., 2012).

5. Pulmonary system.
   a. The potential for posttransplant pulmonary complications in the immunosuppressed host must be evaluated prior to transplantation.
   b. Lung disease can increase the risk of anesthesia and surgery. Fluid overload, ventilator dependency, and pneumonia are all potential complications (G. Danovitch, 2010a).
   c. The prevalence of chronic obstructive pulmonary disease (COPD) among patients with kidney failure is rising, and is associated with higher mortality rates than patients without COPD.
      (1) COPD has been correlated with older age, cardiovascular conditions, malnutrition, cancer, and tobacco use.
      (2) These contribute to morbidity and mortality posttransplant.
      (3) Patients with a history of chronic obstructive lung disease or restrictive lung disease need further evaluation by a pulmonologist.
      (4) Severe COPD may be a contraindication to transplant (Kent et al., 2012).
   d. Pulmonary hypertension (PH) has become a recognized complication of CKD and ESRD, causing increased morbidity and mortality before and after transplantation.
      (1) In these populations, PH is thought to be related to endothelial dysfunction, increased cardiac output, valvular disease, and myocardial dysfunction, elevating left heart filling pressure.
      (2) Also, increased vascular calcification in patients with CKD or kidney failure leads to increased pulmonary vascular resistance, leading to PH.

   (3) High rates of systolic and diastolic heart failure are associated with PH.
   (4) Echocardiogram is used to screen patients for PH, and patients with elevated pulmonary arterial pressure or symptoms such as unexplained dyspnea should undergo right heart catheterization (during "dry" state for patients on dialysis) to determine severity of disease (G. Danovitch, 2010a; Kawar et al., 2013; Sise et al., 2013).

   e. Patients who smoke, chew, or use smokeless tobacco should be encouraged to stop. Some programs do not transplant patients who are currently smoking.
   f. Patients with a positive PPD should be treated prophylactically with INH for 6 months (Khosroshahi et al., 2006).
   g Assessment.
      (1) History and physical examination.
      (2) Chest x-ray, PA, and lateral views.
      (3) Pulmonary function studies, if indicated.
      (4) TB testing, by QuantiFERON® Gold or PPD.
      (5) Pneumococcal pneumonia immunization.
      (6) Evaluation by a pulmonologist, if indicated, and possible right heart catheterization, if indicated.
      (7) Evaluation by an infectious disease specialist, if indicated.

6. Neurologic system.
   a. Patients with a history of CVA, TIA, seizure disorder, or other neurologic event are at risk for increased complications in the perioperative and postoperative periods.
      (1) These patients may require neurologic evaluation prior to listing or receiving a kidney transplant.
      (2) This evaluation may be done in concert with the anesthesia evaluation.
      (3) Risk factors for cerebrovascular events include diabetes mellitus, atrial fibrillation, peripheral vascular disease, and previous myocardial infarction or cerebrovascular events (Aull-Watschinger et al., 2008).
   b. Patients with a history of seizures may require a change in therapy due to potential interaction with immunosuppressives.
      (1) This should be done in collaboration with the patient's neurologist.
      (2) Some transplant recipients are at higher risk of seizures while taking immunosuppressive therapy as calcineurin inhibitors (CNI).
      (3) Corticosteroids are associated with neurotoxicity which can result in seizures.
      (4) The transplant candidate should be

prepared for postoperative monitoring of any seizure disorder by a neurologist and understand the potential need to change therapy (Marco, Ferronato, & Patrizia, 2008).
   c. Assessment.
     (1) History and physical.
     (2) Carotid duplex.
     (3) Brain imaging for PKD patients to rule out cerebral aneurysm.
     (4) Evaluation by a neurologist, if indicated.
7. Gastrointestinal system.
   a. Active peptic ulcer disease, pancreatitis, cholecystitis, and diverticulitis must be medically or surgically treated to prevent complications associated with the use of immunosuppressive medications after transplant.
   b. Active or chronic liver disease must be evaluated.
   c. Liver enzyme elevations must be investigated.
   d. The patient with severe gastroparesis must have a thorough evaluation of his or her gastric emptying ability.
   e. Esophageal infections must be completely treated prior to transplantation.
   f. Colonoscopy must be up to date for patients at high risk for colon cancer or over age 50 (G. Danovitch, 2010a; Pham et al., 2010).
   g. Assessment.
     (1) History and physical examination.
     (2) Stool examination for occult blood.
     (3) Radiologic studies as indicated.
     (4) Depending on age, colonoscopy, and/or barium enema.
     (5) Hepatitis B immunization status.
     (6) Liver function tests and hepatitis B and C screening.
     (7) Evaluation by a gastroenterologist and/or hepatologist, if indicated.
8. Endocrine system.
   a. Evaluation and treatment of hyperparathyroidism is completed prior to transplantation.
     (1) Hyperparathyroidism is associated with vascular calcifications, increasing morbidity and mortality.
     (2) High parathyroid levels are also associated with poorer kidney function posttransplant.
     (3) Posttransplant parathyroidectomy may be complicated by further decline in graft function, in addition to usual postoperative risks (Parikh et al., 2013).
   b. Evaluation of patient with diabetes.
     (1) Discussion of kidney alone vs. combined kidney–pancreas transplant. Note whether patient uses insulin pump and efficacy of therapy.
     (2) History of glucose control, episodes of hypo/hyperglycemia requiring medical attention (G. Danovitch, 2010a; Pham et al., 2010).
     (3) Ophthalmology assessment for presence and degree of retinopathy.
     (4) Evaluation for diabetic neuropathy (peripheral and central).
   c. Assess control of hypertension. Uncontrolled hypertension increases risk of cardiovascular and cerebrovascular events at time of transplant (G. Danovitch, 2010a; Townsend et al., 2012).
   d. Females must have recent (within 12 months) gynecologic examination, PAP smear (if sexually active or > 18 years of age), and mammogram (if 40 or older, or at high risk for breast cancer).
   e. Assessment.
     (1) History and physical examination.
     (2) Parathyroid hormone level, serum calcium, phosphorus, and 25-hydroxy vitamin D level.
     (3) Pap smear.
     (4) Mammogram.
     (5) Assessment of birth control: pregnancy is not recommended for at least 1 year posttransplant, or at any time when a patient is taking mycophenolate mofetil or mycophenolic acid, as these medications have been associated with fetal malformations (Klieger-Grossmann, et al., 2010).
     (6) Serum creatinine should also be stable and preferably less than 2.0 mg/dL at a minimum, and preferably ≤ 1.3 mg/dL.
     (7) Discussion of appropriate birth control with individual patient is dependent upon clinical condition.
     (8) Pregnancy is possible soon after transplantation as hormonal changes occur with more normal kidney function (Hou, 2013).
9. Dental system.
   a. Teeth or gum disease must be resolved prior to transplantation.
     (1) Patients who have CKD or are on dialysis have a higher rate of periodontal disease than the general public.
     (2) This places patients at high risk for infection after transplantation (Borawski et al., 2007; G. Danovitch, 2010a).
   b. Presence of infected teeth or gums may threaten the life of the postoperative immunosuppressed patient due to the high risk for bacteremia.

c. Assessment.
   (1) History and physical examination.
   (2) Written statement from dentist regarding status of teeth and gums.

10. Cancer screening.
   a. Patients with kidney failure have a higher risk of cancer than the general population (Mosconi et al., 2011; Pham et al., 2010).
   b. Patients who underwent immunosuppression for treatment of their original kidney disease or for a prior transplant are at increased risk for cancer (Alberú, 2010).
   c. Prior history of cancer that was treated does not preclude transplant.
      (1) Each patient should be individually evaluated regarding risk of recurrence and time frame for transplantation.
      (2) A waiting period of 2 to 5 years, depending on the malignancy, is recommended.
      (3) No waiting period may be necessary for malignancies with a low chance of metastasis such as basal cell carcinomas, encapsulated renal cell carcinoma, primary CNS tumors, and in-situ tumors (Pham et al., 2010; Ponticelli, 2007; Townsend et al., 2012).
   d. All patients should have routine cancer screenings according to American Cancer Society guidelines.

11. Infection.
   a. Infections are a major cause of morbidity and mortality after transplantation.
   b. An active infection is a contraindication to transplant (Fischer et al., 2009).
   c. Patients with hepatitis B or C may be considered for kidney transplantation after evaluation including viral load and possible liver biopsy. Antiviral therapy prior to transplant may be done. See section on transplantation of the hepatitis C positive patient.
   d. Assessment.
      (1) History and physical examination.
         (a) TB testing by Quantiferon Gold or PPD for all patients, with additional testing for positive skin test, or those who are anergic.
         (b) Special attention should be paid to dialysis access sites.
         (c) Careful history to assess for any active infection.
         (d) Include travel history.
      (2) Viral and fungal screening (CMV, EBV, HIV, and varicella; immunization record in children).
      (3) Hepatitis B and C screening (Fischer et al., 2009).

12. Immunologic system.
   a. A thorough assessment of immunologic status will aid in predicting the graft outcome.
   b. Previous transplants, blood transfusions, and pregnancy may alter the host response to additional foreign antigens (G. Danovitch, 2010b).
   c. Autoimmune diseases must be quiescent before transplantation is undertaken (Segelmark, 2013).
   d. Pretransplant modification of the immune system.
      (1) Splenectomy, total body irradiation, and thoracic lymph duct drainage were once used to decrease the number of circulating lymphocytes. These procedures are rarely used currently.
      (2) Plasmapheresis is sometimes used to decrease the presence of cytotoxic antibodies. This is usually done in the form of an antibody reduction protocol in conjunction with intravenous immuno-globulin and immunosuppression (Sadeghi et al., 2013).
   e. Assessment.
      (1) ABO testing identifies the blood type of the donor and recipient.
      (2) Histocompatibility testing is the detection of antigens on cell membranes or in cell walls that determines the genetic composition and defines whether foreign tissue is accepted or rejected by the host.
      (3) Cytotoxic screening or panel reactive antibodies (PRA).
         (a) PRA is a blood test using lymphocytotoxic antibodies obtained from multiparous females or from recipients of multiple blood transfusions to determine the presence of preformed antibodies to human leukocyte antigens (HLA).
         (b) The results range from 0% to 100% and reflect the percentage of antigens on the test panel against which the potential recipient has preformed antibodies (G. Danovitch, 2010b; Ponticelli, 2007).
      (4) Review of transfusion history since last serum sample submitted for cytotoxic screening. Any transfusion may result in the production of antibodies that may affect the recipient's response to a transplanted kidney.
      (5) Review of status of autoimmune disease (titers).
         (a) Transplantation cannot be performed in the presence of active autoimmune disease processes, which may adversely

affect the transplanted kidney (e.g., if the patient has lupus, it is important to wait until quiescent).
   (b) This is also due to the condition of the patient during a time of active immune mediated-disease, which is usually treated with steroids or other immunosuppressive medications.
   (c) The patient will be more susceptible to infections and other complications during active immune disease (Marinaki et al., 2013; Ponticelli, 2007).
   (6) Review of pregnancy history. Challenges to the immune system (multiple pregnancies) may result in the development of significant cytotoxic antibodies.
   (7) Review of HLA antigens of previous transplants. Exposure to foreign HLA antigens from prior transplants may result in development of specific antibodies (G. Danovitch, 2010b; Ponticelli, 2007).
   (8) A current, positive cytotoxic T cell crossmatch between deceased donor and recipient lymphocytes, indicating the presence of preformed antibodies, is an absolute contraindication to transplantation. There are now pretransplant desensitization protocols at some centers to allow transplantation across HLA barriers with live donor transplantation (Becker et al., 2013).
   (9) Some centers use flow cytometry crossmatches to detect very low levels of circulating antibodies, especially in high-risk patients (e.g., retransplants). False positives may be a limitation of this crossmatch (Bunnapradist & Danovitch, 2007; Ponticelli, 2007).
13. Other medical conditions.
   a. Hypercoagulable state.
      (1) Prevalence of thrombophilia in the CKD population increases the risk of graft loss due to renal vein or renal artery thrombosis (Bunnapradist & Danovitch, 2007).
      (2) History of thrombosis, multiple clotting of AV fistulas or grafts, requires more in-depth coagulation screening and possible referral to a hematologist.
      (3) Assessment.
         (a) Prior history of deep vein thrombosis (DVT).
         (b) Further laboratory tests as indicated.
            i. Antiphospholipid antibodies.
            ii. Lupus anticoagulant.
            iii. Anticardiolipin antibody.
            iv. Protein C.
            v. Protein S.
            vi. Homocysteine.
            vii. Factor V Leiden.
            viii. Prothrombin gene mutation (G20210A).
            ix. Antithrombin III.
            x. Activated Protein C.
         (c) Evaluation by a hematologist, as indicated.
   b. Obesity.
      (1) Obese patients are at greater risk for delayed graft function, surgical and wound complications, posttransplant diabetes mellitus, and cardiovascular disease (Lentine, Santos et al., 2012).
      (2) A BMI (Body Mass Index) of > 30 kg/m² is considered a contraindication to transplant at some centers, although many centers consider it up to 35, or look at the patient on a case-by-case basis.
      (3) Weight loss is recommended.
      (4) Bariatric surgery for those morbidly obese may be considered (Lentine, Santos et al., 2012; Teta, 2010).
   c. Diabetes.
      (1) Transplantation is the preferred kidney replacement therapy to improve glycemic control, improve quality of life, and potentially decrease the incidence of macrovascular and microvascular complications of diabetes as compared to remaining on dialysis.
      (2) Consider simultaneous kidney/pancreas transplantation for type I diabetics to prevent recurrence of diabetic complications in the renal graft and prevent or delay other secondary complications of diabetes (Eller et al., 2013).
      (3) Assessment.
         (a) Meticulous assessment of cardiac function.
            i. Stress testing.
            ii. Cardiac catheterization (some centers do even if stress test is normal).
            iii. Cardiology evaluation (Eller et al., 2013; Lentine, Costa et al., 2012).
         (b) Ophthalmologic examination (protocols vary).
         (c) Neurologic evaluation. Determine extent of diabetic neuropathy.
         (d) Gastrointestinal evaluation. Evaluate for gastroparesis or other GI motility concerns prior to transplantation.
         (e) Urologic evaluation. Evaluate for any evidence of neurogenic bladder.

14. Psychosocial system.
    a. Social work interview with patient and family provides information about the patient's illness history, coping ability, and support system, all of which can impact transplant outcome.
    b. Should determine patient's ability to provide informed consent.
    c. Patient and staff should use the pretransplant period to plan for transplant surgery and posttransplant needs.
       (1) Getting to the hospital for transplant.
       (2) Assistance at home after surgery.
       (3) Transportation to follow-up clinic visits.
       (4) Adequate medical insurance and coverage for the cost of medications.
    d. Assessment.
       (1) Adjustment and understanding of present illness and therapy options.
       (2) Living situation.
       (3) Educational background.
       (4) Employment history.
       (5) Lifestyle prior to illness.
       (6) Adherence to treatment regimen.
          (a) Dialyzes as scheduled or misses treatments and/or doctors' appointments?
          (b) Takes medications as prescribed?
          (c) Follows diet?
       (7) History of substance abuse.
       (8) History of psychiatric illness.
       (9) Identify factors warranting further education or therapeutic interventions prior to decision for transplant candidacy.
       (10) Medical insurance and drug coverage for transplant medications.
       (11) Financial resources.
       (12) The financial coordinator gives financial clearance for the transplant and frequently works in tandem with the social worker regarding the last two issues (Dobbels et al., 2008; Maldonado et al., 2012).
15. Role of the referring physician.
    a. May perform the candidate evaluation using local consultants and resources in collaboration with the transplant center.
    b. Communication between referring physician and transplant center is essential.
    c. Transplant center must provide written and verbal reports of hospitalizations and transplant clinic visits.

V. Immediate preoperative care of the kidney transplant recipient.

A. Preparation for surgery.
   1. Communication with referring physician regarding patient's candidacy.
      a. Any current illnesses (infections, malignancies) that may preclude transplantation.
      b. Determine when patient was last dialyzed.
   2. NPO for 6–8 hours preoperatively to prevent perioperative aspiration and postoperative nausea and vomiting.
   3. History and physical are performed to determine that there are no current medical contraindications to transplantation.
   4. Laboratory testing. Pretransplant hematology, chemistries, viral titers, and urine culture are performed to detect any abnormalities and provide baseline data for postoperative comparisons.
   5. Chest x-ray to assess for fluid overload, pneumonia, or new lesions.
   6. EKG obtained to document cardiac function.
   7. Vital signs and baseline weight.
   8. Skin preparation in OR and prophylactic antibiotic dosage prior to surgery.
   9. Vascular access or peritoneal dialysis catheter exit site assessment and effluent culture to assure the absence of infection.
   10. Insertion of intravenous lines, peripheral, and/or central lines.
   11. Immunosuppression may be ordered to be given prior to the surgery.
   12. Patient and family education.
   13. A final cytotoxic crossmatch is performed.
   14. Pretransplant dialysis may be necessary for hyperkalemia or fluid overload to permit safe induction of general anesthesia.
   15. Placement of a foley catheter in operating room (OR) prior to surgery.

VI. The kidney transplant surgical procedure.

A. The surgical procedure is essentially unchanged since the first transplant was performed in 1954.
   1. The kidney is usually placed in the anterior iliac fossa, extraperitoneally (see Figure 3.1).
   2. Preference is given to placement in the right iliac fossa due to the accessibility of the iliac vein.
   3. The renal vein is anastomosed to the iliac vein to minimize leg ischemia and establish outflow for subsequent renal artery anastomosis.
   4. The renal artery is anastomosed to the external iliac artery.
   5. To minimize warm ischemia during anastomosis, the kidney is covered with gauze with crushed iced saline.

6. The ureter is tunneled into the bladder or anastomosed end-to-side to recipient's native ureter or anastomosed to previously created ileal conduit.
    a. In most cases a stent should be placed to decrease the urinary complication rate (Mangus & Haag, 2004).
    b. Stents are generally removed 3 to 4 weeks after transplantation to avoid infection.
    c. It is vital to track and document stent insertion and removal due to the potential for future complications with retained stents (Veale et al., 2010).
7. A Jackson-Pratt or Penrose drain may be placed in the perirenal space to:
    a. Drain blood or lymph.
    b. Detect a urine leak from the ureteral anastomosis.
    c. Reduce the formation of lymphoceles.
    d. Drains are generally removed when output is less than 100 mL/day (Veale et al., 2010).
8. Special considerations.
    a. Inserting adult kidneys into infants or small children (less than 10–12 kg) generally requires intraperitoneal placement. To prevent vascular thrombosis, the venous anastomosis is made to the vena cava while the arterial is to the aorta.
    b. In patients with type 1 diabetes who may be future candidates for pancreas after kidney (PAK) transplant, the kidney is placed in the left iliac fossa in anticipation of future pancreas placement on the right (Veale et al., 2010).

B. The anatomic placement of the graft in the iliac fossa assists in the ease of patient assessment.
    1. Ease of vascular and ureteral placement.
    2. Facilitates diagnosis of rejection.
        a. Graft tenderness is easily assessed.
        b. Easy access for percutaneous needle biopsy to diagnose kidney allograft dysfunction.
    3. Obviates need for pretransplant native nephrectomy.

VII. Postoperative management of the kidney transplant recipient.

A. Maintain circulatory function.
    1. Frequent monitoring of vital signs per center protocol (blood pressure, temperature, pulse, respirations, central venous pressure).
    2. Monitor femoral, popliteal, and pedal pulses bilaterally. Report to credentialed practitioner any diminished flow, especially on side of transplanted kidney.
    3. Monitor cardiac status. Deep vein thrombosis (DVT) prevention per center protocol.
        a. Sequential compression stockings with early

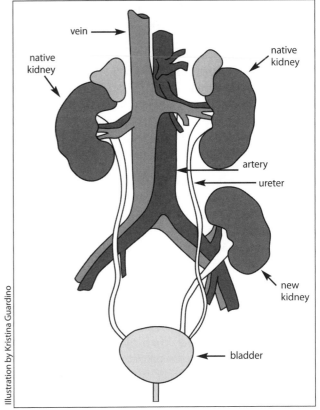

Illustration by Kristina Guardino

Figure 3.1. Kidney transplant placement.

initiation of low-dose aspirin for all nonallergic recipients.
    b. Subcutaneous heparin injections (dose based on kidney function) in high-risk recipients (Veale et al., 2010).
    4. Assess arteriovenous fistula (AVF) or arteriovenous graft (AVG) for function every 4 hours (Wilkinson, 2010).

B. Maintain pulmonary function.
    1. Turn, cough, and deep breathe hourly while awake.
    2. Encourage use of incentive spirometer hourly while awake.
    3. Early ambulation 3 to 4 times daily.

C. Monitor fluid and electrolyte balance per center protocol.
    1. Daily weight.
    2. Monitor fluid intake and urine output per center protocol.
    3. Replace fluids based on urine output per protocol.
    4. Monitor urinary catheter for blood clots which can obstruct the flow of urine and obtain order for gentle irrigation as indicated (Wilkinson, 2010).
    5. Daily laboratory testing to evaluate potassium, creatinine, phosphorus, CBC, etc.
    6. Assess for fluid volume impairment.

a. Fluid volume deficit: hypotension, dry mucous membranes, poor skin turgor (tenting), concentrated urine, decreased central venous pressure (CVP).

b. Fluid volume excess: shortness of breath, crackles, increased CVP, presence of edema.

7. Administer diuretics as prescribed and monitor urine output.

8. Maintain mean arterial pressure above 80 mm Hg to perfuse transplanted kidney and to decrease risk of arterial or venous thrombosis and graft loss (Veale et al., 2010).

D. Prevention of infection.
   1. Pulmonary toilet.
   2. Careful hand washing before and after patient contact.
   3. Promote adequate nutrition for wound healing.
   4. Aseptic care of intravenous lines, wound, and urinary catheter.
   5. Isolate infected patients.
   6. Facilitate oral and skin hygiene.
   7. Modified protective isolation for recipient with leukopenia.
   8. Assess patients for signs and symptoms of infection.
   9. Administer prophylactic antiviral agents and antibiotics as prescribed.

E. Provide and monitor immunosuppressive regimen.

F. Administer pain medication as needed and evaluate effectiveness.

G. Assess and assist with treatment for complications.
   1. Short-term complications.
      a. Rejection.
         (1) Accelerated acute rejection.
            (a) Hyperacute rejection.
            (b) Delayed hyperacute rejection.
         (2) Early cell-mediated rejection (10% or less incidence at many centers).
         (3) Antibody-mediated rejection (Wilkinson, 2010).
      b. Renal artery thrombosis.
         (1) Uncommon, usually occurs in first 2 to 3 days postop. Risk factors: hypercoagulable disorders, multiple arteries, significant atherosclerosis in donor or recipient vessels (Veale et al., 2010).
         (2) Requires early detection for treatment (emergent arteriotomy and thrombectomy) to be effective. Majority require nephrectomy (Veale et al., 2010).
         (3) Signs and symptoms: sudden anuria, graft tenderness.
      c. Renal vein thrombosis.

   (1) Symptoms include decreased urine output, proteinuria, hematuria, graft tenderness, and swelling of graft, thigh, and leg.
   (2) Treated with anticoagulation therapy or attempted thrombectomy with revision of the anastomosis.
   (3) Often requires nephrectomy (Veale et al., 2010).
      d. Urologic complications.
         (1) Urine leak results from ureteral leakage, ureteral disruption, or leak from the bladder.
         (2) Usually a result of poor tissue healing, most often seen in patients with diabetes or in patients taking sirolimus (Rapamune®), ureteral stenosis, or distal ureteric ischemia (Veale et al., 2010).
      e. Delayed graft function (DGF).
         (1) Differential diagnosis.
            (a) Acute tubular necrosis: most frequent cause of DGF.
            (b) Intravascular volume contraction.
            (c) Arterial or venous thrombosis of graft.
            (d) Ureteric or catheter obstruction.
            (e) Urine leak.
            (f) Nephrotoxicity.
            (g) Thrombotic microangiopathy.
            (h) Hyperacute rejection (Wilkinson, 2010).
         (2) Symptoms.
            (a) Decreased urine volume.
            (b) Elevated BUN and creatinine.
         (3) Treatment.
            (a) Dialysis may be indicated for hyperkalemia or volume overload.
            (b) Decrease dietary potassium.
            (c) Avoid nephrotoxic medications and delay use of calcineurin inhibitors.
            (d) All medications should be dosed based on eGFR.
      f. Acute tubular necrosis (ATN).
         (1) Etiology.
            (a) Usually an ischemic injury: prolonged cold or warm ischemic time.
            (b) Deceased donor hypotension or dehydration.
            (c) May be more common with use of expanded criteria donor kidneys (ECDs) and donation after circulatory death (DCD).
            (d) Rare in living donor transplants (Wilkinson, 2010).
         (2) Symptoms are similar to DGF.
            (a) Decreased urine output.
            (b) Elevated BUN and creatinine.
            (c) Nonoliguric ATN (high urine volume with low creatinine clearance).

(3) Treatment as for DGF.
g. Wound complications.
  (1) Patients who are obese are at greater risk (Wilkinson, 2010).
  (2) Include perinephric hematomas, urinomas, lymphoceles, and abscesses which can mechanically compress the kidney or ureters and result in deterioration of kidney function.
  (3) Wound infection: uncommon due to prophylactic antibiotics and improved surgical techniques (Wilkinson, 2010).
  (4) Signs and symptoms.
    (a) Redness, tenderness, swelling, and/or drainage at transplant incision site.
    (b) Fever.
    (c) Elevated WBC.
    (d) Lower extremity edema on same side as the transplant.
h. Urinary tract infection (UTI).
  (1) Most UTIs in the immediate posttransplant period are related to the surgical instrumentation of the urinary tract, the urinary catheter, ureteral stenting, possible anatomic variations post-operatively (e.g., ureteral stricture, vesicoureteric reflux, ureterovesicular stenosis), recipient with preexisting diabetes, and/or neurogenic bladder (Pegues et al., 2010).
  (2) The UTI may cause no symptoms, but more often the following symptoms are present: fever, urinary frequency, urgency, foul-smelling, and/or cloudy urine. Patients with diabetes may experience nausea and/or vomiting with any episode of infection.
  (3) UTIs are the most frequent cause of secondary bacteremia in a kidney transplant recipient. Prompt diagnosis by urinalysis, urine culture, and sensitivity, along with treatment with antibiotics is essential to prevent bacteremia, morbidity, and possible mortality (Pegues et al., 2010).
  (4) Early catheter removal and antibiotic prophylaxis for 6 months after transplantation decreases the incidence of UTIs (Pegues et al., 2010).
i. Metabolic complications include immunosuppression-induced diabetes mellitus (DMT2), Cushingoid effects, and disorders of calcium and phosphorus metabolism.
j. Psychosocial issues include anxiety, depression, sexual dysfunction, coping with body changes, and adjustment to wellness (Danovitch, 2010).
2. Long-term complications.
a. Chronic renal allograft nephropathy (CAN) or chronic allograft failure (CAF), formerly known as chronic rejection (Wilkinson & Kasiske, 2010). Revised Banff 2005 Classification System renamed CAN as "interstitial fibrosis and tubular atrophy (IFTA) without evidence of any specific etiology" (Solez et al., 2007).
  (1) The most common cause of kidney transplant failure after the first year following transplant (Vella & Brennan, 2013).
  (2) Slow, variable rate of decreasing GFR.
  (3) Proteinuria and hypertension.
  (4) Other causes of graft dysfunction need to be ruled out by biopsy.
  (5) Biopsy findings graded by Banff grading system I to III (Solez et al., 2007). Main findings are interstitial fibrosis with tubular loss and atrophy.
    (a) Grade I – mild fibrosis of interstitium.
    (b) Grade II – moderate interstitial fibrosis.
    (c) Grade III – severe interstitial fibrosis.
    (d) May be associated with humoral anti-donor antibodies and C4d complement deposition (Worthington et al., 2007).
  (6) Risk factors.
    (a) Use of expanded criteria donor kidneys (ECDs).
    (b) Prolonged ischemic time.
    (c) Delayed graft function.
    (d) Acute rejection episodes (Wilkinson & Kasiske, 2010).
    (e) Calcineurin inhibitor toxicity.
    (f) Infection (e.g., CMV, polyomaviruses).
    (g) Medication nonadherence.
    (h) Hyperlipidemia.
    (i) Cigarette smoking.
    (j) Suboptimal immunosuppression.
    (k) Poorly controlled diabetes and/or hypertension.
  (7) May delay progression by control of blood pressure and blood glucose, treatment of hyperlipidemia, and avoidance of acute rejection, ACEIs/ARBs to decrease proteinuria. Immunosuppressive regimens may be altered (calcineurin avoidance). Plasmapheresis and immune globulin regimen for anti-donor antibodies (Klein & Brennan, 2013).
b. Recurrence of original disease in the transplant.
c. Gastrointestinal issues such as ulcers, liver disease, cholecystitis, and/or pancreatitis.
d. Ophthalmic problems including cataracts, glaucoma, and/or visual disturbances. Annual dilated eye exam by an ophthamologist is encouraged.
e. Metabolic conditions such as hypertension, immunosupression-induced diabetes mellitus,

secondary hyperparathyroidism, and Cushingoid effects.

f. Transplant renal artery stenosis (TRAS).
   (1) Usually occurs 3 months to 2 years after transplant, but can occur later (Bruno et al., 2004).
   (2) Signs/symptoms: uncontrolled hypertension with multiple medications, new bruit over graft.
   (3) Kidney dysfunction may occur, particularly after addition of an ACEI or ARB.
   (4) Can be diagnosed with ultrasound, but magnetic resonance arteriography or CT angiography is definitive.
   (5) Treatment includes antihypertensive therapy, surgical repair, or balloon angioplasty.

g. Cardiovascular complications can include hypertension, congestive heart failure, coronary artery disease, cerebral vascular disease, and/or peripheral vascular disease.

h. Infections.
   (1) Overview.
      (a) Approximately 80% of infections in kidney transplant recipients are bacterial.
      (b) Kidney transplant recipients are at high risk of infection due to multiple factors including long-term use of immuno-suppressive medications, metabolic abnormalities such as hyperglycemia, uremia, and/or malnutrition, and the use of invasive medical devices such as urinary and central venous catheters (Pegues et al., 2010).
      (c) Routine immunization with inactivated vaccines is safe and recommended for transplant recipients including 23-valent unconjugated and 7-valent conjugated pneumococcal and annual influenza A and B vaccines (Pegues et al., 2010).
      (d) A detailed discussion of infections in transplant recipients is beyond the scope of this chapter, but an excellent discussion can be found in Danovitch's *Handbook of Kidney Transplantation*, Chapter 1, by David Pegues et al.
   (2) UTI.
      (a) Recipients with diabetes and/or with neurogenic bladders may experience recurrent UTIs long-term (Wilkinson et al., 2010).
      (b) In addition, female recipients may experience recurrent UTIs due to sexual intercourse and/or inadequate perineal hygiene.

   (3) Cytomegalovirus (CMV).
      (a) An opportunistic viral infection acquired either from the donor kidney, from reactivation of the latent virus within the recipient, through blood products, or via sexual contact (Pegues et al., 2010).
      (b) Active disease may develop the first month after transplantation or at any time thereafter and is related to the "net state of immunosuppression" of the recipient (i.e., interaction between amount of immunosuppressive medications and recipient's level of immunodeficiency or immune competence).
      (c) The CMV antibody status of donor and recipient are determined at the time of transplant. Primary CMV infections are the most serious (CMV donor (+) kidneys to CMV (-) recipient) and can be life-threatening.
      (d) Signs and symptoms of CMV infection include fever, leukopenia, fatigue, and graft dysfunction.
      (e) With primary infections in particular, CMV invasive disease may occur and is manifested by hepatitis, pneumonitis, colitis, and/or allograft infection.
      (f) Oral or intravenous antiviral agents:
         i. Are initiated early in the posttransplant period and during episodes of rescue therapy.
         ii. Are used to prevent or treat infection and are generally quite efficacious.
         iii. Some centers may use CMV Immune Globulin (CMVIG) in addition to IV or oral antiviral agents to treat active CMV disease. (Pegues et al., 2010).
   (4) BK Virus.
      (a) An opportunistic virus of the polyomavirus family which also includes the JC virus.
      (b) BK virus is latent (60-80% of adults are seropositive) and may reactivate during more intensive dosing of immunosuppressive medications (induction or rescue therapy).
      (c) It may cause tubulointerstitial nephritis, ureteral stenosis or stricture, and/or graft dysfunction.
      (d) Per center protocol, urinary or plasma DNA PCR is screened at center-specified intervals.

(e) Treatment includes reduction of immunosuppressive medications while closely assessing for signs of rejection.
   i. Leflunomide has both antiviral and immunosuppressive properties and is not nephrotoxic, thus is a first line agent for treatment of BK nephropathy.
   ii. Cidofovir (limited by its nephrotoxic side effects), IVIG, and corticosteroids may be helpful (Pegues et al., 2010).

(5) Pneumocystosis. *P. jiroveci* (formerly carinii).
   (a) Although bacterial pneumonia is seen more commonly and is the most frequent life-threatening infection in patients with renal transplants, pneumocystosis carries a risk for serious morbidity and mortality.
   (b) Symptoms include fever, nonproductive cough, hypoxemia, and interstitial infiltration or focal air space consolidation on chest x-ray.
   (c) The risk is highest the first 2 to 6 months posttransplantation and is generally preventable with the use of prophylactic antibiotics.
      i. Trimethoprim sulfamethoxazole (TMP-SMX) single strength.
      ii. Dapsone (for those with allergy to TMP-SMX).
      iii. Aerosolized pentamidine.
   (d) Prophylactic dosing is continued for variable lengths of time, per center protocol. However, dosing should be resumed during periods of increased immunosuppression, such as during rescue therapy (Pegues et al., 2010).

i. Malignancy. Squamous cell skin cancer (most common), solid organ tumors, and lymphomas. Several are virally mediated, such as posttransplant lymphoproliferative disorder (PTLD) due to Epstein Barr virus and squamous cell skin cancer due to human papillomavirus (HPV).

j. Osteoporosis.
   (1) Risk of osteoporosis is quite high due to preexisting bone disease, secondary hyperparathyroidism, and use of long-term glucocorticosteroids.
   (2) Screen with bone density scan (DEXA) at baseline, 6 months posttransplant, and intervals as indicated by risk factors (Wilkinson & Kasiske, 2010).
   (3) Use calcium with vitamin D supplements (in patients with normal calcium levels).
   (4) Use bisphosphonates or calcitonin depending on kidney function.
   (5) Encourage weight-bearing exercise.

k. Posttransplant chronic kidney disease.
   (1) Almost all patients have stage 2 or greater kidney disease.
   (2) Use the same management guidelines as for nontransplant patients with CKD.
   (3) Reduce immunosuppression whenever possible (especially calcineurin inhibitors) (Wilkinson & Kasiske, 2010).

l. Pregnancy after transplantation.
   (1) Patient can have a successful pregnancy after transplantation, but not all programs recommend, and pregnancy is considered high-risk.
   (2) Usually encourage patient to wait at least 1 year after transplant and when kidney function is stable (< 2.0 mg/dL, preferably 1.3 mg/dL) (Wilkinson & Kasiske, 2010).
   (3) Counsel patients on contraception as fertility usually returns after transplant.
   (4) Prepregnancy planning includes evaluation of immunosuppression and other medications to avoid teratogenic medications (mycophenolate mofetil [FDA warning against pregnancy], ACEIs).
   (5) Close monitoring is required by high risk obstetrician during pregnancy and at the time of delivery.

m. Obesity.
   (1) Very common due to medications, liberalization of dietary restrictions, pretransplant unhealthy diet, and sedentary lifestyle.
   (2) Associated with inferior long-term cardiac outcomes posttransplant (Lentine et al., 2008).
   (3) Work in collaboration with patient and dietitian to help maintain a healthy weight.

H. Discharge planning.
   1. Patient/family education begins in the early posttransplant period. Provide simple written information with verbal explanations.
      a. General postoperative care.
      b. Medications: name, dose, action, frequency, and side effects.
      c. Signs and symptoms of rejection: how and when to report.
      d. Follow-up tests and visits to clinic: frequency and purpose.
      e. Recordkeeping: intake and output; daily weight, temperature and blood pressure monitoring; and home glucose monitoring.
      f. Diet.
      g. Posttransplant activity: when to drive, resuming

sexual activity, birth control, and exercise.
  h. Prevention of infection.
  i. Arranging for administration of outpatient medications and treatments.
  j. Education and counseling regarding lifetime commitment to health care and necessity of lifetime immunosuppressive medications.
  k. Importance of meticulous adherence with prescribed therapy.
  2. Scheduling for posttransplant patient follow-up.
  a. Local laboratory testing and clinic visits.
  b. Monitor for short-term and long-term complications.
  3. Communicate with referring physician.
  4. Rehabilitation if indicated.
  a. Facilitate return to pre-illness level of activity.
  b. Vocational rehabilitation: local, state, and federal resources.
  c. Disincentives to rehabilitation.
    (1) Hiring practices of employers: fear of increased time off for illness and follow-up care.
    (2) Added insurance burden to employer.
    (3) Potential lack of disability income (Rifkin, 2010).

I. Miscellaneous considerations.
  1. Changes in family relationships.
  a. Role reversal: dependency to independence.
  b. Recovery from illness.
  2. Body image changes.
  3. Sexual concerns (Wilkinson & Kasiske, 2010).
  4. Economic concerns.
  a. Copays and cost of medications and follow-up (especially when Medicare benefits stop).
  b. Return to employment.
  c. State and local financial assistance (Rifkin, 2010).
  5. Ongoing concerns about graft failure and return to dialysis or death.
  a. First 12 months require close monitoring.
  b. Long-term potential for chronic allograft nephropathy.
  c. Preparation for possible return to dialysis or retransplantation.
  d. Counseling and psychiatric support as indicated (Rifkin, 2010).

Part 4. Immunobiology of Organ Transplant Rejection

Rejection is the process by which the recipient's immune system recognizes and mounts an immune response to eliminate foreign antigens on transplanted tissue. The transplanted tissue or organ is destroyed in the process.

I. Terminology – components of the immune response.

A. Major histocompatibility complex (MHC) – a cluster of genes that are present on the sixth human chromosome that controls the molecules expressed on the surface of cells (HLA molecules).
  1. Two classes of MHC molecules that are important in transplantation.
    a. Class I: HLA-A, HLA-B, and HLA-C.
    b. Class II: HLA-DR, HLA-DP, and HLA-DQ.
  2. Closely matched transplants are not as likely to be recognized and attacked by the immune system.

B. Human leukocyte antigen (HLA) – the primary antigens that help the body recognize "self from nonself."
  1. Expressed on white blood cells and most easily isolated from lymph nodes.
  2. When possible, lymph nodes are procured from a potential deceased donor to isolate the WBCs needed for the crossmatch before transplantation.

C. Antigen – any molecule that can be recognized by the immune system and elicit an immune (antibody) response.
  1. With future exposures, the same antigen stimulates a more rapid and robust antibody response.
  2. This is known as immunologic memory.

D. Antibody – a protein produced by lymphocytes in response to an antigen.
  1. Antibodies are long-lasting, difficult to completely remove, and tend to recur over time (have memory).
  2. They play an important role in transplant immunobiology; they are formed in response to previous transplants, blood transfusions, viral infections, or pregnancy.

E. T lymphocytes.
  1. Responsible for cell-mediated immunity.
  2. Examples are helper and cytotoxic (killer) T cells.

F. B lymphocytes.
  1. Component of the humoral response.
  2. Present foreign antigens to T-cells.
  3. Generate antibody formation.

G. Antigen presenting cells (APCs) – activate antigen specific T-cells.

H. Dendritic cells.
   1. Specialized macrophages that function as APCs.
   2. Initiate the immune response by presenting foreign antigens to T cells.

I. Macrophage.
   1. A phagocytic cell.
   2. Engulfs and destroys infectious organisms and other particles.

J. Cytokines – important to transplant immunobiology.
   1. Interleukin 1 (IL-1) secreted by macrophages, endothelial cells, and some epithelial cells.
   2. Interleukin 2 (IL-2) secreted by T cells.
   3. Responsible for inflammation, proliferation of T cells and natural killer T cells, increased cytokine synthesis, proliferation of B cells, and antibody synthesis (Abbas et al., 2010).

K. Crossmatch – recipient blood cells are combined with donor cells to determine the presence of antibody from the recipient toward the donor.
   1. A positive crossmatch indicates that the patient will have immediate graft rejection.
   2. Flow cytometry crossmatch can detect very low levels of circulating antibodies (Cecka et al., 2010).

II. Immune response to the transplanted kidney.

A. The main function of the immune system, evolved over several thousand years, is to defend against infections and subsequent disease.

B. In transplantation, the immune system is responsible for direct recognition of foreign HLAs (see Figure 3.2).
   1. Donor tissue is first recognized by circulating T–cells. The surgical process itself (dissecting and reattaching blood vessels, restoring blood flow to the ischemic organ) leads to the production of inflammatory cytokines and attraction of macrophages into the graft. An immune response is initiated immediately (Mandelbrot & Sayegh, 2010).
   2. Helper T lymphocytes release cytokines such as interleukin 2 and interferon-gamma to activate cytotoxic T cells.
   3. The T lymphocytes then regulate the gene expression for IL-1 and IL-2 receptors.
   4. IL-2 stimulates T and B lymphocyte proliferation and activation of other lymphocytes.
   5. The activated T cells release other inflammatory cytokines that result in cell damage and allograft injury.
   6. This pathway is important in the acute rejection process (Madelbrot & Sayegh, 2010).

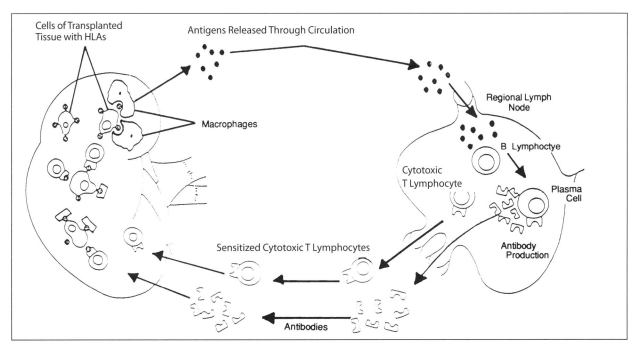

Figure 3.2. Mechanisms of transplanted tissue rejection. Macrophages recognize and process foreign HLAs, and antigenic material is released into the circulation. Lymphocytes in lymph nodes produce activated cytotoxic T lymphocytes and antibodies, which then destroy the transplanted tissue. (See text for details.)

C. Indirect recognition of foreign HLAs.
1. APCs of the recipient take up circulating MHCs shed from the donor cells. This then activates recipient lymphocytes.
2. More important in the process of chronic rejection.

III. Types of rejection.

Kidney transplant biopsy is the gold standard for diagnosis of acute and chronic allograft nephropathy (CAN). Interstitial fibrosis and tubular atrophy (IFTA) describes the characteristic abnormalities seen on biopsy, and this newer terminology may be used interchangeably with CAN.

A. Hyperacute rejection. Rarely occurs due to more sensitive crossmatching techniques; i.e., flow cytometry.
1. Onset is minutes or may be delayed up to 3 days after transplantation (Nast & Cohen, 2010).
2. Recipient has preformed cytotoxic antidonor antibodies and complement.
3. This process usually involves memory B lymphocytes and antibodies.
4. Irreversible and untreatable.
5. Circulating preformed antibodies recognize antigen and bind with antigen in the endothelium.
   a. The complement and coagulation systems are activated by antigen-antibody binding.
   b. As a result of this process, ischemia, hypoxia, and acidosis occur in the endothelium, leading to tissue ischemia and destruction and graft loss.
6. Generally can be prevented by performing crossmatch before transplant.
7. Transplant nephrectomy is necessary.

B. Accelerated rejection. Occurs rarely today due to more sensitive crossmatching techniques (i.e., flow cytometry) and the potency of the induction immunosuppressive regimen.
1. Onset is days.
2. Caused by preformed cytotoxic antibodies, similar to hyperacute rejection.
3. At the time of the transplant, the number of circulating preformed antibodies is insufficient to mount a rejection episode. Over a few days they proliferate rapidly and cause rejection.
4. Clinical signs and symptoms.
   a. Profound oliguria.
   b. Fever.
   c. Rapid loss of transplanted kidney function.
   d. Graft is swollen, tender, and firm.
5. Generally can be prevented by performing crossmatch prior to transplant.
6. Transplant nephrectomy may be necessary for treatment, although plasmapheresis is sometimes attempted.

C. Acute rejection. With improved immunosuppression regimens, there is a 10% or less incidence rate at many centers (Wilkinson, 2010). Two types: cell-mediated and antibody-mediated (humoral).
1. Cell-mediated (T-cell): most common form of early rejection.
   a. Onset is generally days to weeks, but can occur at any time.
   b. Caused by activation of T lymphocytes.
   c. Signs and symptoms.
      (1) Asymptomatic increase in serum creatinine or failure of creatinine to decline below an elevated level.
      (2) Mild or absent: graft tenderness, decreased urine output, edema, electrolyte imbalances, fever, and elevated leukocyte count (Wilkinson, 2010).
   d. Lymphocytes accumulate inside the transplanted organ and migrate into the interstitial spaces.
      (1) Lymphokines are released and attract and cause multiplication of other inflammatory-immune cells.
      (2) Pronounced edema, perivascular hemorrhages, and tubular damage result from the immune attack on the transplanted organ.
      (3) If untreated or treatment is delayed, thrombosis of blood vessels and organ necrosis occur.
   e. Acute rejection can usually be treated with increased immunosuppression. Glucocorticoids are first-line.
2. Antibody-mediated.
   a. On biopsy, diffuse peritubular capillary staining for the complement component C4d is seen.
      (1) Presence of C4d is a marker for the presence of antibody-mediated rejection (Nast & Cohen, 2010).
      (2) Most often occurs in patients with high levels of antibodies (preexisting sensitization).
   b. Generally not responsive to increased immunosuppression. Treated with intravenous human immune globulin, plasma exchange and/or rituximab (an anti-CD20 B-cell antibody) (Wilkinson, 2010).

D. Interstitial fibrosis and tubular atrophy (IFTA).
1. Onset is months to years; it is the most common cause of long-term allograft loss.
2. Many chronic causes affect allograft: calcineurin inhibitor toxicity, hypertension, nephrosclerosis, chronic obstruction, viral infections, recurrent diseases, and chronic rejection. These causes often can be differentiated on biopsy, and treatment varies based on the cause.
3. Chronic rejection is likely a combination of T and

B lymphocyte-mediated rejection.
4. Chronic rejection primarily affects cells in the renal cortex.
   a. Scattered interstitial fibrosis with lymphocyte, plasma cell, and mast cell infiltrates are seen along with tubular atrophy.
   b. Events of the inflammatory immune response cause damage to blood vessel endothelial lining and glomeruli (chronic transplant glomerulopathy).
   c. Gradual ischemia causes chronic tissue fibrosis and attempts at repair by fibroblast proliferation and collagen deposition which causes scarring.
   d. The interstitium is filled with collagen, and blood vessels are blocked by proliferation of intima.
5. There is no successful treatment for chronic rejection.
   a. The patient should be well managed as a patient with CKD in order to prolong kidney function.
   b. However, for other causes of nephropathy such as calcineurin inhibitor toxicity and viral infections, changes in immunosuppression or the addition of antiviral therapies may improve kidney function.

Part 5. Immunosuppressive Therapy

I. **Overview.** See Table 3.1.

A. The goal of immunosuppressive therapy is to modify the immune system enough to prevent rejection, but not so much as to allow infection, malignancies, and other side effects.
   1. In spite of incredible advances, most immunosuppressive agents are not specific to the alloimmune (organ transplant rejection) response.
   2. The net effect of these agents is an overall suppression of the immune response, leading to an unfortunate increase in bacterial and viral infections as well as certain types of cancers.

B. The majority of transplant centers use induction therapy.
   1. Induction therapy is started in the perioperative period.
   2. Depending on the specific agent, it may be administered immediately prior to, during, and/or after transplantation.
   3. Induction therapy is more potent than maintenance immunosuppression since the immune response is heightened in the early postoperative period due to increased inflammation from surgery, ischemia-reperfusion insult, and initial antigen exposure.

4. The goal of induction immunosuppression is to significantly decrease the T cell response to the allograft (Adams et al., 2012).

C. Induction immunosuppression is tapered to achieve stable maintenance immunosuppression within the therapeutic targets determined by each center's protocol.
   1. The most common maintenance immunosuppressive regimen in the United States is mycophenolate mofetil in combination with tacrolimus (85%) either with (58%) or without (42%) glucocorticoids (SRTR, 2011).
   2. Agents used to combat an acute rejection episode are termed rescue agents, and several are the same as those used for induction.

II. Mycophenolate mofetil (CellCept®), mycophenolic acid (Myfortic®).

A. Action.
   1. Mycophenolic acid is an antimetabolite that selectively inhibits the proliferation of T and B lymphocytes by interfering with purine nucleotide synthesis. Both inhibit antibody formation and cytotoxic T cell clonal expansion (Adams et al., 2012).
      a. Mycophenolate mofetil is a prodrug which is converted to mycophenolic acid in vivo.
      b. EC mycophenolic acid is an enteric-coated form of the drug that allows delayed absorption at a higher pH in the gastrointestinal tract. Otherwise, they are essentially the same medication.
   2. These drugs have replaced azathioprine as a maintenance agent because of the significantly decreased incidence of acute rejection (Sollinger, 1995).
   3. Both drugs are largely metabolized in the liver and eliminated through the kidney.
      a. The elimination half-life is approximately 12 hours (G. Danovitch, 2010b).
      b. Usually taken twice daily.
   4. Females of reproductive potential must be made aware of the increased risk of first trimester pregnancy loss and congenital malformations and must be counseled regarding pregnancy prevention and planning (FDA Medwatch, 2013).

B. Nursing implications.
   1. Ensure counseling regarding pregnancy prevention and planning has been done prior to first administration.
   2. Administer as prescribed.
   3. Monitor the white blood cell (WBC) count.
   4. Observe for side effects (see Table 3.1).

Table 3.1

Immunosuppressive Medications

Name of Agent	Purpose	Dose	Method of Administration	Side Effects
Alemtuzumab (Campath®) Recombinant DNA-derived humanized monoclonal antibody (unlabeled use in transplant)	Induction therapy	30 mg	Intravenously over 2 hours as a single dose at the time of transplant. Premedicate with diphenhydramine 50 mg and acetaminophen 500–1000 mg 30 minutes before each infusion. Currently only available through Campath® distribution program.	*Rare:* Anaphylactoid/hypersensitivity reaction Flu-like symptoms Anemia Leukopenia Thrombocytopenia Dizziness Hyper/hypotension Headache Nausea Dyspepsia Stomatitis Skin irritation Opportunistic infections
Antithymocyte globulin (Thymoglobulin®) (rabbit) Polyclonal antibody preparation	Induction or rescue therapy (unlabeled use)	Based on adequacy of WBC/platelet/lymphocyte count. Induction: 1.5–2.5 mg/kg daily for 5–10 days or per center protocol. Treatment of acute rejection: 1.5 mg/kg/day for 7–14 days or per center protocol.	Premedicate with diphenhydramine and acetaminophen and, for first dose, with corticosteroids. Intravenous infusion with in-line 0.22 micron filter over 6 hours (first dose) through central line. Subsequent doses may be given over 4 hours. May be given at a slow rate peripherally when mixed with heparin and hydrocortisone.	Anaphylaxis Cytokine release syndrome Fever and hyperpyrexia Hypo/hypertension Opportunistic infections Increased incidence of malignancy Hematologic toxicity: neutropenia; thrombocytopenia

Azathioprine (Imuran®)
Generic available
	Maintenance immunosuppression	1–3 mg/kg/day orally maintenance
		50 mg tablets
		100 mg vials for IV use
			Orally
			IV as indicated
				Bone marrow suppression:
				  anemia
				  thrombocytopenia
				  bleeding
				  leukopenia
				Hair thinning and loss
				Infections
				Gastrointestinal problems
				Mouth ulcers
				Hepatic dysfunction; hepatitis
				Malignancies

Basiliximab (Simulect®) Anti-Interleukin-2 receptor humanized monoclonal antibody	Induction therapy	20 mg	Intravenously through a peripheral vein. Administered day of transplant and postop day 4.	*Rare:* Anaphylactoid/hypersensitivity reaction Flu-like syndrome Opportunistic infections Increased incidence of diabetes
Belatacept (Nulojix®) Selective T-cell costimulation blocker.	Maintenance therapy	Dosing based on actual body weight at time of transplantation. If change in weight is > 10%, dosing will change. Prescribed dose must be evenly divisible by 12.5 mg. Initial phase: 10/mg/kg/dose on Day 1 and Day 5, Week 2, 4, 8, and 12 following transplantation. Maintenance phase: 5 mg/kg/dose q 4 weeks beginning at Week 16.	IV infusion over 30 minutes using a 0.2–1.2 micron low protein-binding filter.	Increased incidence of lymphoproliferative disorders, and therefore contraindicated in EBV negative patients. Increased incidence of other malignancy and infections Anemia Leukopenia Constipation Diarrhea Nausea, vomiting Fever Headache Hyper/hypotension Hyper/hypokalemia Peripheral edema Urinary tract infection *Rare:* hypersensitivity reactions

Table continues

Table 3.1

Immunosuppressive Medications (page 2 of 3)

Name of Agent	Purpose	Dose	Method of Administration	Side Effects
Cyclophosphamide (Cytoxan®) (Rarely used)	Maintenance immunosuppression if unable to tolerate azathioprine or mycophenolic acid. Used in nontransplant patients with immune-mediated disease.	50–75 mg/day	Orally once a day in the morning. Available as intravenous solution.	Leukopenia Thrombocytopenia Bladder fibrosis GI disturbances Hemorrhagic cystitis Bladder cancer (periodic cystoscopic screening per center protocol)
Cyclosporine Generics available Modified: Neoral®, Gengraf® Cyclosporine modified-micro-emulsion allowing for more consistent absorption. Nonmodified: Sandimmune® Variable rate of absorption. Use same dose to convert from one formulation to another and adjust dose to attain appro-priate therapeutic trough level. (Lexicomp, 2013)	Maintenance immunosuppression	Adjusted to serum drug levels per center protocol; usually 3–4 mg/kg as maintenance dose. 25 mg and 100 mg capsules Also available in oral and intravenous solutions	Usually twice daily dosing based on trough level	Nephrotoxicity Hepatotoxicity Hand tremors Hypertrichosis Gingival hyperplasia Seizures Flushing Hyperesthesia Nausea/vomiting Anorexia Diarrhea Feeling of fullness Headaches Mild anemia Hyperkalemia Hypertension Malignancies Hirsutism Hyperlipidemia
Methylprednisolone Prednisone	Oral maintenance and IV induction and rescue immunosuppression	Oral maintenance: 0.2 mg/kg Methylprednisolone: 4 mg, 8 mg, 16 mg, 32 mg tablets Prednisone: 2.5 mg, 5 mg, 10 mg, 20 mg, 50 mg tablets IV induction and rescue dosing per center protocol	Intravenous for induction or rescue. Oral taper in divided doses, then daily for maintenance.	Cushingoid appearance Increased appetite Na^+/H_2O retention Hypertension Peptic ulcers Easy bruising Impaired wound healing Acne Diaphoresis Infections Hyperlipidemia Osteoporosis Avascular joint necrosis Diabetes Cataracts Pancreatitis Anemia Thrombocytopenia Leukopenia Mood lability Increased incidence of malignancies
Mycophenolate mofetil (CellCept®) Generics available Mycophenolic acid delayed release (Myfortic ®) Generic available	Maintenance immunosuppression	Based on GI tolerance and WBC. Mycophenolate mofetil 250 mg, 500 mg capsules 1000–1500 mg twice daily Also available in an oral suspension 200 mg/mL. Mycophenolic acid delayed release 180 mg, 360 mg tablets 720–1040 mg twice daily	Orally twice daily	Bone marrow suppression: anemia leukopenia thrombocytopenia GI distress

Table continues

Table 3.1

Immunosuppressive Medications (page 3 of 3)

Name of Agent	Purpose	Dose	Method of Administration	Side Effects
Rituximab (Rituxan®)	Treatment of antibody-mediated acute rejection (unlabeled use)	Per center protocol. Approximately 375 mg/m².	Pretreatment with acetaminophen and diphenhydramine is recommended. Start infusion at 50 mg/hr, if no reaction, increase rate by 50 mg/hr increments every 30 minutes, to maximum rate of 400 mg/hour	Infusion hypersensitivity reactions (occasionally fatal) Serious and potentially fatal infections Bowel obstruction/perforation Hepatitis B virus reactivation Mucocutaneous reactions Progressive multifocal leukoencephalopathy Peripheral edema Hyper/hypotension Fever, chills Fatigue Headache Nausea, diarrhea
Sirolimus (Rapamune®)	Maintenance immunosuppression	Adjust to serum trough concentrations per center protocol. 0.5 mg, 1 mg and 2 mg tablets Available in oral solution 1 mg/mL	Orally once daily.	Hyperlipidemia Hypercholesterolemia Diarrhea Anemia Arthralgia Acne Thrombocytopenia Delayed wound healing Mouth sores Rash
Tacrolimus (Prograf®, Hecoria®) Immediate release Generics available	Maintenance immunosuppression	Adjusted to trough level per center protocol. 0.1-0.2 mg/kg in two divided doses 0.5 mg, 1 mg, 5 mg capsules Available in an intravenous solution	Orally twice daily.	Nephrotoxicity Hypertension Diabetes Infections Neurotoxicity Tremors Tingling in hands or feet Paresthesias Insomnia Headache Tinnitus
Tacrolimus extended release (Astagraf XL®)		Adjusted to trough level per center protocol 0.15–0.2 mg/kg/once daily 0.5 mg, 1 mg, 5 mg capsules	Orally once daily in the morning.	Visual light sensitivity Sleep disturbances/nightmares Mood changes Increased incidence of malignancies

Source: Lexicomp®, 2013

III. Azathioprine (Imuran®). This medication is no longer used in de novo transplants. Female transplant recipients who desire pregnancy may be converted to azathioprine from mycophenolate mofetil. Mycophenolate mofetil (Cellcept®) was approved by the FDA in 1995 and is significantly more effective at preventing acute rejection than azathioprine (G. Danovitch, 2010b).

A. Action.
1. Azathioprine is an antimetabolite that interferes with deoxyribonucleic acid (DNA) synthesis, thus decreasing the division of rapidly reproducing cells, including leukocytes.
2. Used in conjunction with other immunosuppressive medications.
3. Taken once daily.

B. Nursing implications.
1. Administer as prescribed.
2. Monitor WBC and liver function tests.
3. Observe for side effects (see Table 3.1).

IV. Calcineurin inhibitor: Tacrolimus (Prograf®) and tacrolimus extended release (Astagraf XL®). About 80% of patients receive tacrolimus upon hospital discharge in the United States and Europe (G. Danovitch, 2010b). This is due to a more tolerable side-effect profile as well as studies showing a significantly decreased incidence of biopsy proven acute rejection episodes (Pirsch et al., 1997).

A. Action.
1. Tacrolimus inhibits T cell and cytokine activation and proliferation primarily by impairing the

activation or induction of gene coding for interleukin-2 (IL-2), IL-4, and tumor necrosis factor and gamma interferon (G. Danovitch, 2010b).
2. Long-acting formulation of tacrolimus approved by FDA in July 2013.
   a. Taken daily.
   b. The half-life ranges from approximately 25 to 30 hours (Astellas Pharma US, Inc., 2013).

B. Nursing implications.
1. Administer as prescribed.
2. Observe for side effects (see Table 3.1).
3. Metabolized via cytochrome P-450 III A (CYP3A) pathway.
4. Calcineurin inhibitors have multiple drug interactions which may cause subtherapeutic or supertherapeutic drug levels leading to either under immunosuppression or drug toxicities (e.g., nephrotoxicity, hyperkalemia, and hypertension).
5. Narrow therapeutic index drug. Monitor trough levels for target range based on center specific protocols.

V. Calcineurin inhibitor: Cyclosporine (Sandimmune®, Neoral®, Gengraf®).
Less commonly used in de novo transplants than tacrolimus.

A. Action.
1. Cyclosporine acts by interfering with the production of interleukin-2 and cytotoxic T lymphocytes.
2. As a result, even though macrophages and T lymphocytes can recognize the transplanted tissue as foreign, the lymphocytes cannot mount an immune response.

B. Nursing implications.
1. Administer as prescribed.
2. Observe for side effects (see Table 3.1).
3. Metabolized via cytochrome P450 III A pathway.
4. Calcineurin inhibitors have multiple drug interactions which may cause subtherapeutic or supertherapeutic drug levels leading to either under-immunosuppression or drug toxicities (e.g., nephrotoxicity, hyperkalemia, and hypertension).
5. Narrow therapeutic index drug. Monitor levels for target range based on center specific protocols.

Nursing implication note: Changing between generic and brand name immunosuppressive medications may result in altered serum drug levels, requiring more frequent monitoring of drug levels per center-specific protocols.

VI. Glucocorticoids. May be used for induction only, or for induction and maintenance. Usually first line treatment for rescue from an acute rejection. Most centers use for several days followed by a rapid taper in the perioperative period. When possible, long-term use is avoided due to serious adverse effects (see Table 3.1).

A. Most commonly used forms are prednisone and methylprednisolone.

B. Dosage and schedule of administration varies widely based on concurrent use of other immunosuppressive therapies.

C. Peak blood concentration is reached in 1 to 2 hours. Biologic effects persist 12 to 24 hours.

D. Action.
1. There has been recent explanation of the exact mechanism of action of corticosteroids in altering the immune response (Rhen & Cidlowski, 2005).
2. Corticosteroids prevent transcription of interleukin-1 and tumor necrosis factor (TNF) by APCs, thus preventing MHC expression. The net effect is decreased antigenicity of transplanted tissue.
3. Corticosteroids exert antiinflammatory effects that result in a decreased inflammatory reaction at the transplant site through decreased cytokine activation and T cell activation. The results are an overall decrease in edema, capillary permeability, leukocyte migration, deposition of a fibrin mesh, and phagocytosis.

E. Nursing implications.
1. Administer as prescribed.
2. Usually taken once daily with food.
3. Observe for side effects (see Table 3.1).
4. Administer H2 antagonists or proton pump inhibitors as ordered to prevent gastrointestinal ulcers.
5. Administer antifungal medications (either systemic or mouthwashes) as prescribed.
6. Encourage early and frequent ambulation to minimize muscle weakness.
7. Monitor blood glucose levels.
8. Provide emotional support to assist patient to adapt to changing body image.

VII. Mammilian target of rapamycin (mTOR) inhibitors: sirolimus (Rapamune®), everolimus (Zortress®). Macrolide antibiotic compound with structural similarities to tacrolimus. Everolimus is a derivative of sirolimus and has similar action and adverse effects.

A. Action.
 1. Sirolimus binds to a cytoplasm-binding protein (the same one that binds tacrolimus, FKBP). Inhibits cytokine-dependent cellular proliferation and T lymphocyte activation by a mechanism that is distinct from that of other immunosuppressive medications (inhibits mTOR) (G. Danovitch, 2010b).
 2. This drug also inhibits antibody production.
 3. Nonnephrotoxic agent.
  a. May cause proteinuria.
  b. May prolong delayed graft function and should be withheld until kidney function commences.
  c. It potentiates the nephrotoxicity of the calcineurin inhibitors.
 4. Sometimes used instead of a calcineurin inhibitor when there is evidence of calcineurin inhibitor nephrotoxicity on biopsy.

B. Nursing implications.
 1. Administer as prescribed.
 2. Observe for side effects (see Table 3.1).
 3. Metabolized via same pathway and same drug interactions as calcineurin inhibitors.
 4. Narrow therapeutic index drug. Monitor trough levels for target range based on center specific protocols.

VIII. Polyclonal antibody preparation: antithymocyte globulin (rabbit) (Thymoglobulin®). Used for induction and rescue therapy per center protocol.

A. Method of preparation.
 1. An animal (rabbit) is injected with human lymphocytes.
 2. The animal then produces antibodies to the foreign human white blood cells.
 3. The globulin, which is the part of the serum containing the antibodies, is separated from the plasma, purified, and stored.
 4. The antithymocyte globulin (ATG) which contains the antibodies is then administered to the organ transplant recipient.

B. Action.
 1. Contains cytotoxic antibodies that act specifically against T lymphocytes and decreases their activity and number by coating T lymphocytes and rendering them ineffective.
 2. In addition, ATG forms blocking antibodies and destroys T lymphocytes by direct antigen-antibody complex formation.

C. Nursing implications.
 1. Administer as prescribed through a central line with a 0.22 micron inline filter to prevent sclerosis

of peripheral veins. Per center specific protocol, administer acetaminophen and diphenhydramine and induction glucocorticoid dose prior to first one to two doses to prevent rigors.
 2. Observe for side effects (see Table 3.1).
 3. May be used for induction or for rescue therapy for those rejections which are refractory to steroid pulses.

IX. Alemtuzumab (Campath1H®). Recombinant DNA-derived humanized monoclonal antibody (MAB) approved for use in chronic lymphocytic leukemia, but not for use in clinical transplantation (G. Danovitch, 2010b). Administered per center protocol. Only available through Campath Distribution Program.

A. Action.
 1. Antibody action directed against cell surface glycoprotein CD52.
 2. Induces a rapid and extensive depletion of peripheral and central lymphoid cells, which lasts for several months (G. Danovitch, 2010b).

B. Nursing implications.
 1. Administer as prescribed.
 2. Observe for side effects (see Table 3.1).

X. Anti-interleukin-2 receptor monoclonal antibody: basiliximab (Simulect®).

A. Action.
 1. Basiliximab (mouse-human chimeric) is a monoclonal antibody that binds to the CD25 or Tac subunit of the IL-2 receptor expressed on activated T lymphocytes, thereby inhibiting IL-2 mediated activation and proliferation.
 2. Has a long half-life secondary to decreased inactivation of human antibodies.

B. Nursing implications.
 1. Administer as prescribed through a peripheral or central line.
 2. Observe for side effects (see Table 3.1).

XI. Selective T-Cell Costimulation Blocker: Belatacept (Nulojix®).

A. Action.
 1. A fusion protein derived from CTLA-4 (a cell surface molecule expressed on activated T cells) and human IgG which was developed to block CD28-CD80-CD86 interactions impairing co-stimulation and T cell activation (Adams et al., 2012).
 2. Requires monthly IV infusions.

B. Nursing implications
1. Help patient schedule monthly IV infusions at an infusion center.
2. Observe for side effects (see Table 3.1).
3. Indicated for prevention of organ rejection and given with basiliximab induction, mycophenolate, and corticosteroids in Epstein-Barr virus (EBV) seropositive kidney transplant recipients (http://online.lexi.com/lco/action/doc/retrieve/do cid/essential_ashp/4489847).

XII. Agents used for rescue therapy for antibody-mediated acute rejection.

A. Intravenous immune globulin (IVIG).
1. Neutralizes circulating auto antibodies and alloantibodies and down regulates antibody production (Adams et al., 2012).
2. May be used in conjunction with plasmapheresis to remove circulating antibodies.
3. May also be used prior to transplantation in a highly sensitized recipient to reduce the panel of reactive antibodies (PRA) and prevent a positive crossmatch.

B. Rituximab (Rituxan®).
1. Anti-CD20 chimeric monoclonal antibody also used to treat posttransplant lymphoproliferative disorder (PTLD) and many other autoimmune disorders (Adams et al., 2012).
2. Binds to CD20 on B cells and causes depletion.
3. Low incidence of infusion reactions.
4. May be used in conjunction with plasmapheresis and IVIG administration.

SECTION B
Simultaneous Kidney–Pancreas Transplantation
Jean Colaneri

I. Historical perspectives of pancreas transplantation.

A. First human whole pancreas transplant performed by Kelly and Lillehei at the University of Minnesota in 1966. The recipient survived 2 months, and then died of sepsis and rejection (Gruessner & Gruessner, 2013).

B. Early pancreas transplant graft survival was less than 10%, and patient survival was less than 50% at 1 year. These failures were attributed to technical difficulties and postoperative complications, including graft thrombosis, fistula formation, necrosis from poor preservation, and difficulties in balancing immunosuppression therapy to control rejection and prevent infection (Squifflet, 2013).

C. Graft survival has continued to increase and is attributed to advancements in surgical techniques and immunosuppressive therapy.

D. Several surgical techniques have been used to manage pancreas graft exocrine secretions.
1. Enteric drainage of pancreatic secretions was used in the earliest transplants.
   a. In later years, bladder drainage of the pancreas became more popular, as this allowed early diagnosis of rejection by measuring the amylase content of the urine.
   b. Bladder drainage avoids possible bacterial contamination from enteric drainage leaks.
   c. From 1987 to 1997, over 90% of the pancreas transplants done in the United States were bladder-drained.
   d. Bladder drainage creates large loss of bicarbonate through the urine, causing hyperchloremic metabolic acidosis and dehydration.
      (1) The alkaline change in the urine predisposes patients to urinary tract infections, and the caustic nature of the pancreatic secretions may cause cystitis, urethritis, and hematuria.
      (2) For these reasons, most kidney–pancreas transplants are done now with enteric drainage of pancreatic secretions (G. Danovitch, 2010a; Gruessner & Gruessner, 2013).
2. Enteric drainage of pancreas secretions has been associated with far fewer urologic complications (Gruessner & Gruessner, 2013).
3. In the kidney–pancreas transplant recipient, the majority of pancreas rejection episodes occur after or simultaneously with kidney allograft rejection, and therefore the serum creatinine is the marker used for suspicion of rejection.

E. There are currently 173 centers that perform kidney–pancreas transplants in the United States (UNOS, 2013).

F. In 2012, there were 801 kidney–pancreas transplants reported to UNOS in the United States. The total number of kidney–pancreas transplants in the US since 1988 is 19,521 (UNOS, 2013b).

G. As of September 20, 2013, there were 2,122 candidates on the UNOS waiting list for a simultaneous pancreas–kidney transplant.

H. UNOS reports national graft and patient survival statistics.
   1. From 1997 to 2004, the graft survival at 1 year, 3 years, and 5 years for primary SPK was 91.7%, 84.1%, and 76.3%, respectively.
   2. Repeat SPK transplant graft survival was 85.2%, 64.1%, and 59.4% at 1 year, 3 years, and 5 years, respectively (UNOS, 2013b).

I. Patient survival for SPK performed in the United States between 1997 and 2004 at 1, 3, and 5 years, was reported to be 94.8%, 90%, and 85.5% respectively (UNOS, 2013b).

II. Basic concepts and goals of pancreas transplantation.

A. The American Diabetes Association (ADA) reports that diabetes mellitus (DM) is an endocrine disease that has been diagnosed in 18.8 million Americans.
   1. However, 7.0 million are unaware they have diabetes.
   2. In 2010, 1.9 million new cases of diabetes were diagnosed in adults 20 years of age or older (ADA, 2013).

B. The ADA reports that the total yearly economic cost of diabetes was $245 billion in 2012 (ADA, 2013).

C. The ADA has classified two types of diabetes. Type 1 diabetes accounts for 5–10% of those diagnosed with diabetes. Type 2, the most frequent type of diabetes, accounts for 90–95% of diabetes.

D. Type 1 diabetes.
   1. Those with type 1 diabetes secrete little or no insulin from the beta cells of the pancreas.
   2. People with type 1 diabetes depend on exogenous insulin for the control of carbohydrate metabolism and prevention of ketoacidosis and wide fluctuations in plasma glucose levels.
   3. Patients with long-term type 1 DM lose their ability to sense the early signs of hypoglycemia (sweating, shaking, tachycardia) and can become unconscious or have seizures due to this hypoglycemic unawareness.
   4. High glucose levels can result in hypotonic fluid loss, dehydration, and electrolyte depletion (Hall, 2012).
   5. Type 1 diabetes is associated with other diseases such as retinopathy, neuropathy, nephropathy, and cardiovascular diseases (angina, myocardial infarction, cerebral vascular accident; these are often grouped together as macrovascular disease) (ADA, 2013; Hall 2012).
      a. In adults ages 20 to 75, diabetes is the leading cause of new cases of blindness every year.
      b. As the leading cause of chronic kidney disease, diabetes accounted for 44% of the new diagnoses in 2008.
      c. Heart disease death rates and the risk of stroke are 2 to 4 times higher in adults with diabetes.
      d. About 60–70% experience mild to severe neuropathy and more than 60% of nontraumatic lower-limb amputations occur in people with diabetes (ADA, 2013).

E. Pancreas transplantation is primarily performed to treat type 1 diabetes and to restore a euglycemic state for the transplant recipient.
   1. Some transplant centers will consider pancreas transplantation in patients with type 2 diabetes in specific circumstances such as severe hypoglycemic unawareness.
   2. Patient survival following simultaneous pancreas–kidney (SPK) transplantation is excellent and has increased incrementally since 1995 (UNOS, 2013b).
   3. As with any treatment option, risk vs. benefit of transplantation/immunosuppression or insulin independence must be carefully evaluated to determine the best choice available for each patient.

F. The ADA position on pancreas transplantation (2004) states that pancreas transplantation "should be considered an acceptable therapeutic alternative to continued insulin therapy in diabetic patients with imminent or established end-stage renal disease who have had or plan to have a kidney transplant" (ADA, 2007).

G. Questions to consider when evaluating a patient as a potential kidney–pancreas transplant candidate.
   1. Is a pancreas transplant the optimal choice for replacement of pancreas endocrine function?
   2. What is the best timing for pancreas transplantation related to progression of nephropathy and the other diseases associated with diabetes?
   3. Do the benefits of a pancreas transplant and immunosuppression outweigh the risks of the long-term complications of diabetes and insulin management?
   4. What is the likelihood that pancreas transplantation will prevent and/or stop the progression of retinopathy, neuropathy, nephropathy, cardiac, and vascular diseases associated with type 1 diabetes?

H. Research indicates that patients who receive a kidney–pancreas transplant report a better quality of life and improved physical and psychological well-being after transplantation.

1. The benefits of having a normal blood sugar, no insulin shots or constant fear of hypoglycemic reactions, and no diabetic diet have contributed to kidney–pancreas transplant recipients reporting feeling more positive and hopeful about the future.
2. Because of the success rates, the decrease in diabetic complications after kidney–pancreas transplantation, and reports of improved quality of life, kidney–pancreas transplantation is a viable and worthwhile treatment of patients with kidney disease and type 1 diabetes (ADA, 2013; Gruessner & Gruessner, 2013).

I. Simultaneous kidney–pancreas transplant (SPK) offers the patient with diabetes and kidney failure the option of correcting uremia and becoming euglycemic, thereby preventing or ameliorating the secondary complications of diabetes (Gruessner & Gruesnner, 2013).
   1. The goal is to perform the procedure in the early stages of kidney failure, and before the other associated diseases of diabetes have occurred. Patients do not accumulate wait time points from UNOS until their glomerular filtration rate (GFR) is ≤ 20 mL/min.
   2. Kidney and pancreas from the same deceased donor are transplanted into a person with diabetes and CKD during one surgical procedure.
   3. Addition of the pancreas does not jeopardize the transplanted kidney's long-term survival or function.
   4. The new pancreas may improve the recipient's long-term survival since many of the medical complications related to diabetes may be eliminated or significantly improved (Lipshutz, 2010).
   5. SPK transplantation outcome is improved if the dual transplant is done early in the course of kidney failure.
      a. This does not often happen due to the long waiting times for organs.
      b. Some regions require that patients be on dialysis before being listed for a transplant, and then list candidates together with those waiting for a kidney only. These patients can wait several years before getting a simultaneous pancreas–kidney donor.
   6. Patients listed for a simultaneous pancreas–kidney transplant remain eligible to receive a kidney transplant alone should an acceptable kidney become available without the pancreas. If a kidney transplant alone occurs, patients may still be eligible for reevaluation for a pancreas after kidney transplant.

III. Evaluation of the candidate for simultaneous pancreas–kidney (SPK) transplant.

A. Refer to the section on kidney transplantation for general guidelines for candidate criteria and recipient evaluation. This section includes the specific assessment of the patient with diabetes who is being evaluated for SPK transplantation.

B. Candidate criteria and assessment for pancreas transplantation.
   1. Age.
      a. Emphasis on complications of diabetes rather than chronologic age.
      b. Some programs require recipients to be at least 18 years of age and not older than 60 years.
   2. Laboratory assessment of potential recipients may include, in addition to routine studies for kidney transplant:
      a. Metabolic studies.
         (1) Serum C-peptide levels.
         (2) Glycosylated hemoglobin.
         (3) Antibodies to islet cells.
      b. Thyroid function studies.
      c. Serum amylase and lipase.
      d. Lipoprotein profile.
   3. Cardiovascular system assessment.
      a. Most attention is given to this system in preoperative evaluation owing to the incidence and risks of macrovascular and microvascular disease in persons with type 1 diabetes. Persons with diabetic neuropathy can have significant coronary artery disease without angina (Eller et al., 2013).
      b. The more advanced the cardiovascular or peripheral vascular disease in the potential recipient, the more likely the candidate is to have a higher morbidity and mortality rate following pancreas transplantation.
      c. Some centers will transplant recipients with previous myocardial infarction or cardiovascular disease once the potential candidate undergoes coronary artery bypass grafting or angioplasty.
      d. Workup for the cardiovascular system in diabetic patients is center specific due to the poor predictive value of noninvasive imaging in diabetics, but includes:
         (1) Electrocardiogram (EKG).
         (2) Nuclear stress test with follow-up coronary angiogram if the stress test is positive or there is a history of angina or myocardial infarction, or
         (3) Dobutamine stress echocardiography.
            (a) Any patient with a positive study should be referred to cardiology.

(b) Many programs have a designated cardiologist to address these patients (G. Danovitch, 2010a; Levine, 2012).

    (4) Peripheral vascular studies, including Doppler examination of the lower extremities and assessment of carotid vessels.

4. Neurologic system workup.
   a. A referral to a neurologist is recommended if the patient has a history of cerebrovascular events or other neuropathic conditions that may affect the outcome of transplant surgery or the long-term success of transplant.
   b. Cognitive dysfunction that interferes with the patient's ability to manage self-care should be addressed before transplantation.
5. Urinary tract assessment.
   a. Diabetes is frequently associated with neurogenic bladder dysfunction, which can lead to infections and/or urinary obstruction posttransplant.
   b. Urologic assessment for bladder function should be scrutinized carefully.
      (1) Urinalysis and culture.
      (2) Urine protein studies.
      (3) Voiding cystourethrography with postvoid films.
      (4) Urodynamic studies as prescribed by urologist (G. Danovitch, 2010a; Townsend et al., 2012).
6. Ophthalmologic studies.
   a. Retinopathy and blindness are major complications of type 1 diabetes and indicative of microvascular disease.
   b. It is recommended that patients seeking a kidney–pancreas transplant see their ophthalmologist regularly before and after transplantation.
7. Psychosocial assessment (social worker, psychologist, and/or psychiatrist). See psychosocial assessment for kidney transplantation.
8. Gastrointestinal, endocrine, pulmonary, dental, and immunologic systems assessment is similar to what is discussed in the kidney transplantation section.
9. SPK transplantation is usually contraindicated in any of the following:
   a. Inoperable cardiovascular or peripheral vascular disease.
   b. Incapacitating neuropathies.
   c. Active peptic ulcer disease.
   d. Active malignancy.
   e. Acute infectious process.
   f. Active alcohol or drug addiction.
   g. Untreated psychiatric disease.
   h. Body mass index (BMI) greater than 35.

10. SPK ideal candidate.
    a. 18 to 50 years of age.
    b. BMI 25 to 30, depending on transplant center.
    c. Nonsmoker.
    d. No history of heart disease.
    e. Functional vision.
    f. No peripheral vascular disease.
11. SPK higher risk candidate.
    a. 50 to 60 years of age.
    b. BMI > 30.
    c. Previous myocardial infarction.
    d. Previous stroke.
    e. Significant peripheral vascular disease (G. Danovitch, 2010a; Pham et al., 2010).

IV. Organ procurement process for pancreas transplantation.

A. Pancreas or kidney–pancreas organs for transplantation are largely obtained from deceased donors.
   1. The usual range for acceptable pancreas donation is 10 to 45 years of age, although research continues into the use of older donors to expand the donor pool.
   2. The lower age limit relates to the size of the pancreatic arterial vasculature.
   3. Smaller vessels are associated with higher risk of thrombosis during the anastomotic procedure.
   4. Other considerations for pancreatic donation are similar to kidney donors (G. Danovitch, 2010a).

B. Organ procurement process (G. Danovitch, 2010a; Townsend et al., 2012).
   1. During procurement, amphotericin B solution may be given through a nasogastric tube inserted into the duodenum to decrease the risk of fungal infection.
   2. The pancreas is handled as little as possible during procurement and transplantation. It is a fragile organ, and is susceptible to injury with handling.
   3. The donor spleen is mobilized to use as a handle to decrease manipulation and potential trauma to the pancreas during procurement.
      a. The pancreas and its respective vessels are mobilized.
      b. A portion of the duodenum is transected with the pancreas, and the pancreas is removed with spleen attached.
      c. At many centers, the liver, pancreas, and spleen are removed en bloc and then separated.
   4. The pancreas is flushed with preservation solution to prevent ion flux across the cell membranes. The duodenal section may be flushed again with amphotericin B or preservation solution, depending on center protocols.
   5. Variation of this procedure may include removal

of several abdominal organs with dissection and preservation ex vivo.

6. Pancreas cold ischemic time may be up to 24 hours, if necessary. The goal is to transplant the graft in less than 24 hours.

V. Simultaneous pancreas–kidney transplant.

A. The exocrine function of the native pancreas is not affected by diabetes, so the recipient's pancreas is left in to continue its exocrine function.

B. The transplanted pancreas also maintains its exocrine function, leading to the high risk of fluid and bicarbonate losses, fistula formation, and related infection.
   1. Exocrine drainage management is the most difficult technical aspect of pancreas transplantation.
   2. Currently, in the United States there are two surgical options for pancreas transplantation (G. Danovitch, 2010a; Gruessner & Gruessner, 2013).
      a. Bladder drainage.
         (1) Was the standard approach in the United States.
         (2) Exocrine secretions are drained through the bladder via a small segment of the donor duodenum.
         (3) The pancreas is transplanted with a duodenal cuff from the donor, which is sutured to the recipient's bladder in a side-to-side anastomosis, or duodenocystostomy.
         (4) Pancreatic enzymes are secreted in a largely inactive form, so they do not damage the bladder.
         (5) Measurement of urinary amylase can then assist with detection of pancreas function and rejection after this procedure.
         (6) There is a reduced chance of infection and fistula formation related to other methods of anastomoses because the urinary tract is free from bacteria.
         (7) Complications.
            (a) Metabolic acidosis due to normal losses of bicarbonate via the transplanted pancreas and the bladder's inability to reabsorb the bicarbonate.
            (b) Cystitis related to irritation of the bladder with exocrine enzymes.
            (c) Bleeding of the duodenal cuff.
            (d) Fluid losses through the pancreas with dehydration and hypotension (G. Danovitch, 2010a; Gruessner & Gruessner, 2013).
      b. Enteric drainage.
         (1) Because of the complications of bladder drainage, along with the decreased

rejection rate, pancreas biopsy techniques, and better radiologic studies, the majority of institutions in the United States are using enteric drainage.
         (2) Exocrine function is managed by anastomosis of the graft to the jejunum with or without a Roux-en-Y loop.
         (3) This is the most physiologic method of handling exocrine function.
         (4) Exocrine secretions can be absorbed, and metabolic imbalances are theoretically reduced.
         (5) Complications leading to repeat laparotomy include graft thrombosis, infection, and duodenal leak.
         (6) Some centers use the superior mesenteric vein for venous drainage (G. Danovitch, 2010a; Gruessner & Gruessner, 2013).

C. Operative procedure for SPK transplant differs from a kidney transplant alone (G. Danovitch, 2010a; Townsend et al., 2012).
   1. For a kidney transplant alone, the incision is along the groin area with the kidney being placed outside the abdominal cavity.
   2. For an SPK transplant, the incision is down the middle of the abdomen with the pancreas and kidney being placed within the iliac fossa of the abdominal cavity.
   3. The kidney is first transplanted to protect the pancreas from unnecessary trauma. It is placed in the left iliac fossa to save the right fossa for the pancreas. (Refer to the section on kidney transplantation for further information on the operative procedure for kidney transplantation.)
   4. The pancreas is placed in the right iliac fossa because there is less chance of portal vein kinking after venous anastomosis when it is placed on the right side.
   5. The pancreas can be placed intraperitoneally to prevent deep wound infections, although it is easier to place the pancreas extraperitoneally.
   6. The donor spleen may be removed either before transplantation, during the transplant procedure, or just before closing the abdomen.
   7. Exocrine management occurs as previously described

VI. Complications of pancreas transplantation. See Table 3.2.

A. Postoperative arterial or venous thrombosis.
   1. May occur related to poor preservation, prolonged preservation time, recipient hypercoagulable states, hypotension, or decreased blood flow after ligation of the splenic artery.
   2. Thrombosis is the most frequent cause of early

Table 3.2

Surgical Complications
of Pancreas Transplantation

Thrombosis of vessels supplying and draining pancreas (arterial or venous thrombosis)
Bleeding from vessel
Hematuria (bladder drained)
Infection
Anastomotic leak (both bladder and enteric drained)
Enteric fistula formation (enteric drained)
Graft pancreatitis

graft loss, seen in 10–20% of recipients within a week posttransplant (Lipshutz, 2010).

3. The following interventions are used to prevent and diagnose thrombosis.
   a. Heparin or low molecular weight heparin subcutaneously.
      (1) This is converted to low dose acetylsalicylic acid (aspirin) or antiplatelet therapy which is continued for variable lengths of time.
      (2) Clotting times (INR and partial thromboplastin time [PTT]) are monitored as well as signs and symptoms of bleeding.
      (3) Systemic heparinization may result in bleeding and is generally avoided.
   b. Hypotension is avoided by meticulous attention to fluid management.
   c. Postoperative bed rest may be necessary for 1 to 3 days to protect the vascular anastomoses.
4. Potential signs and symptoms.
   a. A sudden rise in serum glucose levels and decreased urinary amylase and hematuria in bladder-drained pancreata may indicate arterial thrombosis (Lipshutz, 2010).
   b. Sudden abdominal pain and hyperamylasemia may indicate venous thrombosis. Upon surgical reexploration, the pancreas appears large, engorged, and dark blue.
5. Diagnosis is made with Doppler ultrasound, computed tomography (CT) angiogram, or magnetic resonance (MR) angiogram.
6. Prompt surgical intervention is required to prevent serious infection; usually the graft is lost with either arterial or venous thrombosis.

B. Bleeding related to anastomosic complication or anticoagulation therapy.
   1. With bladder-drained pancreata, bleeding may

occur from the duodenal cuff, which is sutured to the dome of the bladder.
   2. The resultant hematuria may require copious, vigorous bladder irrigation using sterile normal saline to prevent bladder outlet obstruction by blood clots. Cystoscopy may be required for obstructive clot evacuation (Lipshutz, 2010).
   3. Anticoagulation therapy may need to be discontinued.
   4. Significant postoperative bleeding may require surgical reexploration.

C. Infection.
   1. May be seen as a superficial wound infection, infected peripancreatic fluid collection, CMV infection, or urinary tract infection (UTI).
   2. Superficial wound infection rates have decreased dramatically due to antibiotic prophylaxis and improved surgical techniques.
   3. Likewise, CMV infections have decreased due to antiviral prophylaxis.
   4. Many peripancreatic fluid collections resolve with percutaneous drains and IV antibiotics and antifungals.
      a. Unresolved infected peripancreatic fluid collections may result in mycotic aneurysms and serious bleeding.
      b. Will necessitate a pancreatectomy (Lipshutz, 2010).
   5. Since diabetic recipients have a higher incidence of neurogenic bladder with incomplete emptying, intermittent self-catheterization may be necessary to prevent chronic UTIs.

D. Anastomotic leaks.
   1. One of the most common complications that occur within the first 3 months after transplantation (Lipshutz, 2010).
   2. Bladder drained pancreata (less commonly performed).
      a. Symptoms include lower abdominal pain, fever, leukocytosis, and elevation of serum amylase.
      b. Diagnosis is made by cystogram or nuclear medicine imaging.
      c. Foley catheter is used to keep the bladder decompressed and prevent further leakage.
      d. Leaks that occur late after transplantation in bladder-drained pancreas transplants may necessitate conversion to enteric drainage.
   3. Enteric drained pancreata.
      a. Leaks can cause fistula or abscess formation.
      b. Smaller anastomotic leaks may be treated with drain placement and IV antibiotics and antifungals.
      c. Surgical reexploration of large infected fluid collections may be required to prevent secondary complications such as sepsis.

E. Early allograft pancreatitis.
  1. Can be related to a preservation injury, ischemia, surgical handling, or other technical complications.
  2. It generally resolves within the first several postoperative days.
  3. Signs and symptoms.
    a. Can include elevated serum amylase, perigraft fluid collections, graft tenderness, and glycemic disregulation.
    b. Serum amylase levels generally peak within 3 days of the pancreas transplant and usually begin to decrease by postoperative day 5.
    c. A consistent rise in serum amylase and/or graft site tenderness may be indicative of rejection, which needs to be ruled out.
    d. Pancreatitis may occur later due to an anastomotic stricture.
    e. Reflux pancreatitis in bladder-drained pancreata may result from neurogenic, distended bladders in diabetic recipients and may require enteric conversion if persistent (Lipshutz, 2010).

F. Sepsis (i.e., peritonitis, bacteremia).
  1. Occurs more frequently in pancreas transplantation than in any other transplant and is a common cause of mortality (Lipshutz, 2010).
  2. Digestive enzymes, amylase and lipase, may cause septic pancreatitis.
  3. Symptoms include fever, abdominal tenderness, and increased blood glucose levels.
  4. Requires aggressive intravenous antibiotics and monitoring of blood glucose levels.
  5. After imaging studies, may require surgical reexploration or drainage of fluid collections by interventional radiology.

VII. Immunosuppression and rejection after pancreas transplantation.

A. See Section A, Part 4, for further information on immunobiology of organ transplant rejection. The same principles apply for pancreas transplantation.

B. Immunosuppressive protocols for pancreas transplantation have similar combinations as in kidney transplantation.
  1. Depending on the type of pancreas transplant, the risk of rejection is in the range of 10–20% (PAK and PTA at higher rejection risk than SPK) and is higher than kidney transplant alone (Lipshutz, 2010).
  2. A more intense immunosuppressive regimen is needed in pancreas transplantation due to the higher rate of rejection (Schmied et al., 2006).

C. Induction antibody therapy is used in the majority of recipients: SPK 91%, PAK 92%, PTA 96%. Thymoglobulin® is most commonly used (83%), followed by alemtuzumab (Campath®) (16%) (Gruessner & Gruessner, 2013).

D. Maintenance immunosuppression.
  1. The majority of recipients currently receive tacrolimus (Prograf®), mycophenolate mofetil (MMF®), and steroids as their initial maintenance immunosuppression. Sirolimus (Rapamune®), as a first-line agent, is used less frequently (Lipshutz, 2010).
  2. Recent studies are investigating the results and feasibility of steroid-free maintenance immunosuppression in pancreas transplantation (Uemura et al., 2011); 30–40% of SPK and PAK recipients were maintained steroid free (Gruessner & Gruessner, 2013).
  3. Drug dosing varies by each institution's specific protocol and is based on target trough levels.

E. All immunosuppressive medications increase the risk of infection. Each immunosuppressive agent has its unique side-effect profile.
  1. MMF: GI distress (diarrhea, nausea, vomiting) and bone marrow suppression (leukopenia, thrombocytopenia).
  2. Tacrolimus: nephrotoxicity, hypertension, hyperkalemia, diabetes type 2.
  3. Sirolimus: delayed wound healing, diarrhea, thrombocytopenia, hyperlipidemia, and hypercholesterolemia.
  4. Prednisone: increased appetite, GI ulceration, impaired wound healing, hyperlipidemia, easy bruising, Cushingoid appearance, osteoporosis.

F. The goal of immunosuppression is to prevent rejection in the transplanted organ while avoiding overimmunosuppression and subsequent infection.
  1. The least amount of immunosuppressive medications to prevent rejection is used.
  2. Frequent lab work is done to monitor for rejection.
  3. The patient is taught the signs and symptoms of rejection to be able to self-monitor after discharge.

G. Signs and symptoms of pancreas rejection (see Table 3.3), although they lack real specificity, include:
  1. Bladder drained pancreata: low/decreasing urinary amylase/lipase levels.
     Enteric drained pancreata: elevated serum amylase/lipase (Lipshutz, 2010).
  2. Unexplained leukocytosis.
  3. Graft tenderness.
  4. Fever greater than 100° F.

Table 3.3

Signs and Symptoms of Pancreas Rejection

Fever > 100° F
Tenderness at graft site
Decreased urinary amylase (bladder drained pancreas)
Increased serum amylase and lipase
Hyperglycemia (late)

5. Hyperglycemia: a very late sign of rejection and may herald the need for pancreatectomy.

H. With SPK, the kidney is the sentinel organ to monitor for rejection and may require a kidney biopsy. Signs and symptoms include:
1. Increased serum creatinine and blood urea nitrogen.
2. Decreased urine output.
3. Tenderness over graft site.
4. Weight gain, greater than 2 pounds over 24 hours.
5. Hypertension.
6. Fever greater than 100° F.

I. The kidney allows for an earlier diagnosis and treatment of rejection, thereby accounting for the improved graft survival of SPK, followed by PAK, then PTA.

J. Detecting rejection after pancreas transplantation is still considered one of the major problems of pancreas transplantation because of its nonspecific signs and symptoms (see Table 3.4).
1. Rejection can only be confirmed with a biopsy, which is invasive and carries risks such as bleeding and infection.

2. Various institutions use various methods, and continued research is being conducted to create a standardized, noninvasive test for detecting pancreas rejection.
3. With simultaneous pancreas–kidney transplants, rejection may be detected by kidney rejection and by the signs and symptoms of pancreas rejection listed above.
4. Transcytoscopic biopsy of the head of the pancreas is another option for bladder-drained transplants (Lipshutz, 2010).
   a. Complications may include hematuria after biopsy, treated with bladder irrigation until clear.
   b. Other postbiopsy complications reported include clot retention and transient hyperamylasemia.
5. Percutaneous ultrasound or CT guided pancreas biopsy is an option to diagnose rejection in enteric-drained pancreata. Complications may include bleeding, graft pancreatitis, pancreatic fistula, or pseudocyst formation.
6. Reliable techniques or laboratory studies for noninvasive diagnosis of rejection are being researched.
   a. Serum amylase remains a poor indicator of rejection because it may also rise in pancreatitis after pancreas transplantation.
   b. Studies have been performed on contrast-enhanced ultrasound in the detection of pancreas rejection with promising results in a small, single-center study. However, further studies need to be performed to ensure differentiation between rejection and other posttransplant complications (Kersting et al., 2013).

K. Treatment for rejection.
1. Generally requires treatment with antibody therapy, antithymocyte globulin.
2. Pancreas rejection is frequently refractory to treatment with high-dose steroids, as they are not long-lasting (Lipshutz, 2010).

Table 3.4

Detection of Rejection in Pancreas Transplantation

Noninvasive methods	Assessment for signs and symptoms of rejection in either the kidney or pancreas (Table 3.3)
	Experimental techniques
	Studies have been performed on contrast-enhanced ultrasound (Kersting et al., 2013)
Invasive methods	Percutaneous pancreas biopsy
	Cystoscopic transduodenal pancreas biopsy

VIII. Postoperative nursing management of the pancreas transplant recipient.

A. General information.
1. In general, pancreas transplant recipients no longer require intensive care monitoring postoperatively.
2. Depending upon each individual transplant program's protocol, once extubated, patients may be moved from the recovery room to a specialized transplant/surgery nursing unit.
3. A regular insulin infusion is administered intraoperatively.
   a. May be discontinued in the recovery room due to the immediate function of the newly transplanted pancreas.
   b. Other programs continue the infusion to allow the newly transplanted pancreas a chance to recuperate (Lipshutz, 2010).

B. Immediate postoperative nursing care.
1. Hemodynamic and fluid status monitoring.
   a. Vital signs.
      (1) Blood pressure monitoring.
         (a) A decrease in systolic blood pressure from patient's baseline may signify dehydration or bleeding.
         (b) A systolic BP less than 90 mmHg is reportable at once (Smeltzer et al., 2008).
         (c) Hypotension must be avoided; it will increase the risk of vascular thrombosis (Lipshutz, 2010).
      (2) Cardiac monitoring: tachycardia, a heart rate over 90, may indicate dehydration, bleeding, fever, stress, and/or pain.
      (3) Central venous pressure (CVP) may be monitored by central line.
      (4) Noninvasive oxygen saturation: maintain over 92% or per center protocol.
   b. Observe for bleeding.
      (1) The urine may be bloody. Monitor for clots and irrigate bladder as ordered.
      (2) Jackson Pratt (JP) drain(s) may be in place. Monitor output and assess amount and color of drainage.
      (3) Observe for drainage on bandages. Circle, date, and time drainage and continue to monitor at assessment intervals.
      (4) Monitor hematocrit as ordered for sudden decrease or downward trend.
      (5) For enteric drained pancreata, assess for GI bleeding, melenic stool (Lipshutz, 2010).
   c. Monitor fluid and electrolyte status. Osmotic diuresis may occur posttransplantation.
      (1) Assess for signs of dehydration.
      (2) Monitor for electrolyte imbalance related to diuresis.

2. High risk for vascular thrombosis.
   a. Signs and symptoms: unilateral lower extremity edema on side of pancreas transplant (usually the right side).
   b. May be maintained on bed rest for short interval after transplantation with no hip flexion to preserve integrity of the vessel anastomoses and prevent thrombosis.
   c. Administer low-molecular-weight or standard subcutaneous heparin with conversion to enteric-coated aspirin for thrombosis prophylaxis.
3. Monitor for anastomotic leakage.
   a. Maintain patency of urinary catheter for bladder decompression and decreased tension on sutures.
   b. Observe quantity and quality of drainage from JP drain(s).
4. Maintain patency of nasogastric tube.
   a. Decreased bowel motility is attributed to intraperitoneal placement of the pancreas and the high incidence of diabetic gastroparesis in recipients.
   b. Assess patient for bowel sounds, flatus, and return of bowel function.
5. Monitor metabolic function related to pancreas function.
   a. For bladder drained pancreata, monitor urinary amylase daily. Urine amylase should be 10,000 to 200,000 IU/L.
   b. Monitor blood glucose levels every 1 to 2 hours.
   c. Due to the use of high dose corticosteroids in the early postoperative period, regular insulin infusion may be used to maintain euglycemia. Chronic hyperglycemia is detrimental to wound healing and promotes infection.
   d. If not on insulin and the newly transplanted pancreas is functioning well, monitor for hypoglycemia. The patient may require high-concentration dextrose infusions to compensate for an initial outpouring of insulin.
   e. Monitor serum amylase for signs of pancreatitis immediately postoperatively and per center protocol.
   f. Monitor immunologic function via white blood cell counts and body temperature.
6. Infection prophylaxis.
   a. Intravenous antibiotics and antifungals are generally continued for 48 hours or longer.
   b. Pneumocystosis (*P. jiroveci* [formerly *carinii*]) and cytomegalovirus (CMV) prophylaxis is started per center protocol.
   c. Coach patient to turn, cough, deep breathe, and use incentive spirometer hourly while awake.

C. Intermediate care.
1. There is a decreased need for hemodynamic monitoring 24 hours after surgery as long as the patient remains stable.
   a. Frequent noninvasive blood pressure monitoring continues per center protocol until the patient has stable fluid balance.
   b. Drains and tubes are discontinued as soon as possible because of the risk of infection and subsequent sepsis.
2. Metabolic monitoring continues, but less frequently than in the first 24 hours as long as the patient is stable.
   a. Blood glucose levels can be monitored when the patient is fasting, and then every 4 to 6 hours, depending on stability and results.
   b. Urine and serum amylase levels are done once daily.
3. Catheters and drains:
   a. For bladder-drained pancreata, the urinary catheter is left in up to 5 days to decompress the bladder and drain exocrine secretions from the pancreas.
   b. Per center protocol, if JP drains are used, they are left in for several days until there is a negative ultrasound (about postop day 5 or per center protocol). No fluid collections should be noted around the pancreas or the kidney (if a kidney transplant was also done).
   c. The nasogastric tube is taken out when there are bowel sounds present, the patient passes flatus, or gastric drainage diminishes. The patient is gradually allowed clear liquids and progresses slowly to a regular diet. Continue monitoring for:
      (1) Pancreatitis secondary to preservation injury, handling of the pancreas during the time of transplantation, or inflammation postoperatively.
      (2) Gastroparesis secondary to diabetes, stress of surgical experience, or potential infection.
4. Ambulation 3 to 4 times per day is encouraged to prevent DVT and prevent pneumonia.
   a. Assess for orthostatic hypotension the first several times that the patient gets out of bed.
   b. Orthostatic hypotension can either be caused by fluid depletion or be secondary to autonomic neuropathy related to diabetes (Lipshutz, 2010).
5. Infection and immunologic assessments.
   a. Temperature every 4 hours.
   b. Wound site every 8 hours.
   c. White blood cell count monitoring daily.
   d. Cultures of JP fluid and urine, as indicated.
   e. CMV antigenemia, if indicated.

f. With temperatures greater than 100° F, urine and blood cultures and a chest x-ray may be done per center protocol.

D. Rehabilitation to discharge.
1. Metabolic effects of the pancreas transplant continue to be monitored.
   a. Glycosylated hemoglobin (HbA1C) should fall to normal values within 3 to 4 months.
   b. C peptide reflects secretory function of the beta cells in the transplanted pancreas.
   c. Blood glucose levels continue to be monitored because of the effects of steroids on glucose metabolism.
   d. Urine amylase continues to be monitored to assist with the diagnosis of pancreatitis or rejection. In patients with enteric drainage of the pancreas, serum lipase levels are followed.
2. Discharge preparation is done through multimedia patient teaching (see Tables 3.5 and 3.6) and includes:
   a. Medications, including names, indications, doses, times taken, and side effects.
      (1) Provide written information at a 6th grade readability level (Dewalt et al., 2010). Additional verbal explanations and opportunity for questions should be provided.
      (2) A written medication schedule with medications, doses, and times to take the medications is helpful for the patient to initially learn and then to review medications.
      (3) Placing medications at the bedside for the patient to prepare and have checked by the nurse reinforces learning through practice and repetition.
      (4) Cues for reminding patients include using cell phone alarms, pill boxes, and placing medications within view.
   b. Signs and symptoms of rejection and infection.
   c. Immunization history and immunizations allowed.
   d. Hygiene, infection prevention, and self-care are stressed, with emphasis on emptying bladder and prevention of UTIs.
   e. Good foot care.
   f. Follow-up clinic appointments are made before discharge.
   g. Other issues are also discussed (see Tables 3.5 and 3.6).
   h. Average length of stay has decreased to 5 to 10 days.

Table 3.5

Patient Outcomes – Combined Kidney/Pancreas Transplant

☐ 1. Can state rationale for taking daily temperatures.

☐ 2. Can recognize fever (temperature greater than 38.5° C or 101° F).

☐ 3. Can take and record oral temperature (has thermometer).

☐ 4. Can explain susceptibility to infection.

☐ 5. Can describe signs and symptoms of infection and appropriate action to take.

☐ 6. Can explain need to take and record weight daily (has scale).

☐ 7. Can recognize weight gain (greater than 2 lb/day or 4 lb/week).

☐ 8. Can explain rationale for measuring and recording intake and output, if needed.

☐ 9. Can measure and record intake and output, if needed.

☐ 10. Can correctly perform and record blood glucose (has blood glucose monitoring machine).

☐ 11. Can state blood glucose parameters that require physician notification.

☐ 12. Can measure and record urine pH (has urine test strips), if bladder drainage.

☐ 13. Can state urine pH parameters that require physician notification, if bladder drainage.

☐ 14. Can state precautions to avoid trauma to transplanted kidney/pancreas.

☐ 15. Can describe typical changes in sexual functioning following transplant.

☐ 16. Can explain importance of avoiding pregnancy for at least 1 to 2 years after transplant.

☐ 17. Can describe signs and symptoms of rejection and appropriate action to take.

☐ 18. Can state actions, dosages, and side effects of medications.

☐ 19. Can explain routine for immunosuppressive blood test monitoring.

☐ 20. Can state how to ensure medication supply.

☐ 21. Can describe identification patient will carry as a transplant recipient.

☐ 22. Can describe dietary and fluid prescriptions.

☐ 23. Has Kidney/Pancreas Transplant Book.

☐ 24. Has written medication instructions that have been reviewed with nurse.

☐ 25. Has rejection and infection cards.

☐ 26. Has written dietary and fluid instructions.

☐ 27. Has arranged for physical therapy consult, if needed.

☐ 28. Has arranged for social service consult.

☐ 29. Has all appropriate telephone numbers for emergencies (physician, clinical nurse specialist, transplant office, transplant unit).

☐ 30. Has follow-up appointment.

Primary Nurse Signature _____

Discharging Nurse Signature _____

Date of Discharge _____

Source: Bartucci, M.R., Loughman, K.A., & Moir, E.J. (1992). Kidney-pancreas transplantation: A treatment option for ESRD and type 1 diabetes. *ANNA Journal, 19*(5), 471. Used with permission.

Table 3.6

What Patients Need to Know about Their Medications Before Leaving the Hospital

- Names of all medications (brand, generic, and common nicknames)

- The rationale for the medication

- Frequency, times, and whether the medication can be taken with food or with other medications

- Instructions for taking medications when blood is to be drawn

- How long the patient can expect to be on the medication

- Common side effects

- What to do if a dose is missed

- What to do in the event the patient cannot take the medication

- Where to store the medication

- How to get a refill

- How much it costs and what insurance will/will not cover

Source: Conway, P., Davis, C., Hartel, T., & Russell, G. (1998). Simultaneous kidney pancreas transplantation: Patient issues and nursing interventions. *ANNA Journal, 25*(5), 459. Used with permission.

IX. Long-term benefits of pancreas transplantation. Many of the secondary complications of diabetes are stabilized or improved by normalization of glucose (Sollinger et al., 2009). Most important, patients no longer suffer from life-threatening hypoglycemic unawareness (Becker, 2012).

A. Nephropathy.
   1. Various studies have shown that pancreas transplantation prevents progression of diabetic nephropathy in the transplanted kidney (Lipshutz, 2010).

B. Peripheral and autonomic neuropathy.
   1. Improvements in peripheral neuropathy have been seen in pancreas transplant recipients after 1 year and in autonomic function at 5 years (Lipshutz, 2010).
   2. Improvements are likely due to both euglycemia as well as normalized kidney function.

C. Diabetic retinopathy. No reversal of retinopathy is seen with pancreas transplantation, but data suggests that stabilization occurs (Shipman & Patel, 2009).

D. Gastroenteropathy. Variable improvement is seen after pancreas transplantation and may also be the result of improved kidney function.

E. Vascular disease.
   1. Cardiac function, as measured by normalization of diastolic dysfunction and decreased left ventricular mass, was shown to improve after transplantation.
   2. Less progression of coronary and carotid artery disease is seen with pancreas transplantation than with kidney transplant alone in recipients with type 1 DM (Lipshutz, 2010).

F. Pregnancy. Pregnancy outcomes are followed through the National Transplant Pregnancy Registry database for kidney–pancreas recipients. Concerns with pregnancy are the same as those for kidney transplant recipients (teratogenicity of mycophenolate mofetil, risk of rejection, hypertension, high risk obstetric patient and infant).

G. Quality of life (QOL) after pancreas transplantation.
   1. QOL makes up the physical, social, psychic, and spiritual well-being of an individual, based on his or her subjective perception of these domains. QOL is measured by the patient's perspective of various concepts by administration of validated, reliable questionnaires.
   2. A meta-analysis of 14,750 organ transplant recipients showed results of improved QOL (Dew et al., 1997).
   3. In a single center cross-sectional, longitudinal evaluation study using the Diabetes Quality of Life, Short Form-36 and Quality of Well-Being questionnaires, diabetes-related quality of life was significantly better in type 1 diabetics following SPK compared to those who remained on the waiting list. This improved diabetes QOL was sustained longitudinally, but an overall improvement in general Quality of Well-Being was not shown in this study. Study limitations included relatively few patients in each study group (Suresh et al., 2005).

X. Islet cell transplantation.

A. Background information.
   1. Regretfully, the promise of islet cell transplantation has not come to fruition in the current era.
   2. The encouraging initial results from the Edmonton protocol in the late 1990s have not shown long-term success in maintaining an insulin-free state for recipients of islet cell transplants.
   3. The number of patients receiving islet transplants has declined over the years, and the procedure is considered experimental in the United States.
      a. The therapy is only available at sites approved by the FDA for clinical research of islet transplantation for type 1 diabetes.

b. The hope for a less invasive, safer, and more cost-effective treatment for type 1 diabetes has not yet been realized, but research is ongoing in multiple sites.

4. In 2009, data from the Collaborative Islet Transplant Registry (CITR) indicated that 70% of adults with type 1 diabetes who received islet transplantation were insulin independent at 1 year, 55% at 2 years, and 35% at 3 years (CITR, 2014). These results are notably inferior to those for SPK as cited at the beginning of this section.

B. Historical perspectives of pancreas transplantation.
1. In 1894, portions of sheep pancreas were transplanted into diabetic patients with no success.
2. In 1972, Ballinger and Lacy achieved success in a rat model.
3. In the 1980s, the first short-term successful islet transplant was performed, but without long-term success.
4. In late 1990s, a small series of successful islet transplants in seven patients, the Edmonton protocol, sparked hope for a successful cure for type 1 diabetes (Shapiro et al., 2000). The success of this protocol was unable to be duplicated subsequently.

C. Basic concepts of islet cell transplantation.
1. The islets of Langerhans are clusters of endocrine cells scattered throughout the pancreas that are responsible for glucose metabolism in the body.
2. Beta cells, located in the islets, secrete insulin in response to hyperglycemia.
3. The pancreas contains approximately 1 million islets which is 2–3% of total pancreatic volume.
4. Islets are isolated from procured pancreata from deceased donors.
   a. Pancreatic duct is cannulated and collagenase is infused to separate islets from exocrine and ductal tissue.
   b. Islets are then centrifuged to remove cellular debris.
   c. Purified islets are infused via catheter to the portal vein and travel to the liver sinusoids.
   d. To achieve adequate numbers of islets, from one to four donor pancreata may be required. Most recipients require more than one islet cell infusion.

D. Recipient selection.
1. Recipients of kidney transplants with type 1 diabetes. See recipient selection for pancreas transplantation.
2. Nonuremic patients with type 1 diabetes with hypoglycemic unawareness or inability to achieve glycemic stability despite intensive efforts.

E. Potential complications.
1. Although less invasive, bleeding, portal vein thrombosis, and portal hypertension may occur.
2. Risks associated with chronic immunosuppression.

F. Future research for pancreatic islet cell transplantation.
1. Improvements in islet harvest to maximize cells to be transplanted (Mineo et al., 2009).
2. Enhanced portal engraftment.
3. Alternative sites to liver for engraftment: peritoneal cavity and omentum.
4. Improved immunosuppression with fewer toxicities.
5. Techniques to promote immune tolerance.
6. Biomarkers for monitoring islet cell function prior to occurrence of hyperglycemia, which is a late indicator of failure.
7. Microencapsulation of islet cells.
8. Use of human embryonic stem cells.

Section C
Chronic Kidney Disease in Transplant Recipients
Clara Neyhart

Part 1. Chronic Kidney Disease in Liver Disease and Liver Transplantation

I. The presence of kidney disease in the patient with cirrhosis.

A. Background information.
1. Kidney disease markedly increases the morbidity and mortality of liver disease.
2. The Model for End-Stage Liver Disease (MELD) score was introduced in 2002 to assist in organ allocation for patients with liver failure.
   a. Prior to the MELD score, patients with kidney failure were considered too sick for liver transplantation, and they would frequently die before transplant.
   b. This score takes into account the serum bilirubin, international normalized ratio of prothrombin time (INR), and serum creatinine to establish severity of illness among those awaiting liver transplantation.
3. The use of the MELD score has resulted in more patients with CKD receiving liver transplants, and has reduced the mortality rate prior to liver transplant.
   a. With increasing numbers of patients with CKD

receiving liver transplants, there are, of course, more patients with CKD posttransplant.
   b. It is important to understand the principles of kidney disease in the context of liver disease (Ginès & Schrier, 2009).

B. Kidney sodium and water retention in liver disease.
   1. Frequent complication of end-stage liver disease (ESLD).
      a. The mechanisms involved in these processes are not completely understood.
      b. Eventually leads to sequelae such as ascites, spontaneous bacterial peritonitis, portal hypertension, varices and variceal bleeding, and hepatorenal syndrome (HRS).
   2. These sequelae are major causes of morbidity and mortality before transplantation and also complicate the care of patients after transplantation.
   3. The causes of sodium and water retention and kidney dysfunction in ESLD are due to pathophysiology of the circulatory system that results in splanchnic and systemic vasodilatation, followed by sodium retention and kidney vasoconstriction.
   4. There are three theories for sodium and water retention in ESLD. These theories overlap but differ in the origin and order of events leading to kidney dysfunction (Friedman & Keefe, 2012).
      a. The underfilling theory suggested that as ascites formation begins and fluid moves into the peritoneal cavity, the intravascular volume contracts.
         (1) Increased plasma oncotic pressure and decreased portal venous pressure cause an "underfilled state."
         (2) The kidneys recognize the decreased blood volume and respond by sodium and water retention (Friedman & Keeffe, 2012).
      b. The overfilling theory suggested that inappropriate sodium and water retention by the kidneys in the absence of volume depletion leads to expanded plasma volume, and therefore directly causes the development of ascites (Zervos & Rosemurgy, 2001).
      c. The peripheral arterial vasodilation theory has replaced these two theories – the underfilling theory and the overfilling theory.
         (1) The peripheral arterial vasodilation theory includes ideas from both the previous two theories.
         (2) This theory suggests that portal hypertension results in splanchnic arterial vasodilation.
            (a) Results in a decrease in the effective circulating arterial blood volume.
            (b) Thus causes an activation of the sympathetic nervous system, the renin

angiotensin system, and antidiuretic hormone, causing vasoconstriction.
            (c) The systemic vasoconstriction leads to renal vasoconstriction followed by renal ischemia (Weber et al., 2012).

C. Ascites.
   1. Defined as collection of free fluid in the peritoneal space.
   2. The ascitic fluid comes from the vascular space of the hepatic circulation and is derived from the liver and intestines.
   3. The constant formation of ascites is due to salt and water retention, which shows there is a relationship between the formation of ascites and the onset of urinary sodium retention.
   4. Once portal hypertension develops and the patient's albumin decreases, fluid moves from the sinusoids and hepatic circulation to the peritoneal cavity.
      a. This causes a decrease in the amount of useful blood volume, causing a decrease in the vascular space.
      b. The renal tubule is then stimulated to reabsorb sodium and water (Friedman & Keeffe, 2012).

D. Electrolyte imbalances.
   1. Hyponatremia.
      a. Usually due to dilution by large amounts of body water.
      b. ADH levels are increased due to nonosmotic stimulation brought on by a decrease in blood volume to the kidneys.
         (1) Hyponatremia tends to worsen as the liver disease progresses.
         (2) The increase in ADH secretion (and water retention) correlates with the severity of liver disease (Heuman et al., 2004).
      c. The best therapy is prevention.
         (1) Serial monitoring of electrolytes and response to diuretics.
         (2) Restriction of water intake in patients with severe hyponatremia may be prescribed.
            (a) This is difficult because to raise the serum sodium significantly, the total fluid intake would need to be lower than the urine volume.
            (b) There is not much data to support fluid restriction unless the patient has neurologic symptoms of hyponatremia (Sterns & Runyon, 2013).
         (3) Generally, hypertonic saline is not a recommended therapy.
            (a) Most patients with ESLD have decreased intravascular oncotic pressure and are not responsive to diuretic therapy.
            (b) Extremely rapid correction of

hyponatremia may result in
neurologic injury.
- (c) In patients who are within hours of
liver transplantation, partial correction
of hyponatremia with cautious use of
hypertonic saline may be helpful
(Sterns & Runyon, 2013).
- (4) Complications of hyponatremia include
confusion, delirium, seizures, lethargy,
weakness, and cerebral edema.
2. Hypernatremia.
   a. Usually due to dehydration or decrease in total
   body water.
   b. Often caused by lactulose that is the hallmark
   treatment for hepatic encephalopathy.
      (1) Due to the osmotic effect in which water
      moves from the plasma to the bowel and
      causes diarrhea.
      (2) More water than sodium is excreted since
      sodium is absorbed by the colon (Lukens et
      al., 2011).
   c. Also occurs in hospitalized patients due to
   insensible water losses from sepsis, fever,
   tachypnea, and dehydration associated with
   diuresis.
   d. The best therapy is prevention.
      (1) Monitor fluid balance.
      (2) Monitor electrolytes.
      (3) Decrease lactulose as appropriate.

E. Acid-base imbalances (Ahya et al., 2006).
1. Respiratory alkalosis.
   a. The cause of respiratory alkalosis in ESLD is
   not well defined.
   b. It may be caused by hypoxemia associated with
   ascites and ventilation-perfusion imbalances,
   increased ammonia levels, and anemia.
   c. Another cause may be intracellular acidosis,
   which can cause hyperventilation.
2. Metabolic alkalosis.
   a. Usually due to iatrogenic or extrarenal causes.
   b. Diuretics may cause a secondary aldosteronism,
   which can result in alkalosis due to increased
   urinary hydrogen loss. This is usually
   accompanied by hypokalemia.
   c. Metabolic alkalosis may also occur due to
   vomiting.
3. Metabolic acidosis.
   a. Lactic acidosis usually occurs in combination
   with factors such as bleeding or sepsis that
   decrease the hepatic blood flow.
   b. Diminishes the use of lactate by the liver and
   kidneys or causes an increase in the formation
   of lactate.
   c. Other causative factors include alcohol use,
   medications, hypotension, and hyperventilation.
4. Respiratory acidosis.

a. Respiratory acidosis is very common in liver
disease.
b. It usually occurs in association with severe
restrictive lung disease due to massive ascites
and pleural effusion.
c. Respiratory failure may ensue with the
associated respiratory muscle weakness that is
due to hypokalemia or respiratory depression
from the drugs that the liver usually detoxifies.

F. Hepatorenal syndrome (HRS).
1. Characterized by a decrease in kidney blood flow
and GFR in which there is no abnormality of the
kidney and no other identified causes of kidney
failure (Nadim et al., 2012; Weber et al., 2012).
2. Other causes of kidney failure must first be ruled
out, including nephritis, obstruction, acute
tubular necrosis, or dehydration.
3. Types of HRS.
   a. Type 1 HRS.
      (1) Rapid deterioration of kidney function.
      (2) The serum creatinine increases more than
      100% from baseline to > 2.5 mg/dL in a
      2-week period.
   b. Type 2 HRS.
      (1) There is a more moderate decrease in renal
      function.
      (2) Defined by (Weber et al., 2012; Nadim et
      al., 2012)
         (a) GFR < 60 mL/min and/or serum
         creatinine > 1.5 mg/dL.
         (b) Urine sodium concentration < 10
         mEq/L.
         (c) Urine-to-plasma osmolality ratio > 1.
         (d) No urinary sediment.
         (e) Negative proteinuria.
         (f) No kidney improvement after albumin
         or saline administration.
         (g) No other cause of kidney failure.
4. Potential causes.
   a. Severe renal vasoconstriction due to portal
   hypertension, peripheral arteriolar
   vasodilatation, increased plasma volume,
   arterial hypotension, activation of the
   sympathetic nervous system, activation of the
   renin–angiotensin system, and oversecretion of
   ADH (Friedman & Keefe, 2012).
   b. Impaired liver metabolism, with or without
   adequate volume, may also lead to HRS.
      (1) The mechanisms leading to HRS are
      independent of volume status and are not
      triggered by volume stimuli and may
      decrease peripheral vascular resistance.
      (2) This causes vasodilatation, a decrease in
      systemic blood pressure, and effective
      blood volume.

(3) May then cause efferent stimulation and renal vasoconstriction (Friedman & Keefe, 2012).

c. Mechanisms to protect glomerular capillary pressures and decrease renal vasoconstriction are lost or reduced in patients with HRS.
(1) This can occur despite having a decreased blood volume.
(2) This may also lead to a further decrease in the GFR.

d. Decrease in "effective" blood volume is another cause of HRS.
(1) Ascites is formed when the splanchnic vessels and hepatic sinusoids create an overabundance of lymph to such an extent that it cannot be returned to circulation.
(2) The lymph accumulates in the peritoneal space, which leads to a decrease in the blood volume.
(3) As the ascites continues to develop, plasma volume is constantly redistributed.
(4) Patients who retain water and sodium have a decreased total peripheral resistance.
(a) Even though there is an increase in total plasma volume, the amount of available blood is decreased.
(b) The total extracellular fluid volume is moved to other fluid compartments, leading to a decrease in effective blood volume (Weber et al., 2012).

e. Other factors that play a role in HRS.
(1) Changes in the renin–angiotensin system and increased sympathetic nervous system (SNS) stimulation.
(2) The renin–angiotensin system helps to maintain the vasoconstriction associated with HRS.
(3) Patients with ESLD have elevated plasma renin levels that may be due to the inability of the liver to inactivate renin or, more likely, due to the continued renal secretion of renin.
(4) This may occur due to decreased perfusion of the kidney leading to stimulation of the renin–angiotensin system or a secondary response to a decrease in blood volume.
(5) Additionally, the secretion of the angiotensin II causes a more profound decrease in perfusion and GFR (Ginès & Schrier, 2009).

f. An increase in the SNS stimulation may also contribute to the cause of HRS.
(1) A decrease in blood volume is recognized as a decrease in arterial pressure.
(2) Through a chain of events, the sympathetic nervous system is activated, which produces renal vasoconstriction and a decreased GFR (Weber et al., 2012).

5. Management of hepatorenal syndrome.
a. Treatment of underlying liver disease as possible, (i.e., antiviral therapy), and/or liver transplantation.
b. Focus should be on prevention and support of the kidneys.

II. Chronic kidney disease after liver transplantation.

Patients who had some degree of renal insufficiency before transplantation are at a greater risk for morbidity and mortality than those who had normal function. Determination of cause and treatment can be difficult in these patients. Therefore, it is best to follow a general approach and then move to possible specific causes of renal impairment such as drug toxicities.

A. Intraoperative and postoperative events may contribute to renal insufficiency.
1. These events include hemorrhage, hypotension, hypovolemia, infection, graft failure, and antibiotic and immunosuppressant use.
2. Usually there are multiple causative factors.
3. In most patients, these factors lead to acute tubular necrosis (ATN) for a short time that usually resolves in less than a month if there is adequate liver function.
4. Routine assessment of serum creatinine, creatinine clearance, and drug levels is necessary (Giusto et al., 2013).

B. As with other patients on calcineurin inhibitors, careful monitoring of drug levels is required with adjustment of dosage as needed.
1. Dosage should be tailored to individual patient.
2. Routine monitoring of the trough level is integral to maintaining adequate immunosuppression, yet it may be inadequate in minimizing nephrotoxic effects (G. Danovitch, 2010b).
3. Avoidance of intravenous calcineurin inhibitors, if possible.
4. Strict monitoring of hemodynamic status postoperatively and maintenance of euvolemia are essential to prevent compromise that would require aggressive use of vasopressor or diuretic medications, since their use enhances the renal toxicity associated with calcineurin inhibitors (Ponticelli, 2007).
5. Reduction in the dose with early, mild kidney function impairment, whenever possible. Change of immunosuppressive medication regimen may be necessary when calcineurin inhibitor toxicity occurs (G. Danovitch, 2012b; Ponticelli, 2007).

III. Chronic kidney disease after liver transplantation: other treatment strategies.

A. Conservative measures.
1. Correct disorders of electrolyte imbalance (sodium and potassium), acid-base balance, and hypovolemia.
2. Careful calculation of intake and urinary output.
3. Detect and correct graft dysfunction and infection immediately.
4. Meticulous wound care.
5. Avoid over immunosuppression which can lead to infection and sepsis.
6. If antibiotics are needed, facilitate the use of nonnephrotoxic agents.
7. Use care in administering agents that increase the blood level of cyclosporine or tacrolimus. Educate patients to avoid these agents.
8. Use the same recommendations as for any patient with CKD (e.g., control of blood pressure, diabetes, treatment of anemia, hyperlipidemia, etc.) (G. Danovitch, 2010a; Ponticelli, 2007; Townsend et al., 2012).

B. Kidney replacement therapy.
1. Initiate kidney replacement therapy as for any patient with CKD stage 5.
2. Careful monitoring for infection with early intervention because of immunosuppressed state.
3. Very little data on dialysis outcomes for liver transplant recipients, but mortality is higher in transplant recipient compared to the nontransplant patient.
4. If the transplanted liver is not functioning well, the patient is more susceptible to bleeding disorders since the liver synthesizes many of the clotting factors.
   a. Abnormal bleeding time, prothrombin time, and disseminated intravascular clotting are all possible.
   b. A patient with a nonfunctional liver transplant and kidney failure is likely to be hemodynamically unstable and may require continuous dialysis in an intensive care unit setting. Low blood-flow rate, frequent flushing, and heparin-free dialysis may be ordered, although type and condition of access will determine these parameters (Hensen & Carpenter, 2010).
5. Patients with liver disease tend to have very low serum protein levels, which will cause third spacing of fluid into the interstitial space. The patient should be monitored carefully for hypotension.
6. Avoid dehydration with dialysis, as this is likely to delay or prevent kidney recovery.

Part 2. Chronic Kidney Disease in Heart Disease and Heart Transplantation

I. Chronic kidney disease with left ventricular dysfunction.

A. Abnormalities in kidney function frequently occur in patients with chronic left ventricular systolic dysfunction.

B. Intrinsic kidney disease may be caused most often by:
1. Advanced age.
2. Atherosclerosis or renovascular disease.
3. Hypertension, which causes lower effective renal plasma flow and higher mean renovascular resistance.
4. Diabetes mellitus, which results in diabetic nephropathy (Anand, 2013).

C. Hemodynamic abnormalities that diminish kidney function are decreased cardiac output and renal blood flow and an elevation in renal vein pressure secondary to an elevated right atrial pressure and tricuspid regurgitation.
1. Hypotension may result in poor renal perfusion (Anand, 2013).
2. Atrial fibrillation leads to atrial structure changes (electrical and mechanical remodeling) and atrial natriuretic peptide release, which influences renal volume. Loss of atrial kick may decrease cardiac output and affect renal perfusion (Lenihan et al., 2013).

D. Neurohormonal abnormalities lead to vasoconstriction from increased concentrations or enhanced responsiveness to norepinephrine, endothelin, and angiotensin II. Neurohormonal abnormalities prevent the release of endogenous vasodilators or diminish their responsiveness (natriuretic peptides and nitric oxide) (Anand, 2013).
1. Initially, angiotensin II causes an increase in efferent glomerular arterial resistance, leading to maintenance of glomerular filtration rate when renal blood flow is reduced. Over time, glomerular filtration rate may fall (Mann & Hilgers, 2013).
2. Markedly elevated plasma renin levels and hyponatremia are signs of great risk for worsening kidney function during ACE inhibitor therapy since maintenance of glomerular filtration rate is dependent on angiotensin II (Colucci, 2013).
3. *Cardiorenal syndrome* is the term used to describe the combination of kidney dysfunction and heart failure that may originate in either organ. The classification of cardiorenal syndrome is as follows (Anand, 2013).

a. Type 1: acute heart failure with declining kidney function.
b. Type 2: chronic heart failure with declining kidney function.
c. Type 3: acute renal failure leads to worsening heart failure.
d. Type 4: chronic renal failure leads to worsening heart failure.
e. Type 5: systemic conditions cause simultaneous renal and cardiac dysfunction.

E. Therapies for heart failure may influence kidney function.
1. ACE inhibitors and angiotensin II receptor blockers decrease the glomerular filtration rate by inhibiting efferent renal arteriolar resistance, thus reducing glomerular blood flow. Serum creatinine rises, leading to kidney dysfunction (Mann & Hilgers, 2013).
   a. The effect of ACE inhibitors and angiotensin II receptor blockers on kidney function is unpredictable. It is influenced by volume status, serum sodium level, and concurrent medications. A rise in serum creatinine and blood urea nitrogen of 10–20% is not unlikely (Colucci, 2013).
   b. Rises in serum creatinine to 3 mg/dL or higher do not preclude the continuation of therapy as long as the serum creatinine is stabilized and hyperkalemia does not occur (Colucci, 2013).
2. Diuretic therapy (all classes) depletes sodium and volume, leading to decreased renal blood flow.
   a. Loop diuretics directly activate neuroendocrine systems (sympathetic nervous system, renin–angiotensin system, and antidiuretic hormone), leading to an imbalance between renal sympathetic activation, angiotensin II, and natriuretic peptides.
   b. During aggressive diuresis with loop diuretics and in the presence of angiotensin-converting enzyme inhibitors, natriuretic peptide levels are reduced, and angiotensin II is diminished. In addition, sympathetic activation and increased vasopressin levels alter the glomerular filtration rate, resulting in kidney function deterioration (Colucci & Sterns, 2013).
3. Beta-blocker therapy appears to be renoprotective. Beta-blocker therapy lowers plasma renin level activity, which will decrease dependence on angiotensin II for maintaining glomerular filtration rate (Colucci, 2013).

II. Collaborative management of chronic kidney disease prior to cardiac transplantation.

A. Permanent discontinuation of ACE inhibitors is rarely necessary when creatinine is moderately elevated. Decreases in kidney function, which lead to interruption in therapy, might prevent optimization of afterload and preload, potentially leading to further compromise of left ventricular function and perpetuation of symptoms (Colucci, 2013).

B. Patients who develop an elevated serum creatinine from ACE inhibitor or angiotensin II receptor-blocking therapies may derive the greatest benefit from the therapies, especially when left ventricular systolic dysfunction is advanced (Hawwa et al., 2013).

C. Beta-blocker therapy is initiated and maintained whenever possible.

D. If atrial fibrillation develops, attempts to restore normal sinus rhythm are a priority (Lenihan et al., 2013).

E. Renal insufficiency serves as a marker for more advanced heart failure. Measurement of GFR (not baseline serum creatinine level) should be monitored, especially when there is an increase in the blood urea nitrogen/serum creatinine ratio, suggesting prerenal failure. Creatinine is not as good a marker since decreased muscle mass is common in the patient with chronic heart failure and/or immediately following surgery (Bloom, 2013).

F. Since comorbid conditions influence the prevalence of renal insufficiency, treatment should reflect current consensus recommendations.

G. Kidney replacement therapies improve prognosis when kidney dysfunction occurs as a result of heart failure and/or the therapies used to treat the condition while awaiting cardiac transplantation, rather than kidney disease present prior to heart failure.
1. Therapies allow for controlled removal of excess sodium and volume, even when diuretic resistance occurs.
2. Therapies replace kidney function when conventional fluid removal with diuretics leads to prerenal depletion and impaired kidney function (Hawwa et al., 2013).
3. Continuous kidney replacement therapies are the first choice during periods of hemodynamic instability.

III. Chronic kidney disease after cardiac transplantation: incidence, definition, outcomes.

A. Early acute kidney injury refers to the immediate postoperative period of 0 to 30 days. The incidence is approximately 25–30% (Gude et al., 2010).
1. Predisposing factors (Bloom, 2013; Gude et al., 2010).

a. Use of calcineurin inhibitors (cyclosporine or tacrolimus) in the early postoperative period. The incidence increases with intravenous dosing or higher drug trough levels.

b. Preoperative kidney dysfunction.

c. Preoperative cardiovascular compromise (presence of hypotension), requiring continuous intravenous vasopressor support.

d. Any hospitalization before transplantation.

e. Perioperative hemodynamic compromise.

f. Sepsis.

2. Signs that suggest severe kidney hypoperfusion with intact tubular function.

a. Oliguria or anuria.

b. High serum creatinine, which peaks 4 to 5 days postoperatively (BUN not reliable indicator as steroids can significantly increase BUN postoperatively); elevated BUN/creatinine ratio.

c. Low urine sodium (less than 10 mEq/L), but this may be inaccurate if the patient is receiving diuretics.

d. Hyponatremia.

e. Low fractional excretion of sodium (less than 1%).

f. Metabolic acidosis.

g. Hyperkalemia disproportionate to elevated serum creatinine.

h. Normal urine sediment (Bloom, 2013).

3. Outcome.

a. If calcineurin inhibitor use was the only factor that produced the decrease in kidney function, and the dosage is reduced, the outcome is usually favorable with a spontaneous recovery in 7 to 10 days (Gude et al., 2010).

b. Irreversible kidney failure may ensue if kidney failure lasts beyond 7 to 10 days and is complicated by septicemia or surgery, or calcineurin inhibitor dose cannot be reduced (Bloom, 2013).

B. Late acute kidney injury occurs after 30 days and has a low incidence of 1 to 2%. The first 6 to 8 weeks after transplantation are when the greatest risk of nephrotoxic effects occur (Gude et al., 2010).

1. Predisposing factors.

a. Use of nephrotoxic drugs together with calcineurin inhibitor, causing a synergistic toxic effect, i.e., amphotericin, ganciclovir, and NSAIDs.

b. Use of drugs that interact with and increase the blood levels of calcineurin inhibitors, causing kidney dysfunction and increasing risk of severe infection.

c. Multisystem organ failure syndrome.

d. Hypertension and hyperlipidemia have been suggested as potential factors that may lead to accelerated atherosclerosis.

2. Signs.

a. Elevation of serum creatinine with or without oliguria. Significant deterioration noted after the third month posttransplant.

b. Low fractional excretion of sodium in the absence of heart failure (Fatehi & Hsu, 2013).

c. No relation has been found between calcineurin inhibitor dose and trough levels and the incidence of acute kidney dysfunction (G. Danovitch, 2010b).

3. Outcome is favorable if there is no heart failure.

IV. Chronic kidney disease after cardiac transplantation: Injury characteristics.

A. Kidney biopsy findings in patients with calcineurin inhibitor toxicity.

1. Tubulointerstitial damage: interstitial fibrosis with tubular atrophy (most frequent finding) (Ponticelli, 2007).

2. Microvascular changes from vasoconstriction of the afferent arterioles cause obliterative vasculopathy, endothelial swelling, and microthrombi from deposition of protein material in necrotic arterial walls (second most common finding).

3. In later stages, fibrous endarteritis occurs (Ponticelli, 2007).

4. Arterial changes lead to an occlusive disorder of the afferent arterioles and ischemic damage to nephrons, causing obliteration and retraction of the affected glomerulus (not common) (Ponticelli, 2007).

B. Electron microscopy.

1. Vacuolization of the proximal tubular cells with destruction of apical microvilli.

2. Giant mitochondria.

3. Dilation of the ergastoplasmic cisternae.

4. Numerous lysosomes (G. Danovitch, 2010a; Ponticelli, 2007).

C. Physiologic findings.

1. Increased renal vascular resistance from persistent renal vasoconstriction, cortical renal artery spasm, and ischemia. These findings are related to:

a. Loss of vasodilatory effects of prostanoids.

b. Altered levels of circulating catecholamines.

c. Alteration in efferent sympathetic signals to the kidney and possibly by the stimulation of endothelin-1 (a potent vasoconstricting peptide that is derived from the endothelium) (Ponticelli, 2007).

2. Decreased glomerular filtration rate and renal plasma flow (G. Danovitch, 2010a; Ponticelli, 2007).

V. Chronic kidney disease after cardiac transplantation: Minimizing nephrotoxic effects of calcineurin inhibitors.

A. Dosage should be tailored to individual patient.

B. Routine monitoring of the trough level is integral to maintaining adequate immunosuppression, yet it may be inadequate in minimizing nephrotoxic effects.

C. Avoidance of intravenous calcineurin inhibitors, if possible.

D. Strict monitoring of hemodynamic status postoperatively and maintenance of euvolemia are essential to prevent compromise that would require aggressive use of vasopressor or diuretic medications, since their use enhances the renal toxicity associated with calcineurin inhibitors.

E. Reduction in the dose with early, mild kidney function impairment, whenever possible.

F. Specific drug therapies when calcineurin nephrotoxicity occurs (G. Danovitch, 2010b).
1. Minimize vasoconstriction effects by administration of calcium channel blockers. Careful monitoring for hemodynamic compromise is necessary since these agents have negative inotropic properties.
2. Other drugs that minimize calcineurin inhibitor effects are atrial natriuretic peptide, cilastatin, dopamine (at low dopaminergic dose), pentoxifylline, and dietary antioxidant supplementation.
3. Consider change in immunosuppressive regimen.

VI. Chronic kidney disease after cardiac transplantation: other treatment strategies.

A. Conservative measures.
1. Correct disorders of electrolyte imbalance (sodium and potassium), acid-base balance, and hypovolemia.
2. Careful calculation of intake and urinary output.
3. Detect and correct graft dysfunction and infection immediately. Optimal wound care in the early postoperative period.
4. Avoid overimmunosuppression (which can lead to infection and sepsis).
5. If antibiotics are needed, facilitate the use of nonnephrotoxic agents.
6. Use care in administering agents that increase the blood level of cyclosporine or tacrolimus (see Table 3.7). Educate patients to avoid these agents.
7. Use the same recommendations as for any patient with CKD (e.g., control of blood pressure,

Table 3.7

Drug Interactions Affecting Calcineurin Inhibitors (Cyclosporine and Tacrolimus) *

Increased Blood Levels	Decreased Blood Levels	Increased Nephrotoxicity
acetazolamide	carbamazepine	acyclovir
azithromycin	cholestyramine	aminoglycosides
cimetidine	glutethimide	amphotericin B
clarithromycin	isoniazid	cimetidine
corticosteroids	phenobarbital	ciprofloxacin
• methylprednisolone	phenytoin	cephalosporins
• prednisolone	primidone	diclofenac
diltiazem	rifampin	lovastatin
erythromycin	IV sulfatrimethoprim	melphalan
fluconazole	IV trimethoprim/sulfamethoxazole	NSAIDs
imipenem-cilastatin	warfarin	pravastatin
itraconazole		ranitidine
ketoconazole		simvastatin
nicardipine		trimethoprim/sulfamethoxazole
verapamil		
grapefruit juice		

IV = intravenous; NSAIDs = nonsteroidal antiinflammatory drugs

* Please note that new medications are always being approved and will not be listed in this table. Consult a current drug reference such as Lexicomp® or the Physician's Desk Reference® as to whether the medication has interactions with the calcineurin inhibitors.

diabetes, treatment of anemia, hyperlipidemia, etc.) (Gustafsson & Ross, 2009).

B. Kidney replacement therapy (KRT).
1. Initiate KRT as for any patient with CKD stage 5.
2. Careful monitoring for infection with early intervention because of immunosuppressed state.
3. Very little data on dialysis outcomes for cardiac transplant recipients, but hemodialysis appears to be preferable to peritoneal dialysis.
4. Consider kidney transplantation, if possible.

Part 3. Chronic Kidney Disease in Lung Transplantation

I. Background information.

A. The reported incidence of CKD in recipients of lung transplants varies widely from 15% to over 60%, due in part to inconsistent classifications of CKD.

B. Roughly 25% of lung transplant recipients develop CKD within 1 year posttransplant, and 40% to 50% by 5 years.

C. Some studies reported CKD as a glomerular filtration (GFR) < 60 mL/min while others used a lower GFR to designate CKD.

D. In any case, the presence and severity of acute kidney injury (AKI) before or after lung transplant is associated with the development of CKD and its comorbidities.

E. The most common diagnoses leading to lung transplant are chronic obstructive pulmonary disease, idiopathic pulmonary fibrosis, cystic fibrosis, and pulmonary hypertension.

F. Sarcoidosis, Alpha 1 antitrypsin deficiency, and obliterative bronchiolitis are other less common diagnoses in patients waiting for lung transplant.

G. 4% to 7% of lung transplant recipients develop kidney failure over the long term (Jacques et al., 2012; Paradela de la Morena et al., 2010; Pham et al., 2009; Wehbe et al., 2012).

II. Acute kidney injury (AKI) after lung transplant.

A. AKI is associated with increased risk of CKD and mortality.

B. Risk factors for developing AKI perioperatively Pham et al., 2009; Robinson et al., 2013).

1. Cardiopulmonary bypass.
2. Ventricular dysfunction.
3. Volume contraction, such as with aggressive diuresis.
4. Acute tubular necrosis from sepsis or hypotension.
5. Calcineurin inhibitors.
6. Nephrotoxic drugs such as antibiotics or antivirals.

III. Patients requiring dialysis have an increased risk for long-term morbidity and mortality (Robinson et al., 2013; Wehbe et al., 2012).

IV. Complications after lung transplant that may impact the dialysis prescription.

A. Impaired gas exchange.
1. Patients remain ventilated for a period of time until stabilized, with impaired delivery of oxygen and CO_2 elimination.
2. Some patients will require extracorporeal membrane oxygenation, particularly with primary graft dysfunction.

B. Edema.
1. Lung transplant patients are frequently fluid overloaded in the immediate postoperative period and may require hemofiltration.
2. Pulmonary edema may be associated with reperfusion of the transplanted lung(s) or heart failure.

C. Possible problems with airway clearance related to denervated transplanted lung(s), resulting in pooling of secretions.

D. Arrythmias. Atrial fibrillation associated with heart failure is not uncommon after lung transplantation

E. Hemodynamic instability is not unusual in the immediate postoperative period or with infection, rejection, or primary graft dysfunction.

F. Coagulopathy in lung transplantation may occur related to use cardiopulmonary bypass and systemic fibrinolytic therapy (Jaksch et al., 2010; Pham et al., 2009).

V. Factors contributing to CKD in the long term after lung transplantation include:

A. Abnormal pretransplant kidney function.

B. Significant history of nephrotoxic medications such as aminoglycosides or amphotericin.

C. Calcineurin inhibitor toxicity.

D. Ischemic insults such as prolonged hypotension, dehydration, or infection.

E. Hypertension.

F. Diabetes.

G. History of acute kidney injury.

H. Dyslipidemia.

I. History of IV inotropic medications (Paradela de la Morena et al., 2010; Pham et al., 2009).

VI. Prevention of CKD progression is attempted through:

A. Avoidance of nephrotoxic agents when possible.

B. Stabilization of calcineurin inhibitor at lowest most effective dose or consider change in immuno-suppression regimen. Sirolimus has been used in small groups of lung transplant recipients.

C. Optimization of hypertension control.

D. Control of diabetes.

E. Control of hyperlipidemia.

F. Maintenance of adequate hydration.

G. Avoidance and prompt treatment of further kidney insults, such as infection or hypotension.

SECTION D
Care of the Kidney Transplant Recipient Who is HIV positive
Laurie Carlson

Kidney transplantation in patients with HIV infection has evolved from an absolute contraindication to a viable option for patients with well-controlled HIV.

I. Historical events.

A. Until 2000, people living with HIV were excluded from evaluation for organ transplantation.

B. Exclusion was based on the concern that immuno-suppression would exacerbate an already immune compromised state and result in poorer outcomes.

C. Increasing the demand for a limited pool of donor organs in a population with a limited expectancy for survival was another concern.

D. The advent of Highly Active Anti-Retroviral Therapy (HAART) and improved prophylaxis against opportunistic infections resulted in decreased

morbidity and mortality and improved life expectancy in people with HIV.

E. HIV infection has changed from a rapidly progressive disease to a chronic condition.

F. People with HIV are dying less often from HIV/AIDS. However, they are now at risk for developing kidney failure and either dying from organ failure or living on dialysis (Palella et al., 1998; Stock & Roland, 2007).

II. Results of kidney transplantation in the HAART era.

A. Early results from prospective pilot studies of kidney transplantation in HIV-infected patients suggest that transplantation is a safe and effective procedure.

B. One-year patient and graft survival were comparable with HIV negative patients.

C. HIV disease progression was not found to be an issue.

D. Acute rejection emerged as a larger problem than anticipated, and rejection rates were reported to be about 50%, double the rate seen in HIV negative patients.

E. Other retrospective studies report similar results to those reported in the pilot prospective studies.

F. A large multicenter, prospective study was indicated (Abbott et al., 2004; Kumar et al., 2002; Pelletier et al., 2004; Stock & Roland, 2007; Stock et al., 2003).

III. NIH Grant: Solid organ transplantation in people with HIV infection: design and outcomes.

A. Between November 2003 and June 2009, 150 HIV-infected patients received kidney transplants through this study. This was a prospective, nonrandomized multicenter study.

B. Study inclusion criteria.
   1. Center specific criteria for transplantation must have been met.
   2. HIV RNA undetectable.
   3. CD4+ T cells > 200 cm.

C. Living and deceased donor organs were included.

D. Immunosuppression included glucocorticoids, cyclosporine or tacrolimus, and mycophenolate mofetil.

E. Induction therapy with thymoglobulin or interleukin-2 receptor blocker was allowed.

F. Routine prophylaxis against opportunistic infections was followed. The duration of therapy was longer and prophylaxis was influenced by CD4 count and previous opportunistic infection history (AI052748, 2003-2013; Stock et al., 2010).

IV. Patient and graft survival.

A. Patient survival rates at 1 and 3 years were 94.6% and 88.2%.

B. Mean graft survival rates at 1 and 3 years were 90.4% and 73.7%.

C. These rates fall between those reported for all kidney transplant recipients and those reported for older (> 65 years) kidney transplant recipients (Stock et al., 2010).

V. Incidence of rejection.

A. An unexpectedly high rate of rejection was observed in the HIV-infected population.

B. The cumulative incidence of rejection at 1 and 3 years was 31% and 41%.

C. In comparison, 1-year SRTR rejection rates are reported at 12.3%.

D. 49 patients (33%) had 67 acute rejection episodes.
   1. 42 (63%) experienced acute rejection episodes.
   2. 4 (6%) experienced acute vascular rejection.
   3. 7 (10%) experienced acute cellular and vascular rejection.
   4. 4 (6%) experienced acute and chronic rejection.

E. In the multivariate analysis the variables associated with an increased risk of rejection were the use of a kidney from a deceased donor and cyclosporine used (Stock et al., 2010).

VI. Effects on HIV.

A. Overall no significant HIV disease progression was reported as a result of transplantation or transplant immunosuppression.

B. HIV RNA generally remained suppressed.

C. CD4+ T-cell counts remained relatively stable.

D. Few incidences of opportunistic infections occurred.

E. Pretransplant, 52 patients (19%) had a history of a previous opportunistic infection (OI).
   1. PCP (30).
   2. CMV (8).
   3. MAC (7).
   4. KS (3).

F. Posttransplant, 13 patients (5%) developed an opportunistic infection.
   1. Cutaneous KS (4).
   2. PCP (2).
   3. Cryptosporidiosis (1).
   4. Candida (6).

G. Of note, there were no recurrences of opportunistic infections in patients with a pretransplant history of an OI.

H. No survival differences based on previous OI history were reported (Stock et al., 2010).

VII. Incidence of infectious and neoplastic complications.

A. 57 (38%) of the 150 kidney transplant recipients had a total of 140 reported infections that required hospitalization.
   1. Bacterial 69%.
   2. Fungal 9%.
   3. Viral 6%.
   4. Protozal 1%.

B. The most common organisms cultured were:
   1. *Escherichia coli* (21).
   2. *Enterococcus* (17).
   3. *Staphylococcus aureus* (12).
   4. *Staphylocccus epidermidis* (11).
   5. *Klebsiella* (8).

C. The most common sites of infection were:
   1. Genitourinary tract (26%).
   2. Respiratory tract (20%)
   3. Blood (19%).

D. About 60% of the serious infections were reported during the first 6 months posttransplant. Nine neoplasms were reported. They include:
   1. Renal cell carcinoma (2).
   2. Kaposi's sarcoma (2).
   3. Oral squamous cell carcinoma (2).
   4. Squamous cell skin cancer, basal cell skin cancer, and cancer of the thyroid gland (1 case each) (Stock et al., 2010).

VIII. Recommended screening and selection criteria.

A. All individuals with CKD and HIV infection must meet standard center-specific clinical criteria for transplantation.

B. They should receive a series of vaccinations that are recommended for all transplant recipients.
   1. Pneumonia vaccination (Pneumovax®) within 5 years of transplant.
   2. Hepatitis A vaccinations.
   3. Hepatitis B vaccinations.
   4. PPD or QuantiFERON®. Patients with a history of a positive PPD must receive 9 to 12 months of treatment.
   5. Anal and cervical examinations to detect the human papillomavirus (HPV) (Carlson, 2008).

IX. HIV-specific criteria.

A. Potential HIV-infected recipients should be evaluated by an HIV specialist to ensure that all HIV-associated issues have been considered.

B. A complete HIV medical history screening performed by an HIV physician or nurse practitioner is recommended and should include:
   1. CD4+ T-cell count history including nadir CD4+ T cell count.
   2. History of AIDs-related opportunistic infections or neoplasms.
   3. Antiretroviral medication history of resistance testing.
   4. History of hepatitis A, B, or C, syphilis, or toxoplasmosis.
   5. Any relevant past medical or surgical history.
   6. Drug allergies.
   7. Any history of abnormal anal or cervical Pap smear.
   8. History of PPD.
   9. Vaccination history (Bartlett, 2008; Carlson, 2008; Mellors et al., 1996, 1997).

C. They should also meet the following HIV-specific criteria.
   1. CD4+ T-Cell count >/= 200 μL within 3 months of transplant.
   2. HIV-1 RNA less than 50 copies.
   3. CD4+ T cells and HIV-1RNA should be monitored every 3 months while waiting for a transplant, and this monitoring frequency should continue posttransplant.
   4. Patients must be on a stable HIV-medication regimen.
   5. A patient with a previous history of an opportunistic infection or neoplasm may be considered if the patient has received appropriate acute and maintenance therapy and there is no evidence of active disease at the time of transplant (AI052748, 2003-2013; Carlson, 2008).
   6. Patients with the history of an infectious complication or neoplasm where effective treatment is not available would be considered high risk and not recommended as a transplant candidate.

D. Progressive multifocal leukoencephalopathy (PML).

E. Chronic intestinal cryptosporidiosis of > 1 month duration.

F. Primary CNS lymphoma.

G. Documented multidrug-resistant fungal infections not expected to respond to oral therapy.

H. Documented influenza or RSV in the 30 days prior to transplant.

I. Any neoplasm is an exclusion except for cutaneous Kaposi sarcoma, in situ anogenital carcinoma, adequately treated basal or squamous cell cancer of the skin, or solid tumors treated with curative therapy and disease free for more than 5 years (AI052748, 2003-2013).

X. Posttransplant management.

A. Drug management is one of the most challenging and complicated tasks posttransplant.

B. The HIV-positive kidney transplant recipient must take both antiretroviral (ARV) medications and immunosuppressive medications concomitantly and lifelong.

C. The ARVs and immunosuppressive medications are metabolized through the same enzyme system (cytochrome P-450 enzyme system).

D. Multiple complex interactions occur between these three classes of drugs and require significant dose adjustments.
   1. In general, ARVs do not need to be adjusted when given with immunosuppressive medications.
   2. Immunosuppression, specifically the calcineurin inhibitors and mTor drugs, require significant dose adjustments when given with ARVs (Carlson, 2008; Frassetto et al., 2007).

XI. Immunosuppressive medication recommendations.

A. Induction therapy may include:
   1. IL-2 receptor inhibitor (anti-CD25 antibody).
   2. Thymoglobulin.

B. Maintenance immunosuppression regimen will include:
   1. Tacrolimus, cyclosporine, or sirolimus/everolimus.
   2. Mycophenolate mofetil (MMF) or mycophenolic acid (MPA).
   3. Prednisone.

C. Based on the results of the NIH trial, the calcineurin inhibitor (CI) recommended is tacrolimus (Stock et al., 2010).

D. Dosing of the calcineurin inhibitor is influenced by the class of antiviral medication (ARV) the patient is taking.
   1. Protease inhibitor regimens require a significant reduction in the dose of CI, i.e., tacrolimus dose would be 1 mg PO once to twice a week. Cyclosporine dose with a PI would be 25 to 50 mg twice a day (Frassetto et al., 2003, 2004, 2007).
   2. Nonnucleoside reverse transcriptase inhibitor-based regimens typically require an increase in the dose of CI. A typical dose of tacrolimus would be 1 to 4 mg PO BID and cyclosporine dose would be 200 to 450 mg PO BID (Frassetto et al., 2003, 2004, 2007).

E. Frequent monitoring and adjusting of CI doses are necessary in the early posttransplant period due to the complex interactions between the CI and the ARV.

F. Mycophenolate mofetil does not require dose adjusting based on the ARV regimen. Standard dose would be 1000 mg PO BID and modified based on toxicity (neutropenia, GI) and clinical judgment.

G. Steroid induction, taper, and maintenance will be according to local site practice (AI052748, 2003-2013; Carlson, 2008; Stock et al., 2010).

H. If patient is treated with thymoglobulin for induction or as a treatment for rejection, a CD4+ T-cell count must be obtained following the first dose. If CD4+ T-cell count is below 75 cells/μL (which it will always be), patient must be started on azithromycin 1200 mg PO once a week.

XII. Antiviral medication regimen recommendations.

A. Initially no recommendations for a specific HIV-medication regimen were made. As long as the regimen was effective in suppressing the virus, the specific regimen did not matter.

B. Current recommendation as a result of the NIH study is to switch patients if possible to an integrase inhibitor-based regimen (raltegravir), which does not affect dosing of calcineurin inhibitors.

C. Changes in the ARV regimen must be discussed with the patient's HIV physician before making any changes.

XIII. Administration and dosing of medications. Holding and restarting ARV therapy posttransplant.

A. All ARV medications must be stopped and restarted at the same time. Restarting only one or two, missing doses of medications, or starting and then stopping can lead to viral resistance to the medications.

B. It is preferable to hold ARV medications for several days or a week and restart when the patient is clinically stable and the GI tract is functioning well.

C. This can be done without risk of HIV disease progression.

D. Frequent blood monitoring and dose adjustments are required to ensure adequate immunosuppressive drug levels are achieved.

E. Some ARVs need to be adjusted based on kidney function.

F. Several ARVs (tenofovir, norvir) can contribute to kidney dysfunction and require careful evaluation and monitoring (Carlson, 2008; Roling et al., 2006).

XIV. HIV surveillance recommended posttransplant.

A. The patient should be evaluated by the primary HIV provider 1 month posttransplant.

B. The HIV provider and recipient must be informed to contact the transplant team before changing the ARV regimen or beginning any new medications as this may interfere with the immunosuppression drug levels.

C. CD4+ T-cell count and HIV-1RNA should be monitored 1 month posttransplant and then every 3 months.

D. Yearly screening, depending on risk factors, is recommended for PPD, cancers, and infections.

XV. Acute rejection.

A. There is a higher incidence of acute rejection in HIV-positive transplant recipients.

B. Maintenance therapy with tacrolimus is recommended.

C. Treatment for rejection is based on biopsy finding.

D. Thymoglobulin and OKT3 have been effective in reversing rejection. Begin appropriate opportunistic prophylaxis with rejection therapy (see below).

E. Antibody-mediated rejection has been managed with standard, recommended therapy.

XVI. Opportunistic infection prophylaxis recommended posttransplant.

A. Background information.
   1. The use of prophylactic medications has significantly improved the survival rates in both transplant recipients and people with HIV.
   2. Both populations are susceptible to the same opportunistic infections and require similar medications to prevent them.
   3. The duration, previous opportunistic infection history, and CD4+ T-cell count are additional variables that must be considered for the HIV-infected transplant recipient. Current prophylaxis recommendations can be seen below (CDC, 2014).

B. *Pneumocystis jiroveci* (formerly *carinii*) pneumonia.
   1. Indicated for all patients: lifelong and should start immediately posttransplant.
   2. Preferred regimen with Bactrim 1 double strength (160 mg trimethoprim/800 sulfamethoxale) PO daily or single-strength PO daily.
   3. Alternatives: dapsone 100 mg PO QD (contraindicated if G6PD deficient), atovaquone 1500 mg PO daily, or aerosolized pentamidine 300 mg monthly.

C. Toxoplasmosis.
   1. Indications: primary prophylaxis for Toxo IgG positive patients with CD4+ T-cell count < 200 cells µL.
   2. Preferred regimen: Bactrim DS 1 tab PO daily.
   3. Alternatives: Bactrim SS 1 PO daily, dapsone 100 mg PO daily + pryimethamine 50 mg PO daily and leucovorin 25 mg PO daily or atovaquone 1500 mg PO daily.
   4. Secondary prophylaxis for patients with a prior history of toxoplasmosis must be reinstituted

immediately posttransplant for 1 month, during the treatment of acute rejection for 1 month, or when the CD4 T-cell count drops below 200 cells µL.

D. Mycobacterium avium complex (MAC).
   1. Prophylaxis is indicated for patients with no prior history of MAC when CD4+ T-cell count is < 75 cells µL. Prophylaxis may be discontinued when the CD4+ T-cell count is above 100 cells/µL for 6 months.
   2. Preferred regimen is azithromycin 1200 mg PO weekly.
   3. Prophylaxis must be started on every patient who receives Thymoglobulin.
   4. Alternative regimen: clarithromycin 500 mg PO BID. Consider drug interactions with immunosuppressive medications.
   5. Patients with a pretransplant history of MAC must begin prophylaxis immediately posttransplant for 1 month, during treatment of acute rejection for 1 month, and when CD4+ T-cell count drops below 75 cells/µL.
      a. Preferred regimen: azithromax 600 mg PO daily and ethambutol 15 mg/kg/day.
      b. Alternative regimen: clarithromycin 500 mg PO BID plus ethambutol 15 mg/kg/day.

E. Cytomegalovirus (CMV).
   1. Patients with no prior history of CMV should follow transplant program's standard of care.
   2. Patients with a prior history of CMV require secondary prophylaxis immediately posttransplant, during the treatment of acute rejection for 1 month, and whenever CD4+ T-cell count drops below 100 cells/µL. Prophylaxis may be discontinued when CD4+ T-cell count is above 200 cells/µL for 6 months.
   3. Preferred regimen: valganciclovir 900 mg PO daily for 6 months.
   4. Alternative regimen: ganciclovir 1 gram PO TID for 6 months.

F. Epstein-Barr virus (EBV).
   1. Indicated for EBV-negative recipient with an EBV positive donor.
   2. Preferred regimen: ganciclovir 5 mg/kg/IV daily while hospitalized and changed to ganciclovir 1 gram PO TID for 1 year.

G. Candidiasis.
   1. Recommended prophylaxis with fluconazole 100 mg PO once a week for 3 months.
   2. Severe toxicity from CI may result if daily fluconazole is required. Careful monitoring of drug levels is necessary. Dose reduction of the CI by 50% is recommended.

H. Cryptococcosis, extrapulmonary.
   1. No prophylaxis indicated in patients without a prior history.
   2. Patients with a prior history of cryptococcosis require prophylaxis immediately posttransplant for 1 month, during the treatment of acute rejection for 1 month, and whenever the CD4+ T-cell count drops below 200 cell/μL. Prophylaxis may be discontinued when CD4+ T cell count is above 200 cells/μL for 6 months.
   3. Preferred regimen is fluconazole 200 mg PO daily.
   4. Carefully monitor and adjust dose of calcineurin inhibitors when taking daily fluconazole.

I. Histoplasmosis.
   1. No prophylaxis is indicated in patients without a prior history.
   2. All patients with a prior history regardless of CD4+ T-cell count require prophylaxis.
   3. Preferred regimen is itraconazole 200 mg PO BID taken with food.
   4. Alternative regimen: fluconazole 400 mg PO daily.

J. PPD testing and TB prophylaxis.
   1. PPD testing is recommended to be done at screening for transplant and every 12 months.
   2. Patients who have a PPD that cannot be interpreted (history of BCG vaccination or are anergic) should have a chest x-ray.
   3. If a positive PPD is noted prior to transplant, prophylaxis/treatment should be instituted pretransplant and continued in the posttransplant period.
   4. Preferred regimen.
      a. INH 300 mg PO daily and pyridoxine 50 mg PO daily x 9 months, or
      b. INH 900 mg + pyrodixine 100 mg BIW x 9 months.
   5. Alternative regimens: (only if absolute contraindications to INH regimens).
      a. Rifampin 600 mg PO daily x 4 months.
      b. Rifabutin 300 mg PO daily x 4 months.
      c. Rifampin should not be used in patients on a protease inhibitor or a nonnucleoside reverse transcriptase inhibitor.

XVII. Human papillomavirus (HPV) screening.

A. Background information.
   1. Both HIV-infected individuals and solid organ transplant recipients are at increased risk for HPV-associated cancers.
   2. HIV-positive patients have a high prevalence of anogenital human papillomavirus (HPV) infection and anal cancer precursors, known as anal intraepithelial neoplasia (AIN) 2 or 3

(AI052748, 2003-2013; Holly et al., 2001; Palefsky et al., 2001).

B. HIV-positive transplant patients may be at especially high risk of anal cancer.

C. Since HIV-positive solid-organ transplant patients are at risk for anal cancer, it is recommended that, at a minimum, all patients receive routine digital rectal exams (DRE) to screen for rectal cancers. If possible, it is best if anal Pap smears can be performed with referral to undergo an anoscopy if there are any abnormal results.

D. Anal Pap tests are a screening test for anal cancer and precancerous lesions. These precancerous lesions are known by various names such as anal intraepithelial neoplasia (AIN), anal dysplasia, or anal squamous intraepithelial lesions (ASIL).

E. In the United States, the Bethesda classification system is generally used for anogential cytology as follows.
   1. Unsatisfactory for evaluation (state reason).
   2. Negative for intraepithelial lesion or malignancy.
   3. Atypical squamous cells of uncertain significance (ASC-US).
   4. Atypical squamous cells – cannot exclude high grade SIL (ASC-H).
   5. Low-grade squamous intraepithelial lesions (LSIL).
   6. High-grade squamous intraepithelial lesions (HSIL).
   7. Cancer.
   8. Other interpretation.

F. Anal cancer is diagnosed when the abnormal cells lining the anus have invaded below the basement membrane layer (bottom) of the epithelium and begins to spread into the tissues below. Anal cancer may arise inside the anal canal or outside the opening of the anus. If not caught early, anal cancer can be fatal.

G. Anal cytology is used to determine who needs to undergo the next step in the evaluation: high-resolution anoscopy (HRA).

H. Anal LSIL and HSIL are very common among men who have sex with men (MSM), and even more common in MSM with HIV infection. Data from earlier studies showed that at the first visit, 36% of HIV-positive MSM had LSIL or HSIL compared to 7% of HIV-negative MSM. But 36% of the HIV-negative men developed LSIL or HSIL within 2 years.

I. Other groups of people are at risk of anal HPV infection and anal SIL. HIV+ women have been shown to have more anal HPV infection than cervical HPV infection and to be at high risk of having an anal cytology abnormality. Similarly, HIV-positive men who have no history of anal intercourse have been shown to have high rates of anal HPV infection and anal SIL (Palefsky et al., 2001).

J. Follow-up.
1. If cytology showed LSIL, this may indicate a transient change. All patients with LSIL will be referred to the consulting anoscopist for HRA.
2. If the cytology tests obtained show HSIL, refer the patient for high-resolution anoscopy and biopsy.
3. Treatment of HSIL is controversial, and the decision on whether or not to treat the lesion is an individual one. Treatment consists of destruction of the abnormal lesions. This can be done by freezing, burning, or application of a corrosive substance such as trichloroacetic acid (TCA) to the lesion (AI052748, 2003-2013; Holly et al., 2001).

XVIII. Posttransplant management – long-term.

A. Background information.
1. Although data on long-term posttransplant complications in HIV-positive recipients have not been reported, it is highly likely that these issues will begin to emerge as increasing numbers of recipients are living longer.
2. Transplant recipients and people living with HIV experience similar long-term complications and therefore could be at the same risk or greater risk for developing these complications.

B. Cardiovascular disease.
1. Cardiovascular disease is the most common cause of morbidity and mortality posttransplant.
2. 75% to 85% of recipients are hypertensive posttransplant.
3. 60% develop hyperlipidemia.
4. Incidence of cardiovascular disease in HIV is also significant.
5. 30% of people living with HIV are hypertensive.
6. Risk factors include:
   a. Dyslipidemia.
   b. Diabetes mellitus.
   c. Metabolic syndrome.
   d. Smoking.
7. Management of cardiovascular disease includes:
   a. Modify risk behaviors: exercise, smoking cessation, and dietary interventions.
   b. Antihypertensive medications.
   c. Pharmacologic intervention for blood sugar, cholesterol, and triglyceride management (Carlson, 2008; Gazi et al., 2006; Ostovan et al., 2006).

C. Bone disorders.
1. Factors contributing to the incidence of osteopenia, osteoporosis, and osteonecrosis in patients with kidney failure include:
   a. Pretransplant renal insufficiency.
   b. Hyperparathyroidism.
   c. Smoking.
   d. Poor dietary calcium intake.
2. Factors contributing to the incidence of osteopenia, osteoporosis, and osteonecrosis in patients with HIV include:
   a. Corticosteroid use.
   b. Coagulopathy.
   c. Alcohol intake.
   d. Smoking.
   e. Prolonged use of protease inhibitor antiviral medications.
   f. Lipodystrophy.
   g. Lack of weight bearing exercise.
   h. Body weight < 20% or > 20% above ideal body weight.
3. Management of bone disease.
   a. Monitor with thyroid function tests, serum calcium, parathyroid hormone, vitamin D, and testosterone levels.
   b. Bone density scans (DEXA).
   c. Behavioral interventions including exercise, smoking cessation, dietary intervention, and limited alcohol consumption.
   d. Pharmacologic interventions to include alendronate , calcium, vitamin D therapy, and hormone or testosterone replacement therapy (Allison et al., 2003; Carlson, 2008; Morse et al., 2007).

D. Cancers.
1. Malignancies can be a serious problem posttransplant.
2. Common malignancies include:
   a. Skin cancers (squamous and basal cell).
   b. Gynecologic cancers (cervical, uterine, vulvar, and perineum).
   c. Human papillomavirus (HPV) associated cancers.
3. All recipients should be screened yearly and referred appropriately.
4. Women should have a cervical Pap or colposcopy every 6 to 12 months.
5. Both men and women should be screened with anal Pap smears for detection of HPV disease yearly.
6. Routine self-examinations (Carlson, 2008).

XIX. HCV, HIV, and kidney transplantation.

A. Currently there are no recommendations regarding transplantation in the HIV/HCV co-infected kidney transplant candidate, including:
   1. Pretransplant or posttransplant HCV treatment.
   2. Most effective HCV regimen to recommend.

B. A finding of cirrhosis on pretransplant liver biopsy would exclude the patient from transplant consideration.

C. Outcomes of HIV/HCV kidney transplant recipients reported in the NIH study.
   1. 7 deaths occurred among 122 HIV/HCV negative patients (6%) and 4 among 28 HIV/HCV-positive patients (14%).
   2. Patient survival and graft survival at 1 year for HIV/HCV-positive recipients was 88.6% and 88.3% compared with 96.1% and 90.9% for HIV/HCV negative recipients.
   3. HIV/HCV-positive patients experienced a higher average rate of serious infections per follow-up year compared with HIV/HCV negative patients (0.8 vs. 0.5) (Stock et al., 2010).

D. HIV/HCV co-infected patients requiring both a kidney and liver transplant would not be recommended due to poor outcomes reported in the NIH study.

E. HIV/HCV co-infected patients must be selected carefully and monitored closely to obtain information about how best to treat and to optimize outcomes (Carlson, 2008).

XX. Quality of life.

A. Quality of life has become an important factor to consider in addition to the standard clinical measures of patient and graft survival.

B. This may be due to that fact that many treatments for chronic disease frequently fail to cure and that the benefits gained may be at the expense of taking toxic or unpleasant medications and adhering to a complex and lifelong therapeutic regimen.

C. Data on quality of life using the SF 36 instrument were obtained on the HIV-positive kidney transplant recipients participating in the NIH trial.

D. SF36 questionnaires were completed at 4 time points: pretransplant, year 1, year 2, and year 5.

E. In the mental and physical component scores, minimal change was noted pre and posttransplant in the HIV kidney transplant recipients.

F. In both subscales, HIV kidney transplant recipients scored similar to the general population pretransplant and posttransplant.

G. Self-reported measurements of quality of life were maintained in the HIV kidney transplant recipient. It is difficult to show improvement when the scores pretransplant are normal. However, it is significant to know that scores did not decline posttransplant considering some unique challenges HIV-positive kidney transplant recipients face. The unique challenges include:
   1. Managing two complex medical regimens.
   2. Taking multiple medications with significant drug interactions.
   3. Managing and coping with side effects.
   4. Adjusting pretransplant expectations to posttransplant realities that result from overestimating benefits, unmet expectations, and the practice of minimizing complications.
   5. Emotional adjustment.

SECTION E
Hepatitis C Infection and Kidney Transplantation
Laurie Carlson

I. Introduction.

A. Liver disease as a result of chronic hepatitis C virus (HCV) infection is an important cause of morbidity and mortality in dialysis and kidney transplant recipients (Aljumah et al., 2012).

B. The annual incidence of HCV infection is reported to range from 0.2% to 6.2% (Liu & Kao 2011; Terrault & Adey, 2007).

C. The reported prevalence rates of chronic HCV infection among patients with CKD ranges from 3.4% to 80% depending on geographic variation.

D. The prevalence of HCV infection in kidney transplant recipients ranges between 7% and 40% with wide demographic and geographic variation (KDIGO, 2008).

E. Kidney transplant recipients who are HCV-positive have a reduced survival rate (Terrault & Adey, 2007).

F. Patients who are HCV-positive pretransplant have a significantly increased risk of posttransplant liver disease. Chronic active hepatitis and an unusual form of severe cholestatis and rapidly progressive liver failure have been described in HCV-positive kidney transplant recipients (Natov & Pereira, 2013).

G. Approximately 40% of kidney transplant recipients who are HCV-positive will have progressive liver fibrosis within 5 years posttransplant (Terrault & Adey, 2007).

H. HCV-infected patients with CKD who are treated with HCV therapies pretransplant and achieve a sustained viral response typically remained HCV negative posttransplant (Terrault & Adey, 2007).

I. HCV eradication pretransplant reduces the risk for posttransplant liver- and renal-associated complications.

II. Several types of kidney diseases are associated with HCV disease, including (Kamar, 2013):

A. Mixed cryoglobinemia.

B. Membranoproliferative glomerulonephritis (MPGN).

C. Membranous nephropathy.

D. Polyarteritis nodosa.

E. Crescentic glomerulonephritis may be superimposed on any of these glomerular lesions.

III. HCV diagnosis in CKD patients. All kidney transplant patients should be screened for HCV during the pretransplant evaluation phase. The diagnosis of HCV is determined by the following tests (Liu & Kao, 2011).

A. Serological assays: detection of anti-HCV antibodies by third generation enzyme immunoassay.
   1. Enzyme immunoassay (EIA) – third generation, fewer false positives with this assay.
   2. Recombinant immunoblotting assay (RIBA).

B. Virological assays.
   1. HCV-RNA is the direct marker of HCV replication.
   2. It is used to measure the level of viral replication in the liver and to monitor the effectiveness of treatment.
   3. Nucleic acid testing (NAT) is based on qualitative HCV RNA detection or on HCV RNA quantitation.

C. Biochemical assays.
   1. ALT.
   2. Aminotransferases.

D. Invasive tests to evaluate liver histology.
   1. Percutaneous liver biopsy is the gold standard to assess liver histology.

2. Limitations in the CKD population include:
   a. Poor patient acceptance.
   b. Risk of serious bleeding post biopsy.
   c. Sampling and interpretation error.

E. HCV-infected patients should be routinely screened for:
   1. Proteinuria.
   2. Hematuria.
   3. Hypertension.
   4. Kidney function.
   5. Cryoglobulinemia.
   6. Complement.
   7. Rheumatoid factors.

F. Indications for treatment.
   1. Moderate to severe disease evidenced by nephrotic syndrome, elevated serum creatinine levels, new hypertension, fibrosis, or tubulointerstitial disease on biopsy.
   2. Progressive disease.
   3. Decision to treat is based on potential of benefits and risks of therapy (KDIGO, 2008).

IV. Evaluation of the HCV-positive kidney transplant recipient. The following tests make up a recommended and standard pretransplant workup.

A. Liver enzymes (albumin, T bilirubin, AST, ALT, alkaline phosphatase).

B. HCV antibody confirmation, HCV RNA, HCV genotyping, IL28.

C. Abdominal ultrasound.

D. Liver biopsy per institutional protocol. Results of the biopsy determine whether patient requires an evaluation for a liver transplant.

E. Evaluation by a hepatologist.

F. Consideration of pretransplant treatment for HCV.

V. Pretransplant treatment of HCV.

A. Treatment of HCV prior to transplant is advisable in patients who are otherwise good candidates for kidney transplantation.
   1. Pretransplant treatment is recommended as interferon therapy posttransplant is still contraindicated due to an increased risk of severe rejection.
   2. The goal of treatment is to decrease liver-related morbidity and mortality.
   3. Sustained viral suppression is defined as the surrogate endpoint of interferon-based therapy.

4. The most important measurement is the SVR, sustained virological response with an undetectable HCV-RNA 24 weeks after the completion of therapy by a sensitive HCV-RNA assay (Aljumah et al., 2012; Liu & Kao 2011).

B. Pretreatment assessment should include:
1. Complete medical history and physical.
2. Psychiatric history.
3. Screening for depression and alcohol use.
4. Biochemical markers for liver disease and hepatic function: ALT, AST, serum albumin, serum bilirubin (total and direct) and prothrombin time.
5. Hemoglobin, hematocrit, WBC with differential, and platelet count.
6. TSH, serum creatinine, serum glucose, uric acid, serum ferritin, iron saturation, and serum ANA.
7. HIV serology.
8. Pregnancy.
9. Serum HbsAG, anti-HBc, anti-HBs, anti-HAV.
10. Quantitative HCV RNA measurement.
11. Previous antiviral therapies and response.
12. Eye exam for retinopathy (KDIGO, 2008; Yee et al., 2012).

C. Recommended treatment.
1. Interferon (standard or pegylated INF) adjusted for creatinine clearance below 50 mL/min.
2. Low-dose ribavirin 200 mg daily or 200 mg thrice weekly (Copegus has been FDA approved for use in CKD or hemodialysis).
3. Administer dose after hemodialysis.
4. Varying rates of sustained viral responses (SVR) have been reported 33–50% (Fabrizi et al., 2010; Gordon et al., 2008).
5. Safety and efficacy data are not yet available on protease inhibitor triple therapy in patients with CKD.
6. Triple therapy for HCV genotype 1 with an oral protease inhibitor (telaprevir or boceprevir) together with pegylated interferon and ribavirin became standard of care in 2011 in patients with liver disease.
   a. Minimal data has yet been reported with this combination therapy in CKD patients.
   b. Small case series and single-center experience with triple therapy are beginning to be reported in the CKD population, showing some promising results.
7. Monitoring recommendations for pretransplant patients on therapy include:
   a. HCV RNA.
   b. CBC with differential (weekly).
   c. Liver function studies.
   d. Renal panel.
   e. Glucose, thyroid stimulating hormone, uric acid.
   f. Fundoscopic exam.
   g. Psychiatric/substance use screening (updated on the management and treatment of HCV infection from the VA).
   h. Frequency of monitoring should be at least every 4 weeks and may need to be increased depending on patient tolerance, response to treatment, blood counts, or other clinical indicators.

VI. HCV-positive deceased donor to HCV-positive kidney transplant recipient.

A. Background information.
1. Studies have shown that kidney transplant recipients who received organs from HCV-positive donors experience higher rates of liver disease but not lower survival rates than transplant recipients who received organs from HCV negative donors.
2. Other studies have reported conflicting results showing both higher rates of liver disease and lower overall patient and graft survival rates.
3. Despite these inconclusive reports, there may be a survival benefit from receiving an HCV-positive donor versus remaining on dialysis. An additional benefit is a shorter wait time on the transplant list (Abbott et al., 2004).

B. To be eligible to receive an HCV-positive organ, the recipient must be confirmed HCV-positive (EIA and NAT testing).

C. The risk of superinfection with a donor HCV genotype different from the genotype of the recipient is unknown. Typically, genotypes 1 and 4 are acceptable. However, in the near future with the advent of the new protease inhibitors and triple therapy, restricting the genotype may no longer be necessary.

D. Recipients with evidence of cirrhosis are not eligible to receive an HCV-positive organ.

E. HCV-positive recipients without HCV viremia should not be excluded from receiving an HCV-positive donor organ.

F. Informed consent must be obtained for acceptance of HCV-positive donor kidney. Patients must be fully informed about the risks and potential benefits of receiving an HCV-positive organ.

G. Recipient acceptance criteria in UNET updated to indicate recipient will accept a hepatitis C donor.

H. On admission for transplant, recipient blood work to include quantitative HCV RNA by PCR in addition to liver function studies (KDOIGO, 2008).

VII. Posttransplant care of HCV-positive recipient.

A. All patients with HCV infection, regardless of treatment or treatment response, should be monitored for HCV-associated morbidities.
1. The focus should be on monitoring liver function and prevention, detection, and treatment of extrahepatic complications (i.e., new onset diabetes after transplant [NODAT]).
2. Selective and cautious treatment with interferon therapy.

B. Repeat quantitative HCV RNA by PCR at regular intervals posttransplant per center-specific criteria.

C. Liver enzymes (ALT, AST, alkaline phosphatase, T bilirubin) should be checked monthly for the first 6 months posttransplant and then quarterly thereafter.

D. Prompt referral to a hepatologist when worsening of liver enzymes occurs.

E. Liver ultrasound.

F. Liver biopsy if clinically indicated.

G. Screen patients with evidence of cirrhosis for hepatocellular carcinoma (HCC) annually with a liver ultrasound and alpha fetal protein level.

H. MPGN is observed in the allograft of HCV-infected recipients.
1. Obtain baseline urine protein to creatinine ratio and urinalysis within the first 2 weeks posttransplant or once stable kidney function is achieved.
2. Monitor for proteinuria every 3 to 6 months in the first year following transplant and every 6 months thereafter.

I. Consideration for posttransplant treatment for HCV (KDIGO, 2008).

VIII. HCV infection and outcome after kidney transplantation.

A. Patients infected with HCV have better survival outcomes with a kidney transplant than remaining on dialysis (Liu & Kao 2011; Terrault & Adey, 2007).

B. However, kidney recipients infected with HCV have worse patient and graft survival compared with the kidney transplant recipients not infected with HCV (KDIGO, 2008; Terrault & Adey, 2007).

C. Patients who are HCV-positive pretransplant have a significantly increased risk of posttransplant liver disease.

D. Disease progression is evidenced by:
1. Increased proliferation of the virus posttransplant, resulting in a 1.0 to 1.5 log IU/mL.
2. Increase in serum viral titers.
3. Elevation of ALT levels in transplant recipients with previously normal liver function tests and increase further in patients who had elevated ALT levels prior to transplant.
4. Risk factors associated with progression of fibrosis include severity of liver disease pretransplant and duration of follow-up posttransplant (Terrault & Adey, 2007).

E. Increased mortality observed in the HCV-positive kidney transplant recipient is due to:
1. Progressive liver disease posttransplant.
2. New onset diabetes posttransplant.
3. Posttransplant glomerulopathies.
4. Sepsis (KDIGO 2008; Terrault & Adey, 2007).

IX. Posttransplant treatment of HCV-positive kidney transplant recipient.

A. Treatment posttransplant is not routinely recommended due to the concerns about interferon (IFN) precipitating an acute rejection, the possibility of severe allograft dysfunction, complications of anemia, and the patient's intolerance of the treatment.

B. While pretransplant treatment for HCV and achievement of viral clearance reduces the risk of recurrent or de novo HCV-associated glomerular diseases, some situations may necessitate the need for HCV treatment posttransplant. Situations such as HCV-associated glomerulonephritides causing progressive kidney disease, patients with cirrhosis, bridging fibrosis, or severe cholestatic hepatitis are examples of clinical situations where the risk benefit assessment would support posttransplant treatment.

C. The decision to treat must be made on a case-by-case basis. When treatment is indicated, therapy must be comanaged with a multidisciplinary team that includes experienced HCV providers and kidney transplant specialists.

D. For many years, pegylated interferon alfa and ribavirin have been the standard of care for HCV infection. They are also the only published guidelines for HCV therapy in patients with kidney transplants. Combination therapy is most likely to achieve a sustained viral response. Recommended doses are:
1. Pegylated interferon alfa 135 micrograms sq weekly.
2. Ribavirin 200/600 mg daily carefully monitored and dose adjusted on the basis of kidney function to decrease the risk of anemia complications.

3. The toxicities observed with HCV therapy posttransplant require frequent monitoring, dose reductions, and aggressive support with growth factor.

E. The recent introduction of direct-acting antivirals (DAAs) revolutionized HCV treatment.

F. In 2011, triple therapy with the first-generation protease inhibitors (telaprevir or boceprevir) in combination with pegylated interferon alpha-2a and/or ribavirin became available. Minimal data is available on this combination therapy in kidney transplantation. However, several small case reports of dialysis and kidney transplant recipients receiving triple therapy are now being reported and show promising results (Aljumah et al., 2012; Dumortier et al., 2013).

G. The second-generation protease inhibitor (Olysio [simprevir] and NS5b polymerase inhibitor, Solvadi [sofosbuvir]) were approved for treatment of HCV infection in late 2013. These new direct-acting antivirals (DAA) have essentially eliminated the use of telaprevir and boceprevir.

H. Sofosbuvir has not been studied in patients on dialysis or with a CRCL < 30. Current studies are in progress.

I. Clinical studies in HCV liver transplant have demonstrated that there are no interactions between sofosbuvir or simprevir and the calcineurin inhibitors/mTORs, making them attractive agents to use in transplant recipients.

J. Treatment guidelines for the use of new DAA in kidney transplant recipients have not yet been developed. But some academic institutions have developed their own treatment guidelines based on AASLD-published guidelines in this rapidly evolving field.

K. There are already third-generation DAAs currently in phase 2 and 3 clinical trials, as well as new agents that target different areas of the HCV viral cycle that have been submitted to the FDA and are awaiting approval. As the field of HCV treatment is dynamic and rapidly changing, the AASLD and the Infectious Diseases Society of America (IDSA) are partnering together to establish consensus and HCV guidelines that will be updated in a timely manner as developments in this field progress over the next several years (AASLD, 2014).

References

AASLD, IDSA, IAS–USA (American Association for the Study of Liver Diseases, Infectious Diseases Society of America, International Antiviral Society–USA). (2014). *Recommendations for testing, managing, and treating hepatitis C*. Retrieved from http://www.hcvguidelines.org

Abbas, A.K., Lichtman, A.H., & Pillai, S. (2010). *Cellular and molecular immunology* (6th ed.). Philadelphia: Saunders-Elsevier.

Abbott, K.C., Swanson, S.J., Agodoa, L.Y., & Kimmel, P.L. (2004). Human immunodeficiency virus infection and kidney transplantation in the era of highly active antiretroviral therapy and modern immunosuppression. *Journal of the American Society of Nephrology, 15*(6), 1633-9. doi:10.1097/01.ASN.0000127987.19470.3A

Abecassis, M., Bartlett, S.T., Collins, A.J., Davis, C.L., Delmonico, F.L., Friedewald, J.J., … Gaston, R.S. (2008). Kidney transplantation as primary therapy for end-stage renal disease: A National Kidney Foundation/Kidney Disease Outcomes Quality Initiative (NKF/KDOQI) conference. *Clinical Journal of the American Society of Nephrology, 3*(2), 471-480. doi:10.2215/CJN.05021107

Adams, A., Kirk, A., & Larsen, C. (2012). Transplantation immunobiology and immunosuppression. In C.M. Townsend, Jr., R.D. Beauchamp, B.M. Evers, & K.L. Mattox (Eds.), *Sabiston textbook of surgery: The biological basis of modern surgical practice* (19th ed., pp. 617-654). Philadelphia: Saunders-Elsevier.

Ahya, S.N., Soler, M.J., Levitsky, J., & Batile, D. (2006). Acid-base and potassium disorders in liver disease. *Seminars in Nephrology, 26*, 466-470. doi:10.1016/j.semnephrol.2006.11.001

AI052748 (2003-2013) Solid Organ Transplantation in HIV: Multi-Site Study. NIAID, NCT00074386.

Alberú, J. (2010). Clinical insights for cancer outcomes in renal transplant patients. *Transplantation Proceedings, 42*, S36-S40. doi:10.1016/j.transproceed.2010.07.006

Aljumah, A.A., Saeed, M.A., Al Flaiw, A.I., Al Traif, I.H., Al Alwan, A.M., Al Qurashi, S.H., … Al Sayyari, A.A. (2012). Efficacy and safety of treatment of hepatitis C virus infection in renal transplant recipients. *World Journal of Gastroenterology, 18*(1), 55-63. doi:10.3748/wjg.v18.i1.55

Allison, G.T., Bostrom, M.P., & Glesby, M.J. (2003). Osteonecrosis in HIV disease: epidemiology, etiologies, and clinical management. *AIDS, 17*, 1-9. doi:10.1097/01.aids.0000042940.55529.9300002030-200301030-00003

American Diabetes Association (ADA). (2007). Pancreas transplantation in Type 1 Diabetes. *Diabetes Care, 27*(Suppl. 1), S105. doi:10.2337/diacare.25.2007.S111

American Diabetes Association (ADA). (2013). Data from the 2011 *National Diabetes Fact Sheet*. Retrieved from http://www.diabetes.org/diabetes-basics/statistics

Anand, I.S. (2013). Cardiorenal syndrome: A cardiologist's perspective of pathophysiology. *Clinical Journal of the American Society of Nephrology, 8*, 1-8. doi:10.2215/CJN.04090413

Astellas Pharma US, Inc. (n.d.). *Astagraf XL package insert*. Retrieved from http://dailymed.nlm.nih.gov/dailymed/lookup.cfm?setid=550a5cd4-fbf2-4c09-b577-6bde8fcbdf6e

Aull-Watschinger, S., Konstantin, H., Demetriou, D., Schillinger, M., Habicht, A., Hörl, W.H., & Watschinger, B. (2008). Pre-transplant predictors of cerebrovascular events after kidney transplantation. *Nephrology, Dialysis and Transplantation, 23*, 1429-1435. doi:10.1093/ndt/gfm766

Bartlett, J.G. (2008). *Factors affecting HIV progression*. Retrieved from http://www.uptodate.com/contents/factors-affecting-hiv-progression

Becker, L.E., Süsal, C., & Morath, C. (2013). Kidney transplantation across HLA and ABO antibody barriers. *Current opinions in*

organ transplantation, 18, 445-454. doi:10.1097/MOT
.0b013e3283636c20

Becker, Y. (2012). Kidney and pancreas transplantation. In C.M.
Townsend, Jr., R.D. Beauchamp, B.M. Evers, & K.L. Mattox (Eds.),
*Sabiston textbook of surgery: The biological basis of modern
surgical practice* (19th ed., pp. 666-681). Philadelphia: Saunders-
Elsevier.

Bloom, R.D. (2013). *Renal function and nonrenal solid organ
transplantation.* Retrieved from http://www.uptodate.com/
contents/renal-function-and-nonrenal-solid-organ-
transplantation

Borawski, J., Wilczyńska-Borawska, M., Stokowska, W., & Myśliwiec,
M. (2007). The periodontal status of pre-dialysis chronic kidney
disease and maintenance dialysis patients. *Nephrology Dialysis
Transplantation, 22,* 457-464. doi:10.1093/ndt/gfl676

Brar, A., Jindal, R.M., Elster, E.A., Tedla, F., John, D., Sumrani, N., &
Salifu, M.O. (2013). Effect of peripheral vascular disease on
kidney allograft outcomes: A study of the U.S. Renal Data System.
Transplantation, 95, 810-815. doi:10.1097/TP.0b013e31827eef36.

Bruno, S., Remuzzi, G., & Ruggenenti, P. (2004). Transplant renal
artery stenosis. *Journal of the American Society of Nephrology,
15*(1), 134.

Bunnapradist, S., & Danovitch, G. (2007) Evaluation of adult kidney
transplant candidates. *American Journal of Kidney Diseases, 50*(5),
890-898).

Canaud, G., Audard, V., Kofman, T., Lang, P., Legendre, C., &
Grimbert, P. (2012). Recurrence from primary and secondary
glomerulopathy after renal transplant. *Transplant International,
25,* 812-824. doi:10.1111/j.1432-2277.2012.01483.x

Carlson, L. (2008). Clinical management of the HIV-positive kidney
transplant recipient. *Nephrology Nursing Journal, 35*(6), 559-567.
Retrieved from http://www.prolibraries.com/anna/?select=session
&sessionID=1067

Cecka, J.M., Rajalingam, R., Zhang, J., & Reed, E.F. (2010). Chapter
3-histocompatibility testing, crossmatching, and immune
monitoring. In G.M. Danovitch (Ed.), *Handbook of kidney
transplantation* (5th ed.). Philadelphia: Lippincott Williams &
Wilkins.

Centers for Disease Control (CDC). (2014). *Recommended
immunizations for adults by medical condition.* Retrieved from
http://www.cdc.gov/vaccines/schedules/downloads/adult/adult-
schedule-easy-read.pdf

Centers for Medicare & Medicaid Services (CMS). (2008, Tuesday,
April 15). Final rule. Conditions of coverage for end stage renal
disease facilities. Medicare and Medicaid Programs, *Federal
Register, 73,* 20369-20484. Retrieved from
http://www.cms.gov/Regulations-and-Guidance/Legislation/
CFCsAndCoPs/downloads/esrdfinalrule0415.pdf

Collaborative Islet Transplant Registry (CITR). (n.d.). *Main page.*
Retrieved from http://www.citregistry.com

Colucci, W.S., & Sterns, R.H. (2013). *Use of diuretics in patients with
heart failure.* Retrieved from http://www.uptodate.com/contents/
use-of-diuretics-in-patients-with-heart-failure

Colucci, W.S. (2013). *Renal effects of ACE inhibitors in heart failure.*
Retrieved from http://www.uptodate.com/contents/renal-effects-
of-ace-inhibitors-in-heart-failure

Danovitch, G.M. (2010a). *Handbook of kidney transplantation.*
Philadelphia: Lippincott Williams & Wilkins.

Danovitch, G.M. (2010b). Immunosuppressive medications and
protocols for kidney transplantation. In G. Danovitch (Ed.),
Handbook of kidney transplantation (5th ed., pp. 77-126).
Philadelphia: Lippincott Williams & Wilkins.

Danovitch, I. (2010). Psychiatric aspects of kidney transplantation. In
G. Danovitch (Ed.), *Handbook of kidney transplantation* (5th ed.,
pp. 389-408). Philadelphia: Lippincott Williams & Wilkins.

Delmonico, F.L., & Dew, M.A. (2007). Living donor kidney
transplantation in a global environment. *Kidney International,
71*(7), 608-614. doi:1038/sj.ki.5002125

Dew, M.A., Jacobs, C.L., Jowsey, S.G., Hanto, R., Miller, C., &
Delmonico, F.L. (2007). Guidelines for the psychosocial
evaluation of living unrelated kidney donors in the United States.
American Journal of Transplantation, 7, 1047-1054.
doi:10.1111/j.1600-6143.2007.01751.x

Dew, M.A., Switzer, G.E., Goycoolea, J.M., Allen, A.S., DiMartini, A.,
Kormos, R.L., & Griffith, B.P. (1997). Does transplantation
produce quality of life benefits? A quantitative analysis of the
literature. *Transplantation, 64,* 1261.

DeWalt DA, Callahan LF, Hawk VH, Broucksou KA, Hink A, Rudd
R, Brach C. April 2010. Health Literacy Universal Precautions
Toolkit. (Prepared by North Carolina Network Consortium, The
Cecil G. Sheps Center for Health Services Research, The
University of North Carolina at Chapel Hill, under Contract No.
HHSA290200710014.) AHRQ Publication No. 10-0046-EF)
Rockville, MD. Agency for Healthcare Research and Quality.

Dobbels, F., Skeans, M.A., Snyder, J.J., Tuomari., A.V., Maclean, J.R.,
& Kasiske, B.L. (2008). Depressive disorder in renal
transplantation: an analysis of Medicare claims. *American Journal
of Kidney Diseases, 51*(5), 819-828. doi:10.1053/j.ajkd.2008.01.010

Dumortier, J., Guillaud, O., Gagnieu, M.C., Janbon, B., Juillard, L.,
Morelon, E., & Leroy, V. (2013). Anti-viral triple therapy with
telaprevir in haemodialysed HCV patients: Is it feasible? *Journal
of Clinical Virology, 56*(2), 146-149. doi:10.1016/j.jcv.2012.10.009

Eller, K., Kniepeiss, D., & Rosenkranz, A.R. (2013). Preoperative risk
evaluation: Where is the limit for recipients of a pancreatic graft?
Current Opinion in Organ Transplantation, 18, 97-101.
doi:10.1097/MOT.0b013e32835c9666

Fabrizi, F., Dixit, V., Messa, P., & Martin, P. (2010). Pegylated
interferon monotherapy of chronic hepatitis C in dialysis patients:
Meta-analysis of clinical trials. *Journal of Medical Virology, 82*(5),
768-75. doi:10.1002/jmv.21542

Fatehi, P., & Hsu, C. (2013). *Diagnostic approach to the patient with
acute kidney injury or chronic kidney disease.* Retrieved from
http://www.uptodate.com/contents/diagnostic-approach-to-the-
patient-with-acute-kidney-injury-acute-renal-failure-or-chronic-
kidney-disease

Fischer, S.A., Avery, R.K., & the AST Infectious Disease Community
of Practice. (2009). Screening of donor and recipient prior to solid
organ transplantation. *American Journal of Transplantation,
9*(Suppl. 4), S7-S18).

Frassetto, L.A., Browne, M., Cheng, A., Wolfe, A.R., Roland, M.E.,
Stock, P.G., … Benet, L.Z. (2007). Immunosuppressant
pharmacokinetics and dosing modifications in HIV-1 infected
liver and kidney transplant recipients. *American Journal of
Transplantation, 7*(12), 2816-20. doi:10.1111/j.1600-
6143.2007.02007.x

Frassetto L.A, Chen, W., Kansal, N., Levi M., Carlson L., Roland,
M.E., … Benet L.Z. (2004). Immunosuppressant adjustments of
doses and dosing intervals in HIV-infected kidney and liver
transplant patients. In *TransplantAsia,* December 1–4, 2004;
Singapore.

Frassetto, L., Thai, T., Aggarwal A.M., Bucher P., Jacobsen W.,
Christians, U., … Floren, L.C. (2003). Pharmacokinetic
interactions between cyclosporine and protease inhibitors in
HIV+ subjects. *Drug Metabolism and Pharmacokinetics, 18*(2),
114-120. doi:10.2133/dmpk.18.114

Friedman, L.S., & Keefe, E.B. (2012). *Handbook of liver disease* (3rd
ed.). Philadelphia: Saunders-Elsevier.

Gazi, I.F., Liberopoulos, E.N., Athyros, V.G., Elisaf, M., &
Mikhailidis, D.P. (2006). Statins and solid organ transplantation.
Current Pharmaceutical Design, 12(36), 4771-83.

doi:10.2174/138161206779026308

Ginès, P., & Schrier, R.W. (2009). Renal failure in cirrhosis. *The New England Journal of Medicine, 361*, 1279-1290. doi:10.1056/NEJMra0809139

Giusto, M., Berenguer, M., Merkel, C., Aguilera, V., Rubin, A., Corradini, S.G., ... Merli, M. (2013). Chronic kidney disease after liver transplantation: Pretransplantation risk factors and predictors during follow-up. *Transplantation, 95*(9), 1148-1153. doi:10.1097/TP.0b013e3182884890

Gordon, C.E., Uhlig, K., Lau, J., Schmid, C.H., Levey, A.S., & Wong, J.B. (2008). Interferon treatment in hemodialysis patients with chronic hepatitis C virus infection: A systematic review of the literature and meta-analysis of treatment efficacy and harms. *American Journal of Kidney Diseases, 51*(2), 263-77. doi:10.1053/j.ajkd.2007.11.003

Gruessner, R.W.G, & Gruessner, A.C. (2013). The current state of pancreas transplantation. *Nature Reviews/Endocrinology, 9*,566-562. doi:10.1038/nrendo.2013.138OI

Gude, E., Andreassen, A.K., Arora, S., Gullestad, L., Grov, I., Hartmann, S., ... Simonsen, S. (2010). Acute renal failure early after heart transplantation: risk factors and clinical consequences. *Clinical Transplantation 24*, E207-E213. doi:10.1111/j.13990012.2010.01225.x

Guerra, G., Ilahe, A., & Ciancio, G. (2012). Diabetes and kidney transplantation: Past, present and future. *Current Diabetes Reports, 12*, 597-603. doi:10.1007/s11892-012-0306-3

Gustafsson, F., & Ross, H.J. (2009). Renal sparing strategies in cardiac transplantation. *Current Opinions in Organ Transplantation, 14*, 566-570. doi:10.MOT.0b013e32832e6f7b

Hall, J.E. (2012). Insulin, glucagon and diabetes mellitus. In J.E. Hall & A.C. Guyton (Eds.), *Pocket companion to Guyton and Hall textbook of medical physiology* (pp. 591-599). Philadelphia: Saunders-Elsevier.

Hawwa, N., Schreiber, M.J., Jr., & Tang, W.H. (2013). Pharmacologic management of chronic reno-cardiac syndrome. *Current Heart Failure Reports, 10*, 54-62. doi:10.1007/s11897-012-0122-8

Henson, A., & Carpenter, S. (2010). Intra-operative hemodialysis during liver transplantation: An expanded role of the nephrology nurse. *Nephrology Nursing Journal, 37*(4), 351-356.

Heuman, D.M., Abou-Assi, S.G., Habib, A., Williams, L.M., Stravitz, R.T., Sanval, A.J., ... Mihas, A.A. (2004). Persistant ascites and low serum sodium identify patients with cirrhosis and low MELD scores who are at high risk for early death. *Hepatology, 40*(4), 802-810. doi:10.1002/hep.20405

Holly, E.A., Ralston, M.L., Darragh, T.M., Greenblatt, R.M., Jay, N., & Palefsky, J.M. (2001). Prevalence and risk factors for anal squamous intraepithelial lesions in women. *Journal of the National Cancer Institute, 93*(11), 843-849. doi:10.1093/jnci/93.11.843

Hou, S. (2013). Pregnancy in renal transplant patients. *Advances in Chronic Kidney Disease, 20*(3), 253-259. doi:10.1053/j.ackd.2013.01.011

Jacques, F., El-Hamamsy, I., Fortier, A., Maltais, S., Perrault, L.P., Liberman, M., ... Ferraro, P. (2012). Acute renal failure following lung transplantation: Risk factors, mortality, and long-term consequences. *European Journal of Cardio-Thoracic Surgery, 41*, 193-199. doi:10.1016/j.ejcts.2011.04.034

Jaksch, P., Koinig, H., & Klepetco, W. (2010). Critical care management. In W.T. Vigneswaran & Garrity, E. (Eds.), *Lung transplantation* (pp. 224-236). London: Informa Healthcare of Informa, UK, Ltd.

Karam, G., & Giessing, M. (2011). Bladder dysfunction following renal transplantation: is it predictable? *Transplantation Proceedings, 43*, 387-390. doi: 10.1016/j.transproceed.2010.12.017

Kawar, B., Ellam, T., Jackson, C., & Kiely, D.G. (2013). Pulmonary

hypertension in renal disease: Epidemiology, potential mechanisms and implications. *American Journal of Nephrology, 37*, 281-290. doi:10.1159/000348804

Keith, D.S. (2013). Transplantation in the elderly patient. *Clinics in Geriatric Medicine, 29*(3), 707-719. doi:10.1016/j.cger.2013.05.010

Kent, B.D., Eltayeb, E.E., Woodman, A., Mutwali, A., Nguyen, H.T., & Stack, A.G. (2012). The impact of chronic obstructive pulmonary disease and smoking on mortality and kidney transplantation in end-stage kidney disease. *American Journal of Nephrology, 36*(3), 287-295. doi: 10.1159/000342207

Kersting, S., Ludwig, S., Ehehalt, F., Volk, A., & Bunk, A. (2013). Contrast-enhanced ultrasonography in pancreas transplantation. *Transplantation; 95*(1), 209-214. doi:10.1097/TP.0b013e31827864df

Khosroshahi, H.T, Shoja, E.A., Beiglu, L.G., & Hassan, A.P. (2006). Tuberculin testing of kidney allograft recipients and donors before transplantation. *Transplantation Proceedings, 38*, 1982-1984. doi:10.1016/j.transproceed.2006.06.016

Kidney Disease Improving Global Outcomes (KDIGO). (2008). KDIGO Guideline for the Prevention, Diagnosis, Evaluation and Treatment of Hepatitis C in Chronic Kidney Disease. *Kidney Disease Improving Global Outcomes, 73*(Suppl. 109). Retrieved from http://kdigo.org/home/hepatitis-c-in-ckd

Klein, C., & Brennan, D. (2013). *C4d staining in renal allografts and treatment of antibody mediated rejection.* Retrieved from http://www.uptodate.com/contents/c4d-staining-in-renal-allografts-and-treatment-of-antibody-mediated-rejection

Klieger-Grossmann, C., Chitayat, D., Lavign, S., Kao, K., Garcia-Bournissen, F., Quinn, D.... & Koren, G. (2010). *Journal of Obstetrics and Gynaecology Canada, 32*(8), 794-797.

Kosmadakis, G., Daikos, G.L., Pavlopoulou, A., Kostakis,A., Tzanatou-Exarchou, H., & Bolentis, J.N. (2013). Infectious complications in the first year post renal transplantation. *Transplantation Proceedings, 45*, 1579-1583. doi:10.1016/j.transproceed.2012.10.047

Kumar, M., Damask, A., Roland, M., Stock, P., Gold, M., Fyfe, B., ... Swartz, C. (2002). Kidney transplantation (KTX) in HIV-positive end stage renal disease (ESRD) patients – A prospective study. *American Transplant Congress 2003*, Washington, DC.

Lenihan, C.R., Montez-Rath, M.E., Scandling, J.D., Turakhia, M.P., & Winkelmayer, W.C. (2013). Outcomes after kidney transplantation of patients previously diagnosed with atrial fibrillation. *American Journal of Transplantation, 13*(6), 1566-1575. doi:10.1111/ajt.12197.

Lentine, K., Brennan, D., & Schnitzler, M.A. (2005). Incidence and prevalence of myocardial infarction after kidney transplantation. *Journal of the American Society of Nephrology, 16*, 496-506. doi:10.1681/ASN.2004070580

Lentine, K., Rocca-Rey, L.A., Bacchi, G., Wasi, N., Schmitz, L., Salvalaggio, P.R., ... Brennan, D.C. (2008). Obesity and cardiac risk after kidney transplantation: Experience at one center and comprehensive literature review. *Transplantation, 86*(2), 303-312.

Lentine, K.L., Costa, S.P., Weir, M.R., Robb, J.F., Fleisher, L.A., Kasiske, B.L., ... Eagle, K.A.(2012). Cardiac disease evaluation and management among kidney and liver transplantation candidates. *Journal of the American College of Cardiology, 60*(5), 434-480. doi:10.1016/j.jacc.2012.05.008

Lentine, K.L., Santos, R.D., Axelrod, D., Schnitzler, M.A., Brennan, D.C., & Tuttle-Newhall, J.E. (2012). Obesity and kidney transplant candidates: How big is too big for transplantation? *American Journal of Nephrology. 36*, 575-586. doi:10.1159/000345476

Lipshutz, G. (2010). Kidney and pancreas transplantation in the diabetic patient. In G.M. Danovitch (Ed.), *Handbook of kidney transplantation* (5th ed., pp. 330-354). Philadelphia: Lippincott Williams & Wilkins.

Liu, C.H., & Kao, J.H. (2011). Treatment of hepatitis C virus infection in patients with end-stage renal disease. *Journal of Gastroenterology and Hepatology, 26*(2), 228-239. doi:10.1111/j.1440-1746.2010.06488.x

Lukens, B., Nierman, D.M., & Schiano, T.D. (2011). Lactulose: How many ways can one drug be prescribed? *The American Journal of Gastroenterology, 106*, 1726-1727. doi:10.1038/ajg.2011.182

Mahr, A., Heijl, C., Le Guenno, G., & Faurschou, M. (2013). ANCA-associated vasculitis and malignancy: Current evidence for cause and consequence relationships. *Best Practice & Research Clinical Rheumatology, 27*, 45-56. doi:10.1016/j.berh.2012.12.003

Maldonado, J.R., Dubois, H.C., David, E.E., Sher,Y, Lolak, S., Dyal, J., & Witten, D. (2012). The Stanford integrated psychosocial assessment for transplantation (SIPAT): A new tool for the psychosocial evaluation of pre-transplant candidates. *Psychosomatics, 53*(2), 123-132. doi:10.1016/j.psym.2011.12.012

Mandelbrot, D., & Sayegh, M. (2010). Transplantion immunobiology. In G.M. Danovitch (Ed.), *Handbook of kidney transplantation* (5th ed., pp. 2333-2343). Philadelphia: Lippincott Williams & Wilkins.

Mandelbrot, D.A., Paviakis, M., Danovitch, G., Johnson, S.R., Karp, S.J., Khwaja, K., ... Rodrigue, J.R. (2007). The medical evaluation of living kidney donors: A survey of US transplant centers. *American Journal of Transplantation, 7*, 2333-2343. doi:10.1111/j.1600-6143.2007.01932.x

Mangus, R.S., & Haag, B.W. (2004). Stented vs nonstented extravesical ureteroneocystostomy in renal transplantation: A meta-analysis. *American Journal of Transplantation, 4*, 1889.

Mann, J.F., & Hilgers, K.F. (2013). *Renal effects of ACE inhibitors in hypertension*. Retrieved from http://www.uptodate.com/contents/renal-effects-of-ace-inhibitors-in-hypertension

Marco, S., Ferronato, C., & Patrizia, B. (2008). Neurologic complications after solid organ transplantation. *Transplant International, 22*, 269-278. doi:10.1111/j.1432-2277.2008.00780.x

Marinaki, S., Lionaki, S., &. Boletis, J.N. (2013). Glomerular disease recurrence in the renal allograft: A hurdle but not a barrier for successful kidney transplantation. *Transplantation Proceedings, 45*, 3-9. doi:10.1016/j.transproceed.2012.12.021

Massie, A.B., Montgomery, R.A., & Segev, D.L. (2011). Does the kidney donor index need non-donor factors? *American Transplant Congress Abstracts*. Abstract #32.

Mellors, J.W., Munoz, A., Giorgi, J.V., Margolick, J.B., Tassoni, C.J., Gupta, P., ... Rinaldo, C.R., Jr. (1997). Plasma viral load and CD4+ lymphocytes as prognostic markers of HIV-1 infection. *Annals of Internal Medicine, 126*(12), 946-954. doi:10.7326/0003-4819-126-12-199706150-00003

Mellors, J.W., Rinaldo, C.R., Jr., Gupta, P., White, R.M., Todd, J.A., & Kingsley, L.A. (1996). Prognosis in HIV-1 infection predicted by the quantity of virus in plasma. *Science, 272*(5265), 1167-1170. doi:10.1126/science.272.5265.1167

Mineo, D., Pileggi, A., Alejandro, R., & Ricordi, C. (2009). Point steady progress and current challenges in clinical islet transplantation. *Diabetes Care, 32*(8), 1563-1569.

Moers, C., Smits, J., Maathius, M.J., Treckmann, J., van Gelder, F., Napieralski, B.P., ... Ploeg, R.J. (2009). Machine perfusion or cold storage in deceased donor kidney transplantation. *New England Journal of Medicine, 360*, 7-19.

Montgomery, R.A., Locke, J.E., King, K.E., Segev, D.L., Warren, D.S., Kraus E.S., ... Haas, M. (2009). ABO incompatible renal transplantation: A paradigm ready for broad implementation. *Transplantation, 8*(8), 1246-1255. doi:10.1097/TP.0b013e31819f2024

Morse, C.G., Mican, J.M., Jones, E.C., Joe, G.O., Rick, M.E., Formentini, E., & Kovacs, J.A. (2007). The incidence and natural history of osteonecrosis in HIV-infected adults. *Clinical Infectious Diseases, 44*(5), 739-48. doi:10.1086/511683

Mosconi, G., Stalteri, L., Centofanti, F., Capelli, I., Carretta, E., Persici, E., ... Stefoni, S. (2011). Incidence of cancer in kidney transplantation waiting list patients: A single center experience. *Transplantation Proceedings, 43*, 1003-1005. doi:10.1016/j.transproceed.2011.01.121

Nadim, M.K., Kellum, J.A., Davenport, A., Wong, F., Davis, C., Pannu, N., Tolwani, A., ... Genyk, Y.S. (2012). Hepatorenal syndrome: The 8th international concensus conference of the Acute Dialysis Quality Initiative (ADQI) Group. *Critical Care, 16*(1), 1-17. doi:10.1186/cc11188

Nast, C., & Cohen, A. (2010). Pathology of kidney transplantation. In G.M. Danovitch (Ed.), *Handbook of kidney transplantation* (5th ed., pp. 311-329). Philadelphia: Lippincott Williams & Wilkins

Natov, S., & Pereira, B.J.G. (2013). *Hepatitis C virus infection and renal transplantation*. Retrieved from http://www.uptodate.com/contents/hepatitis-c-virus-infection-and-renal-transplantation

O'Connor, K.J., Delmonico, F.L., Gritsch, H.A., & Danovitch, G.M. (2010). The science of deceased donor kidney transplantation. In G.M. Danovitch (Ed.), *Handbook of kidney transplantation* (5th ed., pp. 61-76). Philadelphia: Lippincott Williams & Wilkins.

Ostovan, M.A., Fazelzadeh, A., Mehdizadeh, A.R., Razmkon, A., & Malek-Hosseini, S.A. (2006). How to decrease cardiovascular mortality in renal transplant recipients. *Transplantation Proceedings, 38*(9), 2887-92. doi:10.1016/j.transproceed.2006.08.091

Palefsky, J.M., Holly, E.A., Ralston, M.L., Da Costa, M., Bonner, H., Jay, N., ... Darragh, T.M. (2001). Effect of highly active antiretroviral therapy on the natural history of anal squamous intraepithelial lesions and anal human papillomavirus infection. *Journal of Acquired Immune Deficiency Syndrome, 28*(5), 422-428. Retrieved from http://www.ncbi.nlm.nih.gov/pubmed/11744829

Palella, F.J., Delaney, K.M., Moorman, A.C., Loveless, M.O., Fuhrer, J., Satten, G.A., ... Holmberg, S.D. (1998). Declining morbidity and mortality among patients with advanced human immunodeficiency virus infection. HIV Outpatient Study Investigators. *New England Journal of Medicine, 338*(13), 853-60. doi:10.1056/NEJM199803263381301

Paradela de la Morena, M., De La Torres Bravos, M., Fernández Prado, R., Delgado Roel, M., García Salcedo, J.A., Fieira Costa, E., ... Borro Maté, J.M. (2010). Chronic kidney disease after lung transplantation: Incidence, risk factors, and treatment. *Transplantation Proceedings, 42*, 3217-3219. doi:10.1016/j.transproceed.2010.05.064

Parikh, S., Nagaraja H., Agarwal A., Samavedi S., Von Visger J., Nori U., ... Singh N. (2013). Impact of post-kidney transplant parathyroidectomy on allograft function. *Clinical transplanatation, 27*, 397-402. doi:10.1111/ctr.12099

Pegues, D.A., Kubak, B.M., Maree, C.L., Gregson, A.L. (2010). Infections in kidney transplantation. In G.M. Danovitch (Ed.), *Handbook of kidney transplantation* (5th ed., pp. 61-76). Philadelphia: Lippincott Williams & Wilkins.

Pelletier, S.J., Norman, S.P., Christensen, L.L., Stock, P.G., Port, F.K., & Merion, R.M. (2004). Review of transplantation in HIV patients during the HAART era. *Clinical Transplantation*, 63-82. Retrieved from http://www.ncbi.nlm.nih.gov/pubmed/16704139

Pham, P.T., Pham, P.A., Pham, P.C., Parikh, S., & Danovitch, G. (2010). Evaluation of adult kidney transplant candidates. *Seminars in Dialysis, 23*(6), 595-605. doi:10.1111/j.1525-139X.2010.00809x

Pham, P.T., Slavov, C., & Pham, P.C. (2009). Acute kidney injury after liver, heart and lung transplants: Dialysis modality, predictors of renal function recovery and impact on survival. *Advances in Chronic Kidney Disease, 16*(4), 256-267.

Pirsch, J.D., Miller, J., Deierhoi, M.H., Vincenti, F., & Filo, R.S. (1997). A comparison of tacrolimus (fk506) and cyclosporine for immunosuppression after cadaveric renal transplantation. FK506 Kidney Transplant Study Group. *Transplantation, 63*(7), 977.

Ponticelli, C. (2007). Medical complications of kidney transplantation. Abingdon, UK: Informa Healthcare.

Ponticelli, C., & Graziani, G. (2012). Education and counseling of renal transplant recipients. *Journal of Nephrology, 25*(6), 879-889. doi:10.5301/jn.5000227

Power, R.E., Hickey, D.P., & Little, D.M. (2004). Urological evaluation prior to renal transplantation. *Transplantation Proceedings, 36*, 2962-2967. doi:10.1016/j.transproceed.2004.11.006

Rhen, T., &. Cidlowski, J.A. (2005). Anti-inflammatory action of glucocorticoids-new mechanisms for old drugs. *New England Journal of Medicine, 353*, 1711-1723

Rifkin, M.H. (2010). Psychosocial and financial aspects of transplantation. In G.M. Danovitch (Ed.), *Handbook of kidney transplantation* (5th ed., pp. 432-440). Philadelphia: Lippincott Williams & Wilkins.

Robinson, P.D., Shroff, R.C., & Spencer, H. (2012). Renal complications following lung and heart-lung transplantation. *Pediatric Nephrology, 28*, 375-386.

Rodelo, J.R., Nieto-Ríos, J.F., Serna-Higuita, L.M., Henao, J.E., García, A., Reino, A.C., … Arbeláez, M. (2013). Survival of renal transplantation patients older than 60 years: A single center experience. *Transplantation Proceedings, 45*, 1402-1409. doi:10.1016/j.transproceed.2012.10.053

Roling, J., Schmid, H., Fischereder, M., Draenert, R., & Goebel, F.D. (2006). HIV-associated renal diseases and highly active antiretroviral therapy-induced nephropathy. *Clinical Infectious Diseases, 42*(10), 1488-95. doi:10.1086/503566

Sadeghi, M., Daniel, V., Wang, H., Zeier, M., Schemmer, P., Mehrabi, A., … Opelz, G. (2013). Plasmapheresis adjusts inflammatory responses in potential kidney transplant recipients. *Transplantation, 95*(8), 1021-1029. doi:10.1097/TP.0b013e318286191b

Schmied, B.M., Muller, S.A., Mehrabi, A., Welsch, T., Buchler, M.W., Zeier, M., & Schmidt, J. (2006). Immunosuppressive standards in simultaneous kidney-pancreas transplantation. *Clinical Transplantation, 20*(Suppl. 17), 44-50. doi:10.1111/j.1399-0012.2006.00599.x

Scientific Registry of Transplant Recipient (SRTR). (2011). *2011 annual data report.* Retrieved from http://srtr.transplant.hrsa.gov/annual_reports/2011

Segelmark, M. (2013, April). Renal transplantation in ANCA-associated vasculitis. *La Presse Medicale, 42*(4 Pt 2), 568-571. doi:10.1159/000347142

Shapiro, A., Lakey, J., Ryan, E., Korbutt, G., Toth, E., Warnock, G., … Rajotte, R. (2000). Islet transplantation in seven patients with type 1 diabetes mellitus using a glucocorticoid-free immunosuppressive regimen. *New England Journal of Medicine, 343*(4), 230-238.

Sharif, A. (2013). Unspecified kidney donation – A review of principles, practice and potential. *Transplantation, 95*(12), 1425-1430. doi:10.1097/TP.0b013e31829282eb.

Shipman, K.E., & Patel, C.K. (2009). The effect of combined renal and pancreatic transplantation on diabetic retinopathy. *Clinical Ophthalmology, 3*, 531-535.

Sise, M.E., Courtwright, A.M., & Channick, R.N. (2013, June 5). Pulmonary hypertension in patients with chronic and end stage kidney disease. *Kidney International*, 1-11. Advance online publication. doi:10.1038/ki.2013.186

Smeltzer, S., Bare, B., Hinkle, J., & Cheever, K. (Eds.). (2008) *Brunner & Suddarth's textbook of medical-surgical nursing* (11th ed.). Philadelphia: Lippincott Williams & Wilkins.

Solez, K. (2010). History of the Banff classification of allograft pathology as it approaches its 20th year. *Current Opinion in Organ Transplantation, 15*(1), 49-51. doi:10.1097/MOT.0b013e328334fedb

Solez, K., Colvin, R.B., Racusen, L.C., Sis, B., Halloran, P.F., Birk, P.E., … Weening, J.J. (2007). Banff '05 meeting report: Differential diagnosis of chronic allograft injury and elimination of chronic allograft nephropathy (CAN). *American Journal of Transplantation, 7*(3), 518–526. doi:10.1111/j.1600-6143.2006.01688.x

Sollinger, H.W. (1995). Mycophenolate mofetil for the prevention of acute rejection in cadaveric renal allograft recipients. U.S. Transplant Mycophenolate Mofetil Study Group. *Transplantation, 60*(3), 225-232.

Sollinger, H., Odorico, J.S., Becker, Y.T., D'Alessandro, A.M., & Pirsch, J.D. (2009). One thousand simultaneous pancreas–kidney transplants at a single center with 22-year follow-up. *Annals of Surgery, 250*, 618-630.

Squifflet, J.P. (2013). Kidney and pancreas transplantation: The history of surgical techniques and immunosuppression. In T. Rath (Ed.), *Current issues and future direction in kidney transplantation* (pp. 249-275), New York: Intech. doi:10.5772/55347

Sterns, R.H., & Runyon, B.A. (2013). Hyponatremia in patients with cirrhosis. Retrieved from http://www.uptodate.com/contents/hyponatremia-in-patients-with-cirrhosis?source=search_result&search=Hyponatremia+in+patients+with+cirrhosis&selectedTitle=1%7E150

Stock, P.G., Barin, B., Murphy, B., Hanto, D., Diego, J.M., Light, J.… & Roland, M.E. (2010). Outcomes of kidney transplantation in HIV-infected recipients. *New England Journal of Medicine, 363*(21), 2004-2014. doi:10.1056/NEJMoa1001197

Stock, P.G., & Roland, M.E. (2007). Evolving clinical strategies for transplantation in the HIV-positive recipient. *Transplantation, 84*(5), 563-571.

Stock, P.G., Roland, M.E., Carlson, L., Freise, C.E., Roberts, J.P., Hirose, R., … Ascher, N.L. (2003). Kidney and liver transplantation in human immunodeficiency virus-infected patients: a pilot safety and efficacy study. *Transplantation 76*(2), 370-375.

Terasaki, P.I. (2012). A personal perspective: 100-year history of the humoral theory of transplantation. *Transplantation, 93* (8), 751-756. doi:10.1097/TP.0b013e3182483713

Terrault, N.A., & Adey, D.B. (2007). The kidney transplant recipient with hepatitis C infection: pre- and posttransplantation treatment. *Clinical Journal of the American Society of Nephrology, 2*(3), 563-75. doi:10.2215/CJN.02930806

Teta, D. (2010). Weight loss in obese patients with chronic kidney disease: Who and how? *Journal of Renal Care, 36*(Suppl. 1), 163-171. doi:10.1111/j.1755-6686.2010.00176.x

Townsend, C.M., Jr., Beauchamp, R.D., Evers, B.M. & Mattox, K.L. (Eds.). (2012). Sabiston textbook of surgery: *The biological basis of modern surgical practice* (19th ed.). Philadelphia: Saunders-Elsevier.

U.S. Food and Drug Administration (FDA) Medwatch. (2014). *CellCept (mycophenolate mofetil) capsules, tablets, oral suspension and CellCept (mycophenolate mofetil hydrochloride) for injection.* Retrieved from http://www.fda.gov/Safety/MedWatch/SafetyInformation/ucm310868.htm

Uemura, T., Ramprasad, V., Matsushima, K., Shike, H., Valania, T., Kwon, O., … Kadry, Z. (2011). Single dose of alemtuzumab induction with steroid-free maintenance immunosuppression in pancreas transplantation. *Transplantation, 92*(6), 678. doi:10.1097/TP.0b013e31822b58be

United Network for Organ Sharing (UNOS). (2013a). *Living kidney donation consent and medical evaluation policies.* Retrieved from

http://optn.transplant.hrsa.gov/contentdocuments/living_kidney
_donor_requirements_faq.pdf

United Network for Organ Sharing. (2013b). *Policy 3.5, Allocation of
kidneys*. Retrieved from optn.transplant.hrsa.gov/
PoliciesandBylaws2/policies/pdfs/policy_7.pdf

Veale, J, Singer, J., & Gritsch, H.A. (2010). The transplant operation
and its surgical complications. In G.M. Danovitch (Ed.),
Handbook of kidney transplantation (5th ed., pp. 181-197).
Philadelphia: Lippincott Williams & Wilkins.

Vella, J., & Brennan, D.C. (2013). *Chronic renal allograft nephropathy*.
Retrieved from http://www.uptodate.com/contents/chronic-
renal-allograft-nephropathy?source=search_result&search=Chro
nic+renal+allograft+nephropathy&selectedTitle=1%7E31

Weber, M.L., Ibrahim, H.N., & Lake, J.R. (2012). Renal dysfunction
in liver transplant recipients: Evaluation of the critical issues.
Liver Transplantation, 18, 1290-1301. doi:10.1002/lt.23522

Wehbe, E., Brock, R., Budev, M., Xu, M., Demirjian, S., Schreiber,
M.J., & Stephany, B. (2012). Short-term and long-term outcomes
of acute kidney injury after lung transplantation. *The Journal of
Heart and Lung Transplantation, 31*, 244-251.

Welsh, R.C., Cockfield, S.M., Campbell, P., Hervas-Malo, M., Gyenes,
G., & Dzavik, V. (2011). Cardiovascular assessment of diabetic
end-stage renal disease patients before renal transplantation.
Transplantation, 91(2), 213-218. doi:10.1097/TP.0b013e381ff4f61

Wilkinson, A. & Kasiske, B.L. (2010). Long-term posttransplantation
management and complications. In G.M. Danovitch (Ed.),
Handbook of kidney transplantation (5th ed., pp. 217-250).
Philadelphia: Lippincott Williams & Wilkins.

Wilkinson, A. (2010). The "first quarter." The first three months after
transplantation. In G.M. Danovitch (Ed.), *Handbook of kidney
transplantation* (5th ed., pp. 198-216). Philadelphia: Lippincott
Williams & Wilkins.

Worthington, J.E., McEwen, A., McWilliam, L.J., Picton, M.L., &
Martin, S. (2007) Association between C4d staining in renal
transplant biopsies, production of donor-specific HLA antibodies,
and graft outcome. *Transplantation; 83*, 398.

Yee, H.S., Chang, M.F., Pocha, C., Lim, J., Ross, D., Morgan, T.R., &
Monto, A. (2012). Update on the management and treatment of
hepatitis C virus infection: Recommendations from the
Department of Veterans Affairs Hepatitis C Resource Center
Program and the National Hepatitis C Program Office. *American
Journal of Gastroenterology, 107*(5), 669-89; quiz 690.
doi:10.1038/ajg.2012.48

Zervos, E.E., & Rosemurgy, A.S. (2001). Management of medically
refractory ascites. *The American Journal of Surgery, 181*, 256-264.
doi:10.1016/S0002-9610(01)00565-7

CHAPTER **2**
Hemodialysis

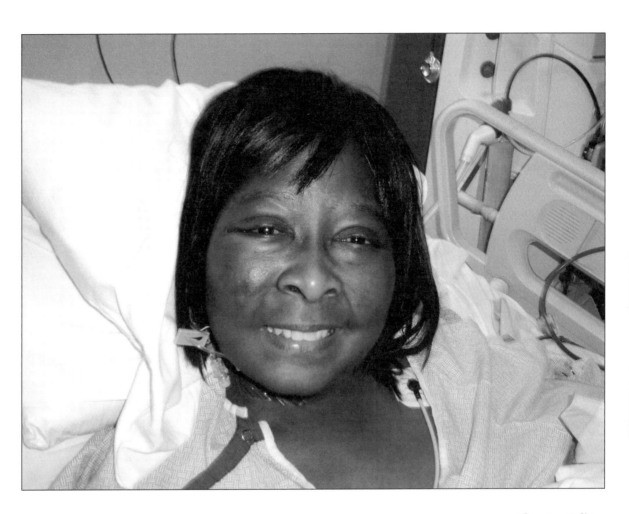

Chapter Editor
Karen C. Robbins, MS, RN, CNN

Authors
Karen C. Robbins, MS, RN, CNN
Deb Castner, MSN, APRN, ACNP, CNN
Darlene Jalbert, BSN, RN, CNN
Judy Kauffman, MSN, RN, CNN
Glenda M. Payne, MS, RN, CNN
Joan E. Speranza-Reid, BSHM, RN, CNN

CHAPTER **2**

Hemodialysis

This offering for **2.6 contact hours** is provided by the American Nephrology Nurses' Association (ANNA).

American Nephrology Nurses' Association is accredited as a provider of continuing nursing education by the American Nurses Credentialing Center Commission on Accreditation.

ANNA is a provider approved by the California Board of Registered Nursing, provider number CEP 00910.

This CNE offering meets the continuing nursing education requirements for certification and recertification by the Nephrology Nursing Certification Commission (NNCC).

To be awarded contact hours for this activity, read this chapter in its entirety. Then complete the CNE evaluation found at **www.annanurse.org/corecne** and submit it; or print it, complete it, and mail it in. Contact hours are not awarded until the evaluation for the activity is complete.

Example of reference for Chapter 2 in APA format. Use author of the section being cited. This example is based on Section F – Dialyzer Reprocessing.

Jalbert, D. (2015). Hemodialysis: Dialyzer reprocessing. In C.S. Counts (Ed.), *Core curriculum for nephrology nursing: Module 3. Treatment options for patients with chronic kidney failure* (6th ed., pp. 69-166). Pitman, NJ: American Nephrology Nurses' Association.

Interpreted: Section author(s). (2015). Title of chapter: Title of section. In ...

Cover photo by Sandra Cook.

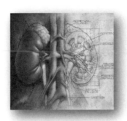

CHAPTER 2

Hemodialysis

Purpose

This chapter describes the chemical principles used during hemodialysis and current technologies available. It focuses on providing hemodialysis treatments that are not only safe and accurate, but are customized for the individual patient. Strategies that can be used to reach desired patient outcomes, while avoiding adverse events, are addressed. Complications associated with the dialysis procedure are explained, including assessment and interventions. Additionally, it discusses how to establish and reach the estimated dry weight of the patient on hemodialysis while minimizing untoward effects.

An overview is provided of hematocrit-based blood volume monitoring, descriptions of the most common equipment options in current use, and suggested strategies for more effective fluid volume management during the hemodialysis process.

Technical aspects for hemodialysis are addressed for water treatment and dialyzer reprocessing, regulatory requirements, and safe practices. The provision of a safe, individualized hemodialysis treatment is an essential component of this chapter. There is a strong emphasis on patient safety starting with a list of safety considerations in hemodialysis and spread throughout the chapter with safety alerts.

Objectives

Upon completion of this chapter, the learner will be able to:
1. List factors affecting the rate of diffusion.
2. Identify factors affecting net flux of solute during hemodialysis.
3. Describe how to calculate the transmembrane pressure to obtain desired ultrafiltration rate during hemodialysis.
4. Discuss the causes and related interventions for managing blood and dialysate compartment alarms.
5. Describe the use of urea kinetic modeling for patients on hemodialysis.
6. Define Kt/V and current target values for hemodialysis adequacy.
7. Compare benefits vs. risks in the use of sodium and ultrafiltration profiles during hemodialysis.
8. Outline the causes, signs and symptoms, prevention, and treatment of complications of the hemodialysis procedure.
9. Recommend strategies to avoid the known potential complications of dialyzer reuse.

Significant Dates in the History of Hemodialysis

1861   Thomas Graham is considered to be the father of modern dialysis. This colloid chemist from London coined the terms *dialysis* and *selective diffusion*.

1890   Bicarbonate peritoneal lavage was used in Europe to treat cholera.

1913   The term *artificial kidney* was coined by John J. Abel, Leonard Rowntree, and B.B. Turner at Johns Hopkins University in Baltimore. They devised a "kidney" using celloidin tubing for membranes and crushed leech heads (hirudin) for anticoagulation. The "kidney" was not efficient enough for humans, and hirudin was toxic to humans.

1923   In Germany, Nicheles used the peritoneal membrane from an ox to make an "artificial kidney."

1924   In Giessen, Germany, Georg Haas performed the first human dialysis.

1935	Heparin was purified and replaced the toxic and expensive hirudin; regenerated cellulose tubing was developed.
1940	Dr. Willem Johan Kolff in Gronigen, Germany, unable to save a young patient dying from uremia, began simple experiments studying the dialyzability of urea using cellophane.
1942-1943	Kolff designed the rotating drum artificial kidney, which was used in Holland for successful treatment of patients with acute renal failure.
1945	Kolff performed the first successful dialysis treatments on a 67-year-old female with acute renal failure who recovered kidney function and lived another 7 years.
1946	Kolff wrote that the artificial kidney should be used for acute renal failure but was not indicated for chronic therapy.
1946	Gordon Murray performed the first hemodialysis in North America. The patient eventually recovered complete renal function and survived.
1946-1947	The events of World War II prevented communication among physicians working around the world on treatment of uremia.
1947	Kolff found effectiveness of hemodialysis superior to peritoneal and intestinal lavage for urea removal. His artificial kidney was shipped to Canada, New York, and London. Kolff came to the United States where he assisted in the initiation of the first dialysis at Mount Sinai Hospital in New York City. Drs. John Merrill and George Thorne were present and made the decision to launch a program in Boston to support a transplant unit they were planning to establish.
1947	Van Garretts (Copenhagen), made a hand-wound coil kidney and used it successfully to treat humans.
Early 1950s	Kolff went to Boston and worked with Edward Olsen, a machinist, and Dr. Carl Walter to modify Kolff's design. The Kolff-Brigham artificial kidney evolved and was the machine used by military physicians of the United States Army.
1950-1953	Drs. Paul E. Teschan, George E. Schreiner, and colleagues used artificial kidneys to treat acute renal failure from battle injuries in Korean War MASH units. The survival rate of patients with acute renal failure improved.
1954-1990	Intravenous iron (iron dextran) became available for treatment of iron deficiency anemia. It was removed from the market in 1990 for quality manufacturing concerns.
1956	Kolff developed a disposable coil dialyzer and gave it to Travenol®; no other company thought it had any practical application. Repeated vascular access remained a significant challenge to chronic therapy.
1957	Dr. Fred Kiil, Norway, developed the first flat plate parallel flow dialyzer that was widely used, employing cuprophane as the dialyzing membrane (MEI, 2013).
1959	After development of the Quinton-Scribner external shunt, the first two patients on chronic maintenance dialysis were started using the Kiil dialyzer.
1960	Dr. David Dillard, a pediatric heart surgeon, implanted the first Scribner shunt developed by Dr. Belding Scribner, to dialyze Clyde Shields in Seattle, Washington, the first person on chronic dialysis. He lived 11 years and succumbed to a heart attack.
1964	Home dialysis was started by Drs. Curtis and Scribner in Seattle; Stanley Shaldon in London; and John Merrill, Eugene Schupak, and Cameron Hampers in Boston.
1965	The internal arteriovenous fistula was developed by Drs. Michael J. Brescia and James E. Cimino in New York, NY.
1967	The first hollow fiber kidney was developed and clinically tested.
1973	Federal support for treatment of end-stage renal disease (ESRD) became available in the United States through the passage of HR-1, a bill that supported payment for patients with ESRD.
1974	Large surface-area dialyzers that allowed a decrease in treatment time became available.
1978	Polytetrafluorethylene (PTFE) was configured into graft material for arteriovenous vascular access.

Late 1970s
Reprocessing of dialyzers was implemented for cost containment.

1970s   Calcitriol was identified and Vitamin D analogs (calcitriol, paricalcitol, doxecalciferol) start coming into use for treatment of renal bone disease, "renal osteodystrophy," now known as chronic kidney disease – mineral bone disorder, CKD-MBD.

1980s   Volumetric hemodialysis machines allowed for more highly permeable membranes to be safely used.

1980s   Automated peritoneal dialysis and continuous ambulatory peritoneal dialysis were widely accepted as maintenance dialysis modalities.

1980s   Hepatitis outbreak occurred as it set the stage for personal protective equipment (PPE).

1989   Recombinant human erythropoietin was commercially available for use in patients with ESRD on dialysis, the first erythropoiesis-stimulating agent (ESA).

Early 1990s
Intravenous forms of vitamin D analogs became commercially available for management of CKD-MBD.

1990s   Noninvasive blood volume monitoring became available for monitoring intravascular volume during hemodialysis.

1990s-2009
Intravenous iron (iron dextran) became available again following its earlier removal from the market due to quality manufacturing concerns. Several new forms of low molecular weight intravenous irons became available (iron sucrose, sodium ferric gluconate, ferumoxytol) as widespread use of ESAs require iron repletion.

1997   National Kidney Foundation published *Dialysis Outcomes Quality Initiative (DOQI) Clinical Practice Guidelines for Adequacy of Hemodialysis, Adequacy of Peritoneal Dialysis, Treatment of Anemia of Chronic Renal Failure*, and *Vascular Access* (NKF, 1997).

Late 1990s into 2000s
Resurgence of interest in return to home hemodialysis with daily or nightly therapy.

2002   National Kidney Foundation published *The Kidney Disease Outcomes Quality Initiative (KDOQI) Clinical Practice Guidelines for Chronic Kidney Disease.* Subsequent revisions and expansions serve as guidelines for the care of patients with all stages of chronic kidney disease including patients on hemodialysis (NKF, 2002).

2005   NxStage® obtaineds FDA approval for their portable home hemodialysis machine.

2006   Roche tried to bring long acting ESA, Micera, to market in the United States but could not due to patent restrictions.

2005-2012
Additional KDOQI Guidelines (Anemia, Transplant, Hypertension, Vascular Access, Diabetes and CKD, Nutrition, Dyslipidemia, and Cardiovascular Care) released and earlier Guidelines revised.

2008   Ongoing Kidney Disease, Improving Global Outcomes (KDIGO), an international organization, published clinical practice guidelines for CKD, Blood Pressure in CKD, Glomerulonephritis, Acute Kidney Injury, Anemia, Chronic Kidney Disease Mineral and Bone Disorder (CKD-MBD), Care of Kidney Transplant Recipients, Glomerulonephritis, Lipids in CKD, and Hepatitis C in CKD (KDIGO, n.d.).

2008   Center for Medicare and Medicaid Services (CMS) published the first revision of the *Conditions for Coverage for ESRD* since its enactment in 1972 (CMS, 2008).

2009   Boston Steering Committee met for the first time since 1989 to review outcomes in ESRD population from current practices; concluded that current models of care are insufficient and more emphasis is needed to manage left ventricular hypertrophy (LVH) to reduce morbity and mortality associated with CKD and ESRD.

2011   Reimbursement for dialysis changed to a prospective payment schedule or "bundled payment" covering cost of dialysis, dialysis-related medications and lab tests, and a quality incentive program.

2012   Affymax released peginesatide (Omontys®), a once-monthly ESA.

2013   Affymax voluntarily removed Omontys® from the market due to unexpected anaphylactic reactions.

2015   Amgen's patent for ESA, Epogen®, expires and Mircera returns to the United States.

2015   Triferic is approved as the first iron replacement drug that is delivered as a dialysate additive.

SECTION A
Principles of Hemodialysis
Deb Castner

I. Principles of hemodialysis.

A. Hemodialysis is made possible through the principles of diffusion, osmosis, and ultrafiltration (convection).
   1. The action of these principles makes it possible to remove and replace electrolytes and buffers as well as remove uremic toxins and excess plasma water.
   2. The artificial dialyzer serves as the semipermeable membrane, a solution pathway for blood, and a fluid compartment for dialyzing fluid (dialysate) (Latham, 2006).
   3. Dialysis restores acid-base, fluid, and electrolyte balance.

B. The hemodialysis procedure replaces only the filtration function of natural kidneys.
   1. It is an intermittent therapy unlike the natural kidney that performs this function in a slow and continuous fashion.
   2. Hemodialysis does not replace the hormonal functions of a kidney. Various medications are used to augment those functions (e.g., BP control, mineral and bone metabolism, and anemia management) (Latham, 2006).

II. Definition of hemodialysis.

A. Hemodialysis is a form of kidney replacement therapy (KRT) in which waste solutes are removed primarily by diffusion from blood flowing on one side of a membrane into dialysate flowing on the other side.

B. Fluid removal that is sufficient to obtain the desired weight loss is achieved by establishing a hydrostatic and osmotic pressure gradient across the membrane. This fluid removal provides some additional waste solute removal, particularly for higher molecular weight solutes (AAMI, 2010, p.16).

C. There are many safety considerations related to hemodialysis; see Table 2.1. There are safety alerts throughout the chapter.

III. Solute removal or mass transfer is the physical process that involves molecular and convective transport of molecules. They include the following processes.

A. Diffusion (conductive dialysis) – the movement of a molecule from a region of higher solute concentration to a region of lower solute

concentration and is the result of random movement of molecules driven by thermal energy (see Figures 2.1 and 2.2).
   1. Diffusion in hemodialysis occurs across the semipermeable membrane that separates the blood compartment from the dialysate compartment.
      a. A semipermeable membrane allows passage of some molecules while restricting or preventing the transit of others.
      b. The dialyzer functions as the semipermeable membrane and bridge between these two components (see Figures 2.3 and 2.4).

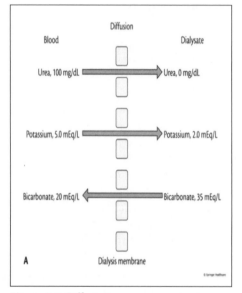

Figure 2.1. Diffusion.
Used with permission from Merck Medicus Springer Healthcare.

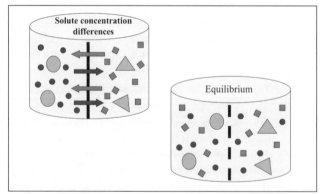

Figure 2.2. Diffusion.
Used with permission from Latham, C. (2006). Hemodialysis technology. In A. Molzahn & E. Butera, (Eds.), *Contemporary nephrology nursing: Principles and practice* (2nd ed., pp. 531-558). Pitman, NJ: American Nephrology Nurses' Association.

Table 2.1

Safety Considerations in Hemodialysis

"Safety is avoiding both short- and long-term harm to people resulting from unsafe acts and preventable adverse events" (The Joint Commission, 2012, p. vii.).

I. Know and follow your facility's policy and procedures for equipment maintenance and recording and reporting machines potentially in need of repair(s).

II. Alarms are present for the safety of patients. Do not clear an alarm without assessing the patient and the equipment to be sure of the cause and correction for the alarm.

III. Do not solely rely on machine alarms. Know and understand the machine response to an alarm situation. For example:
   A. During an abnormal conductivity or temperature range alarm, the dialysate flow should go into the bypass mode. Check the machine to ensure it has performed that safety measure. Know what to do to remedy and protect your patient if the machine alarm condition does not engage, such as removing the dialysate hose connectors manually and taking the machine out of service.
   B. In an alarm condition on the blood side (e.g., a high venous pressure alarm), assess the patient and access as well as observe the machine to ensure the blood pump stopped and the venous clamp is engaged.

IV. Alarm fatigue – exposure to a large number of alarms leading to sensory overload, slow, or nonexistent response to alarms. This can lead to complacency and have an adverse impact on patient safety (Cvach, 2012; Horkan, 2014).
   A. Evaluate the need for each alarm; eliminate unneeded alarms.
   B. Assess whether alarm limits may be altered (to decrease the number of alarms) without putting patients at risk for harm (Horkan, 2014).
   C. Do not override an alarm without determining its cause; do not automatically push "reset."

V. Patient concerns
   A. The vascular access should be visible at all times during the hemodialysis treatment (CMS, 2008a, V407, https://www.cms.gov/Medicare/Provider-Enrollment-and-Certification/GuidanceforLawsAndRegulations/downloads/esrdpgmguidance.pdf
   B. The patient's face must be visible at all times, i.e. head not covered, sunglasses off.
   C. The patient should be visible at all times during the hemodialysis treatment.
   D. Monitor the patient's blood pressure at least every 30 minutes, more often if indicated.
   E. Discourage patients eating while on hemodialysis (e.g., risk of choking, prevent hypotension). If the patient must eat, limit the quantity of food and avoid high carbohydrate meals.

VI. Staff member concerns
   A. All patient care staff should be certified in CPR per facility policy that may include an accredited source (e.g., American Heart Association or American Red Cross).
   B. All patient care staff must be aware of emergency procedures and their respective roles in keeping patients safe and protecting themselves.
   C. Always practice universal precautions and protect patients from cross contamination.
   D. Use proper patient identifiers before performing patient care or administering medications – do not assume you have the patient's identity correct. Familiarity resulting from frequent contact with patients may increase the opportunities for errors – assuming patient identity fosters errors!

VII. Environmental concerns
   A. Clean up any spill immediately.
   B. Minimize clutter to reduce infection control risks and risks for falls.

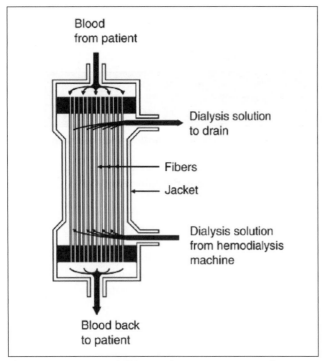

Figure 2.3. Semipermeable membrane: cross-section diagram of a hollow fiber dialyzer.

Retrieved from http:www.kidney.niddhk.nih.gov

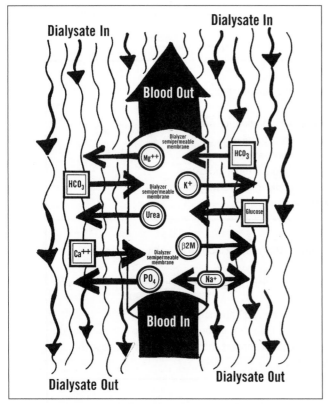

Figure 2.4. Movement of solutes across hemodialyzer membrane.

Used with permission from Latham, C. (2006). Hemodialysis technology. In A. Molzahn & E. Butera, (Eds.), *Contemporary nephrology nursing: Principles and practice* (2nd ed., pp. 531-558). Pitman, NJ: American Nephrology Nurses' Association.

2. Several factors affect the rate of diffusion in hemodialysis.
   a. Molecular size and weight.
      (1) Molecules that are too large to pass through the pores in a semipermeable membrane are nondiffusable.
      (2) Heavier molecules move more slowly. Depending on certain characteristics, they may exert an effect that causes water to move into the compartment that contains the nondiffusable molecule (see Figure 2.5).
   b. Solute charge: Positivity or negativity of charge can affect movement of molecules, either repelling or attracting solutes to move, dependent on their location, across the semipermeable membrane (see Figure 2.6).
   c. Size and number of pores in a semipermeable membrane.
      (1) The greater the number of pores, the faster the diffusion.
      (2) Larger pores allow diffusion of larger molecules.

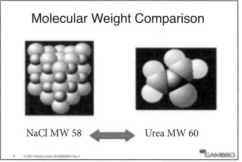

Figure 2.5. Example of molecule size.

Used with permission from Gambro.

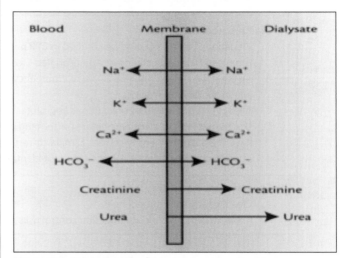

Figure 2.6. Solute transfer flux.

Used with permission from Merck Medicus Springer Healthcare.

d. Surface area of semipermeable membrane: generally the larger the surface area, the more rapid rate of diffusion occurs.

e. Temperature of the solutions on either side of the semipermeable membrane.
   (1) Higher temperature of solutions creates more molecular movement and more rapid diffusion.
   (2) Cooler temperature causes slowing of the molecular movement and a decrease in the rate of diffusion.

f. Concentration of solutes in the blood as compared to concentration of solutes in the dialysate.
   (1) The greater the concentration gradient for a given solute, the more rapidly diffusion occurs, given the above constraints (see Figure 2.7).
   (2) When equilibrium of a solute on the two sides of the membrane is reached, diffusion ceases.
   (3) Diffusion can occur in either direction, depending on the solute concentration in the respective compartments. Back-diffusion occurs when solutes move from the dialysate side into the patient's blood (see Figure 2.8).

g. Thickness of the semipermeable membrane may exert an influence on diffusion rate; thick membranes may decrease the rate of diffusion, but diffusion is not always proportional to membrane thickness.

h. Resistance to diffusion retards the rate at which solutes move to the membrane edge in the blood compartment, across the membrane, and away from the membrane edge into the flowing dialysate stream. A film layer develops on both the blood and dialysate sides of the membrane that can slow the rate of diffusion.

B. Solute drag or convective removal: Solutes move across the semipermeable membrane in conjunction with water movement.
   1. Definition.
      a. The rate at which solutes diffuse through the thin layers of blood, membrane, and dialysate. also known as triple-laminated solution or a three-dimensional finite volume (Eloot, DeWachter, & Verdonck, 2002), is termed *overall permeability*.

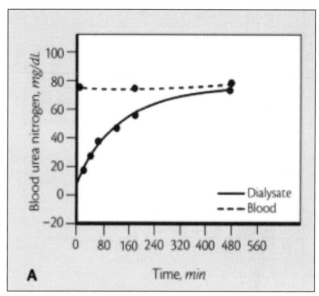

Figure 2.7. Solute transfer over time.
Used with permission from Merck Medicus Springer Healthcare.

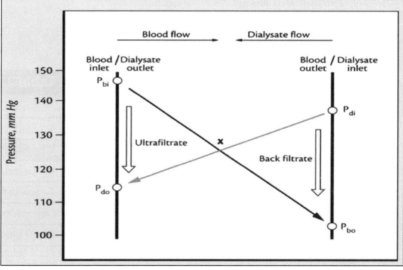

Figure 2.8. Pressure inside the blood compartment and the dialysate compartment with a fixed net zero ultrafiltration rate.
Used with permission from Merck Medicus Springer Healthcare.

   b. Expressed as the overall transport coefficient of Ko in cm²/min.
   2. The Ko is a unique value for each solute; it measures the efficiency of a dialyzer design.
      a. It is the summed value of the reciprocals for each of the resistances found in the blood side, dialyzer membrane, and dialysate.
      b. Net flux:
         (1) Expressed as a product as mL/min. or L/min.
         (2) The amount of solute leaving the blood and entering the dialysate (or opposite, depending on the concentration gradient) per unit of time.

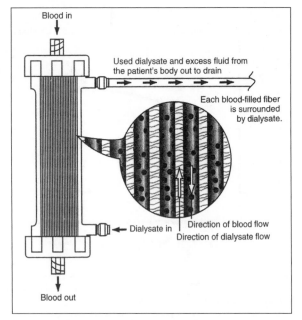

Figure 2.9. Counter current configuration of blood and dialysate.

Used with permission from Latham, C. (2006). Hemodialysis technology. In A. Molzahn & E. Butera, (Eds.), *Contemporary nephrology nursing: Principles and practice* (2nd ed., pp. 531-558). Pitman, NJ: American Nephrology Nurses' Association.

(3) The equation for net flux is measured from either blood side or dialysate side.
3. Factors affecting net flux.
   a. Membrane surface area: net flux generally increases as surface area increases.
   b. Permeability of membrane for a specific solute (molecular size or weight) or Ko. Net flux is generally higher for small molecules and lower for large molecules.
   c. Mean concentration gradient between blood and dialysate.
   d. Net flux is more rapid with large concentration gradients.
   e. Blood-dialysate flow configuration
      (1) Cocurrent or concurrent.
         (a) Blood and dialysate flow in the same direction from dialyzer inlet to outlet.
         (b) Concentration gradient and net flux decrease as blood and dialysate approach the outlet.
         (c) Recommended when optimal solute clearance is not desired or slower clearance is desired to prevent dialysis disequilibrium syndrome (DDS). (See Section E for further information about DDS.)
      (2) Countercurrent flow (see Figure 2.9).
         (a) Blood and dialysate flow in opposite directions.

(b) Maintains an optimal blood-dialysate concentration gradient (high net flux) throughout the dialyzer until blood and dialysate flows approach similar concentrations.
(c) Usually requires 1.5 to 2.0 times higher dialysate flow rate relative to blood flow rate to achieve maximum efficiency.
(d) The flow direction most commonly used; optimizes solute removal.
4. Mass balance: the amount of solute recovered on the dialysate side is equal to the amount of solute lost from the blood side.

C. Clearance.
   1. Expresses the performance of the dialyzer for solute removal. The amount of blood completely cleared of a solute per unit time, usually expressed as mL/min or L/min.
   2. Clearance is not dependent on the incoming blood solute concentration because this is the volume-cleared parameter (constant regardless of

Table 2.2

Formula for Clearance

$K = Qb[(Cbi-Cbo)/Cbi] + Qf(Cbo/Cbi)$
Where:
K = clearance of solute in mL/min
J = solute flux in mg/min
Qbi = blood flow rate into the dialyzer in mL/min
Qbo = blood flow rate leaving the dialyzer in mL/min
Cbi = solute concentration of blood entering the dialyzer in mg/mL
Cbo = solute concentration of blood leaving the dialyzer in mg/mL
Qf = ultrafiltration rate in mL/min
Qdi = dialysate flow rate into the dialyzer in mL/min
Qdo = dialysate flow rate leaving the dialyzer in mL/min
Cdi = solute concentration of dialysate entering the dialyzer in mL/min
Cdo = solute concentration of dialysate leaving the dialyzer in mL/min
Example:
Cbi BUN = 80 mg/dL or 0.8 mg/mL
Cbo BUN = 20 mg/dL or 0.2 mg/mL
Qf = 10 mL/min
Qbi = 300 mL/min
$K = 300[(0.8 - 0.2) / 0.8] + 10(0.2/0.8) = 227.5$ mL/min

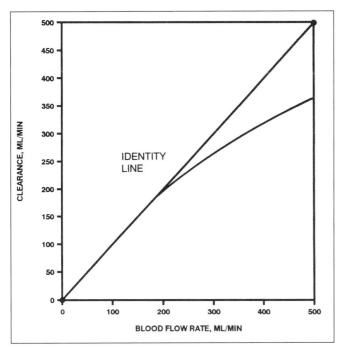

Figure 2.10. The relationship between blood flow (Qb) in mL/min and clearance in mL/min in a typical dialyzer. Clearance increases with blood flow; at some point it diverges from the identity line with Qb as a function of membrane permeability (Ko) and area (A).

Table 2.3

Formula for Dialysance

$D = Qbi[(Cbi - Cbo)/(Cbi - Cdi)] + Qf(Cbo/Cbi)$
Where:
D = dialysance in mL/min
Cbi, Cbo, Qf, etc.: see Table 2.2 (to the left)

incoming blood concentration) while net flux is the mass of solute removed per unit time and is dependent on the clearance-concentration product.

3. The efficiency of a hemodialyzer is largely dependent on its rate of diffusion (Rocco et al., 2006) (see Table 2.2).

4. Factors affecting clearance.
   a. Membrane permeability for a given solute and surface area, KoA (the efficiency of the dialyzer in removing urea).
   b. Blood flow rate: clearance is equal to blood flow rate up to some level at which clearance will be limited by KoA (see Figure 2.10).
   c. Dialysate flow rate and flow configuration.

D. Dialysance: "blood volume in milliliters per unit cleared of a substance by dialysis (as by an artificial kidney)" (http://www.merriam-webster.com/medical/dialysance). Can be used as an expression of dialyzer efficiency when solute concentration in the dialysate is not zero (such as recirculating dialysate systems (see Table 2.3).

E. The formula for dialysance cannot be used in sorbent dialysate systems (e.g., Redy®, Allient® or Nx Stage®) to assess actual effective clearance in recirculating systems; clearance is decreased because of the diminished blood-to-dialysate concentration gradient.

F. In single-pass dialysate systems, where dialysate concentration for many solutes is zero, clearance and dialysance are the same.

G. Factors effecting dialysance are similar to those affecting clearance.

H. Dialyzer specifications – manufacturers provide details regarding dialyzer membrane material, solute and ultrafiltration coefficient numbers, surface area, and clearance with each box of dialyzers purchased at their websites. Some examples are below.
   1. Fresenius – http://fmcna-dialyzers.com/dialyzers-site/products.html
   2. Baxter – http://www.baxter.com/healthcare_professionals/products/dialyzers.html
   3. Gambro – http://www.gambro.com/en/usa/Products/Hemodialysis/Dialyzers/Revaclear/?tab=other2Tab

IV. Fluid removal.

A. Process.
   1. Accomplished using hydrostatic or hydraulic pressures against the dialyzer membrane as well as osmosis.
   2. The body's water compartments consist of the intracellular fluid (cytoplasm) and extracellular fluid composed of blood plasma and fluid in the interstitial tissue (see Figure 2.11).
   3. These compartments exchange water and dissolved solutes (respiratory gases, nutrients, wastes, regulatory and immune defense molecules) using diffusion and other passive transport mechanisms through the semipermeable cell membranes and the cell layers that separate them.
   4. Regulating the composition of these different fluids in the different compartments is crucial to maintaining internal homeostasis.
   5. Dialysis occurs in the plasma (vascular or blood) fluid compartment.
   6. The disconnect of movement of fluid from the

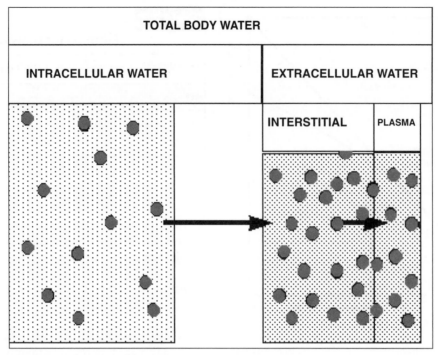

Figure 2.11. Body fluid compartments.

Source: Krane (1998). Retrieved from http://pedsccm.org/FILE-CABINET/Metab/DKA-CEdema.html#overhydration. Used with permission from Dr. Elliott Krane.

interstitial compartment into the blood compartment, as well as the speed of removal from the blood compartment, can cause the symptoms a patient may report during treatment such as muscle cramps, lightheadedness, hypotension, headache, or fatigue (see Figure 2.12).

7. Each patient has an identified target for fluid removal, also referred to as dry weight, ideal weight, estimated dry weight, or target weight. See Section D in this chapter for more extensive discussion.

B. Ultrafiltration or convective transport: the process by which plasma water is removed (expressed in mL/min, mL/hour, or L/hour) resulting from a pressure gradient between the blood and dialysate compartments. There are two types of pressure that may influence ultrafiltration.

1. Osmosis.
   a. The movement of water across a membrane permeable only to water.
   b. Water moves from an area of lesser solute concentration to an area of greater solute concentration to equalize the concentration between the components.

2. Osmotic pressure: the amount of pressure required to exactly oppose this water movement across the semipermeable membrane separating these two compartments with unequal solute concentrations.

3. Oncotic pressure.
   a. During dialysis, plasma proteins exert osmotic

pressure in the blood compartment and oppose water movement out of that compartment.
   b. Expressed as mmHg; usually exerts a relatively small effect during dialysis.

4. Hydraulic pressure.
   a. The actual pressure that forces water out of one compartment into another compartment.
   b. Expressed as mmHg.

5. Ultrafiltration (see Figure 2.13).
   a. The result of net transmembrane pressure (TMP) in the dialyzer.

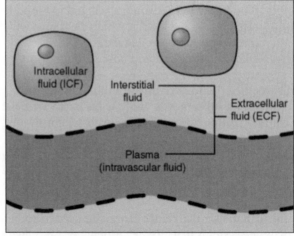

Figure 2.12. Major fluid compartments.

Used with permission from what-when-how, In-Depth Tutorials and Information; http://what-when-how.com/nursing/fluid-and-electrolyte-balance-structure-and-function-nursing-part-1

Table 2.4

Formula for Mean Transmembrane Pressure (TMP)

TMP = [Pbi + Pbo)/2] – [Pdi + Pdo)/2]
Where:
TMP = transmembrane pressure in mmHg
Pbi = inlet blood compartment pressure in mmHg
Pbo = outlet blood compartment pressure in mmHg
Pdi = inlet dialysate compartment pressure in mmHg
Pdo = outlet dialysate compartment pressure in mmHg

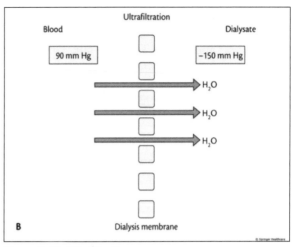

Figure 2.13. Ultrafiltration.

Used with permission from Merck Medicus Springer Healthcare.

b. Moves plasma water from the blood compartment to the dialysate compartment because of the net pressure gradient across the membrane (see Table 2.4).

6. Blood compartment pressure decreases from the inlet to the outlet side of the dialyzer with the typical blood circuit configuration.

7. Dialysate compartment pressure decreases from the inlet side to the outlet side of the dialyzer.
   a. With negative pressure or pulling effect in the compartment, absolute pressure is lower; that is, more negative at Pdo (outlet dialysate compartment in mmHg) than Pdi (inlet dialysate compartment pressure in mmHg).
   b. The same relationship holds with positive pressure or a pushing effect on the dialysate.

8. Can be accomplished with either positive pressure on the blood compartment, negative pressure on the dialysate compartment, or some combination of both; the rate per mmHg is the same in a given dialyzer, independent of the approach used.

9. Backfiltration: the movement of fluid from the dialysate side to the blood side; occurs more commonly with high efficiency/high flux dialyzers (Ford, Ward & Cheung, 2009). Cellulose versus synthetic type dialyzer membranes are associated with backfiltration (Hoenich, 2008).
   a. Backfiltration can occur in situations where the patient has minimal fluid gain/goal for fluid removal and thus low TMP, so pressure on the blood side is lower than dialysate side (Latham, 2006).
   b. *Safety alert.* Risks of backfiltration: the movement of contaminants, endotoxins, and/or fluid into the patient's bloodstream. Long-term exposure to low levels of endotoxin have been implicated in inflammatory responses (Ford, Ward & Cheung, 2009). Backfiltration may prevent reaching the desired UF goal.

10. Factors affecting ultrafiltration.
    a. Transmembrane pressure (TMP), venous resistance plus negative pressure (Hanson, n.d. http://www.hdcn.com/symp/09nant/content/09nant_han/flash/09nant_han.pdf).
    b. Membrane water permeability.
    c. Dialyzer surface area may be decreased with thrombus formation within the dialyzer header or the individual fibers.

11. The ultrafiltration coefficient (KUF in mL/hr/mmHg).
    a. A dialyzer characteristic that expresses relative efficiency of water removal; reflects membrane water permeability and surface area (see Figure 2.14).
    b. TMP is calculated for the length of time ultrafiltration will be done using the known or estimated KUF of the dialyzer.

12. TMP calculation.
    a. UF goal/Number of hours of treatment=UF volume in mL/hour.
       UF volume per hour/UF coefficient of dialyzer (KUF)=TMP (Hanson, n.d., http://www.hdcn.com/symp/09nant/content/09nant_han/flash/09nant_han.pdf).
    b. Example: UF goal 4000 mL/ 4 hours = 1000 mL/hour.
       UF volume per hour 1000/ KUF 50 = TMP 20.
    c. Limitations of formula.
       (1) KUF decreases progressively through the treatment, being maximum in the early period of HD.
       (2) The formula provides no regard for the contribution of oncotic pressure that varies from patient to patient and even within the same patient at different times in the HD treatment (Pedrini, 2011, http://ndt.oxfordjournals.org/content/early/2011/02/18/ndt.gfq795.full).
       (3) Underscores the advantages of using

volumetric HD equipment that measures UF removed and adjusts TMP/UF rate accordingly.

V. Components of a hemodialysis system (see Figure 2.15).

A hemodialysis system consists of the patient's vascular access and the disposable, extracorporeal (blood) circuit that is the dialyzer, blood tubing, blood pump, arterial/venous alarms, and air detector alarm.

The second part of the system is the dialysate circuit composed of the mixing and delivery system within the dialysis machine, the dialysate solution, transmembrane/ ultrafiltration chambers, dialysate heater, conductivity and temperature alarms (Latham, 2006).

Some machine models may have built-in extra features (e.g., automated blood pressure monitoring, fluid and sodium profiling, online clearance, access blood flow testing, and site-of-care charting). Home HD machine models may include a blood loss sensor to detect needle dislodgement or machine parameters telemonitoring (see Figure 2.16).

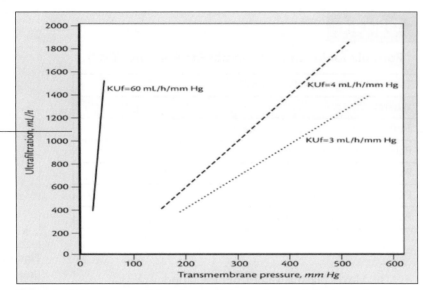

Figure 2.14. Water permeability of a membrane and control of volumetric ultrafiltration in hemodialysis.

Used with permission from Merck Medicus Springer Healthcare.

A. Blood pump.
   1. Pumps blood from the patient's vascular access and through the tubing and dialyzer (extracorporeal circuit).
      a. Resistance in vascular access (needles, arteriovenous fistulae or grafts, or central vein catheters).
      b. Resistance in the extracorporeal circuit is high and prevents passive flow.

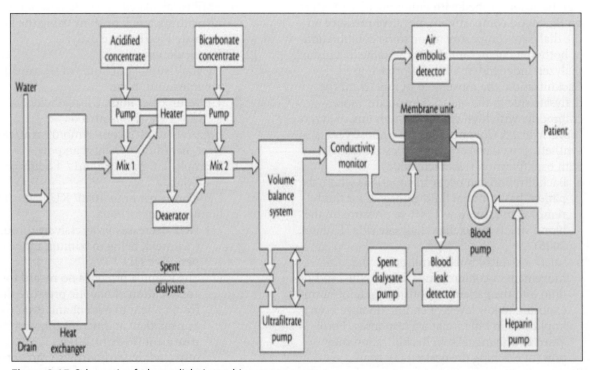

Figure 2.15. Schematic of a hemodialysis machine components.

Used with permission from Merck Medicus Springer Healthcare.

2. Two or more rollers rotate in a closed compartment that compresses the blood pump tubing segment against an enclosed semicircular pump housing wall.
   a. Rollers are self-occluding in most equipment to provide the appropriate compression against the housing to deliver an accurate blood flow rate through the dialyzer.
   b. Pump calibration is checked periodically to assure stable and accurate blood flow rates.
   c. Calibration for the blood tubing is critical to ensure accurate measurement and delivery of blood flow. *Note*: some dialysis machines display the size in mm for which the pump is calibrated. Tubing segment size varies by manufacturer as well as patient population, adult vs. pediatric patients.
3. Factors affecting blood pump functioning.
   a. There must be no extraneous high resistance to flow of blood through blood tubing and dialyzer.
   b. If obstruction exists inside the dialyzer or between the blood outlet of the dialyzer and patient (e.g., dialyzer clotting, venous drip chamber clotting, kinked lines), pressure will increase inside the dialyzer and increase blood compartment pressure. If the pressure exceeds roller occlusion tolerance (+300 to +400 mmHg), retrograde flow across the rollers may occur and decrease effective stroke volume per revolution and, therefore, the blood flow rate.
   c. If obstruction exists between the circulatory access site and the pump (e.g., kinked line, clotted access needle, or catheter), the arterial blood compartment pressure (up to the blood pump) will decrease (become more negative) and exceed maximum specified pressure value.
      (1) High negative pressure may cause a pressure alarm or arterial bloodline collapse or cavitation as a consequence of insufficient flow into the blood pump, decrease stroke volume per roller revolution, and thus diminish effective blood flow rate through the dialyzer.
      (2) If negative pressure is high enough (equal to or greater than -250 mmHg at the needle), subclinical hemolysis may result.
      (3) Blood pump should be stopped until problem(s) is/are corrected.
      (4) *Safety alert.* Always check the patient and vascular access, blood lines for any kinks, and connections when responding to an arterial or venous pressure alarm.

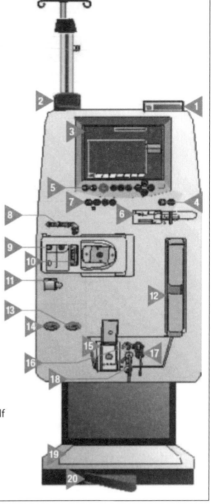

Phoenix System at a Glance

1 Card reader
2 Visual Alarm Indicator
3 Display Screen
4 Heparin Control Panel
5 Main Control Panel
6 Heparin Syringe Holder
7 Blood Pump Control Panel
8 4 Position Line Clamps
9 Pressure Sensors
10 Blood Pump Cover and Latch
11 Air Bubble Detector and Patient Sensor
12 BiCart® Cartridge Holder
13 Arterial Line Clamp/Clip
14 Venous Line Clamp
15 Waste Handling Option Device (WHO)
16 Acid/Acetator Connector
17 Bicarbonate Connector
18 Chemical Connector
19 Concentrate Container Shelf
20 Locking Brake

Figure 2.16. Phoenix system at a glance.
Used with permission from Gambro.

B. Dialyzer.
   1. Description.
      a. Blood and dialysate compartments are discrete areas of the dialyzer and are completely separated by the semipermeable membrane.
      b. The blood contains excess quantities of specific solutes (e.g., metabolic waste products and some electrolytes) and inadequate concentrations of other physiologic solutes (e.g., bicarbonate and calcium).
      c. The dialysate is free of metabolic waste products and generally has a lesser concentration of some electrolytes (e.g., K^+, Mg^{++}) than the blood, although Na^+, HCO_3^- (or acetate), and Ca^{++} content may be higher.
      d. Solutes, electrolytes, and water will cross the semipermeable membrane as a consequence of diffusion and convection according to concentration and hydraulic pressure gradients.
   2. Types of membrane composition (see Table 2.5).

Table 2.5

Dialyzer Membrane Polymers

Membrane Type	Material
Cellulosic	
	Cuprammonium cellulose (Cuprophan®)
	Cuprammonium rayon
	Modified cellulose acetate
	Saponified cellulose ester
	Regenerated cellulose
Modified	
Substituted with acetate	Cellulose diacetate (CA, CDA)
	Cellulose triacetate (CTA)
Cellulosynthetic	DEAE-substituted cellulose and cellulose (Hemophan®)
Coated	Cuprammonium rayon coated with polyethylene glycol (PEG)
	Regenerated cellulose coated with vitamin E
Synthetic	
	Polyacrylonitrile and methacrylate (PAN)
	Polyacrylonitrile and methallyl sulfonate (AN-69®)
	Polyamide, polyarylethersulfone, and polyvinylpyrrolidone (Polyflux)
	Polycarbonate
	Polyethylene polyvinyl alcohol (EVAL)
	Polymethylmethacrylate (PMMA)
	Polysulfone (PS)

Latham, C. (2006). Hemodialysis technology. In A. Molzahn & E. Butera, (Eds.), *Contemporary nephrology nursing: Principles and practice* (2nd ed., pp. 531-558). Pitman, NJ: American Nephrology Nurses' Association.

a. Cellulose.
   (1) Treated by cuprammonium process (Cuprophane®) with or without various agents (e.g., cellulose acetate [CA]; saponified cellulose ester [SCE]); considered symmetric membranes because inside and outside of the membrane looks the same.
   (2) Material induces leukopenia and complement activation (i.e., inflammatory response to membrane material) during dialysis when membrane is new; described as not biocompatible.
b. Modified cellulosic membranes (e.g., cellulose triacetate).
   (1) Generally produced in hollow fiber configuration.
   (2) Induces milder inflammatory response and considered more biocompatible than cellulose.
c. Synthetic membranes include polyacrylonitrile (PAN), and polysulfone (PSF),

polymethylmethacrylate (PMMA), polycarbonate, polyamide.
   (1) Some were made in flat sheets, but primarily used in hollow fiber devices.
   (2) Asymmetric membrane with the thin permeable skin on the blood contacting surface with a thick supporting structure around its skin.
   (3) Described as biocompatible; induces less leukopenia and/or complement activation even when the membrane is new.
3. Factors affecting dialyzer performance.
   a. Dialyzing membrane surface area: the larger the surface area of a given membrane, generally the greater the clearance and ultrafiltration.
   b. Pore size or permeability: pores in the membrane must be large enough to permit uremic toxins, electrolytes, and water to pass through with ease, but small enough to prevent passage of blood cells, proteins, bacteria, endotoxin, and viruses.

c. Pore size distribution: large population of larger pores gives higher clearance of larger solutes; water permeability is less affected by pore size and distribution.

d. Ultrafiltration coefficient and ultrafiltration predictability: ideally predictable and consistent with each treatment.

e. Compliance: the volume of the dialyzer should remain small and relatively constant with changes in TMP as found in fixed geometry dialyzers such as hollow fibers; more compliance is seen in flat plate dialyzers.

f. Blood leak rate/blood recovery: should be negligible and the dialyzer should allow for almost complete return of blood to the patient at the end of dialysis.

g. Resistance to clotting: dialyzer should allow for minimal anticoagulation without resulting in thrombus formation and loss of dialyzer efficiency.

h. Biocompatibility: membrane should be biocompatible (i.e., elicits only mild inflammatory response) (see Section E).

4. Dialyzer configurations. Hollow fiber dialyzer: design most commonly used in the United States (refer to Figure 2.3).

a. Design: Thousands of hollow fibers of cellulosic or synthetic membrane are embedded at each end in potting material; the entire bundle with potting material is encased in hard clear plastic jacket.

b. Flow geometry is generally counter current to optimize clearance; blood flows through the hollow fibers while dialysate flows counter current along the outside of the fibers.

c. Compliance is very small; does not increase with increasing blood flow rate or dialysate pressure.

d. Ultrafiltration is achieved by applying negative pressure to dialysate compartment, positive pressure to the blood compartment, or some combination of both.

5. Categories of dialyzers.

a. Conventional dialyzers.
   (1) Smallest surface area.
   (2) Low KUF.
   (3) Efficient low-molecular-weight clearance up to 5000 daltons.
   (4) Longer treatment time may be needed to achieve adequate dialysis, i.e., clearances and ultrafiltration.
   (5) Membrane material is usually cellulose.

b. High-efficiency dialyzers.
   (1) Larger surface area.
   (2) Medium KUF.
   (3) Efficient low-molecular-weight clearance up to 5000 daltons.

   (4) Membrane material can be modified cellulose or synthetic.

c. High-flux dialyzers.
   (1) Medium to large surface area.
   (2) High KUF.
   (3) High molecular weight cutoffs up to 15,000 daltons.
   (4) Membrane material is synthetic and more biocompatible than other types of membranes.
   (5) Requires use of volumetric ultrafiltration control systems.

C. UF (Ultrafiltration) profile: Volumetric or programmable fluid removal, also known as ultrafiltration (UF) profile, is available on most dialysis machines. Rather than the UF rate remaining the same throughout the treatment, the rate can be set using various patterns such as higher during the beginning of the treatment, and lower toward the end of the treatment, or alternating between low and high UF rates to stabilize the patient and allow for capillary refill and maximum fluid removal (see Figure 2.17).

1. Advantages may include:
   a. Decreased signs and symptoms related to hypovolemia.
   b. Period of plasma filling and refilling.
   c. Achievement of target weight.

2. Allows fluid removal at times when the fluid is more readily available determined by observing the patient and reviewing patient data. A profile would be selected based on when the patient becomes symptomatic, comorbidities, and cardiovascular status.

3. Disadvantages: While an individual profile may seem to emerge, caution must be used as this can vary among HD treatments. This may lead to incorrect fluid removal, i.e. hypovolemia or hypervolemia posttreatment.

4. Factors influencing this profile include, but are not limited to:
   a. Extracellular fluid (ECF) osmolarity related to albumin levels.
   b. Sodium level.
   c. Glucose level.
   d. Tissue hydration.
   e. Medication.
   f. Changes in lean body mass.
   g. Patient comorbidities and cardiovascular status.

5. UF profile that uses intermittently high UF rates may not be tolerated by some patients in that it may cause compensatory vasoconstriction, exhausting the patient and promoting postdialysis fatigue. High UF rates promoted pronounced decrease in blood volume and a high incidence of unwanted side effects (Donauer, Kolbin, Bek, Krause & Bohler, 2000).

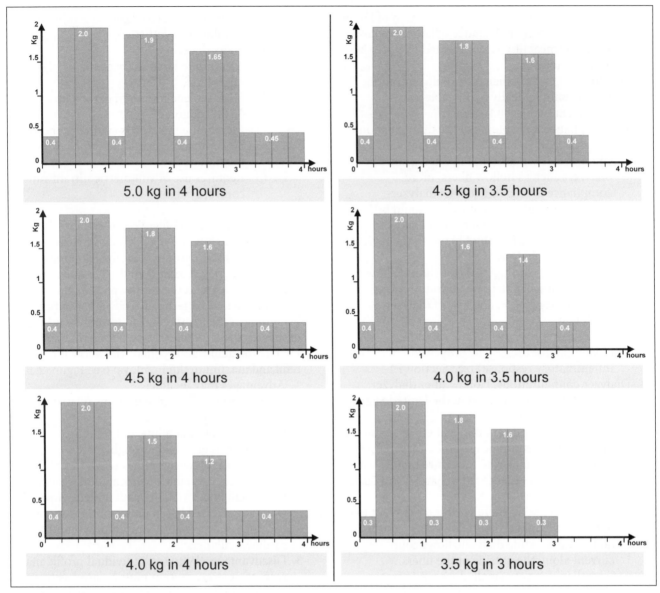

Figure. 2.17. Phoenix sample UF profiles.

Used with permission from Gambro.

6. Sequential UF Profile (also known as Isolated UF or pure ultrafiltration). (See Section D,V.I.4, for more information about this technique.)
   a. A program that uses transmembrane and venous pressures to remove fluid only.
   b. Dialysate is not delivered to the dialyzer.
   c. The intent is easier fluid removal when electrolytes are not being removed simultaneously, but less effectively than during diffusive clearance as occurs during hemodialysis.
   d. It can be used in conjunction with an HD treatment or as an extra treatment when extra fluid removal is the only goal (e.g., an acute episode of heart failure or after a procedure that requires intravenous fluids that would need to be removed). See Fresenius 2008K2

Hemodialysis Machine Operator's Manual for an example of this option at: http://fmcna.com/fmcna/idcplg?IdcService=GET_FILE&allowInterrupt=1&RevisionSelectionMethod=LatestReleased&Rendition=Primary&dDocName=PDF_100050219
   e. Disadvantages.
      (1) Clearance via diffusion does not take place as there is no circulating dialysate.
      (2) Patients may complain of feeling cold since there is no dialysate, hence no exposure to temperature control.
      (3) *Safety alert.* Observe for rebound hyperkalemia.
      (4) May have a high UFR that may not be tolerated by patients with cardiovascular issues.

D. Dialysate delivery system.
   1. Proportioning system (see Figure 2.18).
      a. Definition: a system that mechanically mixes an appropriate amount of water and concentrate to achieve physiologic dialysate composition. Dialysate flow rates range from 300 to 1000 mL/min.
      b. Types of systems.
         (1) A fixed proportioning ratio of water to concentrate.
         (2) A feedback control system that automatically proportions an amount of concentrate relative to water to achieve the desired dialysate composition and conductivity.
      c. With bicarbonate dialysate, two concentrate streams are proportioned to achieve the desired buffer concentration.
      d. Central proportioning unit is a large stationary unit (holding tank) that mixes, heats, monitors, and delivers dialysate for multiple stations or dialyzers at the desired individual flow rate.
         (1) Each station or dialyzer has a unit that may control dialysate flow rate, independently monitor the blood compartment parameters, and provide ultrafiltration capability.
         (2) Advantages: cost and labor efficient, and offers consistent dialysate preparation and monitoring dialysate for multiple patients.
         (3) Disadvantages.
            (a) Equipment failure may disable treatment for all patients.
            (b) Malfunction may deliver unsuitable dialysate to a number of patients.
            (c) No flexibility in electrolyte composition in dialysate unless there is more than one tank present with corresponding portals at dialysis stations.
      e. Individual proportioning unit is a device within the dialysis machine that mixes, heats, monitors, and delivers dialysate for an individual machine.
         (1) Dialysate is prepared by using a container of commercially prepared or manually mixed electrolyte solution.
         (2) Requires electrical and water source with adequate pressure and appropriate drain for spent dialysate.
         (3) Monitors dialysate functions and monitors blood compartment parameters and may incorporate a blood pump and heparin pump.
         (4) Advantages: can individualize dialysate composition; rapid setup and production of suitable dialysate; easy to replace if equipment fails.

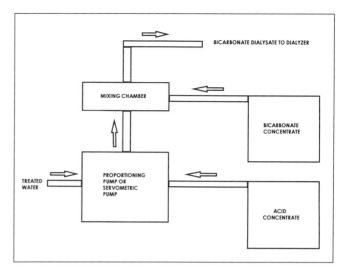

Figure 2.18. Single proportioning system.

         (5) Disadvantage: more equipment to maintain; cost for dialysate and labor.
   2. Regenerative system.
      a. Definition: the use of sorbents packed in a multilayer cartridge to purify and regenerate a constant recirculating volume of dialysate. Used dialysate exiting the dialyzer is filtered through the sorbent material and routed back as new dialysate (see Figure 2.19).
      b. The binding capacity and specificity of the sorbents used will determine the type and amount of uremic solutes and electrolytes removed from the patient and adsorbed by the cartridge.
         (1) Urease, an enzyme, is used to adsorb and degrade urea to ammonium for absorption

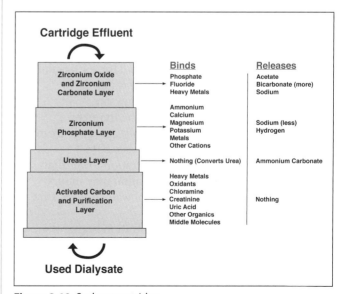

Figure 2.19. Sorbent cartridge.

Used with permission from Medscape, Ash, S.R. (2008). Sorbent dialysis systems: An expert commentary; http://www.medscape.com/viewarticle/576534

by zirconium; produces bicarbonate as a result of the process.

(2) Activated carbon layer that protects the urease from trace metal contamination and chlorine, chloramines, bleach, or solutions used to disinfect the system.

(3) Zirconium phosphate acts as a cation exchanger, while zirconium oxide functions as an anion exchanger and removes phosphate.

(4) Activated charcoal adsorbs nonionic organic solutes, such as creatinine, uric acid, phenols, and other large molecules.

(5) This system is not currently available and is apparently being redesigned by Fresenius as the PAK, for use as a portable dialysis system (http://www.nocturnaldialysis .org/technology_whats_coming.htm) (Agar, 2012).

   c. Advantages: small water requirement for dialysate preparation; does not require water pretreatment; small and portable.

   d. Disadvantages: low efficiency because of the dialysate flow rate of 250 to 300 mL/min; may have an initial drop in dialysate pH; because calcium, magnesium, and potassium are removed, must reinfuse at least calcium and magnesium into the dialysate reservoir using an infusion pump.

3. Portable dialysis equipment: NxStage System One uses one of two systems for dialysate.

   a. Premixed bagged dialysate, or

   b. The Pureflow Purification Pak converts tap or source water to AAMI quality water that is mixed with electrolytes in the Dialysate Sak to generate dialysate (see Figures 2.20, 2.21, and 2.22).

E. Dialysate composition.

1. Sodium.

   a. Major cation of dialysate and the extracellular compartment of total body water.

   b. The range of physiologic dialysate concentration may vary. The frequent concentrations used in dialysate range from 135 to145 mEq/L (Daugirdas, 2014).

   c. Dialysate sodium concentration lower than plasma sodium concentration may induce intracellular movement of water and plasma volume depletion.

   d. Dialysate sodium concentration higher than plasma sodium concentration may induce extracellular movement of water, intracellular dehydration, and stimulation of thirst (Daugirdas, 2014).

   e. The objective in dialysis is to achieve euvolemic status and normal body sodium content at the

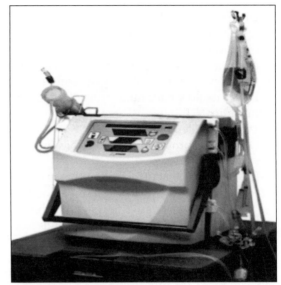

Figure 2.20. Nx Stage System One.
Used with permission from NxStage.

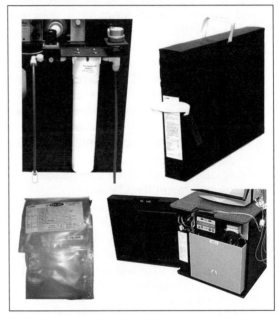

Figure 2.21. Purefow SL Components.
Used with permission from NxStage.

end of the treatment. The sodium concentration required to accomplish this objective may vary depending on salt and water intake or loss during dialysis.

(1) More than 80% of sodium removal is convective with current HD practices and only 15 to 20% is diffusive.

(2) It is estimated that more than three-fourths of patients on conventional HD undergo dialysis with a dialysate sodium concentration above their "set point" (Santos & Peixoto, 2008).

   f. Sodium modeling during dialysis.

(1) Various profiles (e.g., step, linear,

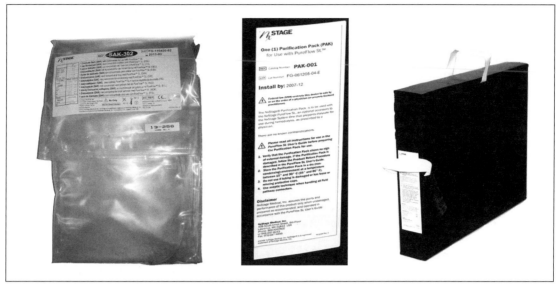

Figure 2.22. Dialysate Sak and Purification Pak.
Used with permission from NxStage.

exponential) have been used to reduce the incidence of intradialytic hypotension in some patients. These profiles deliver a higher sodium at the beginning of dialysis and end at a selected range usually 135 to 140 mEq/l. The net result, regardless of profile used, is a high "time averaged" dialysate sodium concentration in the 140 to 145 mEq/L range (Sergio & Peixoto, 2008). See Fresenius 2008K2 Hemodialysis Machine Operator's Manual at http://fmcna.com/fmcna/idcplg?IdcService =GET_FILE&allowInterrupt=1&RevisionS electionMethod=LatestReleased&Renditio n=Primary&dDocName=PDF_100050219

(2) Higher dialysate sodium or sodium profiles should be avoided due to the increase in extracellular osmolality stimulating thirst, increasing water intake, and increasing inter-dialytic weight gains, especially in patients with poor residual kidney function (RKF).

(3) The NKF-KDOQI Clinical Practice Guidelines for Adequacy recommend that high dialysate sodium concentrations and sodium profiling be avoided. Dietary restriction of sodium and adequate management of ultrafiltration during treatment should be employed to facilitate achieving the patient's true dry weight (NKF 2006a, http://www2.kidney.org/ professionals/KDOQI/guideline_upHD_P D_VA/hd_guide5.htm).

(4) If using a sodium profiling program, evaluate the patient for a change in serum sodium.

(5) Conductivity readings can be used to calculate delivered sodium during dialysis; for instance, a conductivity reading of 13.8 m/cm is roughly equivalent to a sodium of 138.

2. Potassium.
   a. Major intracellular cation in the body.
   b. Dialysate concentration varies from 0 to 4 mEq/L, depending on the need to decrease serum potassium level.
      (1) There are associated risks, particularly when potassium levels are reduced rapidly, due to its effect on the QT interval when dialyzing a patient against a zero or 1 mEq potassium bath (Palmer, 2009).
      (2) *Safety alert*. Zero to 1 mEq potassium bath should only be considered with safety measures in place such as cardiac monitoring or in an intensive patient monitoring environment, even if only used for part of the HD treatment.
   c. Low dialysate potassium concentration has been associated with cardiac dysrhythmias, especially in patients receiving digitalis preparations.
   d. Rapid potassium removal during dialysis is more likely to produce dysrhythmias than total amount removed.
   e. Clinical consequence of low postdialysis serum potassium is not certain, but it may contribute to postdialysis fatigue and muscle cramps.
   f. Studies have associated higher prepotassium levels of 4.6–5.3 mEq/L with better survival. Patients with predialysis potassium levels of

less than 4.0 or greater than 5.6 mEq/L were associated with increased mortality (Palmer, 2009).

3. Magnesium.
   a. An abundant intracellular cation.
   b. Dialysate concentration may vary from 0.5 to 1 mEq/L (Henrich, 2009; Daugirdas, 2014).

4. Calcium.
   a. Concentration varies from 2.5 to 3.0 mEq/L. (Daugirdas, 2014).
   b. Patient lab results parameters to maintain, decrease, or increase calcium levels and medications used should be considered, as ordered by physician/APRN/PA or per facility protocol.
   c. Normal values for serum calcium is 8.4 to 10.2 mg/dL. (Check the lab's specific parameters.)
   d. Medications influencing calcium levels.
      (1) Use of calcium-containing phosphate binders and active vitamin D sterols has led some clinicians to lower dialysate calcium concentration to decrease the calcium load.
      (2) As an alternative, noncalcium containing phosphate binders and/or a calcimimetic agent, such as cinacalcet hydrochloride, may be prescribed to maintain a serum calcium level within target range. See KDOQI Clinical Practice Guidelines for Bone Metabolism and Disease in Chronic Kidney Disease, Guideline 9 (NKF, 2002 http://www2.kidney.org/professionals/KDOQI/guidelines_bone/).

5. Chloride.
   a. Dialysate contains combinations of sodium chloride, potassium chloride, and calcium chloride, and the actual concentration of the various combinations will vary depending on the specific concentration formulations and anion concentrations.
   b. Total dialysate concentration will be in the range of 95 to 105 mEq/L.

6. Glucose.
   a. Glucose is usually added to prevent loss of sizable amounts of glucose. This may be particularly problematic in the patient with diabetes and/or the patient who is fasting.
   b. When present, dialysate glucose concentration ranges from 100 to 250 mg/dL.

7. Buffer.
   a. The most frequent buffer used for acid-base correction for patients on chronic hemodialysis in the United States is bicarbonate; concentrations range from 25 to 40 mEq/L (Schulman, 2008).
   b. Bicarbonate concentration is ordered based on the individualized patient's serum CO_2 level and comorbidities. Normal concentration is in the range of 22 to 29 mEq/L. For patients on HD, the target serum bicarb is around 22 mEq/L predialysis.
   c. If acetate is used as the buffer, concentrations range from 29 to 39 mEq/L.
   d. Acetate requires metabolic activities (the citric acid cycle) to take up a hydrogen ion, thereby repleting body buffer stores.
      (1) The conversion of acetate to bicarbonate occurs in the liver.
      (2) Acetate use is associated with hemodynamic instability and hypotension (Palmer, 2009).
   e. Bicarbonate is a more physiologic buffer, thought to be associated with fewer symptoms and better tolerance than acetate to ultrafiltration during dialysis.
   f. Bicarbonate is available in liquid or powder form that is reconstituted before use.
   g. High dialysate bicarbonate concentrations increase the likelihood of precipitate formation and delivery system malfunction.
   h. Dilute acetic acid or sodium hypochlorite may be used to remove precipitates from the flow path during dialysis equipment cleaning.
   i. *Safety alert.*
      (1) Bicarbonate is more susceptible to bacterial growth because, unlike acetate, the concentrate is not bacteriostatic or bactericidal.
      (2) Bicarbonate is not stable; reconstituted bicarbonate in an open container loses carbon dioxide and solution buffer becomes carbonate (Palmer, 2009; Ward, 2008).

F. Special features – HD machine design has progressed dramatically with the availability of smaller and less costly computerization of electric circuits. The resurgence of home HD therapies has paved the way to improve delivery systems.
   1. Automatic blood pressure monitoring.
      a. BP monitors integrated into the HD machine.
      b. Manually set for readings frequency.
      c. Set high and low BP limits for alarm conditions.
   2. Blood volume monitoring (BVM).
      a. A noninvasive monitor, sometimes integrated into the dialysis machine, that uses a sensor on the arterial blood line chamber.
      b. Uses light or ultrasound to determine blood dilution and thereby blood volume changes during UF.
      c. Produces a wave form on a monitoring screen used to assess accessibility of fluid to be removed, tolerance to UFR, and blood volume changes. Some monitors incorporate pulse

oximetry (pulse ox), access flow, and hematocrit in real-time readings.
   d. A method to determine plasma volume refill. For more information on how to interpret BVM go to http://www.slideshare.net/ringer21/section-2-theory-critline-iii-tqa (Hema-Metrics, 2006). Also see Section D of this chapter for further information.
3. Continuous dialysate monitoring.
   a. Samples of spent dialysate are analyzed in real time.
   b. Determines effectiveness of dialysis, or for precise management of electrolyte and fluid balance.
4. Incorporated site of care computerized charting networks systems.
   a. Integrated into the dialysis machine or stand-alone computer.
   b. Records machine and BP pressure readings, patient observations, standing orders, etc.
   c. Transfers the information to a larger database for record keeping, billing and research.
5. Remote monitoring systems.
   a. Allows for transfer of patient and machine data to a different location for patients who do nocturnal or daily hemodialysis regimens at home.
   b. Allows one provider to oversee several patients in various locations.
6. Blood loss sensors for detection of blood spills.
   a. Used to prevent or detect blood line dislodgement. Can be used for patients on home dialysis or in-center facilities in high risk groups (e.g., patients with dementia or who are restless) (ANNA, n.d., http://www.annanurse.org/resources/venous-needle-dislodgement).
   b. Blood loss sensors can be attached at the juncture of the bloodlines and fistula needles or near the access site.
   c. Sensors work by setting off an alarm for patient or staff members to correct problem or by bluetooth technology that sends signal to machine and clamps venous line and stops blood pump (http://www.news-medical.net/news/20130211/WetAlert-wireless-wetness-detector-from-Fresenius-Medical-Care.aspx).
   d. Useful for patients doing home nocturnal treatments or in patients at risk for needle dislodgement.

VI. Hemodialysis machines monitoring systems
(Gomez, 2011).

A. *Safety alert.*
   1. Ensure that all required HD monitoring systems are placed in the test mode and pass the required safety checks before every HD treatment.

   2. It is imperative that the venous bloodline is placed in the line clamp between the dialyzer and the patient. This ensures the line will be clamped in an alarm condition to protect the patient from potential injury.
B. Blood compartment of the extracorporeal circuit.
   1. Prepump arterial pressure.
      a. Measured in the blood circuit between the patient and the blood pump (prepump). The pressure reading will be negative, or below zero.
      b. Pressure (mmHg) is read on a gauge, meter, light emitting diode (LED), or video screen.
      c. Upper and lower limits may be manually set or set automatically by the equipment or user.
      d. Excursions above or below limits will activate an audible and visual alarm, stop the blood pump, and require user intervention; there will be a temporary cessation of UF until the alarm condition is corrected.
      e. Lower limit of pressure monitor should not exceed -250 mmHg because of possible hemolysis from high vacuum pressure.
      f. Pressure will generally decrease (become more negative) during dialysis with ultrafiltration because of increasing blood viscosity (increasing hematocrit) and/or decreasing cardiac output with plasma volume reduction. Given the same needle gauge, pressure will be lower (more negative) with higher hematocrit and higher blood flow rates.
      g. Conditions causing alarm.
         (1) Low alarm (more negative).
            (a) Hypotension or vasoconstriction.
            (b) Occlusion or insufficiency in arterial supply from the vascular access.
            (c) Compression or kinking of the bloodline between the patient and the arterial monitoring site.
            (d) Malposition or infiltration of the arterial fistula needle.
            (e) Blood pump set at a rate exceeding that which the vascular access can supply, i.e., the pump speed is greater than the access flow rate.
            (f) "Flooding" the transducer monitor or monitoring line so that pressures are not accurately measured.
            (g) Failure to unclamp the monitoring line.
         (2) High alarm (less negative).
            (a) If upper limit is set at some point below zero, separation of the bloodline will cause the pressure to return to zero and activate the high limit alarm.
            (b) Any air leak between the patient and the monitoring site, such as with the

saline infusion line; because pressure is generally negative in this segment, air will be pulled into the circuit and pressure will move toward zero.

 (c) Decrease in blood pump speed.

2. Postpump or predialyzer arterial pressure.
 a. Pressure is measured between the blood pump and the dialyzer. The pressure reading is positive, or above zero.
 b. Readout is in the form of gauge, meter, LED, or video screen in mmHg.
 c. Upper and lower limits may be manually or automatically set by the equipment or user.
 d. Excursions above or below the set limits will activate an audible and visual alarm, stop the blood pump, and require user intervention. In some equipment there will be a temporary cessation of ultrafiltration until alarm condition is corrected.
 e. Primary utility is to monitor clotting in the dialyzer.
 f. Pressure will generally increase during dialysis with ultrafiltration because of increasing blood viscosity. Under some clinical circumstances, such as high hematocrit and/or high blood flow rates, high pressures may be observed (greater than 400 mmHg).
 g. Conditions causing alarm (Gomez, 2011, pp 132-138).
  (1) Low alarm.
   (a) Line separation between monitoring point and downstream circuit to the patient; any leak in this segment of the extracorporeal circuit; because pressure is positive in this segment, blood will leak from this site; lower limit should be set above zero.
   (b) Occlusion in the bloodline between the blood pump and the monitoring site.
   (c) Decrease in blood pump speed.
  (2) High alarm.
   (a) Kink in bloodline between the monitoring site and patient.
   (b) Malposition or infiltration of the venous fistula needle.
   (c) Increase in blood pump speed.
   (d) Clotting in the dialyzer.

3. Venous pressure in the extracorporeal circuit.
 a. Measures pressure and integrity of the extracorporeal circuit from the monitoring site to the venous return to the patient (access).
 b. Readout is in the form of a gauge, meter, LED, or video screen, in mmHg.
 c. Upper and lower limits are manually set or automatically set by the equipment or user.
 d. Excursions above or below the set limits will activate an audible and visual alarm, stop the

blood pump, and require user intervention. In some equipment, there will be a temporary cessation of ultrafiltration until the alarm condition is corrected.
 e. Pressure will generally be greater than zero or positive.
 f. Pressure will generally increase during dialysis with ultrafiltration because of increasing blood viscosity.
 g. Given the same needle gauge, higher pressure will be seen with higher hematocrit or higher blood flow rate.
 h. Initial high pressures may be associated with early access failure due to venous stenosis.
 i. Conditions causing an alarm.
  (1) Low alarm.
   (a) Separation of bloodline from venous fistula needle; leak in this segment of the extracorporeal circuit; because pressure is generally positive in this segment, blood will leak from the site. *Safety alert.* This can be a life-threatening situation if the leak is not detected promptly! Ensure all connections are secure. The vascular access site must be exposed and visible at all times!
   (b) Decrease in blood pump speed.
   (c) Occlusion in bloodline between dialyzer and monitoring site.
   (d) A severely clotted dialyzer may decrease pressure sufficient to trigger low alarm.
   (e) "Flooding" or "wetting" the transducer monitor or monitor line with saline or blood, causing inaccurate low pressure reading.
   (f) Failure to unclamp the monitor line.
  (2) High alarm.
   (a) Occlusion or obstruction in bloodline between the monitoring site and the patient.
   (b) Malposition or infiltration of the venous needle.
   (c) Embolus (sufficient in size to completely or partially occlude the bloodline, fistula needle, or catheter) from dialyzer or venous drip chamber into downstream bloodline.

4. Air detector.
 a. Detects air bubbles and foam in the venous bloodline by change in light transmission to a photoelectric cell or ultrasonic detection device located on or below the venous drip chamber.
 b. Manually armed or automatically set by the equipment when sensor head is in place.
 c. When alarm is activated, blood pump is

automatically stopped and venous bloodline clamp activated below the sensing site; requires user intervention to correct or override.
d. Condition causing alarm: air, foam, or microbubbles at sensing site.

C. Dialysate circuit electronic monitors.
1. Dialysate composition (conductivity).
   a. Continuously measures electrical conductance or conductivity of dialysate, which is dependent on the concentration and mobility of the contained ions; expressed in milliohms; reflects the concentration of sodium salts, the major electrolyte in the dialysate.
   b. Upper and lower limits on the physiologic range of conductivity are usually preset by the manufacturer; upper and lower limits within the physiologic range may be manually set or automatically set as a function of the base conductivity for proportioned dialysate.
   c. When conductivity exceeds the upper or lower limits, system should immediately go into bypass to divert dialysate to drain; should be accompanied by audible and visual alarms.
   d. Conditions causing alarm: incorrect composition of dialysate.
      (1) Low conductivity: too much water, too little concentrate, or only one of the acid or bicarbonate concentrates required for bicarbonate dialysate is available.
      (2) High conductivity: too little water or too much concentrate.
2. Dialysate flow rate.
   a. Measures and displays the dialysate flow rate on the front panel of the delivery system.
   b. Flow rate may be preset by manufacturer. Operator may be able to change flow rate to several settings, decrease flow rate, or turn dialysate flow off.
   c. Divergence from desired rate may decrease dialyzer efficiency or consume more concentrate. Poses no lethal threat to patient.
   d. Conditions causing an alarm.
      (1) Dialysate pump failure.
      (2) Power failure.
      (3) Inadequate water pressure.
      (4) Obstruction in outflow.
      (5) Inadequate availability of concentrate.
3. Dialysate temperature.
   a. Thermostat controls electric heater or hot and cold mixing valve; heat exchanger may be incorporated in dialysate circuit to conserve energy required to heat cold water to normal dialysate temperature setting; thermostat or monitor in dialysate circuit before the dialyzer monitors dialysate temperature.
   b. Range is usually preset by manufacturer.

c. Dialysate temperature.
   (1) High limit of 41°C.
      (a) Protein denaturation and hemolysis can occur at temperatures greater than 42°C (Jepson & Alonso, 2009).
      (b) Warmer dialysate temperatures are associated with higher rates of diffusion (Nissenson, 2008).
   (2) Low limit of 33°C.
      (a) Low dialysate temperature below the patient's temperature (average 36°C, 96°F) may induce chilling in patients and can cause vessel spasm leading to reduced blood flow rates.
      (b) Well recognized that there is a benefit for blood pressure stability with lower dialysate temperature (34° to 36°C) through maintenance of vascular tone (Damasiewicz & Polkinghorne, 2001).
      (c) Lower temperatures are cardioprotective. Patients have reported more energy and reduced recovery time from HD following the use of cooler dialysate temperatures.
      (d) If low temperature is used, dialysis time may need to be increased by 8% for every 3°C below 37°C (Nissenson, 2008).
   d. Excursion above the high temperature limit activates an audible and visual alarm, and opens the bypass valve to divert dialysate to drain until alarm condition is rectified; low temperature may activate an alarm, but may or may not activate the bypass valve.
   e. Conditions causing alarm.
      (1) Mechanical malfunction of heater.
      (2) Power supply failure.
4. Blood leak detector.
   a. Photoelectric cell in the dialysate circuit after the dialyzer which detects light transmission changes in effluent dialysate.
   b. Sensitivity may be preset by manufacturer or may be modified by user; may have several sensitivity settings that can be manually selected.
   c. When blood in effluent dialysate is detected, audible and visual alarms are activated and the blood pump stops; in some equipment, there will be cessation of ultrafiltration.
   d. Validation of blood in effluent may be done with blood leak testing strips, using only those strips designed for that purpose.
   e. Generally requires replacement of the dialyzer.
   f. Conditions causing alarm.
      (1) Membrane leak or rupture.
      (2) Fouling of photoelectric cell from dialysate residue or bicarbonate precipitate.

(3) Excessive air in dialysate stream.

g. Do not reinfuse the patient's blood as there is the potential for direct mixing of the dialysate with the patient's blood.

5. Dialysate pressure or transmembrane pressure (TMP).

a. Measures negative pressure or, in some equipment, the TMP (transmembrane pressure); may be a passive monitor in some equipment; in other delivery systems, it may incorporate the actual mechanism for generating pressure for ultrafiltration.

b. May have upper and lower limits that can be manually set.

c. If limits are in place, will activate an audible and visual alarm; in some equipment, it will stop the blood pump and ultrafiltration, while in other systems, it will stop dialysate flow and ultrafiltration.

d. Conditions causing an alarm.

(1) Mechanical malfunction of the negative pressure pump.

(2) Failure of the pump in a volumetric ultrafiltration control system.

(3) Obstructed blood side transducer; leads to incorrect venous pressure reading and a drift in TMP (usually to the positive side) sufficient to cause alarm.

(4) Power supply failure.

(5) Excursions beyond limits.

e. It is important to maintain a minimum UFR, especially when using a high flux dialyzer, to avoid the risk of reverse ultrafiltration of dialysate with a zero, or near zero UFR. Refer to the dialyzer manufacturer's recommendations for the given configurations of that dialyzer.

6. Blood Volume Monitoring (BVM). (See Section D for more detailed discussion of this technology.)

a. Technologies designed to monitor fluid removal during HD to enhance better control of UFR.

b. Integrated into select dialysis machines by manufacturers (stand-alone and integrated versions).

c. Monitoring functions may include blood volume, hematocrit, oxygen saturation (O_2 sat), and percent blood recirculation in the vascular access.

VII. Urea kinetic modeling.

A. Background and rationale.

1. Urea kinetic modeling (UKM): "The ultimate goal of dialysis treatments is a decrease in solute levels in the patient; measurement of isolated solute levels can be misleading if the solute measured is not representative of all uremic toxins. Because no solute probably qualifies in this respect, it is reasonable to pick as a marker an easily dialyzed solute, such as urea, for which concentrations in the patient decrease significantly during the treatment. Urea clearance determined from a ratio of concentrations, rather than from an absolute value, is a sensitive marker of small-solute diffusion across the dialyzer. Because dialysis most effectively removes small solutes, urea Kt/V is a sensitive measure of the overall dialysis dose" (NKF, 2006b, http://www2.kidney.org/ professionals/KDOQI/guideline_upHD_PD_VA/ hd_guide2.htm).

2. Predialysis and postdialysis serum blood urea nitrogen (BUN) concentrations are collected during a specific treatment. Results are used to develop an appropriate dialysis prescription and can be used as quality measure or as quality improvement targets (NKF, 2006c, http://www2.kidney.org/professionals/KDOQI/ guideline_upHD_PD_VA/hd_guide7.htm).

a. Used to assess the consistency of delivery of that prescription.

b. Reflects changes in the patient's BUN level during a single dialysis treatment and is reported as a percentage (NKF, 2006b, http://www2.kidney.org/professionals/KDOQI/ guideline_upHD_PD_VA/hd_guide2.htm; NKF, 2006c, http://www2.kidney.org/ professionals/KDOQI/guideline_upHD_PD_V A/hd_guide7.htm).

3. Increased protein catabolism has been associated with the severity of clinical manifestations of uremia; urea is the bulk catabolite of protein.

4. BUN can serve as a marker for small molecular weight solutes in patients on dialysis.

a. Can be used to determine the net amount of protein catabolized/day in patients on dialysis.

(1) Urea generation is linearly related to protein catabolism.

(2) With accurate measurement of BUN concentrations and formal mathematical analyses, a reliable estimate of dietary protein intake can be made in stable patients in nitrogen balance.

b. From the calculation of dietary protein intake, phosphate ingestion and hydrogen ion liberation can be calculated (see Figure 2.23).

(1) Phosphate.

(a) Each gram of dietary protein catabolized in a whole-food North American diet contains approximately 15 mg of phosphate.

(b) Dairy protein contains approximately 28 mg of phosphate/gram of catabolized protein.

(c) Most patients on hemodialysis require

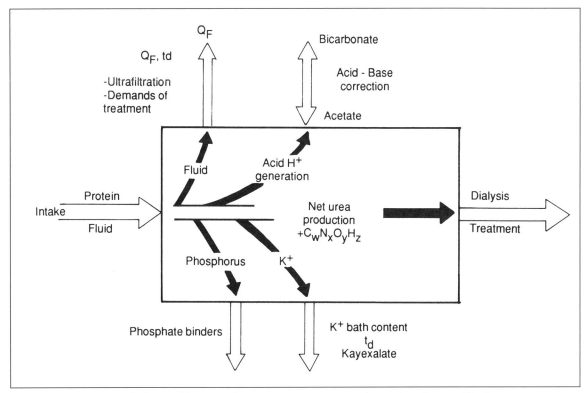

Figure 2.23. Protein catabolism yields urea, other nitrogenous waste products, phosphate, and hydrogen.

phosphate binders to manage phosphate concentrations.
  (2) Hydrogen ion.
      (a) Each gram of protein catabolized liberates 0.75 mEq of hydrogen.
      (b) Large protein intakes are associated with large acid loads which must be buffered from available body base stores including bone.
      (c) Buffer must be repleted during dialysis by dialysate bicarbonate.
  c. Can be used as a marker solute to quantify dialysis therapy and individualize the dialysis dose prescription based on unique patient and treatment parameters.
  d. Can serve as quality improvement tool to determine the dose of dialysis delivered relative to the dose prescribed.

B. Application of the urea kinetic model.
  1. Requires determination of specific patient parameters and an understanding of the interaction between patient and treatment variables.
  2. Most frequently used model is the variable volume, single pool urea model.
     a. The NKF-KDOQI Clinical Practice Guidelines for Hemodialysis Adequacy recommends that (NKF, 2006b, http://www2.kidney.org/professionals/KDOQI/guideline_upHD_PD_VA/hd_guide2.htm):
        (1) The dose of dialysis should be measured and monitored routinely.
        (2) The delivered dose of hemodialysis in adult and pediatric patients should be measured using formal urea kinetic modeling, a single-pool, variable-volume model (NKF, 2006b, http://www2.kidney.org/professionals/KDOQI/guideline_upHD_PD_VA/hd_guide2.htm)
     b. Assumes urea is distributed in a single, well-mixed volume or pool.
  3. Patient parameters of the model are those parameters associated with unique characteristics of each patient.
     a. Urea volume (V) is the body water volume of distribution for urea; considered to be total body water (TBW), expressed in mL or L.
        (1) With normal body composition, it is approximately 58% of body weight; fat tissue contains less water and muscle tissue relatively more water (DePalma & Pittarad, 2001, http://www.hemodialysis-inc.com/articles/bodywater.pdf).
        (2) In obese individuals, TBW may be less than 58%, and may range from 40 to 50% of body weight.
        (3) In lean, muscular males, TBW may be greater than 58%, and range from 60 to 70% of body weight.

(4) Lean, elderly males with relatively little body fat may also have higher TBW, in the range of 60 to 70% of body weight.

b. V (urea volume) in the kinetic model can be calculated in several ways.

(1) From the drop in urea during dialysis with a known dialyzer urea clearance, operated for a known length of time; calculation is complicated and requires computational assistance.

(2) From surface area as a function of height, weight, and gender; and anthropometric measures.

(3) As some fixed percentage of body weight; this is the least accurate method to estimate V.

c. TBW.

(1) Can be accurately determined with radioisotope dilution methods.

(2) Bioelectrical impedance has been proposed as a suitable method to determine TBW.

4. As protein is catabolized, urea is generated and distributed in body water in mg/min.

a. The breakdown of ingested protein produces urea, which is normally excreted by the kidneys.

b. Other products of protein catabolism include creatinine in small amounts, uric acid, phosphate, sulfur, and fecal nitrogen.

c. In the absence of renal excretion of urea, the concentration of BUN increases; rate of increase reflects the net generation of BUN or Gu.

d. Gu can be calculated from the change in body urea content from the end of one dialysis to the beginning of the next dialysis.

e. Computer solution of both V and Gu equations can now be done with a single set of predialysis and postdialysis BUN values and suitable treatment information.

(1) To express concentration in SI units, the BUN multiplied by 0.357 can be used to convert BUN values to urea concentration in mmol/L.

(2) To convert BUN to urea nitrogen values, the BUN multiplied by 0.1667 will give urea nitrogen values in mmol/L.

f. From Gu, the clinician can calculate the net amount of protein catabolized; if the patient is stable or in zero nitrogen balance, this is equal to dietary protein intake.

(1) The equation to calculate net grams of protein catabolized in 24 hours (PCR, g/24 hours) from Gu in the adult patient is as follows: PCR, g/24 hr = 9.35(Gu)+11.04.

(2) If patient is catabolic or anabolic, PCR will not equal dietary protein intake.

(a) If patient is catabolic, PCR will overestimate dietary intake.

(b) If patient is anabolic, PCR will underestimate protein intake.

(3) If residual renal urea clearance is present but not measured, PCR will be underestimated.

5. Normalized protein catabolic rate (NPCR) is the net amount of protein catabolized or ingested per kilogram of normalized body weight per 24 hours; expressed as NPCR in g/kg/day.

a. NPCR is expressed per unit of normalized or ideal body weight; PCR is the total grams of protein catabolized per 24 hours. Protein is prescribed as g/kg of normalized body weight/24 hours.

Example:
Patient #1 is obese with a body weight of 75 kg or V=30 L. The prescribed dietary protein intake would be V/.58 or 30/.58 = ideal body weight of 51 kg. The diet prescription would be 50 to 55 g of protein/24 hours or 1.0 g/kg/24 hours for ideal body weight rather than 75 g/24 hours using actual body weight.

b. The frequent dietary prescription for patients on hemodialysis is 1.0 to 1.2 g/kg/24 hours.

(1) Assures adequate protein nutrition if 2/3 of the protein is high-biologic-value protein (i.e., meat, milk, fish, eggs).

(2) Is considered adequate for nutritional needs, but avoids generating excessive amounts of urea, phosphate, and hydrogen ions, as discussed above.

6. KrU is the residual renal urea clearance in mL/min.

a. Will be a lower value than residual creatinine clearance and is generally about 0.55 to 0.60 of residual renal creatinine clearance.

b. Residual renal urea clearance represents one of the urea removal mechanisms, since it operates 24 hours/day compared to the intermittent removal by hemodialysis.

c. KrU in mL/min is calculated from urine volume (Uv in mL), urine urea concentration (Uu in mg/dL), mean BUN in mg/dL, and time of collection (t in minutes). The calculation is as follows: KrU = (Uu/Mean BUN)(Uv/t).

d. In the patient with chronic kidney disease who does not require dialysis (steady state conditions), Gu can be calculated from the measured KrU and BUN concentrations which bracket the urine collection. Gu in mg/min = (KrU in mL/min)(Mean BUN in mg/dL). PCR can be calculated as shown above from Gu.

7. In the patient on hemodialysis, where BUN

concentration oscillates as a function of the removal during treatment and accumulation between treatments, the BUN concentration in the body is equal to the following: C = (Urea input – Urea output)/V and is a function of V, PCR, KrU, and dialysis dose.
- a. V will influence BUN if input is constant. *Example:* the same amount of protein ingested by a patient with a large V will result in a lower BUN concentration than the same protein load ingested by a patient with a small V.
- b. Input will be represented by PCR or NPCR. Rate of rise in BUN will be dependent on the net amount of protein catabolized between treatments and the V into which urea nitrogen is generated. Higher protein intake will increase the rate of BUN rise relative to a low protein intake in the same patient.
- c. Output will be primarily controlled by urea removal during dialysis.

C. Treatment parameters related to the urea kinetic model are those aspects that constitute the primarily urea removal mechanisms. They generally can be controlled or manipulated.
- 1. K or dialyzer urea clearance: the rate at which available blood through the dialyzer is completely cleared of urea (see dialyzer section).
  - a. K is a function of membrane permeability, size and membrane area (KoA in mL/min), blood flow rate (Qb in mL/min or L/min), and dialysate flow rate (Qd in mL/min); it can be influenced by a change in membrane, Qb, KoA, and Qd.
  - b. K is manipulated to achieve a drop in BUN concentration during dialysis; the desired K will be achieved by manipulation of Qb during dialysis or by selection of a dialyzer (KoA) that will provide the desired clearance.
  - c. The curvilinear drop in BUN concentration that occurs during dialysis follows first order phenomenon. The bulk amount of urea removed (flux) is a function of BUN concentration (although dialyzer urea clearance is constant). As concentration falls, the flux decreases and BUN concentration declines at a slower rate.
- 2. A major parameter that influences the drop in BUN concentration during dialysis is the length of dialysis session or t (time) in minutes.
  - a. A dialyzer with a known urea clearance operated for a specified time will produce a predictable drop in BUN concentration.
  - b. The length of time required to achieve that drop in BUN will be a function of dialyzer urea clearance, and patient V or volume to be cleared.

c. These three parameters, K, t, and V, are integrally related and control the rate at which BUN concentration drops during dialysis as well as the total decrease in BUN concentration that occurs over the hemodialysis treatment.

D. Kt/V is a tool to prescribe the dose of dialysis.
- 1. A treatment prescription can be defined as the use of a specified dialyzer for a prescribed treatment time with prescribed blood and dialysate flow rates.
- 2. A dialysis prescription can be written using Kt/V.
  - a. Kt/V is a dialyzer urea clearance (K in mL or L/min) times the length of dialysis (t in minutes) and the product divided by patient V (V in mL or L).

    Example:
    Dialyzer K is 220 mL/min or .220 L/min;
    Treatment time is 3.5 hours or 210 minutes;
    Patient V is 35 L
    Kt/V = [(.220)(210)]/35 = 1.32.

  - b. NKF-KDOQI Clinical Practice Guidelines for Hemodialysis Adequacy recommend that the prescribed dose of dialysis be at least 1.43 to maximize the chance that a minimum dose of 1.2 per treatment will be attained when a patient dialyzes three times a week; the respective URR would be 70% (NKF, 2006d). See the full clinical practice guideline at thttp://www2.kidney.org/professionals/KDOQI/guideline_upHD_PD_VA/hd_guide2.htm

E. Urea kinetic modeling can be used to assess treatment delivery relative to the prescription.
- 1. Knowledge of the model and application in the development of an appropriate dialysis prescription allows the caregiver to assess adequacy of a given therapy by accepted criteria, and manipulate treatment variables to obtain the desired dialysis prescription.
- 2. Actual treatment delivery can be assessed from predialysis and postdialysis BUN concentrations and patient weights, and treatment information from the specific dialysis.
  - a. With BUN concentrations, weights, dialyzer type, blood and dialysate flow rates, and treatment time, the delivered Kt/V and NPCR can be calculated using rigorous mathematical analysis.
  - b. The NKF-KDOQI Clinical Practice Guidelines for Hemodialysis Adequacy state that all patients on hemodialysis within a facility should have a delivered dose of dialysis measured using the same method (NKF, 2006e, http://www2.kidney.org/professionals/KDOQI/guideline_upHD_PD_VA/).

c. NKF-KDOQI Clinical Practice Guidelines for Hemodialysis Adequacy state that the delivered dose of dialysis should be monitored at least once a month in adult and pediatric patients (NKF, 2006e, http://www2.kidney.org/professionals/KDOQI/ guideline_upHD_PD_VA/).

3. The total drop in BUN concentration during dialysis will be a function of patient size, as represented by the volume of distribution for urea (total body water) or V, the dialyzer urea clearance (K), and the length of time for dialysis (t). The drop in BUN concentration will be inversely related to the V (e.g., given the same treatment conditions, a smaller drop in BUN concentration represents a larger V) (see Figure 2.24).

a. If the drop in BUN concentration during dialysis is less than expected, the prescribed therapy was under delivered or less therapy was given than expected.

b. If the drop in BUN concentration during dialysis is more than expected, the delivered therapy appears to be higher than the prescription.

   (1) May be related to sample error (e.g., as the result of drawing the postdialysis BUN sample from the venous bloodline rather than the arterial line at the end of dialysis).

   (2) May be related to urea rebound.

     (a) During dialysis, BUN concentration disequilibrium exists between two compartments.

     (b) At the end of dialysis, there is rapid equilibrium between the two compartments and BUN concentration rises rapidly.

     (c) This represents the two-pool distribution of urea.

   (3) Disequilibrium may be between the intracellular BUN concentration and the extracellular compartment of which the vascular compartment is one component. This is the result of relatively slow transport of urea from one compartment to the other.

c. The disequilibrium may reflect the relatively low blood flow to the large urea-containing compartment or volume (skin, bone, and muscle) compared to the high blood flow to the smaller urea-containing compartment. This is the flow-volume disequilibrium concept.

d. Equilibration occurs usually within 30 to 60 minutes after the end of dialysis.

e. The magnitude of urea rebound seems to be associated with the rate of urea clearance relative to urea volume (K/V). The magnitude of urea rebound may be as high as 50% of the

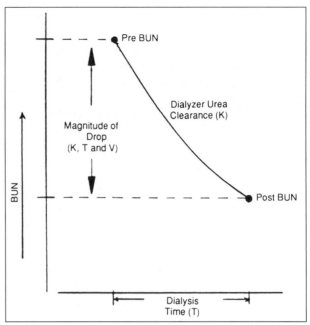

Figure 2.24. Drop in BUN concentration with dialyzer urea clearance (K) and treatment time (T)

postdialysis BUN concentration. For example, if the postdialysis concentration is 20 mg/dL and there is 50% urea rebound, the equilibrated BUN will be 30 mg/dL.

   (1) NKF-KDOQI Clinical Practice Recommendations suggest that women, smaller patients, and patients who are malnourished may need more dialysis to reach target prescription due to possible differences in urea distribution and/or postdialysis rebound (NKF, 2006d, http://www2.kidney.org/professionals/KD OQI/guideline_upHD_PD_VA/hd_guide4. htm).

   (2) Delivered Kt/V may be further complicated by cardiopulmonary recirculation, where well-dialyzed blood is returned to the venous circulation and heart, where this blood reduces the effective systemic BUN concentration coming back to the dialyzer; reduces the effective concentration gradient in the dialyzer; it is usually dissipated within 2 minutes after dialysis.

   (3) NKF-KDOQI Clinical Practice Guidelines for Hemodialysis Adequacy state that predialysis and postdialysis samples should be drawn on the same hemodialysis treatment (NKF, 2006b, http://www2.kidney.org/professionals/KD OQI/guideline_upHD_PD_VA/hd_guide2. htm).

   (4) NKF-KDOQI Clinical Practice Guidelines

for Hemodialysis Adequacy state that the predialysis BUN sample should be drawn just prior to the dialysis treatment, avoiding the dilution of the blood sample by saline or heparin; the postdialysis BUN sample should be drawn using the slow flow/stop pump technique.

(a) At the end of dialysis, the ultrafiltration is stopped, dialysate flow is reduced or discontinued, and the blood pump is reduced to 50 to 100 mL/min. After 15 seconds, the postdialysis BUN sample is drawn from the arterial sample port closest to the patient.

(b) This avoids false low BUN concentration from access recirculation (NKF, 2006f, http://www2.kidney.org/professionals/KDOQI/guideline_upHD_PD_VA/hd_guide3.htm).

4. The dialyzer clearance (K), treatment time (t) information, and predialysis/postdialysis BUN concentrations and weights allow the calculation of effective V (urea volume) to uniquely fit these data. Obviously errors occur in K and t, but calculation of effective V provides useful information.

a. Identifies persistent technical problems (Gomez, 2011, pp. 128-131).

(1) Errors in dialyzer clearance (K).
(a) Fistula recirculation.
(b) Inaccurate estimate of dialyzer performance.
(c) Errors in blood pump setting.
(d) Blood pump calibration errors.
(e) Variability in cross-sectional area of the blood pump tubing segment which affects stroke volume per revolution of the blood pump.
(f) Inadequate dialyzer reprocessing.
(g) Dialysate flow errors.

(2) Treatment time (t) errors.
(a) Treatment time measured by wall clock or personal wristwatch.
(b) Blood pump is gradually increased over the first 15 to 30 minutes of dialysis.
(c) Blood pump speed is reduced for hypotension or muscle cramps.
(d) Frequent extracorporeal blood compartment pressure alarms or dialysate compartment alarms.
(e) Needle manipulation and infiltration.
(f) Dialyzer blood leak.
(g) Treatment time electively changed by patient or care provider.

(3) BUN measurement errors.
(a) Predialysis BUN sample diluted by saline in the fistula needle or lock fluid within central venous catheter.
(b) Predialysis BUN sample drawn after the start of dialysis.
(c) Postdialysis BUN sample drawn from the venous port.
(d) Laboratory error.
(e) Laboratory calibration error.
(f) Analysis of the two samples on different laboratory equipment or different analysis runs.

b. Allows comparison of kinetic V with the anthropometric V (height, weight, gender, and age) as a check on accuracy.
c. Allows calculation of NPCR.
d. Allows quantification of the prescription changes necessary to achieve desired Kt/V.

F. All parameters of the model are integrally related; change or modification in any one of these components may have an effect on the entire model system.

1. Modification in protein intake (input) in a patient will change the rate of urea production and the predialysis BUN value.

2. A reduction in treatment time or clearance (output) will remove less urea during dialysis which will be reflected in a higher postdialysis BUN value; if protein during the interdialystic interval is the same, the next predialysis BUN value will be higher.

3. The parameters that can be manipulated more easily are those associated with dialysis. Protein intake may or may not be amenable to modification.

4. The three variables, BUN, NPCR, and Kt/V, are predictably related.
a. A specific Kt/V with a known NPCR will produce a unique predialysis BUN.
b. As shown in Figure 2.25 on a three-variable plot, if two variables are known, the remaining variable can be determined.

Example:
If measured midweek predialysis BUN is 73 mg/dL; the delivered Kt/V is 1.1; the NPCR that intersects these two points is 0.96 g/kg/24 hours.

c. The three-variable plot for eKt/V is shown in Figure 2.26.

5. Referring back to Figure 2.24, it can be seen that with the same Kt/V of 1.1, midweek predialysis BUN concentration may range from 29 mg/dL (at NPCR 0.5 g/kg/day) to 81 mg/dL with NPCR 1.1 g/kg/day; demonstrates the difficulty of assessing adequacy of dialysis prescription or dialysis delivered dose from a single predialysis BUN concentration.

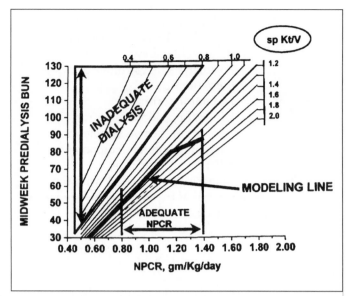

Figure 2.25. Delivered Kt/Vsp therapy plot.

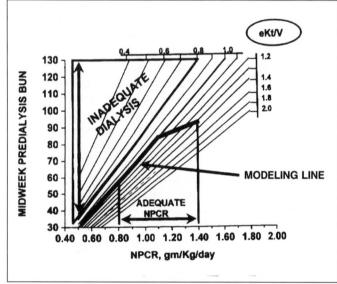

Figure 2.26. Delivered Kt/V therapy plot.

a. A predialysis and postdialysis BUN value measured on a single dialysis session each month, with appropriate treatment information, allows one to determine the actual treatment delivered to the patient compared to that prescribed.
   (1) If NPCR varies, but the actual delivered dialysis dose remains constant, the predialysis BUN concentration will move along one of the diagonal Kt/V treatment lines.
   (2) If NPCR is constant, but therapy delivery varies, the measured predialysis BUN concentration will move vertically and cross different Kt/V lines.

b. This type of graphic display of treatment information will facilitate evaluation of the consistency of treatment delivery as well as provide information about the patient's NPCR.

G. There are several limitations when using formal urea kinetic modeling (NKF, 2006d, http://www2.kidney.org/professionals/KDOQI/guideline_upHD_PD_VA/hd_guide4.htm).
   1. The assumption that urea is distributed in a single, well-mixed volume, when in fact, urea is distributed in two pools.
   2. Formal urea kinetic modeling requires the effort and personnel time to process data. User must be able to understand the patient-dialyzer system to use information; requires comprehensive knowledge of dialysis and clinical events to interpret results of kinetic modeling.

H. Urea reduction ratio (URR) calculation is a simplified approximation of formal urea kinetic modeling that can be used to assess treatment delivery.
   1. URR uses predialysis and postdialysis BUN concentrations to calculate the following:

   URR =
   (Predialysis BUN – Postdialysis BUN/Predialysis BUN in mg/dL) x (100)

   Example:
   Predialysis BUN = 100 mg/dL
   Postdialysis BUN = 30 mg/dL [(100-30)(100) x 100 = 70%

   2. Clinical data and NKF-KDOQI Guidelines state a URR of 70% or greater is needed.
   3. There is a correlation with Kt/V.
   4. It is a simple calculation, requiring only a calculator and two BUN values.
   5. The NPCR cannot be derived from the URR.
   6. Ignores volume changes during the dialytic interval and may lead to some error in actual delivered dose.
   7. Information regarding the quality incentive payments through the prospective payment system (PPS) for hemodialysis can be found at http://www.cms.gov/Medicare/End-Stage-Renal-Disease/ESRDQualityImproveInit/index.html (CMS, 2013).

SECTION B
Water Treatment
Glenda Payne

I. Safe water is critical for patients on hemodialysis (HD).

A. Drinking water is not sterile.
1. Municipal water supplies are treated to be safe for drinking; this does not mean all bacteria are removed.
2. The Environmental Protection Agency (EPA), which sets the limits for drinking water, allows up to 500 colony forming units (CFU) in municipal water cultures (EPA, 2013). This level of microorganisms, while not harmful if consumed by drinking, would be harmful to patients on HD.

B. Patients on HD are routinely exposed to large quantities of water.
1. On average, a healthy adult consumes 10 to 12 liters of water per week.
2. About 97% of the dialysate is water, exposing a patient on HD to 350 to 400 liters per week. Because of the volume of exposure, even trace contamination can be harmful.

C. Patients exposed to the water in dialysate are not protected by their body's normal defense mechanisms because the pathway of exposure differs from water that is ingested.
1. Healthy adults filter ingested water through their gastrointestinal tract, which includes the membranes of the stomach and intestine, and blood circulation through the liver to remove contaminates. Well-functioning kidneys filter out contaminates that may be present in drinking water.
2. Exposure to water by patients on HD is through a thin, semipermeable membrane, where filtration is dependent upon the size of the particle, not on whether that particle might be harmful.
   a. Breaks in the membrane allow for more complete exposure of the patient's blood to any contaminate in the water.
   b. Patients who require HD do not have the protection of well-functioning kidneys to filter out any contaminates.

D. If water or dialysate is unsafe for use, all patients being treated at that time can be harmed or killed simultaneously.
1. In conventional HD, water is centrally delivered to every treatment station. The same bicarbonate concentrate may be used for all patients, while the acid concentrate prescribed may vary, based upon individual needs.
2. *Safety alert.* If the water, bicarbonate, or acid is contaminated, all patients receiving treatment at the time of the exposure are at risk for potential harm.

II. How patients are affected by exposure to unsafe water for HD treatment.

A. Table 2.6 lists the known water contaminates that can affect patients on HD, and the minimum levels known to cause patient injury.

Table 2.6

**Water Contaminates and Lowest Levels
That Can Cause Patient Injury**

Contaminate	Lowest concentration associated with toxicity
Aluminum	0.06 mg/L
Chloramines	0.25
Fluoride	1.0
Copper	0.49
Zinc	0.2
Nitrate	21 (as N)
Sulfate	200
Calcium/Magnesium	88 (Ca++)
Sodium	300

Source: Adapted from Table in Layman-Amato, Curtis & Payne, 2013, p. 385
http://www.prolibraries.com/anna/?select=session&sessionID=2840.

B. The Association for the Advancement of Medical Instrumentation (AAMI) sets maximum levels of these contaminates at one-half of the minimum level known to cause patient injury.

C. The AAMI limits for chemical contaminates are listed in Table 2.7 (AAMI, 2014a).

D. Table 2.8 lists water contaminants and the patient symptoms these contaminants may cause (ANSI/AAMI 13959:2014, Annex A, 2014a).

E. Immediate risks of exposure to contaminated HD water for patients include anemia, hemolysis, bone disease, neurologic deterioration, methemoglobinemia, metabolic acidosis, sepsis, pyrogenic reactions, and death (ANSI/AAMI 13959:2014, Annex A, 2014a).

F. Long-term risks for patients who experience HD with inadequately treated water include chronic inflammatory disease from repeated exposure to low levels of endotoxin and other bacterial-derived products (Layman-Amato, Curtis & Payne, 2013, p 402, http://www.prolibraries.com/anna/?select=session&sessionID=2840).
   1. These patients may not have an overt pyrogenic reaction, but exhibit symptoms over time.
   2. Symptoms may include resistance to erythropoietin, reduced serum albumin, malnutrition, decreased transferrin levels, beta-2 microglobulin amyloidosis (e.g., carpal tunnel syndrome), and accelerated atherosclerosis leading to increased cardiovascular risk and mortality (Layman-Amato, Curtis & Payne, 2013, p 402, http://www.prolibraries.com/anna/?select=session&sessionID=2840).

III. Ensuring the water used for HD is safe.

A. The most important water treatment "component" is the human element.
   1. Selecting and training personnel to recognize the risks presented by water and dialysate to patients is a critical management responsibility.
   2. Staff members assigned to operate or monitor the water treatment system must complete a training program approved by the medical director and the governing body of the outpatient dialysis facility (CMS, 2008b, IG V696).
   3. Audits of the practices related to water treatment and dialysate preparation must be conducted at least annually and more frequently if problems are identified (CMS, 2008b, IG V260). A qualified person must physically observe the water system start-up procedures, the test for hardness, the test for total chlorine, and the acid and bicarbonate mixing to ensure that each person assigned these tasks is following facility policy and performing as expected.

Table 2.7

List of Maximum Allowable Levels of Chemicals

Maximum allowable levels of toxic chemicals and dialysis fluid electrolytes in dialysis water [a]	
Contaminant	**Maximum concentration mg/L[b]**
Contaminants with documented toxicity in hemodialysis	
Aluminum	0.01
Total chlorine	0.1
Copper	0.1
Fluoride	0.2
Lead	0.005
Nitrate (as N)	2
Sulfate	100
Zinc	0.1
Electrolytes normally included in dialysis fluid	
Calcium	2 (0.05 mmol/L)
Magnesium	4 (0.15 mmol/L)
Potassium	8 (0.2 mmol/L)
Sodium	70 (3.0 mmol/L)

[a] The physician has the ultimate responsibility for ensuring the quality of water used for dialysis.
[b] Unless otherwise noted.

Maximum allowable levels of trace elements in dialysis water	
Contaminant	**Maximum concentration mg/L**
Antimony	0.006
Arsenic	0.005
Barium	0.1
Beryllium	0.0004
Cadmium	0.001
Chromium	0.014
Mercury	0.0002
Selenium	0.09
Silver	0.005
Thallium	0.002

Source: Adapted from ANSI/AAMI 13959:2014 (AAMI, 2014a). Used with permission.

Table 2.8

Patient Outcomes Potentially Related to Water

Sign or symptom	Possible H$_2$O cause
Anemia	Aluminum, chloramines, copper, zinc
Bone disease	Aluminum, fluoride
Hemolysis	Chloramines, copper, nitrates
Hypertension	Calcium, sodium
Hypotension	Bacteria, endotoxin, nitrates
Metabolic acidosis	Low pH, sulfates
Muscle weakness	Calcium, magnesium
Nausea, vomiting	Bacteria, calcium, copper, endotoxin, low pH, magnesium, nitrates, sulphates, zinc
Neurodeterioration, encephalopathy	Aluminum

Source: ANSI/AAMI 13959:2014, Annex A, 2014a.

4. Education for all responsible staff members should include the "whys" for each step in the water treatment and dialysate preparation, with emphasis on the reasons that safe water is critical to patient safety. Understanding "why" decreases the risks of staff members altering expected practice or taking shortcuts.

B. Responsibility for safe water and dialysate.
   1. The operator of the equipment is responsible to follow facility procedures and to notify the nurse in charge and technical supervisor if there is any question or problem with the system.
   2. The registered nurse (RN) in charge is responsible to:
      a. Know the basics of water and dialysate safety and to monitor those working with her/him to ensure that tests are performed accurately and results are recorded correctly.
      b. Notify the medical director immediately if problems cannot be resolved quickly, and to ensure the medical director is aware of any issue with the water and dialysate systems.
   3. The nurse manager is responsible to ensure all staff assigned any responsibility for water treatment or dialysate preparation are qualified by training and have documentation of current competency.
   4. The medical director is ultimately responsible for the water and dialysate systems. He/she is responsible for approving a training program (CMS, 2008b, IG V696) that is specific to the water treatment and dialysate preparation systems

in use and for ensuring all persons assigned responsibility for these tasks have completed training and demonstrated competency.

IV. Why drinking water is not safe for HD.

A. All public water systems that provide drinking water must meet Environmental Protection Agency (EPA) standards. EPA standards are set to ensure drinking water safety, but allow levels of contaminants in drinking water that would pose a risk to patients on HD (EPA, 2014, http://water.epa.gov/drink/contaminants/index.cfm).

B. Municipal source water may be from surface water or ground water.
   1. Ground water comes from wells or springs while surface water comes from lakes or rivers.
   2. Both water sources include contaminants that can be classified into inorganic and organic chemicals.
   3. Inorganic contaminates include ionic compounds such as dissolved salts, minerals and metals, and gases.
   4. Organic contaminates include bacteria, viruses, and algae.
   5. Municipal water may also be contaminated with industrial wastes, fertilizers, pesticides, and sewage.

C. Making the water suitable to drink ("potable").
   1. The municipality may add chemicals such as chlorine/chloramines for disinfection, aluminum for clarity, fluoride to prevent dental caries, and

phosphates and other pH adjusters to prevent or slow pipe corrosion.

2. Many of the additives used to treat drinking water are toxic if they remain in the water used for HD.

V. Relevant recommendations and regulations related to safe water and dialysate for HD.

A. AAMI is the organization that sets standards for medical devices and products.
   1. The Renal Disease and Detoxification (RDD) Committee of AAMI is composed of voluntary representatives from the dialysis industry (suppliers, manufacturers, and providers); regulatory agencies including the Centers for Medicare & Medicaid Services (CMS), the Centers for Disease Control (CDC), and the Federal Drug Administration (FDA); and professional organizations such as the American Nephrology Nurses' Association (ANNA), http://www.aami.org/standards/index.html
   2. The RDD Committee develops consensus standards in all areas related to HD (e.g., water and dialysis quality, water treatment equipment, dialysis equipment, and reprocessing).
   3. In the context of this document, the statement "required by AAMI" means that this expectation is present as a recommended or required practice in the AAMI documents related to water and dialysate at the time of publication.

B. CMS adopted a specific AAMI standard for water and dialysate quality as a regulation when the End Stage Renal Disease (ESRD) Conditions for Coverage (CfC) were updated in 2008 (CMS, 2008b).
   1. This standard, RD 52:2004, was updated by AAMI in 2006, replaced in 2011, and updated in 2014: (http://www.aami.org/publications/standards/dialysis.html).
   2. Until CMS updates the ESRD regulations related to water and dialysate quality through a formal, rule-making process, the RD52:2004 document will continue to be the minimum expected practice.
   3. In the context of this document, the statement "required by CMS" means that the expectation at present is a requirement in the CMS 2008 regulations or interpretive guidance.

C. From 2009 to 2011, AAMI adopted a suite of five International Standard Organization (ISO) documents in replacement of RD52:2006 (see Table 2.9). The major change in the ISO documents was to lower the allowable microbiological levels for water (see Table 2.10) and dialysate (see Table 2.11).

D. In 2014, AAMI adopted an updated version of these

Table 2.9

Documents Adopted by AAMI in Replacement of RD 52

Identification #	Title
ANSI/AAMI 11663 (AAMI, 2014, 2014c)	Quality of dialysis fluid for hemodialysis and other related therapies
ANSI/AAMI 13958 (AAMI, 2014, 2014d)	Concentrates for hemodialysis and related therapies
ANSI/AAMI 13959 (AAMI, 2014, 2014a)	Water for hemodialysis and other related therapies
ANSI/AAMI 26722 (AAMI, 2009, 2014, 2014b)	Water treatment equipment for hemodialysis applications and related therapies
ANSI/AAMI 23500 (AAMI, 2014, 2014e)	Guidance for the preparation and quality management of fluids for hemodialysis and related therapies

five documents, with a deviation for the United States. The deviation is to the provisions defining the culture incubation time, temperature, and media to be used. The deviation includes the use of an incubation time of 48 hours at a temperature of 35° C with culture media of trypticase soy agar (known as TSA) or standard methods agar and plate count agar (also known as TGYE). These documents are titled ANSI/AAMI (document number, such as 23500):2014.

VI. Water treatment for hemodialysis.

A. Basic vs. optional components.
   1. Basic components for water treatment systems include:
      a. Two carbon tanks.
      b. Reverse osmosis (RO) system.
      c. A quality monitor.
      d. Deionization (DI) may be used as back-up for the RO, but is not generally used as the primary treatment component for chronic outpatient dialysis centers.
   2. Optional components.
      a. Used to increase the efficiency and effectiveness of the water treatment system.
      b. Selected based upon analysis of the source water to adequately pretreat the water to protect the RO, as well as remove contaminates.
      c. Monitored to ensure they are functioning as expected.

B. Phases of water purification.

Table 2.10

Comparison of RD 52 and AAMI Recommendations for Dialysis Water Microbiological Quality

Contaminant	AAMI Max Level	AAMI Action Level	RD 52 Max Level	RD 52 Action Level
Total viable bacteria count (TVC)	< 100 CFU/mL	50 CFU/mL	< 200 CFU/mL	50 CFU/mL
Endotoxin	< 0.25 EU/mL	0.125 EU/mL	< 2 EU/mL	1 EU/mL

Source: Adapted from ANSI/AAMI 11663:2014 (AAMI, 2014c).

Table 2.11

Comparison of RD 52 and AAMI Recommendations for Dialysis Fluid (Dialysate) Microbiological Quality

Contaminant	AAMI Max Level	AAMI Action Level	RD 52 Max Level	RD 52 Action Level
Total viable bacteria count (TVC)	< 100 CFU/mL	50 CFU/mL	< 200 CFU/mL	50 CFU/mL
Endotoxin	< 0.5 EU/mL	0.25 EU/mL	< 2 EU/mL	1 EU/mL

Source: Adapted from ANSI/AAMI 11663:2014 (AAMI, 2014c).

1. Pretreatment or conditioning the feed water is done to prevent damage to the RO membrane, help the RO to perform optimally, and prevent harm to patients.
2. Purification or treatment of the water is done by the RO or DI system to remove contaminates and prevent harm to patients.
3. Posttreatment components "polish" the water or improve the water quality by ultraviolet irradiation and/or ultrafiltration.
4. Flow diagrams of the water treatment system must be available and each device labeled with its individual operation (CMS, 2008b, IG V696).
5. Include the expected parameters on all logs used to document equipment monitoring to provide ready reference for staff members to identify when a limit has been violated.

C. Pretreatment components for water treatment. See Figure 2.27 for a schematic of a typical pretreatment system layout.
   1. Back flow preventer.
      a. This valve prevents water or disinfectants in the dialysis center water system from flowing back into the city water systems.
      b. Generally required by the municipality, and must be inspected annually by a qualified plumber.
      c. Not required by AAMI or CMS.
   2. Tempering valve.
      a. Functions like the handle in a shower to adjust the temperature of the water.
      b. The feed water temperature should be about 72° to 77°F for the RO to work most efficiently.
      c. Not required by AAMI or CMS.
   3. Booster pump.
      a. Increases the incoming water pressure to ensure sufficient water volume will go through the "cascade" of water treatment components and supply the RO.
      b. Some older pumps may require an expansion tank to equalize pressure in the plumbing; these tanks can be a source of bacterial growth.
      c. Not required by AAMI or CMS.
   4. Pressure gauges.
      a. Placed before and after each water treatment component to monitor the pressure across the component.
      b. If the component is obstructed or clogged, the pressure reading before that component will

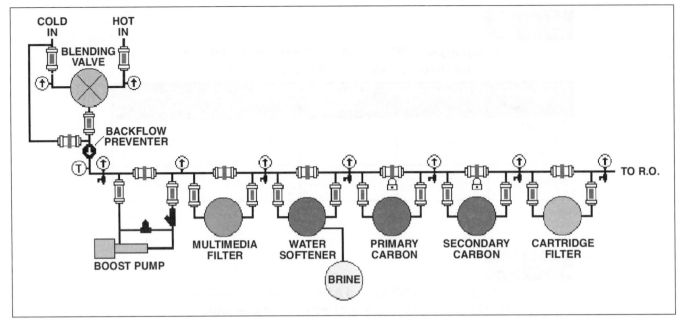

Figure 2.27. Typical pretreatment system.

Used with permission from Layman-Amato, R. Curtis, J., & Payne, G.M. (2013). Water treatment for hemodialysis: An update. *Nephrology Nursing Journal,* *40*(5), 383-404. Available at http://www.prolibraries.com/anna/?select=session&sessionID=2840.

rise above the pressure reading of the gauge following that component, indicating a need to remove the obstruction.

(1) This "change" in pressure is referred to as "Delta P." A triangle, Δ, the Greek symbol for Delta, may be used to symbolize "Delta."

(2) Clearing the obstruction can be done by changing a disposable filter or backwashing the component (allowing water to flow from the exit of the component to the entry to flush the obstruction to drain).

5. Sediment filters: filters are used at various points in the water treatment system to remove particles of various sizes.

a. Multimedia filters.

(1) Placed early in the water treatment cascade, a multimedia or depth filter may be used to remove particulates and colloidal matter larger than 10 microns.

(2) Generally used if the source water has a high sediment rate.

(3) Are tanks filled with varying sized "rocks," gravel, and sand, from larger to quite small; these work by trapping smaller and smaller particles as the water soaks down through the media.

(4) Are maintained by backwashing either on a routine schedule or when changes in pressure ("Δ P") indicate the tank is clogged.

(5) Not required by AAMI or CMS.

b. Disposable filters.

(1) May be placed at various points in the water treatment cascade as a means of removing particulates.

(2) The filter housing should be opaque to prevent the growth of algae.

(3) Monitored by Delta P; an increase in the pressure before the filter from the pressure postfilter indicates the need for replacement.

(4) Not required by AAMI or CMS.

6. Chemical injection systems: used if needed to decrease the pH of the incoming feed water to between 5 and 8 so the RO membrane and carbon tanks can perform optimally, or for chlorine/chloramine reduction. Not required by AAMI or CMS.

a. May use hydrochloric or sulfuric acid for pH alteration, or sodium bisulfite or ascorbic acid for chloramine reduction.

b. If the system is used for chloramines reduction, it does not replace the requirement for two carbon tanks with a 10-minute empty bed contact time (EBCT) (CMS 2008b, IG V 192, http://www.cms.gov/Medicare/Provider-Enrollment-and-Certification/GuidanceforLawsAndRegulations/Downloads/esrdpgmguidance.pdf).

c. Chemical injection systems.

(1) Consists of a reservoir of chemical, a metering pump, and a mixing chamber.

(2) The system must tightly control the amount of chemical injected into the water line.

(3) An automatic injection system must include automated continuous monitoring of the pH after the acid injection site and an alarm to alert the operator of failure.

d. Chemicals used must be compatible with all water treatment components and must be reduced to safe levels prior to the water treated by chemical injection reaching the point of patient use.

e. Chemical injection systems should be followed with a sediment filter as the lower pH will cause dissolved metals in the feed water, such as aluminum and some salts to precipitate. The sediment filter will remove the precipitates (Layman-Amato, Curtis, & Payne, 2013, http://www.prolibraries.com/anna/?select=sessi on&sessionID=2840).

7. Water softener and brine tank. See Figure 2.28 for a typical water softener setup. Softeners remove calcium and magnesium and protect the RO from the scale that these minerals would form on the membrane, which would decrease membrane permeability and function.

a. The softener is filled with resin beads, which exchange sodium for calcium and magnesium.

b. Sodium does not cause scale on the RO membrane and is easily rejected.

c. Water hardness postsoftener must be checked at the end of the treatment day to verify the softener is sufficiently sized to soften the water for a full day of treatment.

d. Facility policy may require monitoring prior to the start of the treatment day to ensure the softener successfully regenerated, i.e., using brine from the tank to recharge the resin with sodium. Monitored by Delta (Δ) P.

e. The brine tank should be kept at least one-half full with clean pelletized salt and steps taken to ensure a "salt bridge" (a solid layer of salt across the tank) does not form, preventing adequate salt saturation of the brine.

f. Not required by AAMI or CMS.

8. Carbon adsorption tanks: Carbon is the primary tool used to remove chlorine and chloramines from the source water. Two tanks, connected in series (i.e., the effluent of the first tank flows into the second tank) with a minimum of 10 minutes of EBCT are required by AAMI and CMS.

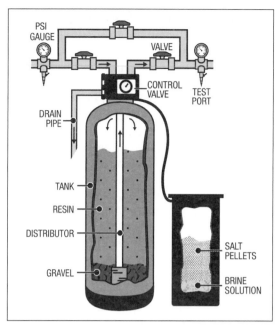

Figure 2.28. Typical water softener setup.

Used with permission from Layman-Amato, R. Curtis, J., & Payne, G.M. (2013). Water treatment for hemodialysis: An update. *Nephrology Nursing Journal, 40*(5), 383-404. Available at http://www.prolibraries.com/anna/?select= session&sessionID=2840.

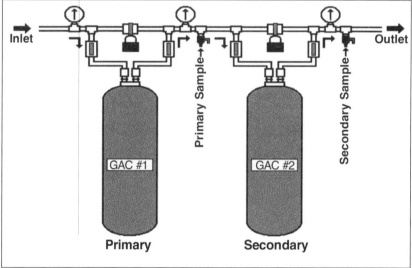

Figure 2.29. Illustration of paired carbon filters.

Used with permission from Layman-Amato, R. Curtis, J., & Payne, G.M. (2013). Water treatment for hemodialysis: An update. *Nephrology Nursing Journal, 40*(5), 383-404. Available at http://www.prolibraries.com/anna/?select= session&sessionID=2840.

(ANSI/AAMI 26722:2014b; CMS 2008b, IG V192). See Figure 2.29 for an illustration of paired carbon filters.

a. Carbon adsorption is a chemical process that allows adherence of chlorine and chloramine to the granular activated (or "charged") carbon (GAC). Carbon also removes organic compounds such as herbicides, pesticides, and industrial solvents. When the pH of the feed water is higher, the charge on the GAC is lowered, reducing the adherence of chlorine and chloramines.

b. GAC used to fill the tanks must have a minimum iodine rating of 900 or equivalent, be virgin carbon (nonregenerated) and have a mesh size of 12 x 40 or smaller.

c. Monitoring the function of the tanks is achieved by testing for total chlorine, with an acceptable test result being less than 0.1 parts per million (ppm). A single test for total chlorine is stipulated to avoid confusion of results when testing for both free and total chlorine are done (AAMI, 2014e, 23500:2014). Patient exposure to higher levels of chloramines and chlorine can cause severe hemolytic anemia, methemo-globinemia, and death. (See Section E.)

(1) *Safety alert.* Monitoring is required prior to every shift of HD treatments, or every 4 hours if there are no set patient shifts.

(2) Testing is performed from a sample taken from a port between the first and second tank.

(a) If this test shows a level of 0.1 ppm or greater, the nurse in charge must be notified and a test done after the second tank.

(b) If the level of total chlorine after the second tank is 0.1 ppm or greater, treatments must be stopped immediately, and the medical director notified.

(c) If the level of total chlorine after the second tank is less than 0.1 ppm, treatment may continue with more frequent testing (e.g., every 1 to 2 hours) and arrangements made to replace the carbon tanks. When possible, the second tank can be rotated into the first position; or both tanks must be changed out.

d. Carbon tanks are maintained by backwashing, which does not regenerate the carbon or "rinse away" the chlorine and chloramines. Backwashing does "rearrange" the carbon, exposing new adsorption sites, and prevents "channeling," where water flow establishes channels through the same areas of carbon.

e. Carbon supports bacterial growth and should be considered a potential source of bioburden for the RO membrane.

f. Banks of tanks may sometimes be necessary to provide sufficient EBCT. Several tanks may be plumbed together as the first bank, or worker tanks, with additional tanks plumbed together as the second bank, or polishers. These tanks should be set up in series, with each tank's effluent flowing into the following tank, so that all the water being treated flows through every tank.

g. Ten minutes EBCT refers to the volume of water in the media space (if the tank was empty of media) that would run the RO for 10 minutes. EBCT is used as an indirect measure of the amount of contact between the carbon and water, and can be calculated using the formula of:

EBCT = (V/Q) X 7.48, using the input flow rate in gallons per minute (gpm) as Q and the volume of carbon media in cubic feet as V, and with 7.48 being the number of gallons in a cubic foot (Layman-Amato, Curtis, & Payne, 2013, http://www.prolibraries.com/anna/?select=session&sessionID=2840).

9. Monitoring the function of each component in the water treatment system is required.

10. *Safety alert.* It is imperative that water testing for total chlorine is performed at prescribed intervals without fail! Notify the nurse in charge and the medical director of any breakthrough and follow facility policies and procedures for safety interventions.

D. Water purification (treatment) components.

1. Reverse osmosis (RO) systems are the most frequently used water purification component. RO systems have a prefilter to remove particulates that may have entered the water during the pretreatment (such as carbon fines), a pump to increase water pressure, stainless steel containers ("vessels") to allow application of pressure, and RO membranes to purify the pretreated water.

a. The RO produces purified water through the use of pressurized water that is forced through a semi-permeable membrane, leaving most of its contaminants behind (overcoming natural osmosis using hydraulic pressure, thus creating "reverse osmosis"). The incoming stream is split into two, with one stream the purified product stream and one the waste stream. See Figure 2.30 for a graphic illustration of an RO System. Also see http://www.prolibraries.com/anna/?select=session&sessionID=2840

b. RO membranes will reject approximately 95% to 99% of charged particles. Contaminants with no charge (bacteria, viruses, endotoxin) that are larger than 200 daltons molecular weight cut-off will be removed by sieving. The pH, temperature, and damage to the RO membrane will change rejection characteristics.

c. RO membranes are made of a spiral wound polyamide material that is damaged by oxidants such as total chlorine and high levels of peracetic acid.

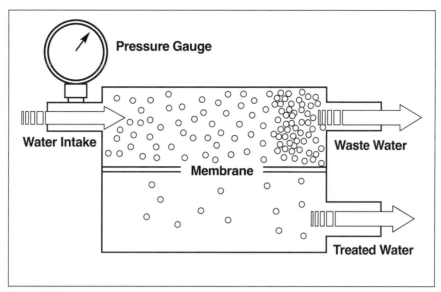

Figure 2.30. Graphic illustration of an RO System.

Used with permission from Layman-Amato, R. Curtis, J., & Payne, G.M. (2013). Water treatment for hemodialysis: An update. *Nephrology Nursing Journal, 40*(5), 383-404. Available at http://www.prolibraries.com/anna/?select= session&sessionID=2840.

d. Final water quality is measured by either conductivity in microsiemens/cm or total dissolved solids (TDS) displayed as mg/L or parts per million (PPM). Each measure indicates the total quantity of ions that remain in the RO product water, not which ions remain.

e. RO membrane performance is measured by percent rejection, which is the percent of charged contaminants that are removed to the waste drain (e.g., 95% rejected). The formula to calculate percent rejection is:

Rejection rate =

$$\frac{\text{Feed water conductivity (TDS)} - \text{Permeate conductivity (TDS)} \times 100}{\text{Feed water conductivity (TDS)}}$$

Most RO systems have a direct reading for percent rejection (CMS 2008 IG, V200; ANSI/AAMI 23500: 2014, 2014e).

f. The percent rejection and conductivity/TDS will vary depending on how well the RO membrane is functioning and the amount of dissolved solids in the feed water.

g. Product water must be continuously monitored, and a visual and audible alarm that can be seen and heard in the patient care area must be included.

h. To validate that the RO provides water that meets CMS requirements and AAMI standards, an AAMI chemical analysis must be done on the product water at least annually and whenever the rejection rate falls below 90% (refer to Table 2.7). Note that some state ESRD licensure rules include more stringent requirements.

i. There must be a set point for the water quality alarm that is based on the characteristics of the source water. If that set point is violated, the system should have an automatic divert-to-drain valve so inadequately purified water is not sent to patient use.

j. Monitoring includes validating the water quality prior to the start of the treatment day, recording and observing for trends in Delta (Δ) P, pump pressure, and the flow rates for both the product and reject streams.

2. Deionization (DI) systems: DI systems may be used as a backup system to an RO, or to polish RO treated water in locations where the source water is difficult to adequately purify for use in HD. At the time of publication of this text, there was an individual HD system on the market that uses DI as the primary purification element in a disposable water treatment system (NxStage Medical, Inc., 2011, http://www.nxstage.com/homehemodialysis/products/fluids).

a. DI has a finite capacity. Once exhausted, it will dump mass quantities of retained ions back into the product water, especially the weakly attracted ones such as aluminum and fluoride. This characteristic presents a serious risk to patients and has caused serious injuries and deaths.

b. DI tanks contain resin beads that remove both positively and negatively charged ions from the water in exchange for hydroxyl (OH^-) and hydrogen (H^+), which combine to form pure water (H_2O).

(1) Mixed bed deionizers contain both cationic and anionic resin beads in the same tank.

(2) Dual bed deionizers consist of multiple tanks with each containing either all cation-attracting or all anion-attracting resins. At least one anion and one cation tank must be used for each installation, and these should be followed by a mixed-bed deionizer.

c. The quality of DI treated water is measured using resistivity (inverse of conductivity). DI treated water must be one megohm/cm or greater specific resistivity at 25°C.

d. AAMI and CMS require that resistivity be continuously monitored with an audible and visual, temperature compensated alarm. The staff must be able to hear the alarm in the patient care area.

e. AAMI and CMS require the DI system to automatically divert the processed water to drain if the resistivity is less than 1 meg-ohm/cm and that the system not be used until the tanks are replaced (CMS, 2008b, IG, V203; ANSI/AAMI 23500:2014, 2014e).

f. Bacteria and endotoxin are not removed by DI as they do not contain an electrical charge. DI tanks tend to grow microbes and should be exchanged regularly.

g. AAMI and CMS require that DI systems are followed by ultrafiltration (UF) to remove both endotoxin and bacteria (ANSI/AAMI 23500:2014, 2014e; CMS, 2008b, IG, V204).

h. DI is not intended to be used instead of an RO for primary purification in centralized treatment water systems used to prepare water for use with multiple patients. DI coupled with UF is unable to remove low-molecular-weight bacterial byproducts such as microcystins (toxins from blue-green algae), which have caused liver failure and death in patients (ANSI/AAMI 23500:2014, 2014e).

i. DI resins used for dialysis must be designated medical or potable water grade and must be regenerated at the supplier separately from other more contaminated resins. The tanks should also be disinfected at the supplier.

j. AAMI and CMS require that carbon filtration precede DI to prevent formation of carcinogenic nitrosamines (ANSI/AAMI 23500:2014, 2014e; CMS, 2008b, IG V204).

k. At least two mixed bed DI tanks must be used in a series configuration, one as the worker, one as a backup.

l. AAMI and CMS require that resistivity be recorded twice daily; Δ P should be monitored and recorded once a day (ANSI/AAMI 23500:2014, 2014e; CMS, 2008b, IG V202).

E. Posttreatment components.
1. Ultraviolet irradiation (UV) uses a low-pressure mercury vapor lamp enclosed in a transparent quartz sleeve that emits a germicidal 254 nm (nanometer) wavelength to deliver a dose of radiant energy to inhibit microbial growth.
   a. UV is able to penetrate the cell wall of bacteria to destroy it or render it unable to replicate.
   b. UV resistant bacteria strains may develop if the equipment is not maintained properly.
   c. UV shall be equipped with an intensity meter that delivers 16 milliwatt-sec/cm^2 or, if the UV has no meter, delivers a radiant dose of at least 30 milliwatt-sec/cm^2.
   d. Endotoxin levels may increase as a result of destruction of microbes.
   e. UV must be followed by ultrafiltration (UF) to remove the particles of endotoxin.
   f. Replace the UV bulb every 8000 hours or annually and clean quartz sleeve routinely. Record radiant output and Δ P daily.
2. Endotoxin retentive filter or ultrafilter (UF): a very fine filter capable of removing bacteria and endotoxin.
   a. May be either a cross-flow design (with a feed stream, a product stream and a waste stream) or a dead-ended design (with one stream that flows in, then out).
   b. AAMI and CMS require that UF must follow DI (CMS 2008 IG, V204; ANSI/AAMI 23500:2014, 2014e).
   c. UF should be validated for medical use.
   d. UF will grow bacteria if not routinely disinfected or replaced.
   e. May be used at points of use (e.g., reprocessing equipment, on dialysate line, etc.) instead of, or in addition to, being used in the central water treatment system.
   f. Δ P should be monitored and recorded at least daily.
      (1) A differential pressure reading of zero might indicate that water is flowing around and not through the filter.
      (2) A high Δ pressure reading would indicate the filter is clogged.

F. Distribution systems.
1. There are two types of distribution systems, direct and indirect.
   a. Direct systems deliver water from the RO directly to the distribution loop for use.
   b. Indirect distribution systems deliver the treated water to a storage tank first.
2. Water storage tanks provide a way to accumulate the product water and deliver it to the distribution loop. Unused product water is recirculated back into the tank.

a. The large surface area in the storage tank is conducive to microbial growth.
b. The following design features are important to reduce microbial growth:
   (1) The tank should be designed with a cone-shaped bottom and a tight fitting lid, vented with a microbial air filter.
   (2) The tank should fill from the top with an internal spray mechanism.
   (3) All parts are to be made of inert material that does not leach contaminants.
c. The tank should be just large enough to meet peak water demand without exceeding it.
d. If a water storage tank is used, an aggressive and frequent disinfection program should be employed.

3. Distribution systems.
   a. Water distribution piping systems should be a continuous loop design where water is returned to the RO or storage tank and designed to minimize biofilm formation.
   b. Made of inert materials only. No copper, brass, aluminum, lead, zinc, or other toxic materials shall be used. Purified water is "aggressive" and will leach chemicals from these materials, re-contaminating the water.
   c. No dead-ends or multiple branches should exist; these add risk for bacterial contamination, as well as providing potential for disinfectants to be inadequately rinsed from the system.
   d. Rough joints must be avoided, as these provide a niche for bacterial growth.

4. Biofilm: Distribution systems are at risk for contamination with biofilm. Biofilm is formed by communities of microorganisms that attach to surfaces and secrete a gelatinous substance (extracellular polymer, glycocalyx) to protect themselves and create an endless supply of food.
   a. To minimize biofilm formation, there should be flow in the piping and through the storage tank during the hours of operation. Velocity of flow has not been found to prevent biofilm formation (AAMI, 2014e).
   b. Biofilm starts to form on wet surfaces almost immediately.
      (1) As biofilm communities grow larger, the flow of water through the distribution system can "break off" a large colony of biofilm and result in a "spike" of positive cultures.
      (2) While some biofilm is unavoidable in water distribution systems, a level of biofilm that prevents achievement of the required limits for microorganisms and endotoxins in the water is referred to as biofouling and must be avoided.

Table 2.12

Mixing Ratios and Symbols

Concentrate type	Acid: Bicarbonate and water	Symbol
35 X	1:34	Square
36.83 X	1:35.83	Circle
45 X	1:44	Triangle
36.1 X	1:35.1	Hexagon

VI. Ensuring dialysate safety: dialysate is prepared from purified water plus acid and bicarbonate concentrates.

A. Basic safety provisions.
   1. Limited variety of acid concentrates: sufficient variety should be provided to meet the needs of the patients without providing so many different solutions that errors are more likely to occur.
   2. Single mixing ratio.
      a. The mixing ratio defines the proportions of water, acid, and bicarbonate that are mixed together by the dialysis machine to make dialysate.
      b. Safe practice requires that all concentrates used in a facility be of the same mixing ratio to prevent mix-ups and potential patient harm from use of components of different mixing ratios.
      c. Each mixing ratio is identified by a specific symbol (see Table 2.12).
      d. All machines in the facility should be set to use the same mixing ratio.
      e. Responsible staff members should be trained to carefully order the specified ratio and to check incoming supplies for a match with that ratio.
   3. Point of use testing.
      a. CMS requires that dialysate testing at the point of use be done before each treatment (CMS, 2008b, IG V250).
      b. Required testing is dependent on the dialysis machine manufacturer's guidance and may include both pH and conductivity.
      c. Each facility must set limits for the acceptable variation between the hand-held and the machine measures for conductivity.
      d. Staff members must be educated to understand the reason for this test (to validate the machine is proportioning the acid, bicarbonate, and water correctly) and the allowable variation.
   4. Acid concentrate: the acid concentrate includes the electrolytes, to include sodium, potassium, magnesium, and calcium. The specific electrolytes

for use in the dialysis of an individual patient are determined by the practitioner's order. A facility may choose to use a standard acid for most patients, but is expected to have options available as needed.

a. Acid concentrate is available in gallon containers, in bulk containers (usually 55 gallon drums), and as a dry powder to be mixed with purified water on site.

b. Storage: acid concentrate is highly acidic, preventing the growth of bacteria. Unless storage time is limited by the manufacturer, it is not restricted.

c. When dry powder is mixed with purified water to form acid concentrate, the acid powder manufacturer's directions must be followed for:
   (1) The amount of water to be used.
   (2) Any specified sequence of mixing if there are multiple packets to be added.
   (3) The testing to be done to validate correct mixing was accomplished.
   (4) The acceptable ranges for those test results.

d. Distribution of acid concentrate may be via individual containers placed on the front of the dialysis machine, or the acid concentrate may be piped to the individual patient station via a central delivery system.

e. Security of concentrate distribution: safety steps should be in place to prevent accidental mix-ups of acid concentrates.
   (1) If there is remote access to the inlet to the acid concentrate storage system (as would be used to allow pumping of concentrate from a truck or drum outside the facility into an interior storage tank), this inlet must be secured to prevent tampering.
   (2) The mixing tank and delivery plumbing should form an integral system.
   (3) If a single mixing system is used to prepare more than one acid concentrate, the system must be thoroughly rinsed of the first concentrate before beginning to mix a different concentrate.

f. Labeling all containers and distribution ports is required. Acid labels should include the color code of red.
   (1) The mixing tank must be labeled as to contents at all times.
   (2) Labeling either the individual container or the outlet port must include sufficient information to accurately identify the critical electrolytes (i.e., potassium and calcium) and the mixing ratio.

5. Bicarbonate concentrate: a standard bicarbonate solution is used for all patients in a facility.
   a. Bicarbonate concentrate is available in gallon containers, as a dry powder to be mixed with

purified water on site, and in powder-filled cartridges or bags that are connected to the individual dialysis machine to prepare bicarbonate concentrate on-line during the patient's treatment.

b. Storage.
   (1) Bicarbonate concentrate supports bacterial growth.
   (2) Storage time must be carefully limited not to exceed that allowed by the manufacturer's guidance (usually 24 hours postdilution) to prevent microbiological contamination.

c. When dry powder is mixed with purified water to form bicarbonate concentrate, the bicarbonate powder manufacturer's guidance must be followed for:
   (1) The amount of water to be used.
   (2) The testing to be done to validate correct mixing was accomplished.
   (3) The acceptable ranges for those test results.

d. Distribution of bicarbonate concentrate may be via individual containers placed on the front of the dialysis machine, or the concentrate may be piped to the individual patient station via a central delivery system.
   (1) Labeling all containers and ports is required. Bicarbonate labels should include the color code of blue.
   (2) The mixing tank contents must be labeled at all times.
   (3) The label on the individual container and/or the outlet port must include sufficient information to accurately identify the contents (e.g., "Bicarb") and the mixing ratio (i.e., numbers or symbol).

VII. Maintain water and dialysate systems safely to prevent microbiological contamination.

A. Routine disinfection of the water and bicarbonate concentrate delivery systems must be done at a frequency to prevent the growth of bacteria, rather than in response to positive cultures or evidence of endotoxin contamination.

1. Cultures and endotoxin testing must be done prior to disinfection.

2. In a "worst case" scenario, samples are taken as distant from the time and date of the last disinfection as possible. Ensure that the timing of sample collection takes into consideration the days of laboratory operation to allow receipt of the samples when the laboratory is open.

3. Unless the dialysis facility has implemented a validation program that has demonstrated that a longer period between disinfection cycles maintains the equipment below the action levels

for bacteria and endotoxin, disinfection of the equipment should be at least every 30 days (AAMI, 23500, 2014e).

B. Disinfection methods include chemical disinfectants, heat, or ozone.
   1. Disinfectants: careful attention to dilution, exposure time, and rinsing free is required. Be aware that some disinfectants may harm the RO membranes.
   2. Heat is being used more commonly because it does not require vigorous rinsing and does not carry the risk of patient exposure to chemicals.
      a. Special plumbing is required to withstand the high temperatures required to disinfect the distribution system with heat.
      b. Temperature (approximately 80°C) and contact time (at least 10 minutes) must be monitored to ensure effectiveness.
   3. Ozone is commonly used to disinfect bicarbonate distribution systems and sometimes used to disinfect water distribution systems.
      a. Requires an ozone generator.
      b. Monitoring must ensure that a sufficient level of ozone for effective disinfection is achieved.
      c. The ozone must be removed to safe levels before the system is used for patient treatment.
   4. Disinfection should include the product side of the RO membrane as well as the distribution system, as bacterial growth can occur through the RO membrane.
   5. Disinfection records must include the dates and times of disinfection and dates and times of sample collection for cultures and endotoxin levels.
   6. Samples sites for cultures and endotoxin levels.
      a. Sites for water samples for microbiologic monitoring should include:
         (1) The start and end of the distribution system.
         (2) The storage tank (if present).
         (3) The water source for the bicarbonate mixing system.
         (4) The reuse equipment.
      b. Repeated results above the action levels require consideration to sample additional sites to determine the source of the contamination.
      c. Dialysate samples for cultures and endotoxin levels must be obtained from at least two machines each month, with a system in place to ensure that each machine is sampled at least every 12 months.
      d. State ESRD licensing rules may require more frequent testing.
      e. Sampled dialysis machines are representative of all machines.
         (1) If repeated test results are above the action

level, the user must presume that other machines may also be contaminated.
         (2) The investigation should address all machines, rather than simply the machines tested that month (AAMI, 23500, 2014e).

C. Ultrapure dialysate.
   1. Patients on HD are in a chronic inflammatory state. Endotoxin exposure has been cited as a possible potentiator of inflammation as well as cardiac stunning.
   2. Ultrapure dialysate requires a maximum allowable level for cultures (total viable count) of less than 0.1 CFU/mL and for endotoxin of less than 0.03 EU/mL. (AAMI, 11663, 2014c).
   3. These levels are only achievable through the use of endotoxin-retentive filters that are validated by the manufacturer as able to deliver this quality of dialysate that are used according to the manufacturer's instructions.

VIII. Quality Assessment Performance Improvement (QAPI) activities for water and dialysate.

A. Technical staff member(s) responsible for the water treatment and dialysate preparation systems should routinely participate in QAPI activities.

B. Routine reports to QAPI should include evidence of monitoring the water treatment and dialysate preparation systems (CMS, 2008b, IG V627).

C. Monitoring includes evidence of daily testing. Log review should include verification that readings and test results are within expected limits or that action is taken.

D. Results of cultures and endotoxin testing should be displayed in a way to allow review of results from each collection site for at least 6 months to facilitate identification of any trends (CMS, 2008b, IG V213).

E. If trends of increasing bacterial counts or endotoxin levels are identified, the medical director is responsible for oversight to develop and implement an action plan to reduce these levels (CMS, 2008b, IG V179).

Resources
ANSI = American National Standards Institute
AAMI = Association for the Advancement of
             Medical Instrumentation
ISO = International Standards Organization (ISO)

Section C
The Hemodialysis Treatment
Joan E. Speranza-Reid

I. Predialysis equipment preparation. The dialysis equipment is prepared and tested to assure a safe and effective dialysis treatment. (CDC, 2013b; http://www.cdc.gov/dialysis/prevention-tools/index.html; Gomez, 2011; Hoenich & Levin, 2007; Misra, 2005)

Refer also to the following resources:
- CDC Infection Training Video and Print Resources for Preventing Bloodstream and Other Infections in Outpatient Hemodialysis Patients, CDC (2013 a) http://www.cdc.gov/dialysis/prevention-tools/training-video.html
- Infection Control Guidelines in Hemodialysis, CDC Dialysis Station Routine Disinfection (2013b) http://www.cdc.gov/dialysis/prevention-tools/index.html
- APIC Guide to Elimination of Infections in Hemodialysis (2010), http://www.apic.org/Resource_/EliminationGuideForm/7966d850-0c5a-48ae-9090-a1da00bcf988/File/APIC-Hemodialysis.pdf
- HRET Infection Control Checklists are resources that should be used by facilities (2010). http://www.hret.org/quality/projects/improving-infection-coontrol-practices-ESRD-facilities.shtml
- National opportunity to improve infection control in ESRD (NOTICE) (2011). http://www.hret.org/quality/projects/resources/infection_control_checklist_11212011.pdf

A. The dialyzer is prepared as follows.
   1. Using aseptic technique, attach bloodlines to appropriate dialyzer ports.
   2. When preparing a dry pack dialyzer, verify and document:
      a. Dialyzer matches prescription.
      b. Membrane integrity is checked.
   3. When preparing a processed (reuse) dialyzer, verify and document dialyzer:
      a. Labeled with correct patient name and other identifying information.
      b. Prescribed dialyzer for this patient.
      c. Membrane integrity is checked.
      d. Positive test for the presence of sterilant prior to the priming procedure.
      e. Negative test for the presence of sterilant after the priming procedure.
      f. Follow facility and Association for the Advancement of Medical Instrumentation

(AAMI) standards for reuse (AAMI, 2011).
      g. *Safety alert.* Document all of the above information and verify with two people (two staff members must document *all* facets of verification; the patient is encouraged to confirm the dialyzer is his/hers and may be one of those documenting that identification).
   4. Rinse extracorporeal circuit with normal saline to remove air, glycerin, sterilants, and/or disinfectants, and any other manufacturing residue, according to manufacturer's recommendations.
   5. Rinse dialysate compartment of dialyzer with prescribed dialysate according to manufacturer's recommendations.
   6. The reprocessed dialyzer must be tested for residual disinfectant or sterilant after the rinsing procedure and before patient use. Testing and results must adhere to manufacturer instructions and recommendations. Document testing results.
   7. Follow manufacturer's recommendations and facility policies and procedures.
   8. Minimize the length of time supplies and extracorporeal system are prepared in advance and recirculated per unit policy. *Editor's note*: At the time of this publication, no documented evidence could be found regarding the appropriate time the extracorporeal system could be safely prepared in advance (Schrauf, 2014, http://www.prolibraries.com/anna/?select=session&sessionID=3017).

B. Delivery system preparation will depend on the specific system used and may also depend on the type of buffer used. Manufacturer recommendations and procedures should be followed.
   1. Ensure dialysis machine has been disinfected per facility protocol.
   2. Any disinfectant/sterilant present in the system must first be rinsed and the system tested to ensure no residual disinfectant/sterilant remains prior to dialyzer preparation.
   3. Dialysate temperature, pH, and conductivity must be within acceptable and safe limits.
   4. Integrity of bloodlines is verified and absent of kinking or other deficiencies. Refer to Figures 2.43 and 2.44 on page 137 to see examples.
   5. All alarms must be tested and functioning correctly.
   6. Hydraulic pressure testing may be performed with volumetric ultrafiltration machines.
   7. Most, if not all steps, should be documented.
   8. The primed dialyzer should be placed in recirculation mode until the patient begins treatment. The recirculation mode is an important step to prevent sterilant rebound from the dialyzer potting compound into the extracorporeal circuit. It is common practice for facilities to dispose of unused bloodlines and discard or reprocess the dialyzer after recirculating normal saline for the

unit specified number of hours per facility policy.

9. If the dialyzer has recirculated with normal saline for a period of time that exceeds the time limit defined by facility policy, the dialyzer should be filled with fresh normal saline prior to treatment initiation or discarded per facility policy.

10. Dialyzer and bloodlines should be free of air at end of priming procedure before initiating hemodialysis treatment.

II. Predialysis patient assessment and preparation

(Daugirdas, 2014; Gomez, 2011; Latham, 2006, Purcell, 2004). (See also fluid assessment parameters in Section D.)

A. The patient is assessed predialysis to ensure a safe and appropriate dialysis treatment. Assessment should include but not be limited to:

1. Weight: Compare estimated dry weight to predialysis and last treatment postweight.
2. Edema: peripheral, facial, periorbital, sacral.
3. Skin: turgor, color, temperature.
4. Jugular venous distention in supine and Fowler's or semi-Fowler's position.
5. Ultrafiltration rate related to dialysis time, patient weight, age, and comorbidities that may affect safe fluid removal. The Dialysis Outcomes and Practice Patterns Study (DOPPS) reported an increase in all-cause mortality for a UFR greater than 10mL/kg/hour (Bragg-Gresham et al., 2006).
6. Blood pressure (sitting and standing as appropriate for patient condition), comparing results to previous dialysis treatments.
7. Continued need for and number of antihypertensive medications and/or dose changes or elimination; assess if patient held dose or changed time for antihypertensive medication pretreatment.
8. Temperature and changes between predialysis and postdialysis results. Average temperature is 96.8° F (36°C).
9. Heart rate/rhythm/sounds: quality, rate, rhythm, pericardial rub, gallop.
10. Respiratory rate, rhythm, quality, breath sounds (wheezes, rales, crackles, diminished breath sounds), oxygen needs.
11. Peripheral pulses and capillary refill.
12. Mental status: orientation, confusion, restlessness, mood, speech, thought processes, changes from baseline.
13. Ambulation: ability, gait changes.
14. General sense of well-being.
15. Reported posttreatment recovery time.
16. Appetite: changes and degree of thirst.
17. Fluid losses related to: bowel dysfunction, ascites, lymphocele, vomiting, draining wounds, nasogastric tube.
18. Changes in abdominal girth measurement.
19. Residual kidney function/urine output.
20. Current complaints of or interdialytic history of: headache, dizziness, blurred vision, nausea, vomiting, diarrhea, constipation, tarry stool, muscle cramps, shortness of breath, dyspnea, chest pain, palpitations, weakness, fatigue, insomnia, pain, fever/chills, bleeding, urgency or frequency of urination, other problems since last treatment.
21. History of injuries, falls, bleeding, unusual bruising, surgical procedures, and menses.
22. Condition and patency of vascular access.
23. Review pertinent laboratory data, such as electrolytes/minerals (calcium, phosphorous, potassium, magnesium, sodium "set point"), blood glucose, serum albumin, hemoglobin/hematocrit.

B. Administer, and adjust as necessary, the prescribed hemodialysis treatment based on predialysis assessment findings. Components of the hemodialysis prescription include:

1. Hemodialysis treatment time.
2. Dialyzer to be used.
3. Blood flow rate.
4. Dialysate flow rate.
5. Dialysate composition.
6. Anticoagulation.
7. Fluid removal plan.
   a. Ultrafiltration rate as appropriate for patient age, weight, comorbidities. Calculate the ultrafiltration rate (UFR) or transmembrane pressure (TMP) as appropriate for dialysis equipment. Calculations will determine the total amount of fluid to be removed during treatment and should include any projected intake or fluid losses during treatment.
   b. Blood or blood products, fluid intake, ice, normal saline expected to be administered, or medications given in some volume of diluents should be included in the projected fluid intake during treatment.
   c. Projected fluid intake will also include the normal saline volume the patient may receive from extracorporeal circuit priming and blood return at end of hemodialysis treatment.
   d. Urinary output or emesis should be considered outputs for the purpose of calculating the total amount of fluid removal during HD.

III. Initiation of Hemodialysis. Basic steps necessary to initiate a dialysis treatment (CDC, 2013c, https://www.youtube.com/watch?v=_0zhY0JMGCA &feature=youtu.be; Gomez, 2011; Latham, 2006).

A. Prepare and cannulate vascular access or access central venous catheter (CVC) according to facility procedure.

B. Obtain blood sampling for laboratory analysis after vascular access cannulation is completed. Ensure sample is not diluted with normal saline from fistula needle (if used for needle preparation) or CVC (previous posttreatment lock).

C. Administer anticoagulant as prescribed and wait 3 to 5 minutes until patient is systemically anticoagulated to reduce potential for thrombus formation in the dialyzer and extracorporeal circuit.

D. If the patient is to receive the equivalent of the normal saline priming volume, flush the extracorporeal circuit with fresh normal saline before connecting the arterial and venous bloodlines to the patient. This will avoid exposure to residual particulate matter from the manufacturing process and any rebound of sterilant during normal saline recirculation.

E. Stop the blood pump; clamp the arterial and venous bloodlines, and saline tubing. Securely attach arterial bloodline end to arterial access, and venous bloodline to venous access, preferably using an interlocking connection (e.g., Luer-Lok). Ensure all clamps are open on dynamic access lines and bloodlines. *Note*: Some facilities apply tape over interlocking connections.

F. Start blood pump at less than 200 mL/min. Ensure pressure monitor lines are unclamped and monitor pressures to assure adequate arterial blood supply and the absence of clamps on bloodlines. Monitor arterial and venous pressures and visually assess for infiltration of vascular access. *Note*: Follow the facility specific procedures.

G. Follow the facility's and manufacturer's procedure for initiation of hemodialysis.

H. On rare occasions (overt pulmonary edema or other medical reason), the normal saline prime volume is discarded to eliminate extra fluid volume to the patient. In this situation, allow patient blood to fill the extracorporeal circuit to beyond the venous drip chamber, then connect the venous bloodline to the venous vascular access. *Safety alert.* This procedure requires great caution and attention due to the risk of accidental exsanguination. Due to the potential for a lethal complication, this practice is restricted to special circumstances or eliminated in most dialysis facilities.

I. Initiate extracorporeal circuit pressure monitoring if not already instituted.

J. Establish desired blood flow rate and note time. This is the start of dialysis treatment time.

K. Set limits on all monitors if necessary or check that they are appropriately set.

L. Set dialysate flow rate according to prescription.

M. Initiate anticoagulation infusion per facility protocol if prescribed.

N. Ensure bloodlines are adequately secured to patient per facility protocol.

IV. Intradialytic patient assessment and management (Daugirdas, 2014; Gomez, 2011). Monitor the patient throughout the hemodialysis treatment to assure a safe and effective treatment and to determine the patient's response to the delivery of the hemodialysis prescription.

A. Patient assessment includes:
   1. Blood pressure (BP) and pulse comparing results to predialysis values and established acceptable parameters.
      a. Follow the facility's policy regarding time intervals for measuring the BP.
      b. Typically every 30 minutes or as indicated by a change in the patient's condition.
   2. Amount of UFR fluid removal and UF time left.
   3. Respiratory rate and quality of respirations.
   4. Temperature, if indicated.
   5. Hemodialysis access (see Chapter 3, Vascular Access, in this module).
      a. Access and connections visible at all times.
      b. Infiltration or hematoma.
      c. Inability to achieve or maintain prescribed blood flow rate.
      d. Arterial or venous pressure outside of established parameters.
      e. Bleeding.
      f. Pain.
   6. Any new complaint reported by the patient which could be an early sign of complication or adverse reaction to the dialysis treatment.
      a. Headache, dizziness, or blurred vision.
      b. Nausea, vomiting.
      c. Fever, chills.
      d. Chest pain or palpitations.
      e. Tachycardia.
      f. Shortness of breath, dyspnea.
      g. Change in mental status (e.g. agitation, confusion, restlessness).
   7. Response to anticoagulation.
      a. Review previous treatment responses to anticoagulation.
      b. Note presence of thrombus formation in dialyzer and/or extracorporeal system.
      c. Note bleeding occurrence from body sites (e.g. eyes, nose, genitourinary system).

B. Once hemodialysis is initiated, assess integrity of the extracorporeal circuit including connections and delivery system alarms.
   1. Bleeding at access site.
   2. Loose access/bloodline connections.
   3. Signs of extracorporeal system clotting.
   4. *Safety alert.* Vascular access must be visible at all times throughout HD treatment (CMS, 2008, V407, https://www.cms.gov/Medicare/Provider-Enrollment-and-Certification/GuidanceforLawsAndRegulations/downloads/esrdpgmguidance.pdf).

C. Patient and equipment monitoring should be completed and documented promptly per facility policy.
   1. Immediately upon treatment initiation.
   2. At regular intervals during the hemodialysis treatment.
   3. Any change in patient condition.
   4. Per facility policy.

D. The patient is educated and encouraged to recognize and report early signs of adverse responses to the hemodialysis treatment so preventive measures can occur.

E. Monitor the patient throughout treatment for signs and symptoms of treatment-related complications.
   1. Air embolism.
   2. Bleach or sterilant exposure.
   3. Dialyzer reaction.
   4. Exsanguination.
   5. Hemolysis.
   6. Pyrogenic reaction.

F. Modify patient treatment plan as indicated through patient assessment to prevent complications.

G. Appropriately treat complications if they occur (see Section E).

H. Administer medications as prescribed per facility policy, procedures, and/or protocols.

V. Discontinuation of hemodialysis. Basic steps required to terminate the hemodialysis treatment in a safe and efficient manner (Gomez, 2011; Latham, 2006; NKF, 2006).

A. Anticoagulation infusion or bolus dosing may be discontinued before termination of hemodialysis depending upon facility procedure and prescription. This may shorten postdialysis bleeding from needle sites.

B. All patient and extracorporeal circuit parameters are documented.

1. If a postdialysis blood sample is to be drawn, reduce the blood pump speed to 100 mL/min.
2. The NKF-DOQI Clinical Practice Guidelines for Hemodialysis Adequacy recommend the postdialysis blood sample for determining treatment adequacy be drawn from the arterial bloodline injection site approximately 15 seconds after blood pump speed has been reduced to 50 to 100 mL/min at the end of the hemodialysis treatment (NKF, 2006f, http://www2.kidney.org/professionals/KDOQI/guideline_upHD_PD_VA/hd_guide3.htm).

C. Stop blood pump, obtain blood sample if appropriate, and return blood to patient with normal saline per facility procedure.

D. Continue blood compartment monitoring until a patient circuit is terminated. The air detector should remain armed until the venous bloodline is disconnected from the patient.

E. See Chapter 3 in this module for postdialysis management of the vascular access.

VI. Postdialysis patient assessment. The patient is assessed after the dialysis treatment to determine the patient's response to the delivered hemodialysis prescription (CDC, 2013c, https://www.youtube.com/watch?v=_0zhY0JMGCA&feature=youtube; Gomez, 2011, NKF, 2006).

A. The assessment should include but not be limited to:
   1. Blood pressure (sitting and standing as appropriate for patient) and pulse comparing results to predialysis values and to establish acceptable parameters for the patient.
   2. Temperature, comparing to predialysis value.
   3. Access condition and any difficulty achieving homeostasis after needle removal.
   4. Mental status: orientation, confusion, restlessness, mood, speech, thought processes, change from baseline.
   5. Patient condition upon completion of treatment and before leaving the facility.
   6. Method of departure from the facility (e.g., ambulatory, walker, wheelchair, etc.).
   7. Weight: Compare postdialysis weight to targeted posttreatment weight and ordered dry weight and adjust as indicated and prescribed per physician/APRN/PA. Document Plan of Care changes to address attaining dry weight.
   8. If blood volume monitoring is used, conduct plasma refill at end of treatment to assess if there is accessible fluid still available to be removed.

B. All predialysis, intradialysis, and postdialysis assessment information should be documented, compared, and interpreted. Additional treatments, interventions, and teaching should be initiated as appropriate.

C. Treatment adequacy may be determined by one or more of the following.
   1. Blood chemistries.
   2. Absence or amelioration of uremic signs and symptoms.
   3. Patient self-report of well-being.
   4. Fluid status.
   5. Morbidity during or between dialysis treatment.
   6. Quantification of the delivered dialysis dose (see Section A for urea kinetic modeling (NKF, 2006f, http://www2.kidney.org/professionals/KDOQI/ guideline_upHD_PD_VA/hd_guide5.htm).

D. Delivery system is rinsed and/or cleaned and sterilized according to manufacturer's recommendations.

VII. Anticoagulation during hemodialysis

(Davenport, Lai, Hertel, & Caruana, 2014; Fischer, 2007; Gomez, 2011; Koster et al., 2007; Murray et al., 2004).

A. Rationale for anticoagulation during hemodialysis.
   1. Uremic toxin accumulation causes disruptions in the coagulation system.
   2. As blood comes into contact with foreign surfaces (bloodlines, dialyzer membrane, air [in drip chambers]), the clotting mechanism is activated.
   3. The clotting mechanism starts with a coating of plasma proteins on the surfaces followed by platelet adherence and aggregation (thromboxane A2 generation) and the activation of the intrinsic coagulation cascade.
   4. The clotting cascade may continue on to significant thrombus formation, fibrin deposition, and clotting in the extracorporeal circuit.
   5. Additional factors affecting the clotting cascade.
      a. Low blood flow through the dialyzer.
      b. Access recirculation.
      c. High hematocrit leading to hemoconcentration and increased blood viscosity.
      d. High ultrafiltration rate.
      e. Intradialytic administration of blood and blood products.
      f. Intradialytic administration of lipid infusion.
      g. The length, diameter, and composition of bloodlines may affect intradialytic clotting.
   6. Anticoagulation agents and methods are part of each hemodialysis prescription.
   7. Anticoagulation with heparin is the most common method to prevent clotting in the extracorporeal system.

B. Pharmacology of heparin.
   1. Derived from porcine intestinal mucosa (mucosal heparin) or beef lung (beef heparin). *Note*: beef heparin may be unavailable.
   2. Acts by accelerating the activity of antithrombin binding to thrombin. It is most effective in thrombosis prophylaxis, and more heparin is required if thrombosis has developed. Heparin has little inhibitory effect on platelet-surface interaction.
   3. In commercial preparation, heparin is a heterogeneous material of active and inactive species with varying molecular size. A more homogenous heparin preparation has been developed and used for anticoagulation in this patient population (low-molecular weight heparin).
   4. Removed from the circulation through the reticuloendothelial system at a low but constant rate, metabolized in the liver and excreted in the urine.
   5. Adverse side effects of heparin administration include allergy, excessive bleeding, hyperlipidemia, hypoaldosteronism and exacerbation of hyperkalemia, osteoporosis, pruritus, and thrombocytopenia.

C. Methods of heparin administration.
   1. Continuous: Heparin is continuously infused into the extracorporeal circuit during dialysis with a calibrated infusion pump. It is usually infused into the arterial bloodline side of the extracorporeal circuit after the blood pump to avoid excessive infusion due to the negative prepump pressure of the arterial circuit. This may be combined with a bolus loading dose before dialysis initiation.
      a. For patients not receiving treatment using a central venous catheter (CVC), heparin infusion is usually terminated 1 hour before end of treatment since the average half-life of heparin in a dialysis patient is 1 hour. In patients with a CVC, heparin infusion is not terminated until end of treatment.
      b. If used for "tight" heparinization (minimal anticoagulation, sufficient only to prevent clotting of the extracorporeal system), the infusion is not terminated until end of treatment.
   2. Intermittent: A bolus loading dose of heparin is administered to the patient 3 to 5 minutes before treatment initiation per provider order and/or unit policy and procedure. Additional bolus doses of heparin may be administered during dialysis.
   3. Bolus: A bolus loading dose of heparin is administered to the patient 3 to 5 minutes before

treatment initiation per provider order and/or unit policy and procedure with no further heparin administered.

D. Anticoagulation approaches.
  1. Systemic routine heparinization.
     a. Used for patients at normal risk for bleeding and not for those considered to be at an unusually high risk for bleeding.
     b. The objective is to achieve some designated prolongation of a patient's clotting time to prevent thrombus formation in the extracorporeal circuit.
     c. Anticoagulation is initially achieved with a bolus dose before initiation of dialysis. Three to five minutes is needed before initiation of dialysis to ensure systemic effect of anticoagulant. A constant heparin infusion may also be necessary to reduce clotting.
     d. Heparin administration may occur in a standard dosing regimen for all patients or given as individualized doses.
  2. Fractional, tight, or minimal heparinization.
     a. Prescribed for patients who are at slight risk for bleeding.
     b. The objective is to only slightly prolong the patient's clotting time without inducing thrombus formation in the extracorporeal circuit while utilizing judicious heparin dosing.
     c. Small doses of heparin are administered. Clotting times may be measured frequently.
     d. Usually administered with an initial bolus of heparin at treatment initiation followed by a constant infusion.
  3. Target clotting times during hemodialysis.
     a. Activated clotting time (ACT) target is 80% above baseline at start of treatment and 40% above baseline at end of treatment or 40% above baseline during and at the end of treatment (tight).
     b. Whole blood activated partial thromboplastin time (WBPTT) target is 80% above baseline at start of treatment and 40% above baseline at end of treatment, or 40% above baseline during and at the end of treatment (tight).
  4. Alternative methods for anticoagulation with patients at risk for bleeding or heparin allergy.
     a. Regional citrate anticoagulation: Infusion of sodium citrate into the arterial bloodline to form a complex with calcium to prevent activation of the clotting cascade. Calcium is infused into the venous bloodline to restore serum calcium to normal value.
        (1) Must use calcium-free dialysate.
        (2) Complication may occur due to hypocalcemia and citrate toxicity. Overt

symptoms may include nausea, muscle cramps, parathesias, and tetany.
     b. Heparin-free dialysis.
        (1) High blood flow rates equal to or greater than 300 mL/minute must be used.
        (2) Intermittent rapid normal saline flush through the dialyzer at regular intervals are required.
           (a) Generally 100 to 200 mL every 30 minutes.
           (b) Used to observe for and prevent clotting, or to identify the need to change the extracorporeal system if clotting is seen or seems likely.
        (3) Dialysis has been successfully performed with no heparin or alternative anticoagulant.
        (4) The equivalent volume of normal saline administered must be removed by ultrafiltration during the dialysis treatment unless the patient was at or below the prescribed dry weight.
        (5) Indications: pericarditis, surgery, thrombocytopenia, active bleeding, and/or clotting disorders.
     c. Use of a bicarbonate dialysis solution with low concentration citric acid (Citrasate®) has been shown to inhibit blood coagulation and platelet activation on the dialyzer membrane surface and can be used as part of an alternative anticoagulation strategy.
     d. Additional medications such as argatroban and lepirudin are costly alternatives that may be used by physicians for patients unable to receive heparin.

E. Assessing anticoagulation therapy outcomes.
  1. Assess the patient predialysis for any interdialytic changes in condition or events, signs of bleeding, or risk of bleeding.
     a. Open or closed injuries.
     b. Falls.
     c. Bruising or contusions.
     d. Hemorrhage, including the eye.
     e. Surgical, dental, or biopsy procedures that have been or will be performed.
     f. Signs and symptoms of pericarditis.
     g. Medication history that may affect anticoagulation including over-the-counter medications.
     h. Menses.
  2. Intradialytic inspection of the dialyzer and extracorporeal circuit for visual signs of clotting.
     a. Extremely dark blood, shadows, or dark/black streaks in the dialyzer.
     b. Clot formation in drip chambers and/or arterial dialyzer header.

c. Rapid filling of venous chamber and/or transducer filters with blood.

d. Changes in arterial or venous pressures, depending on where clot formation has occurred.

e. Blood in the postdialyzer venous bloodline unable to enter the venous blood chamber (falls back into line segment versus entering chamber).

3. Technical factors that may result in increased clotting.

a. Dialyzer priming.

(1) Air retained in dialyzer due to inadequate priming or poor priming technique.

(2) Lack of or insufficient priming of heparin infusion line.

b. Heparin administration.

(1) Incorrect heparin pump setting.

(2) Incorrect loading dose.

(3) Delayed initiation of heparin pump at start of treatment.

(4) Failure to unclamp heparin infusion line.

(5) Insufficient wait time between administration of loading dose to start of treatment.

c. Vascular access.

(1) Inadequate blood flow rate.

(2) Excessive access recirculation.

(3) Hypovolemia.

(4) Frequent interruption of blood flow due to machine alarm situations or poor/inadequate blood flow.

4. Postdialysis inspection of the dialyzer and extracorporeal circuit for visual signs of clotting.

a. Large amounts of clotting indicate a need for an increase in anticoagulation.

b. Decrease in total dialyzer cell volume (in dialyzer reprocessing program) can indicate dialyzer clotting.

c. Activated clotting time (ACT).

d. Whole blood activated partial thromboplastin time (WBPTT).

e. Plasma partial thromboplastin time (PTT).

f. Lee-White clotting time (LWCT).

5. Platelets.

a. Heparin-induced thrombocytopenia type II is a complication of heparin therapy occurring in 5 to 10% of patients treated with heparin.

b. Related to the presence of heparin-induced antiplatelet antibodies.

c. Initially presents as thrombocytopenia (a reduction in platelet count to 30 to 50% of baseline value). Associated with venous and/or arterial bloodline thrombosis formation in 20 to 50% of cases.

D. Federal regulations have constrained the ability to perform anticoagulation monitoring in the dialysis facility by staff.

1. Dialysis staff can perform anticoagulation monitoring only by using laboratory certified methods which are subjected to regular laboratory quality control.

2. In the absence of facility heparin monitoring, less quantitative methods of anticoagulation monitoring are used (e.g., visual inspection of the extracorporeal circuit for thrombus formation).

VIII. Red blood cell transfusion (Ashton, 2014; Carson et al., 2012; Fishbane & Shah 2014; Shaz & Hillyer, 2011; Tanhehco & Berns, 2012).

A. Red blood cell transfusions were frequently required prior to the introduction of erythropoiesis-stimulating agents (ESAs) when iron supplementation and anabolic steroids were not successful in improving anemia symptoms. Patient hemoglobin (Hgb) levels greatly improved with administration of ESAs, significantly decreasing transfusion needs. Changes in anemia management have resulted in an increase in transfusions in this patient population. *Note:* Patients awaiting transplant or planning transplantation should avoid red blood cell transfusion whenever possible to prevent tissue antigen exposure and possible antibody formation, which may reduce the likelihood of transplantation.

B. The American Association of Blood Banks (AABB) lists four clinical guideline recommendations for red blood cell transfusion (Carson et al., 2012).

1. Adhere to a restrictive transfusion strategy (7 to 8 g/dL) in stable patients.

2. Adhere to a restrictive transfusion strategy in patients with preexisting cardiovascular disease and consider transfusion for patient symptoms or Hgb equal to or greater than 8 g/dL.

3. Transfusion decisions should be influenced by symptoms as well as Hgb levels.

4. No recommendation for or against a liberal or restrictive transfusion threshold for hemodynamically stable patients with acute coronary syndrome.

C. Transfusion related adverse events are classified as acute (within 6 hours of administration) or delayed (days to years). *Safety alert.* For any adverse event(s) that requires the infusion be stopped, follow the facility procedure(s) to report the reaction, including notification of the blood bank, in an effort to identify the etiology of the event and avoid subsequent, similar events. These adverse events include:

1. Febrile nonhemolytic transfusion reactions.

a. Caused by donor leukocytes interacting with patient white blood cell (WBC) antibodies.

b. Temperature increase equal to or greater than 1°C and/or chills/rigors not attributed to other factors.

c. If febrile reaction is suspected, stop transfusion immediately and administer symptomatic care.
2. Allergic reactions.
   a. Caused by an allergen interaction with a preformed antibody.
   b. Wide range of symptoms, mild to life-threatening.
      (1) Urticaria with or without generalized pruritus or flushing.
      (2) Hoarseness.
      (3) Stridor.
      (4) Wheezing.
      (5) Dyspnea.
      (6) Hypotension.
      (7) GI symptoms.
      (8) Shock.
   c. Mild reactions can be treated with antihistamines, with more severe reactions treated with epinephrine and steroids.
   d. Premedication with antihistamine decreases allergic reaction incidence but should not be used in patients without allergic reaction history; administer per physician/APRN/PA order or per facility protocol.
3. Acute hemolytic transfusion reaction (AHTR).
   a. Caused by antigen-antibody complexes activating complement cascade.
   b. ABO incompatible red blood cell transfusion most often associated with transfusion event (e.g., "wrong patient receives wrong blood").
   c. Signs and symptoms include:
      (1) Anxiety.
      (2) Chest and abdominal pain.
      (3) Chills/rigors.
      (4) Dyspnea.
      (5) Fever.
      (6) Flank and back pain.
      (7) Hemoglobinuria.
      (8) Nausea/vomiting.
      (9) Oliguria/anuria.
4. Delayed hemolytic transfusion reaction (DHTR).
   a. Caused by alloantibody formation.
   b. Symptoms usually appear 3 to 10 days after transfusion and include:
      (1) Less than expected increase in Hgb posttransfusion.
      (2) Back pain.
      (3) Chills.
      (4) Fever.
      (5) Jaundice.
      (6) Malaise.
   c. Patients should receive antigen negative red blood cells for future transfusions.
5. Transfusion-associated circulatory overload (TACO).
   a. Caused by circulatory overload posttransfusion.
   b. Symptoms.
      (1) Chest tightness.
      (2) Cough.
      (3) Cyanosis.
      (4) Dyspnea.
      (5) Headache.
      (6) Hypertension.
      (7) Orthopnea.
   c. Treatment includes:
      (1) Discontinue transfusion.
      (2) Administer diuretics if patient has residual kidney function, otherwise institute fluid removal via hemodialysis.
      (3) Administer oxygen.
      (4) Place patient in sitting position.
6. Transfusion-related acute lung injury (TRALI).
   a. Caused by activation of complement cascade and cytokine release.
   b. Symptoms.
      (1) Bilateral pulmonary edema.
      (2) Fever.
      (3) Hypotension.
      (4) Hypoxemia.
      (5) Respiratory failure.
   c. Treatment includes:
      (1) Discontinue transfusion.
      (2) Supportive care for symptoms.
7. Posttransfusion purpura (PTP).
   a. Caused by antiplatelet antibody formation due to an antigen in the transfused blood.
   b. Symptoms occur 2 to 14 days posttransfusion and include:
      (1) Purpuric rash.
      (2) Bruising.
      (3) Mucosal bleeding.
   c. Treatment is intravenous (IV) immunoglobulin.
8. Transfusion-associated graft versus host disease (TA-GVHD).
   a. Caused by donor leukocytes attacking recipient cells.
   b. Rare reaction that usually occurs in severely immunocompromised patients.
   c. Greater than 90% mortality rate.
   d. Symptoms occur 3 to 30 days posttransfusion and include:
      (1) Diarrhea.
      (2) Fever.
      (3) Liver dysfunction.
      (4) Pancytopenia.
      (5) Rash.
   e. Treatment has rare success, and prevention through use of irradiated blood components is advised.
9. Iron overload.
   a. Occurs in patients transfused chronically, especially those with thalassemia and sickle cell

disease. One unit of red blood cells contains 200 to 250 mg iron.
   b. May occur in patients receiving recurrent IV iron dosing.
   c. Signs and symptoms include:
      (1) Cardiomyopathy.
      (2) Cirrhosis.
      (3) Congestive heart failure.
      (4) Endocrine dysfunction.
      (5) Hepatomegaly.
   d. Treatment is administration of iron-chelating medications.
10. Alloimmunization.
   a. Can occur against RBC or HLA antigens.
   b. HLA alloimmunization reduces the likelihood of transplantation.
11. Transfusion infection risks.
   a. Infectious risks are greatly reduced due to improved screening methods.
   b. Infectious agents include:
      (1) HIV.
      (2) Hepatitis C.
      (3) Hepatitis B.
      (4) Human T-cell lymphotropic virus (HTLV).
      (5) CMV.
      (6) West Nile virus (WNV).
      (7) Babesiosis.
      (8) Variant Creutzfeldt-Jakob disease (vCJD).
      (9) Ebola virus disease (EBV).
   c. Bacterial and parasite contamination is now a greater risk than viral contamination.
12. Hyperkalemia.
   a. Red blood cells undergo various changes during storage, one of which increases potassium (K^+) concentration.
   b. Fresh blood product (less than 5 days old) will have a lower K^+ concentration.
   c. Lysis of some transfused red blood cells occurs in the first 2 hours posttransfusion.
   d. Hyperkalemia can be a problem for patients receiving dialysis with infusion of large volumes or rapid infusions.

D. Red blood cell transfusion procedure (Ashton, 2014).
   1. Follow state regulations and facility policy and procedure for blood transfusion.
   2. Ensure blood component is correct for patient per facility policy.
   3. Ensure date on bag of red blood cells is not past expiration date.
   4. Inspect blood component for abnormalities.
   5. Obtain patient consent and educate patient on signs and symptoms of adverse reactions.
   6. Obtain blood pressure, pulse, temperature, and respiratory rate prior to transfusion administration, 15 minutes after initiation of transfusion, every 30 minutes, and posttrans-

fusion, noting any changes. Document results.
   7. The tubing from the blood product attaches to the automated infusion pump, then attaches to the medication port on the arterial bloodline. If a separate infusion pump is not available, attach the tubing from the blood product directly to the arterial bloodline.
   8. Administer at slow rate (equal to or less than 2 mL/min) for first 15 minutes of infusion and observe for adverse reaction.
   9. If no adverse reaction, increase transfusion rate to 250 to 400 mL/min to complete transfusion. *Note*: Include blood component volume into fluid removal target loss.
   10. Document patient response to transfusion in medical record.
   11. One unit of packed red blood cells is expected to increase the Hgb. by approximately 1 g/dL.

SECTION D
Fluid Removal: Obtaining the Estimated Dry Weight During Hemodialysis
Judy Kauffman

I. Definition of true dry weight.

A. The body's weight when fluid volume is optimal.

B. May be referred to as "ideal body weight" (IBW), target weight, estimated dry weight (EDW), true dry weight.

C. The ultrafiltration component of the hemodialysis prescription should be optimized with a goal to render the patient euvolemic and normotensive (while on few blood pressure medications), avoiding symptoms, maintaining organ perfusion and residual urine output (CMS, 2008).

II. Significance of obtaining the dry weight
(National Kidney Foundation [NKF], 2006a, http://www2.kidney.org/professionals/KDOQI/guideline_upHD_PD_VA/hd_guide5.htm; Parker et al., 2013; Purcell et al., 2004; Rodriguez et al., 2005; Shoji et al., 2004).

A. Extra fluid that accumulates in the various body compartments must be safely removed during hemodialysis (HD) with ultrafiltration (UF).
   1. Hypervolemia, the most common cause of the combination of hypertension, left ventricular hypertrophy (LVH), and cardiovascular disease (CVD), contributes to the mortality rate of patients on HD.
   2. Inaccurate overestimation of dry weight has significant consequences.

3. Hypovolemia can cause intradialytic morbidities (IDMs), ischemia, damage to vital organs (e.g., brain, heart), loss of residual kidney function (RKF), and increases mortality rate.

B. The most common admitting diagnoses for patients with chronic kidney disease (CKD) stage 3 are:
1 Pulmonary edema.
2. Acute coronary syndrome.

C. The goal is to obtain normovolemia without IDMs. This combined with solute clearances equals adequacy of dialysis (NKF, 2006a, http://www.kidney.org/professionals/kdoqi/guideline_uphd_pd_va/hd_guide5.htm).

D. The 2008 Fluid Management Guidelines from the Centers for Medicare and Medicare Services (CMS), address the significance of optimal fluid volume management (CMS, 2008). Changes to the Interpretive Guidelines serve to hold hemodialysis facilities more accountable for improving fluid management outcomes. These guidelines (494.90: Plan of Care V543) are much more specific and actually define estimated dry weight (EDW) and the inter/intradialytic measures that will be used to evaluate the outcomes.
1. Patients at their EDW should be asymptomatic and normotensive on minimum blood pressure medications, while preserving organ perfusion and maintaining existing residual kidney function.
2. Patients at their EDW attain normotension for most of their interdialytic period, while avoiding orthostatic hypotension or postural symptoms either during or after dialysis. Excess fluid accumulation may have adverse effects (e.g. hypertension, LVH, cardiovascular complications, and hospitalizations).

III. Patient outcome: The patient will maintain optimal fluid volume status that is euvolemic and normotensive.

A. Nursing management.
1. Fluid assessment parameters (Gomez, 2011).
   a. Weight: predialysis and postdialysis.
   b. Blood pressure (sitting and standing, if appropriate and possible for patient's condition), comparing those to previous HD (normotension is desired), predialysis, intradialysis, and postdialysis.
   c. Apical and peripheral pulses: quality, rate, rhythm.
   d. Respiratory rate and quality; O_2 saturation if available.
   e. Temperature: predialysis and postdialysis with the goal of isothermia.
   f. Neck vein distention, jugular venous pressure.
   g. Capillary refill.
   h. Heart sounds.
   i. Breath sounds.
   j. Dependent and peripheral edema (*Note*: A patient can have fluid excess in the absence of gross clinical evidence of volume expansion, a phenomenon termed "silent overhydration" or "silent volume").
   k. Skin turgor and mucous membranes.
   l. Residual kidney function (RKF) – assess at least every 2 months if urinary output is greater than 100 mL/day.
   m. Fluid intake (oral, parenteral, and intradialytic) and degree of thirst.
   n. Sodium intake (include water source because soft water is created by exchanging calcium for sodium).
   o. Changes in appetite, when and what the patient ate prior to dialysis.
   p. Mental status changes.
   q. General sense of well-being.
   r. Medication regimen and types.
      (1) Ingestion of some medications may stimulate thirst and/or fluid retention (i.e., calcium channel blockers, clonidine, and other vasodilator medications such as narcotics, analgesics, or beta blockers).
      (2) Physicians/APRNs/PAs instruct most patients to hold antihypertensive medications until after HD.
      (3) As patient nears "ideal" dry weight, adjustment of BP medications is paramount.
      (4) Diuretic therapy is effective only when RKF is high enough to provide daily urine output of at least 100 mL.
   s. Measure abdominal girth. Assess abdominal distention caused by extravasation of fluids related to bowel dysfunction, ascites, and lymphocele posttransplant.
   t. Assess for comorbities that may affect fluid removal during hemodialysis (e.g., diabetes, autonomic neuropathy, sepsis, high output kidney failure, ileostomy, cardiac disease, carnitine deficiency).
   u. Assess previous and/or current adherence to prescribed plan of care in consultation with the multidisciplinary team and/or family.
   v. Review previous treatment record, paying special attention to pretreatment and posttreatment, BPs, and intradialytic morbidities.
      (1) Note any interventions for hypotension or other intradialytic morbidities.
      (2) National Kidney Foundation Kidney Disease Outcomes Quality Inititiative (NKF-KDOQI) Clinical Practice Guidelines suggest that a dialysis log summarizing the relevant information such

as body weights, blood pressures, and IDMs is essential to provide a longitudinal dynamic view of ECF volume and blood pressure changes (NKF, 2006a, http://www.kidney.org/professionals/kdoqi/guideline_uphd_pd_va/hd_guide5.htm).

w. Assess patient's knowledge of:
   (1) Fluid ingestion quantification (e.g., liquids, "wet" foods, ice) and individual fluid allowance; generally recommend urinary output plus 1000 mL per day (four 8-ounce glasses).
   (2) Recommended weight gains (not to exceed 1 kg between dialyses during the week; 1.5 to 2 kg during the weekend) (Daugirdas, 2014; NKF, 2006a, http://www2.kidney.org/professionals/KDOQI/guideline_upHD_PD_VA/hd_guide5.htm).
   (3) Sodium restriction (no more than 2.0 grams with a more stringent limitation of 1 to 1.5 g sodium for patients on HD who are hypertensive).

x. Assess amount of daily exercise.

y. Consider recent hospitalizations, current stressors, season, and holidays as indications for possible weight adjustments.

2. Laboratory test results.
   a. Hemoglobin/hematocrit.
   b. BUN, serum creatinine.
   c. Sodium or osmotic sodium set-point.
   d. Blood glucose.
   e. Serum albumin.
   f. Atrial natriuretic peptide and brain natriuretic peptide (ANP/BNP) (acute treatments only).
   g. CO_2 (serum bicarbonate) levels.
   h. Carnitine levels if indicated.
   i. Angiotension levels (elevated levels increase thirst).

3. Interdialytic concerns.
   a. Complaints such as weakness, fatigue, prolonged postdialysis recovery time, dizziness, gastrointestinal (GI) symptoms (e.g., appetite changes, nausea, vomiting, diarrhea, constipation), respiratory difficulties (e.g., shortness of breath at rest, dyspnea on exertion, orthopnea, orthostatic hypotension).
   b. How and when patient resumes BP medications posttreatment.
   c. Fluid losses related to draining wounds, nasogastric tube, fever, vomiting, diarrhea (greater than 5 to 6 loose stools a day), diaphoresis, hyperventilation, and dialysis ultrafiltrate.
   d. Changes in amount of residual urine output.

4. Intradialytic complaints or symptoms (e.g., cramping, hypotension, tachycardia, nausea, vomiting, dizziness) and root cause analysis of symptoms.

5. Intervention.
   a. Determine degree of ultrafiltration (UF) for each HD treatment and feasibility of reaching UF goal safely, without inducing hypotension, based upon patient age, weight, and comorbidity(ies).
   b. DOPPS reported an increase in all-cause mortality associated with a UFR greater than 10 mL/kg/hour (Bragg-Gresham et al., 2006).
   c. Monitor and adjust UF based on patient's response.
      (1) Achieving true dry weight through ultrafiltration should be accomplished gradually over a number of dialysis treatments.
      (2) While decreasing the patient's fluid volume, net fluid loss ideally should not exceed 1 to 2 kg/wk.
      (3) More fluid may be removed during hematocrit-based blood volume monitoring (Hct-based BVM) since the patient's plasma refill rate relative to the current UFR can be observed via the display (see Section V).
   d. Administer fluids according to treatment plan and prescription. Avoid hypertonic injections the last 1/2 hour of treatment and prevent the need for administration of extra fluids and volume expanders during the last 1/2 hour other than the amount for reinfusion.
   e. Sodium modeling requires a physician/APRN/PA order; use cautiously and with discretion for patients with reduced plasma osmolality.
      (1) Ensure return to baseline sodium level individualized for the patient's sodium set-point (average predialysis sodium levels over 3 to 4 months) for the last 1/2 hour as the patient's postdialysis serum sodium is a function of the time-averaged dialysate level, not the terminal level of sodium in the dialysate (see sodium profiling module).
      (2) The NKF-KDOQI Clinical Practice Guidelines do not support the use of sodium profiling or high dialysate sodium levels. UF profiling can be combined with cold dialysate (34–35.5°C) to manage intradialytic hypotension (NKF, 2006a, http://www.kidney.org/professionals/kdoqi/guideline_uphd_pd_va/hd_guide5.htm).
         (a) Avoid their use to avoid thirst, fluid gains, and hypertension.
         (b) Uncertain benefits and possible risk of hypotension have been reported.
         (c) Satisfactory experiences have been reported with a dialysate sodium of 138 mmol/L.

f. Slow UF techniques to probe for dry weight can be combined with cool dialysate, 34° to 36°C, to prevent and manage intradialytic hypotension (Damasiewicz & Polkinghorne, 2011; http://onlinelibrary.wiley.com/doi/10.1111/j.1440-1797.2010.01362.x/full#ss2

g. Recommend changes in estimated dry weight as indicated. *Note*: True dry weight is subject to change related to conditions that cause a loss or gain of nonfluid body tissue.

h. Collaborate with physician/APRN/PA and renal dietitian in planning appropriate fluid and sodium intake and medication prescription.

i. Encourage fluid and dietary management according to prescription.

j. Identify resources to assist patient to achieve goals of fluid management.

k. Initiate consultations as needed.

l. Prolonging treatments (adjusting for longer, or shorter more frequent HD time) may be necessary.

m. Obtain ideal dry weight through Hct-based BVM and refill assessment.

n. Use thermal control (isothermal dialysis) to realize the benefit of blood pressure stability enhanced with lower dialysate temperature, 34 to 36°C, through maintenance of vascular tone (Damasiewicz & Polkinghorne, 2011; http://onlinelibrary.wiley.com/doi/10.1111/j.1440-1797.2010.01362.x/full#ss2

o. Modified Trendelenburg.

p. Reassess medication list monthly or more often if the patient is symptomatic.

q. Treat hypoxemia.

6. Patient/family education on fluid management would include instruction on the following.

   a. Kidney function and relationship to fluid balance.

   b. Diet and fluid management.
      (1) Thirst.
         (a) Relationships between fluid and sodium intake, blood sugar, elevated angiotension levels, and medications.
         (b) Avoid drinking water purified by a water softener which exchanges calcium for sodium. *Note*: attempts at water restriction are futile if sodium limitation is not taught and observed simultaneously (Charra, 2007).
         (c) Use antithirst agents like gum or sugar-free sour hard candy. Suck on a lemon wedge that stimulates the salivary glands. Eat frozen fruit or grapes, peaches, or pineapple (count as fruit allowance in the diet).
         (d) Avoid or limit use of oral care products that contain alcohol or have a drying effect on the oral mucosa. Instead, use oral care products designated to be moisturizing and/or prevent drying of the oral mucosa.
      (2) Review sodium restrictions and how to achieve it, preferred low-sodium foods, how to read food labels, and use of alternate seasonings.
      (3) Individual fluid allowance: generally urinary output plus 1000 mL per day (four 8-ounce glasses).
      (4) Weight changes: 1 kg between treatments during the week; 1.5 to 2 kg during the weekend.
      (5) Provide rationale for eating a small protein meal (vs. large carbohydrate meal) an hour before and/or after hemodialysis. The risk of eating during the hemodialysis treatment is related to the need for blood and oxygen shifting to the gut for digestion that may lead to vomiting, hypotension, and the need to reduce the UF rate/goal. Refer to the facility's policies and procedures to guide unit practice.
      (6) *Safety alert* about eating during HD:
         (a) Risk of choking may be of concern for some patients – evaluate individually.
         (b) Be attuned to infection control risks if patients are eating in the facility.
         (c) Ensure hand hygiene is available for patients prior to handling food.

   c. Signs, symptoms, and management of hypervolemia and hypovolemia.

   d. Importance of preventing IDMs to avoid long-term complications.

   e. Differentiation between solid weight gain (body mass) and fluid weight gain.

   f. Frequent causes of IDM unrelated to fluid removal (e.g., UFR, medications, increasing core temperature, posture, hypoxemia, eating during dialysis, and especially large amounts of food).

   g. Patients can experience an IDM even though they are not at their dry weight due to intravascular hypovolemia or hypervolemia, and the tissues may still have fluid.

   h. Three compartmental fluid shifts occurring during dialysis (extracellular, intracellular, and intravascular).

   i. The meaning of plasma refill.

   j. The causes, effects, and treatment of hypoxemia (possible need for oxygen administration).

   k. Rationale for thermal control vs. dialysate temperature that exceeds patient temperature.

l. Positive effects of exercise in between treatments to prevent fluid gain, and during the last hour of dialysis to prevent IDMs.

m. Self-monitoring of blood pressure and weight measurements.

n. Blood pressure parameters: normotensive pretreatment without antihypertensive medications.

o. Parameters for when to take or hold BP medications predialysis and postdialysis.

p. Effects of posture change.

q. Report changes in prescribed and over-the-counter medications; interdialytic symptoms.

IV. Principles of fluid removal.

A. The Guyton curve (see Figure 2.31).
Note: The Guyton curve is an approximation of fluid dynamics and is patient specific.

1. The Guyton curve (Hema Metrics, 2006, http://www.slideshare.net/ringer21/section-2-theory-critline-iii-tqa).
   a. Illustrates the approximate relationship between extracellular fluid volume and blood volume.
   b. Demonstrates a limit to blood volume as fluid levels continue to increase past a normal range.
   c. As fluid volume is added or removed, the body will distribute its fluid load according to this curve.

2. At ideal dry weight, the average 70 kg adult has approximately 5 liters of blood volume in the intravascular space (Hlebovy, 2006).
   a. This corresponds to a normal extracellular (tissue) fluid level of approximately 17 liters on the Guyton curve for the 70 kg adult.
   b. Approximately 23 liters of fluid are in the intracellular space.

3. "Silent volume" phenomenon.
   a. A person can have fluid excess (10% above dry weight) in the absence of gross clinical evidence of volume expansion.
   b. An excess of even 3 to 5 liters does not cause clinical signs or complaints in some patients.

4. When fluid is added and not removed (as between HD treatments):
   a. When the intravascular capacity of approximately 7 liters is reached, the extracellular tissue space will have expanded from 17 liters to approximately 22 liters.
   b. The presence of edema can be clinically assessed when this amount of expansion has occurred as plasma refill rate, PRR, is at a lesser rate than the UFR.
   c. All additional fluid thereafter expands into the extracellular tissue space.
   d. This area of edema is noted as "A" on the Guyton curve as seen in Figure 2.31.

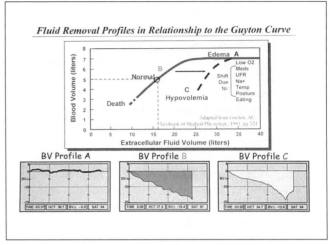

Figure 2.31. Fluid removal profiles in relationship to the Guyton curve.

Used with permission from Hema Metrics.

5. The extracellular tissue spaces can hold as much as 20 to 40 liters, sometimes referred to as "third spacing."

6. The goal of fluid removal is to gently reduce the patient's blood volume down the knee of the Guyton curve to "normal" (normovolemia or euvolemia).
   a. The blood volume is normovolemic and the tissues are at the patient's true dry state (ideal dry weight).
   b. This slow, steady area of descent is noted as "B" on the Guyton curve, as shown on the illustration Figure 2.32.
      (1) This is a pediatric patient with a central venous line for hemodialysis. The O_2 saturation goal for a CVC is greater than 60% and greater than 90% with a fistula.
      (2) The B profile demonstrates appropriate O_2 saturation for the patient's type of vascular access and the dotted line indicates the alarm limit.
      (3) Based upon this profile, no changes should be considered for this patient during the treatment because all parameters are acceptable.
      (4) *Safety alert.* This data must be used in the context of the assessment of all patient parameters and not used exclusively to determine the course of treatment.

7. Symptoms occurring below "normal" are considered a "dry" crash. Both the tissue and intravascular spaces area below "normal" and the patient is hypovolemic.

8. Symptoms occurring on the edema section of the Guyton curve, when the patient is still overloaded, are considered a "wet" crash. This is noted as "C" on the Guyton curve as seen in Figure 2.31.

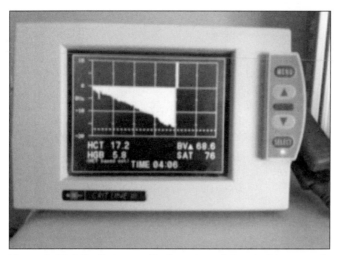

Figure 2.32. B Profile in a pediatric patient dialyzed with a central vein catheter.

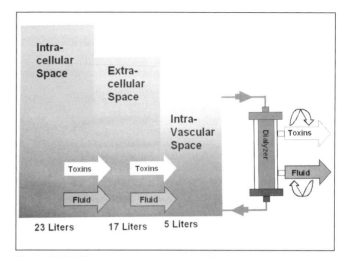

Figure 2.33. Three-compartmental model.

9. Causes of a crash can include, but are not limited to:
   a. Hypoxemia.
   b. Medications.
   c. Incorrect or high ultrafiltration rate (UFR).
   d. Sudden change in position.
   e. Temperature elevation of the patient and/or dialysate.
   f. Decreased plasma osmolality.
   g. Eating, causing splanchnic vasodilitation.
   h. Anemia.
   i. Unstable cardiac status/poor perfusion.
   j. Arrhythmia.
   k. Electrolyte/acid-base imbalance.
   l. Sepsis.
   m. Third spacing (e.g. postoperative, ascites).
   n. Hypovolemia.
10. The areas noted as "A," "B," and "C" on the Guyton curve corresponds to the "A," "B," and "C" profiles described with "Hct-based blood volume monitoring."

B. Plasma refill rate.
   1. During the dialysis process, fluid is removed directly from the intravascular space through ultrafiltration.
      a. Refer to the Three Compartment Model in Figure 2.33.
      b. Volumes listed under each compartment are for the average 70 kg adult at ideal dry weight.
      c. Volumes increase with fluid gains as described with the Guyton curve above.
   2. Fluid removal from the plasma decreases hydrostatic pressure and increases plasma oncotic pressure. This combination enables fluid to move from the extracellular (tissue) space into the intravascular space.

3. The rate of this process is known as the plasma refill rate (PRR).
   a. Plasma refill continues for 30 to 60 minutes after ultrafiltration has been set to minimum or postdialysis.
   b. The majority takes place within 10 minutes.
4. Maintenance of blood volume depends upon rapid refilling of the intravascular space as plasma volume is removed.
   a. Hypotension eventually occurs when the UFR exceeds PRR and plasma volume falls below normal (hypovolemia).
   b. *Safety alert.* A change in blood volume greater than 8% in any hour ("C profile") is an indication of impending hypovolemia unless there is an intervention, as the PRR is at a significantly lesser rate than the UFR, depleting the intravascular space.
5. It was thought the average adult patient could tolerate 500 to 1000 mL of ultrafiltration/hour in the absence of preexisting complications (e.g., serious cardiovascular disease, autonomic dysfunction, and acetate intolerance). The DOPPS study reported an increase in all-cause mortality for a UFR greater than 10 mL/kg/hour (Bragg-Gresham et al., 2006).
   a. The PRR is capable of replacing the blood volume removed to prevent hypovolemia as long as the UFR does not significantly exceed the PRR.
   b. A change in blood volume of –1.33% to –8% per hour up to a total of approximately –8% to –16% ("B profile") is generally well tolerated in the average patient who is overloaded on chronic HD. This suggests the PRR is comparable to the UFR. The ideal percent change is not fixed and will vary among patients, depending upon individual

characteristics, cardiovascular status, and other comorbidities; and may vary from one treatment to the next.

6. The plasma refill rate may be impaired in patients with:
   a. Reduced plasma osmolality.
   b. Low serum albumin.
   c. Hypoxemia.
   d. Ischemia.
   e. Cardiac dysfunction/cardiomyopathy.
   f. Arrhythmias.
   g. Low predialytic diastolic blood pressure.
   h. Increased temperature.
   i. Septicemia.
   j. The use of antihypertensive medications or any medication that causes vasodilatation.
   k. Conditions leading to third spacing, (e.g., surgery, ascites).
   l. Venous pooling (positioning with legs down).
   m. Lower extremity amputation (decreased reserve).
   n. Autonomic dysfunction/neuropathy.
   o. Diabetes.
   p. Splanchnic vasodilatation (eating).
   q. Poor compensatory mechanisms.
   r. Electrolyte/acid-base imbalances.
   s. Anemia.
   t. Residual urine output.
   u. Volume loss from any source (e.g., ileostomy, wound drainage).
   v. Other patient variables.

7. PRR diminishes as the patient approaches dry weight (Schroeder, Sallustio, & Ross, 2004, http://ndt.oxfordjournals.org/content/19/3/652.short).
   a. Frequency of IDMs increase toward the end of HD.
   b. With linear (constant) UFR, frequency can be up to 10 times higher than at the start of treatment.

8. During the first hour, plasma osmolality is highest related to initial concentrations of plasma proteins, urea, atrial natremic protein (ANP), and middle molecules.
   a. Blood sugar is generally higher and core body temperature lower in the first hour.
   b. All of these conditions during the first hour promote plasma refill.
   c. Optimal time to remove excess fluid for the patients on chronic dialysis with adequate compensatory mechanisms, little or no residual urine output, and without known cardiomyopathy. These are the patients who may tolerate a decrease of 8% blood volume change in the first hour of dialysis with an additional BV change of less than –4% the following hours, up to maximum of –16%.

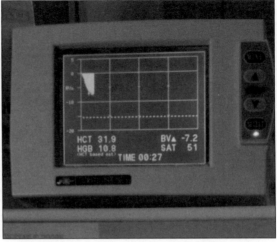

Figure 2.34. C profile. This image demonstrates a C profile in a pediatric patient whose access is a central venous catheter (CVC).

9. Ultrafiltration may be less tolerated and the patient may have symptoms of decreased plasma volume such as cramping and hypovolemia, despite still being fluid overloaded (a "wet" crash) (see Figure 2.34).
   a. The patient could still be on the edema ("A") section of the Guyton curve.
   b. No change in blood volume (a flat line), or a positive change with the UFR greater than minimum is an indication of fluid overload and is referred to as an "A" profile. This indicates that the patient's PRR is occurring at the same (flat line) or greater rate (positive change) than ultrafiltration and suggests that the UFR might be increased without immediate risk of intradialytic symptoms.
   c. Figure 2.34 demonstrates the following.
      (1) This C profile is in a pediatric patient whose access is a central venous catheter (CVC). The oxygen saturation with a CVC should be greater than 60%.
      (2) This patient required oxygen via nasal cannula for the saturation of 51%.
      (3) The ultrafiltration was decreased to achieve a B profile.
      (4) A refill check was performed at the end of the treatment; no PRR was present.
      (5) The patient clinically presented with persistent edema, and the decision was made to extend the duration of the next treatment.
      (6) This demonstrates the need to assess all clinical parameters in the context of the blood volume profile (e.g., oxygen saturation, BP, lung sounds, jugular vein distention).

10. For the above reasons, using the occurrence of signs and symptoms of hypovolemia/hypotension

may result in inappropriate high dry weight estimation. Patients with cardiomyopathy may actually start with a low BP that drops if PRR is greater than UFR and intravascular volume increases.

11. Based on the average refill rate noted above, the minimum UFR for an adult is equal to or less than 400 mL/hour.

12. Putting the patient in minimum UFR for 10 to 15 minutes at any time during the treatment and watching for refill on a BVM can assist in determining true or "ideal" dry weight (IDW). A blood volume increase greater than or equal to 1.55 suggests positive refill, indicating additional fluid may be available for UF during remainder of current or next treatment.

C. The Starling curve.
   1. The most common causes of IDM: a rapid decrease in blood volume or reduced peripheral vascular resistance (PVR).
   2. Measurements/data (Barth et al., 2003).
      a. BP = cardiac output (CO) x peripheral vascular resistance (PVR).
      b. Cardiac output = stroke volume (SV) x heart rate (HR).
      c. BP = SV x HR x PVR.
   3. Hypotension is a consequence of reduction in CO and/or PVR. Any minor decrease in PVR can precipitate a drop in BP as the CO cannot increase to compensate during blood volume depletion.
   4. Loss of the ability to vasoconstrict the resistance vessels (decreasing PVR) is a significant cause of UF-induced hypotension, more so than hypovolemia.
   5. PVR may be affected by:
      a. Antihypertensive and other medications.
      b. Hypoxemia.
      c. Dialysate temperature at or above 36°C.
      d. Dialysate pH/acidotic blood pH, pO_2, pCO_2.
      e. Neural tone/sympathetic nerve activity.
      f. Neuropathies from diabetes or other causes.
      g. Cardiovascular disease (CVD).
      h. Other comorbidities.
      i. Viscosity of blood/anemia.
      j. Vessel radius.
   6. Splanchnic vasodilatation results from ingestion of food immediately prior to, during, or after HD.
      a. This can cause increase in these blood vessels' capacity, resulting in a decrease in systemic BP.
      b. The food effect lasts at least 2 hours (Kinnel, 2005).
      c. A change of greater than –8% an hour, with accompanying hypoxemia, is generally noted during blood volume monitoring (see Figure 2.35).

7. Effects from blood volume loss (see Figure 2.36 and Table 2.13).
   a. Approximately 10% of the total blood volume can be removed with no significant effect on arterial pressure or cardiac output.
   b. CO begins to fall significantly starting at approximately 15% decrease of blood volume loss.
   c. CO begins to plummet at approximately 20% decrease of blood volume.
   d. BP can be sustained up to 10 to 20 to 40 or more minutes (sometimes referred to as the "Golden Hour") related to compensatory mechanisms (increased heart rate, PVR) before it begins to plummet. The time depends on the individual patient's ability to compensate.
   e. Both CO and BP start falling to zero when approximately 35% to 45% of the total blood volume has been removed. This may be irreversible.
   f. Death occurs with 50% loss of blood volume.
8. BP is a late indicator or postfacto measurement for ensuing IDMs.
   a. The KDOQI Guidelines do not support BP or symptoms of hypotension as an indicator of EDW (NKF, 2006a, http://www2.kidney.org/professionals/KDOQI/guideline_upHD_PD_VA/hd_guide5.htm).
   b. The KDOQI Guidelines, combination of UF techniques, dietary sodium restriction, and lower dialysate sodium concentrations has been instrumental in attaining a true dry weight (NKF, 2006a, http://www2.kidney.org/professionals/KDOQI/guideline_upHD_PD_VA/hd_guide5.htm).

D. The inverse relationship between blood volume and blood pressure (see Figure 2.37).
   1. Increased intravascular volume may increase the tension in the myocardium to such a degree that it cannot pump effectively as described below (see Figure 2.38).
   2. Frank Starling mechanism.
      a. Cardiac output can be decreased when the muscle itself becomes overstretched as occurs with hypervolemia.
      b. The heart cannot contract effectively and stroke volume decreases resulting in heart failure.
      c. Hypotension follows.
   3. Laplace's theorem.
      a. Tension in the wall of the myocardium increases as the radius in the chamber increases with hypervolemia.
      b. Wall tension is directly related to the myocardium's demand for oxygen.
      c. When the radius is dilated to such an extent that the demand for oxygen to the heart can no

longer be met, CO declines and the pump begins to fail.

   d. Hypotension follows.

4. When hypotension develops in this scenario, the tendency is to decrease UF and replace volume while the opposite may be indicated (i.e., contraction of the volume and decreasing left ventricular dilation to increase CO) (Diroll & Hlebovy, 2003).

E. Blood pressure lag time phenomenon (NKF, 2006a, http://www2.kidney.org/professionals/KDOQI/guideline_upHD_PD_VA/hd_guide5.htm).

1. 90% of patients on HD could be normotensive by lowering dry weight. However, the blood pressure response to extracellular volume (ECV) reduction is delayed by some weeks.

2. Days to weeks are required to reach a new steady state in which blood pressure will rise. It will eventually decrease after fluid volume excess (FVE) has been corrected and dry weight is achieved.

3. With gradual removal of FVE, blood pressure begins to decrease in 3 to 4 weeks after lowering dry weight, but it eventually reaches a plateau only after 6 to 12 months (may be sooner with Hct-based BVM).

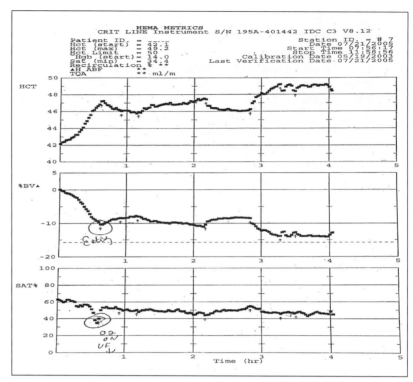

Figure 2.35. The effects of eating. A change of greater than –8% an hour, with accompanying hypoxemia.

Used with permission from Hema Metrics.

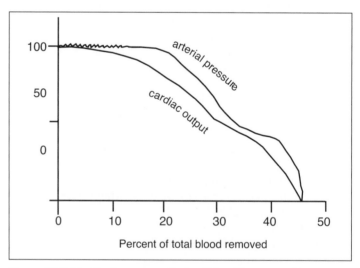

Figure 2.36. The Starling curve effects of blood loss on cardiac output and arterial pressure. BP is a post facto measurement.

Adapted from Guyton, A.C. (1987). *Textbook of medical physiology* (4th ed.), p. 63. Used with permission from Hema Metrics.

Table 2.13

Clinical Result of Hemorrhage

Loss of BV	Likely Result
5–10%	Little change in BP Spontaneous recovery
12–20%	Moderate hypotension Spontaneous recovery
20–30%	Early shock Rapid drop in CO Usually reversible
30–40%	Serious shock May be irreversible

Source: Smith, J.J. (1990). *Textbook of circulatory physiology: The essentials* (3rd ed., p. 267). Baltimore: Lippincott Williams & Wilkins. Used with permission from Hema Metrics.

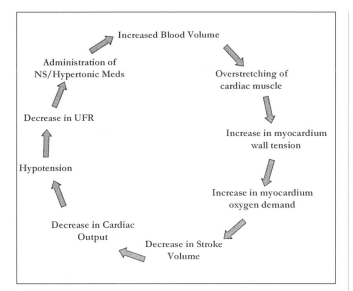

Figure 2.37. Inverse relationship between blood volume and blood pressure.
Used with permission from Hema Metrics.

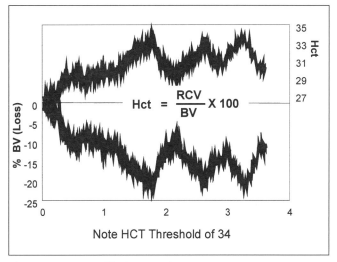

$$Hct = \frac{RCV}{BV} \times 100$$

Note HCT Threshold of 34

Figure 2.38. "A" profile: Positive slope.
Used with permission from Hema Metrics.

4. BP will not increase with increasing body mass.
5. As patients lose excess fluid and their hypertension improves, antihypertensive medications will need to be systematically tapered or discontinued in order to continue removing fluid to obtain dry weight without IDM.
6. The exact mechanism responsible for this lag time is not fully understood. Several explanations for this time lag are offered.
    a. Autoregulation of vascular resistances including functional and structural (remodeling) changes.
    b. Reduced formation or inhibition of vasoactive substances leading to decrease in vascular tone

such as increases in:
    (1) Asymmetric dimethylarginine (ADMA) leading to nitric oxide production.
    (2) Sodium-potassium-adenosine triphosphatase.
    c. Sodium restriction can cause vascular relaxation.
7. Healthcare providers and patients should be aware of the lag time phenomenon and not become discouraged if it takes weeks or months of dry weight adjustments to achieve a lower blood pressure.

F. Hypoxemia.
1. Significant complication of hemodialysis causing periods of ischemia and ensuing intradialytic morbid (IDM) events related to the release of adenosine and subsequent decrease of peripheral vascular resistance (PVR).
2. Adenosine has intrinsic vasodilatory properties and blocks the release of norepinephrine from sympathetic nerve terminals.
3. Symptoms exhibited resemble symptoms of hypovolemia (e.g., nausea, vomiting, restlessness, low blood pressure, cramps).
4. Measurement/data sources.
    a. If available, arterial blood gas analysis for SaO_2, PaO_2; SvO_2 from central venous catheter (CVC), or hemoglobin/hematocrit laboratory result.
    b. Noninvasive: pulse oximetry SpO_2; Crit-Line Monitor® (Fresenius Medical Care).
    c. SaO_2 from fistula or graft.
    d. Venous saturation (SvO_2) from CVC; hemoglobin/hematocrit (Hct).
5. Data.
    a. Oxygen saturation: the percent to which the hemoglobin is filled with oxygen. Circulation of blood volume and hemoglobin from the lungs to tissues must be adequate to prevent tissue hypoxia.
    b. 97% means that 97% of the total amount of hemoglobin in the blood volume is filled with oxygen molecules.
    c. Fewer total hemoglobin molecules cause the total amount of oxygen available to the tissues to be low even though the hemoglobin present is full of oxygen.
    d. The normal range of overall oxygen-carrying capacity is 19 to 20 mL/dL. This is calculated by multiplying 1.39 mL (the amount of oxygen each gram of hemoglobin carries) x hemoglobin x SaO_2 (or SpO_2).
    e. The target predialysis hemoglobin is a minimum of 10 g/dL (Hct 30%). With SaO_2 of 100%, the oxygen carrying capacity would equal 13.9 mL/dL.

6. Arterial blood saturation provides information on how well the lungs are oxygenating the blood.
   a. 90% to 100% is considered normal for arterial saturations (SaO_2).
   b. Mechanisms for intradialytic hypoxemia include:
      (1) Pulmonary edema.
      (2) Chronic obstructive pulmonary disease (COPD).
      (3) Congestive heart failure (CHF).
      (4) Sleep apnea (see Figure 2.39).
      (5) Rebound of reuse agent.
      (6) Bioincompatibility/first use syndrome.
      (7) Pulmonary leukostasis.
      (8) Pulmonary microembolizaton.
      (9) Dialysate composition.
      (10) Alveolar hypoventilation due to CO_2 loss through the dialyzer.
      (11) Warm dialysate temperature greater than 36°C.
      (12) Anemia: Hgb equal to or less than 10 g/dL.
      (13) Hemolysis.
7. SvO_2 is considered a mixed venous sat. Mixture of blood from the upper and lower vena cava caused by rotation of the blood pump (Sodemann & Polascheggm, 2001).
   a. Mixed venous blood saturation (SvO_2) provides information regarding the adequacy of tissue oxygenation.
   b. Tissue oxygen need is met when the amount of oxygen being delivered to the tissues is sufficient to meet the amount of oxygen being consumed. When the oxygen delivery falls below oxygen consumption needs, lactic acidosis develops (SvO_2 less than 30%).
   c. SvO_2 is the measurement of the amount of O_2 returning to the right side of the heart that is left over after tissue needs.
   d. If SvO_2 is normal, both ventilation and circulation are adequate.
   e. 60% to 80% is considered normal for mixed venous saturation levels; less than 60% indicates cardiac dysfunction; less than 50% indicates severe cardiac dysfunction; less than 30% anaerobic metabolism with lactic acidosis beginning.
   f. SvO_2 assists in determining if the CO is adequate to meet tissue O_2 needs. Hence, SvO_2 is used to determine if the CO is providing adequate perfusion.
   g. The continuous monitoring of SvO_2 is a sensitive parameter of continuous CO.
   h. A decreasing CO causes a compensatory rise in oxygen extraction at the tissue level.
      (1) Increased O_2 extraction is the fastest and often the single compensation of the organism following inadequate CO (i.e., a decreased SvO_2 indicates that the CO is not high enough to meet tissue oxygen needs).
      (2) SvO_2 can indicate whether the CO is high enough to meet the need.
   i. A rise in SvO_2 demonstrates a decrease in oxygen extraction, and usually indicates that the cardiac output is meeting the tissue oxygen need.
   j. A return of the SvO_2 to normal, in the presence of a normal or improving lactate, suggests patient improvement.
   k. A rise in SvO_2 (greater than 80%) in the presence of a rising lactate is an inappropriate and ominous finding, suggesting that the tissues are unable to extract oxygen. It can be seen in burns, late septic shock, or in cell poisoning such as cyanide.
   l. SvO_2 can be very helpful when attempting to determine whether a change in therapy is beneficial. Measuring SvO_2 before and after a change can assist in determining whether the therapy made the patient better or worse.
   m. Four causes for a drop in SvO_2.
      (1) The CO is not high enough (CO = heart rate x stroke volume); i.e., heart rate is too fast, too slow, irregular; hypo/hypervolemia; poor ejection fraction.
      (2) The Hgb is too low (i.e., greater to or less than 10 g/dL).
      (3) The SaO_2 is too low.
      (4) The oxygen consumption has increased without an increase in oxygen delivery (not common in HD).

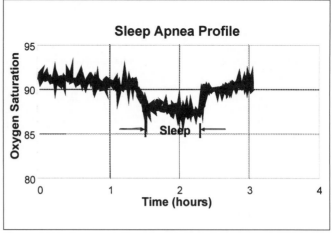

Figure 2.39. Oxygen delivery issues. O_2 Delivery < 50+% of patients on HD have intradialytic hypoxemia, and up to 70% experience sleep apnea

Used with permission from Hema Metrics.

V. Technologies used to obtain dry weight.

A. Volumetric or ultrafiltration-controlled dialysis equipment provides more precise management of fluid removal to reach the ultrafiltration goal set for the patient.

B. Subjective clinical assessment of "dry weight." This method is insensitive and poorly correlates with directly measured ECV. It is the most prevalent technique currently used.

C. Bioimpedence vector analysis (BIVA), management of extracellular fluid, and the assessment of nutritional status (Kalantari et al., 2013).
   1. Noninvasive indicator of total body weight measuring distribution in the intracellular fluid (ICF) and extracellular fluid (ECF) spaces (Peacock, 2010).
   2. Measurements are taken in the calf with electrodes and administering normal saline.

D. Sodium profiling, if ordered by a physician/APRN/PA, is used to enhance PRR by increasing ECF osmolarity through various higher dialysate sodium concentrations.
   1. This technique increases dialysate sodium concentrations early in HD, followed by a progressive decrease to a lower value at the end of the HD session.
   2. Various profiles exist (linear, step, or logarithmic) and offer different changes in the delivered dialysate sodium.
   3. Hypertonic saline has been used in the absence of sodium profiling.
      a. A large portion of sodium is retained even when given 2 hours before the end of the HD.
      b. 78% of hypertonic saline is retained when given even 1 hour prior to the end of therapy.
      c. Hypertonic saline is not used in most facilities, acute and chronic, due to handling and storage regulations related to its hypertonicity.
      d. *Safety alert.*
         (1) The use of hypertonic saline may cause patients to experience increased thirst and the potential for increased interdialytic fluid gains.
         (2) If hypertonic saline is available, it must be stored separately from all other medications due to its hypertonicity, to avoid inadvertent confusion/error/ administration with other medication vials.
   4. Both strategies have been shown to lead to the vicious cycle of increased thirst, increased interdialytic weight gains, hypertension, and the need for excessive UF with the risk for hypotension or muscle cramps.

5. The use of sodium profiling is not supported by KDOQI Guidelines (NKF, 2006a, http://www2.kidney.org/professionals/KDOQI/gu ideline_upHD_PD_VA/hd_guide5.htm).

E. IVC collapse. This technique uses ultrasound and is insensitive and operator dependent. Obesity interferes with results.

F. LA volume. This technique uses ultrasound, is operator dependent, and is affected by overall cardiac function.

G. Biochemical markers. Atrial natriuretic peptide (ANP), nt-Pro-BNP, cyclic guanidine monophosphate (eGMP).
   1. Limitation of markers include that they may be:
      a. Insensitive and nonspecific.
      b. Difficult to use in heart failure and tricuspid/mitral valve disease.
      c. Cannot detect the underhydrated state, normal range, and meaning of a low value.
   2. Predialysis levels of cardiac tropnoin T (cTnT) elevated up to three times above normal levels, suggesting myocardial injury (McIntyre, 2010).

H. UF profiling facilitates movement of fluid from the intravascular space into the dialysate by varying the rate of fluid removal to permit periods of plasma refill.
   1. Goal is to individualize UF rate according to the patient's individual response to HD to avoid hypotension.
   2. An individual profile may seem to emerge but caution must be used as this may need to vary from one HD to the next.
   3. Factors influencing this profile include, but are not limited to:
      a. ECF osmolarity from albumin.
      b. Sodium level.
      c. Glucose levels.
      d. Tissue hydration.
      e. Medication.
      f. Changes in lean body mass.
      g. Cardiac stability.
   4. Varied patient responses to UF profiles.
      a. A UF profile that uses intermittent high UF rates may not be tolerated by some patients. It may cause compensatory vasoconstriction, exhausting the patient and promoting postdialysis fatigue.
      b. *Safety alert.* High UFR may promote pronounced decrease in blood volume and a high incidence of unwanted side effects (Donauer et al., 2000).

I. Isolated ultrafiltration is also referred to as sequential ultrafiltration or pure UF.
   1. Removes iso-osmolar fluid from the systemic circulation via convection; removes excess fluid without changing blood solute concentrations.
   2. Involves bypassing the dialysate solution to drain allowing UF only.
   3. Temperature of the blood returning to the patient is lower with isolated UF than HD since there is no dialysate, hence no temperature control. Patients may complain of feeling cool or cold.
   4. The effects of increasing osmolality, lowering core body temperature, and increase in PVR allow for large amounts of fluid to be removed. The rate is dependent on cardiovascular stability, amount of over hydration and PRR.
   5. Typical prescription is for 1 hour prior to regularly prescribed dialysis time to avoid poor dialysis solute removal adequacy. Clearance via diffusion does not take place as there is no circulating dialysate through the dialyzer.
   6. *Safety alert.* Hyperkalemia and other fatal complications have occurred. Performing HD immediately following isolated UF significantly reduces this risk.

J. Thermal control (isothermic dialysate). A cool dialysate temperature may improve hemodynamic stability by increasing venous tone, oxygenation, PVR, and cardiac contractility. The goal is to keep the patient's pretemperature, intratemperature, and posttemperature the same (isothermia).
   1. Dialysate temperature of 37°C is warmer than the temperature of most patients on HD. The lower body temperature is related to anemia, uremia, immunosuppression, and lowered metabolism. The average patient temperature is 36°C (96.8°F).
   2. Dialysate temperature greater than 36°C adds to the warming of the patient's core and decreasing PVR. Core heating is a powerful vasodilatory stimulus resulting in both venous and arteriolar dilation.
   3. There is a benefit for blood pressure stability with lower dialysate temperature, 34° to 36°C, through maintenance of vascular tone (Damasiewicz & Polkinghorne, 2011, http://onlinelibrary.wiley.com/doi/10.1111/j.1440-1797.2010.01362.x/full#ss2).
   4. Cooler dialysate (34–36° C) appears to dissipate some of heat generated from UF that contributes to vasodilation.
   5. More extracorporeal cooling is necessary with more ultrafiltration to keep patients at a constant temperature (isothermic).
   6. Dialysate temperatures may need to be decreased for patients with a high ultrafiltration to maintain stability.
   7. Cooler dialysate prevents hypoxemia by decreasing oxygen diffusion through the dialyzer; patients report feeling more energetic after HD.
   8. Cooler dialysate can decrease complement activation and the inflammatory process that occurs during HD.
   9. Cooler dialysate is cardioprotective, decreases metabolic needs of the heart, and may prevent or decrease cardiac stunning. Despite it being a well recognized benefit in the literature its use does not seem to be widely accepted.

K. Hct-based BVM: monitoring of blood volume changes that occur over the course of the HD treatment observed using an optical technique to monitor absolute Hct changes, or protein density changes through ultrasound. Blood volume monitoring should be used for all pediatric patients, especially those who weigh less than 35 kg., to evaluate body weight changes for gains in muscle weight vs. fluid overload (CMS, 2008).
   1. Current monitors require a disposable blood chamber to obtain arterial measurements during HD. This technology employs a noninvasive monitor using photo-optical technology to measure the percentage of blood volume change, O_2 saturation, and absolute hemoglobin and hematocrit in real-time, monitoring the blood as it enters the dialyzer.
   2. Oxygen saturation can also be observed through the select BV monitors.
   3. The clinician can observe the maximum Hct and BV achieved without symptoms and guide the following treatments accordingly. Plasma refill checks can be performed to assess availability of extra fluid to be removed during current or next treatment.
   4. Monitors that display an absolute Hct; the value can be used to diagnose and treat anemia and its trend.
   5. The displayed blood volume profile enables the clinician to determine the patient's rate of plasma refill into the intravascular space relative to the current ultrafiltration rate of the dialysis machine.
   6. Proper adjustment of the UFR by the clinician proactively allows reduction in intradialytic hypervolemia and optimizes fluid removal while avoiding intradialytic morbidities. This is based on:
      a. Feedback from the blood volume profile.
      b. The patient's maximum hematocrit.
      c. Result of plasma refill check.
   7. A customized UF profile can be followed based upon the patient's actual PRR during each individual treatment to:
      a. Promote optimization of extracellular fluid status.
      b. Reduce intradialysis and postdialysis morbid complications.

c. Increase improvements in patient well-being.

d. Provide an objective way of assigning ideal, true dry weight through plasma refill or "dry weight check" near treatment end (see Figure 2.40).

8. Any factor that changes the RBC mass and consequently Hct will be reflected in the profile. Examples include:

a. Administration of saline/oral liquids (profile will increase as blood volume increased).

b. Administration of blood (profile will significantly drop during the transfusion from increase in Hct vs. solely volume removal) (see Figure 2.41 on next page).

c. Vascular access recirculation (profile will drop as blood becomes more concentrated).

d. Clotting/kinking in blood tubing (profile will drop).

e. Significant hemolysis (blood volume may increase related to increase in volume released from ruptured cells).

9. Quality outcomes.

a. ECV and Kt/V prescribing is essential to reducing hospitalization rates and readmissions.

b. A nurse could be designated as the fluid manager who could monitor and affect outcomes; maintains normalized fluid balance or ECV control. The nurse would be part of a collaborative interdisciplinary team and responsible for oversight of:

(1) Extra treatments.

(2) Reconciliation of medications and updates.

(3) UFR.

(4) Sodium modeling.

(5) Avoidance of hypoxia.

(6) Root cause analysis of intradialytic morbidities.

(7) ECV target evaluation.

(8) Develop, implement and evaluate care plans to address changes in care to attain dry weight (normovolemia and normotension) to decrease fluid-related hospitalizations, morbidity, and mortality.

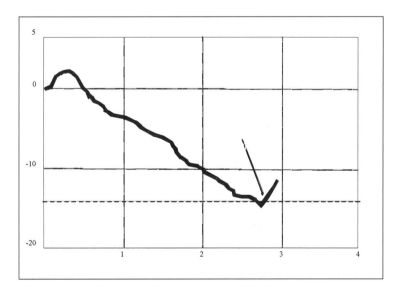

Figure 2.40. "B" profile: linear with dry weight check. Plasma refill is observed (BV does not "level off" when UFR is in minimum and continues to rise by equal to or greater than +1.5%; Hct decreases by equal to or greater than 0.5%). True "ideal" dry weight has not yet been achieved.

Used with permission from Hema Metrics.

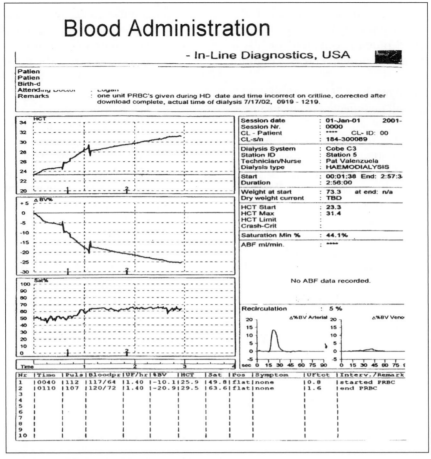

Figure 2.41. Blood administration: Changes in SvO₂ with Hct increase. Blood transfusion started at approximately 50 minutes into the treatment as noted by marker. Note SvO₂ improvements with blood transfusion.

Used with permission from Hema Metrics.

SECTION E

Complications of Hemodialysis: Prevention and Management

Joan E. Speranza-Reid

I.   **Acute hemolysis** (Dutka & Harmon, 2007; Gomez, 2011; Graves, 2001; Jepson & Alonzo, 2009; Sherman et al., 2014; Sweet et al., 1996; Twardowski, 2000).

A. Etiology: Rupture of red blood cells (RBCs) due to problems with composition of the dialysate solution, reprocessing sterilants, insufficient dialysis, hypersplenism, hypophosphatemia, associated diseases, drug induced, or malfunctioning equipment.
  1. Hypertonic or hypotonic dialysate.
     a. Incorrect dialysate composition outside of physiologic parameters caused by dialysate source obstruction, malfunction of concentrate pump, or inaccurate concentrate composition.
     b. Conductivity meter failure due to considerable calibration error, malfunction or dirty probe or meter, improper probe placement, or failure to correct limits on meter.
     c. Inaccurate dialysis machine conductivity calibration.
     d. Mechanical failure bypass caused by equipment malfunction or a retrograde leak across the bypass valve.
  2. Hypertonic or hypotonic IV solutions.
     a. Rapid administration of hypertonic saline (23.4%) has a sizeable osmotic effect and can result in localized hemolysis.
     b. Iatrogenic bolus infusion of distilled water (see Figure 2.42).
  3. Overheated dialysate (greater than 42° C).
     a. Dialysate heater malfunction due to calibration error for high temperature limit, calibration error in dialysate temperature range, or major malfunction in the heater cycle.
     b. Dialysate temperature monitor failure.

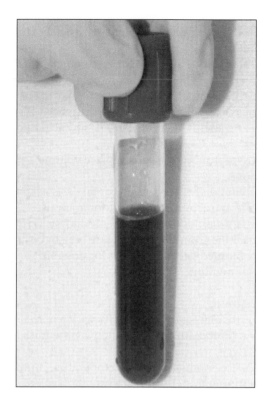

Figure 2.42. A tube containing blood to which tap water was added to demonstrate the appearance of gross hemolysis.

Courtesy of Karen Robbins.

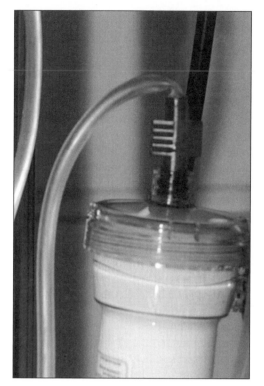

Figure 2.43. A kinked arterial bloodline connected to the hemodialyzer, a potential site to generate hemolysis. This emphasizes the importance of proper set-up of the dialyzer and bloodlines in preparation for every HD treatment.

Courtesy of Karen Robbins.

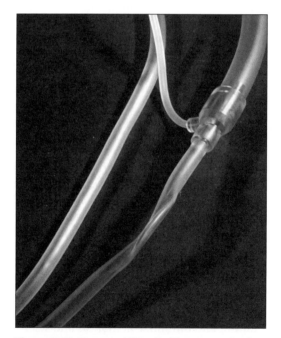

Figure 2.44. Damaged blood tubing as removed from original package; note the kinking and tortuous condition of the arterial bloodline that might lead to hemolysis if actually used for an HD treatment. This finding underscores the need to examine all bloodlines during machine setup and preparation.

Courtesy of Karen Robbins.

c. Mechanical failure bypass caused by equipment malfunction or a retrograde leak across the bypass valve.
4. High negative pressure in the extracorporeal circuit.
   a. Prepump arterial pressure greater than minus 250 mmHg.
   Note: Negative pressure levels resulting in hemolysis are debated in the literature with ranges from –160 mmHg to –250 mmHg.
   b. Access blood flow rate is lower than blood pump rate.
   c. Bloodline kinks immediately before the blood pump or in other segments of the blood pump tubing (see Figure 2.43).
   d. Improperly occluded blood pump roller.
5. Trauma to RBCs as they pass over a defective area in the extracorporeal circuit, narrowed tubing, needle trauma, or catheter malfunction (see Figure 2.44).
6. High blood flow rate through a small gauge needle or catheter lumen.
7. Oxidant hemolysis.
   a. Leaching of copper from copper piping used in dialysis water and concentrate delivery systems

due to low water/dialysate pH. Copper piping is not recommended for reasons cited in Section B of this chapter.

  b. Chloramine breakthrough in dialysis water system when used as a bactericidal agent in water supplies.

  c. Nitrates in well water used for dialysate preparation.

8. Presence of sterilant in dialysate (bleach, formaldehyde, peracetic acid) due to inadequate rinsing of dialyzer, dialysate delivery system, water treatment system, or distribution system.

B. Signs and symptoms.

1. Back and/or abdominal pain that may present with a crescendo of intensity.
2. Chest tightness.
3. Decreased level in serum haptoglobin.
4. Dysrhythmias.
5. Headache.
6. Hyperkalemia.
7. If hyperthermic dialysate is present, the patient will complain of feeling hot.
8. Hypotension.
9. Hypoxemia.
10. Increased levels in LDH, decrease in serum haptoglobin, unconjugated bilirubin, and methemoglobin.
11. Localized burning and pain in the blood return site.
12. Malaise.
13. Nausea/vomiting.
14. Shortness of breath.
15. Venous bloodline becomes translucent, deep burgundy or cherry-red in color. *Note:* This symptom is not always present when hemolysis occurs. Figure 2.42 shows a blood tube with grossly hemolyzed blood.
16. Acute decrease in hemoglobin/hematocrit (Hgb/Hct) (see caution statement under "Hypotension" in this section).
17. When using blood volume monitoring, the blood volume (BV) curve may suddenly become more positive as fluid content of red blood cells (RBCs) is released as a result of hemolysis (Dutka & Harmon, 2007).
18. Pancreatitis and gall stone formation can follow an acute hemolytic episode.
19. Skin pigments may appear deeper in color.

C. Treatment.

1. Discontinue dialysis.
2. Clamp venous line immediately and do not re-infuse the hemolyzed blood.
3. Administer oxygen.
4. Notify physician/APRN/PA.
5. Monitor vital signs and cardiac rhythm. Observe

for dysrhythmias, hypotension, and shortness of breath.

6. Obtain blood samples for unconjugated bilirubin, electrolytes, hemoglobin, haptoglobin, LDH, and methemoglobin. Hyperkalemia may occur due to the release of potassium from ruptured RBCs. Acute anemia may develop if significant hemolysis occurs.
7. If symptoms are severe, replace volume and/or blood.
8. Obtain dialysate samples for analysis as indicated.
9. Save extracorporeal circuit for analysis.
10. *Safety alert.* Remove the hemodialysis (HD) machine from the patient care area to be analyzed by biomedical engineering for possible malfunction.

D. Prevention.

1. Verify dialysate conductivity with external meter and temperature immediately before initiating dialysis.
2. Assure conductivity and temperature monitors are working properly and activate the bypass mechanism to stop dialysate flow to the dialyzer.
3. Clean concentrate containers, lines, and filters per manufacturer recommended processes and frequency and the facility's policies and procedures.
4. Protect all electrical components from corrosive effects of dialysate.
5. Assure routine preventative maintenance of monitors, alarms, and bypass mechanisms.
6. Monitor preblood pump arterial pressures to ensure arterial pressure is not greater than –250 mmHg.
7. Use appropriate blood flow rates and needle gauge for type and size of access.
8. Remove copper piping in water treatment, distribution, and dialysate preparation system.
9. Use charcoal filtration for water supply to remove chloramines and chlorine. Perform chloramine testing per AAMI Guidelines. Verify and document testing results for sterilant presence in water system, dialyzer, and dialysate preparation system.
10. Administer hypertonic saline (23.4%) in limited divided doses (e.g., 10 mL over 30 seconds), and give through the venous chamber to enhance dilution and minimize hemolysis and sclerosing of blood vessels. Use caution with hyperosmolar solutions.
11. The KDOQI Guidelines discourage the increase of sodium balance during dialysis which includes sodium profiling (NKF, 2006a, (http://www .kidney.org/professionals/kdoqi/guideline_uphd_ pd_va/hd_guide5.htm).
12. Assess extracorporeal system to ensure absence of

kinks and other manufacturer defects. See Figures 2.40 and 2.41 for examples of kinked and tortuous bloodlines that could lead to hemolysis.

13. Monitor the patient routinely throughout the treatment for the onset of signs and symptoms of treatment and equipment-related complications.

14. *Safety alert.*
    a. The patient should not be left unattended during the hemodialysis treatment.
    b. It is imperative that carbon tanks are checked for chlorine and chloramine at designated time intervals, without fail! Notify the resource nurse and medical director immediately of any breakthrough, and follow the facility's policies and procedures to ensure patient safety.
    c. Dialysate conductivity must be confirmed with an external meter prior to HD treatment initiation.
    d. Check blood tubing prior to treatment initiation for any kinks or defects; ensure all tubing is free of any twists.

II. Air embolism (Gomez, 2011; Sherman et al., 2014).

A. Etiology. Introduction of a large quantity of air into the venous circulation can be caused by:
1. Defective or disarmed extracorporeal air detector.
2. Loose connections or a disconnection at the arterial blood access site/connector or a small leak before the blood pump, or an open or cracked central venous catheter lumen.
3. Microemboli created by blood passing over a defective area in the extracorporeal circuit.
4. Empty air-vented IV bags and bottles attached to the extracorporeal circuit.
5. Air dissolved in very cold water may exceed the deaeration capacity of the delivery system; air may pass from the dialysate side to the blood side in a dialyzer.

B. Signs and symptoms.
1. Signs and symptoms are dependent upon patient position at the time of the introduction of air.
   a. In seated patients, infused air will travel to the cerebral venous system without entering the heart; can lead to loss of consciousness, convulsions, and even death.
   b. In recumbent patients, infused air tends to travel into the heart, generating foam in the right ventricle, and passing into the lungs, resulting in shortness of breath, cough, chest tightness, and arrhythmias. If air is in the heart, there can be a churning sound on auscultation of the heart.
   c. Patients in Trendelenburg position may have infused air travel to the lower extremities resulting in patchy cyanosis.
2. Visualization of air pockets or foam in the venous bloodline.
3. Patient complains of hearing the "sound of a freight train" or hears "rushing air."
4. Chest pain.
5. Coughing.
6. Cyanosis.
7. Shortness of breath.
8. Arrhythmias.
9. Visual disturbances.
10. Churning sound on auscultation of the heart.
11. Neurologic deficits: confusion, coma, hemiparesis.
12. Death.

C. Treatment.
1. Immediately stop infusion of air, clamp the venous bloodline, and stop the blood pump.
2. Place patient on left side in a recumbent position with the head and chest tilted downward to trap the air in the apex of the right ventricle, away from the pulmonary valve.
3. Provide cardiorespiratory support including the administration of oxygen: 100% oxygen by mask is preferred. Hyperbaric oxygen therapy may be beneficial.
4. It may be necessary to aspirate the air from the atrium or ventricle via a percutaneous needle or heart catheterization.
5. Monitor vital signs.
6. Notify physician/APRN/PA.

D. Prevention.
1. Accurate use of calibrated air foam detector at all times when the patient is on dialysis.
2. Visual inspection of the venous bloodline before connection to access.
3. Visual inspection of vascular access catheter before connection to bloodline.
4. Secure interlocking connections throughout the extracorporeal circuit.
5. Maintain blood pump speed at rate access can deliver (i.e., the blood pump speed should not exceed that of the vascular access).
6. Return the patient's blood with normal saline vs. air rinse back.
7. Use IV solutions in collapsible bags vs. air-vented bottles to avoid possible introduction of air into extracorporeal system. (*Safety alert*: Serum albumin may be delivered via an air-vented bottle.)
8. Remove or clamp empty IV bags, blood bags, or infusion syringes.
9. Heparin infusion should occur after the blood pump (post blood pump).
10. Saline administration line and all stagnant lines should be double clamped.
11. Monitor the patient routinely throughout the treatment for the onset of signs and symptoms of

treatment and equipment-related complications.
12. *Safety alerts.*
   a. The patient should not be left unattended during the hemodialysis treatment.
   b. Ensure all connections are tight and secure.
   c. The air foam detector must remain armed throughout the HD treatment, and until the termination procedure is complete, all blood is returned to the patient, and the blood pump is turned off.

III. Angina/chest pain (Lamiere & Mehta, 2000; Sherman et al., 2014).

A. Etiology.
   1. Occurs in 1% to 4% of all hemodialysis treatments.
   2. Anemia.
   3. Arteriosclerotic cardiovascular disease (ASCVD).
   4. Coronary artery spasm.
   5. Hemolysis.
   6. Hypervolemia and hypovolemia.
   7. Hypoxemia.
   8. Type B dialyzer reaction.
   9. Cardiac (myocardial) stunning.

B. Signs and symptoms.
   1. General: pain or tightness in the chest, back, arm, or jaw.
   2. Women: may be more likely to feel discomfort in the neck, jaw, throat, abdomen, or back.
   3. Patients with diabetes or people who are elderly: shortness of breath is more common.
   4. People who are elderly: signs and symptoms may be masked by weakness, dizziness, and confusion (NHLBI, n.d).
   5. The following links are useful tools for patient education about signs and symptoms of angina (NIH, 2011): http://www.nhlbi.nih.gov/health/health-topics/topics/angina/signs and http://www.nhlbi.nih.gov/health//dci/Diseases/Angina/Angina_SignsAndSymptoms.html).

C. Treatment and prevention (Steps 2 to 10 may occur simultaneously by care team members).
   1. Prevent hypovolemia.
   2. Decrease ultrafiltration rate (UFR) to minimum.
   3. Administer oxygen.
   4. Place in reclining position.
   5. Volume replacement if needed.
   6. Give nitroglycerine per order if blood pressure is within acceptable limits.
   7. Maintain hemoglobin at asymptomatic level.
   8. Cardiac monitoring to assess EKG changes.
   9. Notify physician/APRN/PA.
   10. Discontinue dialysis if chest pain is severe or unresolved.

11. Assess estimated dry weight, ultrafiltration goal, and ultrafiltration rate.
12. Avoid high UF rates.

IV. Bleach exposure (sodium hypochlorite) (Katirci, 2010; Rahmani et al., 2012).

A. Etiology.
   1. Extremely hypertonic solution.
   2. Bleach is cytoxic to all cells in the body.

B. Signs and symptoms.
   1. Bradycardia or tachycardia.
   2. Cardiac arrest.
   3. Chest pain.
   4. Cyanosis.
   5. Hemolysis and resultant hyperkalemia.
   6. Hypotension.
   7. Respiratory distress.
   8. Shock.
   9. Vomiting.
   10. When injected into blood vessels can lead to vessel thrombosis.

C. Treatment.
   1. Discontinue dialysis.
   2. Clamp venous line immediately and do not reinfuse hemolyzed blood.
   3. Monitor oxygen saturation (O_2 sat) and administer oxygen as needed.
   4. Notify physician/APRN/PA.
   5. Monitor vital signs, respiratory status, and cardiac rhythm.
   6. Symptomatic treatment may include cardiac massage and respiratory support.
   7. Obtain blood samples for electrolytes, hemoglobin, haptoglobin, LDH, and methemoglobin. Hyperkalemia may occur due to the release of potassium from ruptured red blood cells. Acute anemia may develop if significant hemolysis occurs, resulting in decreased oxygenation.
   8. Determine source of bleach exposure and whether it is contained to one station/machine or is from a central delivery source.
   9. Obtain dialysate samples for analysis as indicated.
   10. Save extracorporeal circuit for analysis.
   11. Remove the hemodialysis machine from the patient care area to be analyzed by biomedical engineering for possible malfunction.
   12. Follow facility policies and procedures.

D. Prevention/safety alerts.
   1. Appropriate testing for presence of bleach in dialysate and water treatment systems per facility procedure prior to start of patient treatment.
   2. Appropriate testing for presence of bleach in

dialysis equipment per facility procedure prior to start of patient treatment.
3. Prohibit disinfection of dialysate and water treatment systems and dialysis machine while patient is dialyzing.
4. Monitor the patient routinely throughout the treatment for the onset of signs and symptoms of treatment and equipment-related complications.
5. The patient should not be left unattended during the hemodialysis treatment.

V. Cardiac arrest (Herzog, 2004; Pun et al., 2011; Voroneanu & Covic, 2009).

A. Etiology.
   1. Occurs in 4.5 out of 100,000 hemodialysis treatments.
   2. Anemia.
   3. Cardiac tamponade.
   4. Diminished ischemia tolerance/cardiac stunning.
   5. Dysrhythmias.
   6. Electrolyte/acid base imbalance.
   7. Exposure to dialyzer sterilant.
   8. Exsanguination.
   9. Hemolysis.
   10. Hyperthermia/overheated dialysate.
   11. Hypovolemia.
   12. Hypoxemia.
   13. Large air embolism.
   14. Left ventricular hypertrophy.
   15. Myocardial infarction.
   16. Obstructive coronary artery disease.
   17. Obstructive sleep apnea.
   18. Profound shock.
   19. Rapid infusion of cold blood product(s).
   20. Unsafe dialysate composition.

B. Signs and symptoms.
   1. Absence of apical or carotid pulse.
   2. Lack of spontaneous respiratory effort.
   3. Unresponsive.
   4. Asystole or ventricular fibrillation on cardiac monitor.

C. Treatment.
   1. Assess for signs and symptoms noted above.
   2. Begin cardiopulmonary resuscitation and activate emergency resources used for cardiac arrest, in accordance with American Heart Association or American Red Cross standards, or per facility's procedures.
   3. Return blood to patient if confident the arrest was not due to air embolism, hemolysis, or sterilant exposure. Discontinue dialysis if appropriate. Leave access line in place for fluid and medication administration.

4. Use automated external defibrillator (AED) if available to diagnose and treat ventricular arrhythmias.
5. Notify physician/APRN/PA.
6. Remove the hemodialysis machine from the patient care area to be analyzed by biomedical engineering for possible malfunction.
7. Follow facility policies and procedures.

D. Prevention.
   1. Prevent conditions that could lead to cardiac arrest, such as anemia, rapid electrolyte shifts, and profound shock.
   2. Ensure dialysate composition is appropriate for patient.
   3. Adjust UFR to avoid intravascular volume depletion, and hypotension.
   4. Ongoing vigilant assessment during hemodialysis treatment.
   5. Refer patients with dysrhythmias to cardiologist for further evaluation, possible pacemaker, and/or internal defibrillator placement.
   6. EKG/blood volume measurement monitoring during dialysis for patients at risk.
   7. Monitor the patient every 30 minutes or more often as indicated throughout the HD treatment for the onset of signs and symptoms of treatment and equipment-related complications.
   8. *Safety alert.* The patient should not be left unattended during the HD treatment.

VI. Cardiac (myocardial) stunning
(Brown et al., 2015; Burton et al, 2009; Jefferies et al., 2011, http://cjasn.asnjournals.org/content/6/6/1326.full; Kloner et al., 1989, http://www.sciencedirect.com/science/article/pii/0002934389900053; McIntyre, 2010, http://www.karger.com/Article/Pdf/245634).

A. Description.
   1. Prolonged and severe myocardial ischemia can lead to myocyte cell death without the potential for recovery of contractile function of the cells (Kloner, Przyklenk & Patel, 1989, http://www.sciencedirect.com/science/article/pii/0002934389900053).
   2. Left ventricular (LV) dysfunction can result from transient myocardial ischemia even after the return of normal perfusion (McIntyre, 2010, http://www.karger.com/Article/Pdf/245634).
   3. "Hybernating myocardium."
      a. Appears to be a protective mechanism in which the myocardial oxygen demand is reduced in the presence of decreased oxygen supply.
      b. Myocytes may remain viable despite prolonged ischemia and have depressed myocardial contractility (Kloner et al., 1989,

http://www.sciencedirect.com/science/article/pii/0002934389900053).

4. Cardiovascular mortality in patients on HD may be largely attributed to cardiac stunning (Burton, et. al., 2009).

B. Etiology in patients on HD.
1. Recurrent ischemia results from conventional HD as it is a cardiovascular functional stressor leading to functional and structural changes in the myocardium.
2. Fixed systolic dysfunction and heart failure evolve over time from repeated ischemic insults, rendering a poor prognosis (McIntyre, 2010, http://www.karger.com/Article/Pdf/245634).
3. Risk factors.
   a. Intradialytic hypotension.
   b. High volume/rate of ultrafiltration.
   c. Hypovolemia/ischemia.
   d. Patient age.
   e. Predialysis levels of cardiac tropnoin T (cTnT) elevated up to three times above normal levels, suggesting myocardial injury (McIntyre, 2010, http://www.karger.com/Article/Pdf/245634).
   f. Raising dialysate temperature above patient temperature during HD.
   g. Exposure to bioincompatible equipment and endotoxins.

C. Prevention and interventions.
1. Reduced dialysate temperature to avoid vasodilatation and decrease metabolic needs of myocardium.
2. Avoid high UFR. Individualize the UFR based upon patient age, weight, and comorbidities. The Dialysis Outcomes and Practice Patterns Study (DOPPS) reported an increase in all-cause mortality for a UFR greater than 10 mL/kg/hour (Bragg-Gresham et al., 2011).
3. Use blood volume monitoring (BVM) to individualize intravascular fluid removal to PRR with goal of preventing hypovolemia and fast changes in circulating volume.
4. More frequent HD sessions (McIntyre, 2010, http://www.karger.com/Article/Pdf/245634; Jefferies et al., 2011, http://cjasn.asnjournals.org/content/6/6/1326.full).
5. Unknown if introduction of more frequent, less traumatic HD sessions can lead to remodeling of hibernated myocardium (Jefferies et al., 2011, http://cjasn.asnjournals.org/content/6/6/1326.full.
6. Increase length of HD session to reduce UFR.
7. Reassess dry weight at least monthly and adjust the patient's plan of care to address possible need to adjust the weight.

D. Associated concerns.
1. The stress of HD causes ischemia that may be subclinical and can lead to dysregulated blood flow to the heart as well as other vascular beds.
2. Silent cerebral infarct may be associated with the HD induced ischemia.
3. "Gut" stunning may be a pathophysiologic component in malnutrition, inflammation, and other adverse cardiovascular outcomes (McIntyre, 2010, http://www.karger.com/Article/Pdf/245634).

VII. Dialysis disequilibrium syndrome (DDS)
(McIntyre, 2014; Patel et al., 2008; Sherman et al., 2014).

A. Etiology.
1. The rapid removal of urea during HD results in the development of an osmotic gradient between the brain and plasma due to the relatively slow transport of urea across the blood-brain barrier in the cerebral spinal fluid (CSF).
2. CSF osmolality falls more slowly than in plasma, leading to water movement into the brain. Cerebral edema results due to increased brain water content.
3. DDS is most often seen in patients with very high urea plasma concentrations with chronic kidney disease (vs. acute kidney injury) and with rapid urea removal in initial HD treatments. It may be seen in patients who are inadequately dialyzed.
4. DDS is more common in children; patients with a history of head injury, subdural hematoma, stroke, and malignant hypertension; severe metabolic acidosis, and in patients with conditions that predispose to cerebral edema such as hyponatremia.
5. Rapid pH changes and electrolyte shifts may also cause DDS.

B. Signs and symptoms.
1. Usually occur toward the end of the HD treatment but may be delayed for up to 24 hours after the end of treatment.
2. Blurred vision.
3. Cardiac arrhythmia.
4. Headache.
5. Increased pulse pressure.
6. Hypertension.
7. Restlessness.
8. Decreased sensorium.
9. Behavior changes.
10. Muscle cramps.
11. Nausea and vomiting.
12. Seizures.
13. Tremors and restlessness.
14. In severe cases, obtundation, coma, and death can occur.

C. Treatment and prevention.
1. Early identification of mild symptoms.
2. Reduce the efficacy of dialysis by one or more of the following.
   a. Use a less efficient dialyzer (i.e., one with lower clearances/solute removal).
   b. Decrease treatment time.
   c. Decrease blood and dialysate flow rates.
   d. Use concurrent dialysate flow (i.e. blood and dialysate flowing in the same direction).
   e. Bicarbonate dialysate adjusted to individual's serum CO_2 level.
3. Short, more frequent dialysis treatments.
4. Increase dialysate sodium concentration (greater than 140 mEq/L).
5. Administer osmotic agents such as hypertonic saline or glucose to counteract the rapid fall in plasma osmolality.
6. Terminate dialysis treatment if severe or progressive signs and symptoms occur.
7. Review HD treatment orders and plan with physician/APRN/PA for the need for preventive measures, based upon the individual patient's status and comorbidities.

VIII. Dialysis encephalopathy (Rob et al., 2001; Ward & Ing, 2014).

A. Etiology.
1. Neurologic disorder resulting from the accumulation of aluminum in the body.
2. Aluminum toxicity.
   a. Water not properly treated for HD (e.g., acute aluminum intoxication).
   b. Ingestion of large quantities or long-term use of aluminum-containing phosphate binders.
3. Incidence has greatly declined due to water treatment and the use of nonaluminum containing phosphate binders.

B. Signs and symptoms.
1. Ataxia.
2. Dementia.
3. EEG changes.
4. Emotional alterations.
5. Gait changes.
6. Myoclonus.
7. Personality changes.
8. Seizures.
9. Speech disturbances including dyspraxia, dysarthria, aphasia, and stuttering.
10. Trembling.
11. Aluminum related osteomalcia.
12. Anemia.

C. Treatment.
1. Discontinue oral aluminum-based medications.
2. Chelation of aluminum with desferoxamine.
3. Renal transplant.

D. Prevention.
1. Use of appropriately treated water for dialysis.
2. Use of nonaluminum-based phosphate binders.

IX. Dizziness (Roberts et al., 2007; Sherman et al., 2014).

A. Etiology.
1. Anemia.
2. Autonomic neuropathy.
3. Carotid sinus syndrome.
4. Hypoxemia.
5. Medications.
6. Orthostatic/postural hypotension.
7. Vasovagal syncope.
8. Hypovolemia/ischemia.

B. Signs and symptoms.
1. Complaints of dizziness during HD treatment.
2. Complaints of dizziness upon standing.
3. Complaints of interdialytic dizziness.
4. Syncope.

C. Treatment.
1. Assess blood pressure and cardiac rate and rhythm.
2. Volume replacement will be dependent upon severity of symptoms and blood pressure.
3. Normal saline replacement, if severe.
4. Oral fluids, if appropriate, to increase sympathetic tone.
5. Sitting for 10 to 15 minutes to allow for plasma refill.
6. Administer oxygen if needed.
7. Notify physician/APRN/PA if cardiac rhythm is not in normal range for patient.
8. Maintain anemia management goals.
9. *Safety alert.* Ensure the patient and significant others know what to do if the patient experiences these symptoms (e.g., sit down, lie down, elevate feet, and/or drink extra cup of fluid).

D. Prevention.
1. Frequent reassessment of dry weight.
2. Prevent hypovolemia.
3. Adjust UF goal to allow for a reduction of the UFR to the minimum for last 10 to 15 minutes of HD to allow time for plasma refill and start of re-equilibration.
4. Change position slowly at end of treatment.
5. If oxygen was administered during treatment,

leave it on patient until HD treatment is complete and BP has stabilized. Remove before discharge unless patient requires continuous oxygen therapy.
6. Have patient move legs and feet prior to standing to stimulate circulation.
7. Reassess antihypertensive medication as dry weight reductions occur.
8. Instruct patient on blood pressure parameters to resume antihypertensive medications at home after treatment.
9. Add approximately 0.2 to 0.5 kg to estimated dry weight.
10. Maintain anemia management goals.

X. Dysrhythmia (Selby & McIntyre, 2007; Voroneanu & Covic, 2009; Weiner & Sarnak, 2014).

A. Etiology.
1. Electrolyte and pH changes induced by HD.
2. Hyperkalemia/hypokalemia.
3. Hypervolemia/hypovolemia.
4. Rapid infusion of a large bolus of IV solution.
5. Removal of antiarrhythmic medication with HD.
6. Use of incorrect dialysate for patient.
7. Underlying heart disease such as atrial fibrillation.
8. Myocardial stunning.
9. Hypoxemia.
10. High UFR.

B. Signs and symptoms.
1. Chest pain.
2. Dizziness.
3. Fatigue.
4. Irregular, slow, or fast heart rate.
5. Palpitations.
6. Patient complains of anxiety.
7. Syncope.
8. Often asymptomatic.

C. Treatment.
1. Administer oxygen.
2. Reduce UFR to minimum.
3. Reduce dialysate temperature to 34–36°C (Damasiewicz & Polkinghorne, 2011, http://onlinelibrary.wiley.com/doi/10.1111/j.1440-1797.2010.01362.x/full#ss2).
4. Administer antiarrhythmic medications as ordered.
5. Cardiac monitoring for EKG changes.
6. Discontinue HD for severe, symptomatic dysrhythmias.
7. Use of appropriate dialysate electrolyte and bicarbonate concentrates.
8. Use automated external defibrillator (AED), if available, to diagnose and treat ventricular arrhythmias.

9. Notify physician/APRN/PA who may refer the patient to cardiologist for further assessment, possible pacemaker, and/or defibrillator placement.

D. Prevention.
1. If patient is taking digoxin, use a higher dialysate potassium concentration, but never less than 2.0 mEq/L.
2. Reassess serum electrolytes/serum CO_2 monthly to ensure proper concentrate is being used for the individual patient.
3. Administer antiarrhythmic medications as ordered.
4. Monitor heart rate and rhythm, and report changes.
5. Adjust/individualize UFR for the patient's age, weight, and comorbidities to avoid intravascular volume depletion, hypotension, and cardiac stunning. Net fluid loss should not exceed 1 to 2 kg/week unless guided by Hct-based BVM to observe PRR.
6. Limit amount of IV solution given as a bolus.
7. Reinfuse blood at lower blood pump speed during treatment termination.
8. Isothermic dialysate temperature.
9. *Safety alert.*
   a. Ensure the proper dialysate concentrate is used. Notify physician/APRN/PA of changes in laboratory work that may warrant an alteration in the dialysis prescription.
   b. Establish safe practices to confirm additives to dialysate concentrate (e.g., confirm the concentration and additives with two licensed nurses).

XI. Exsanguination (ANNA, n.d.; Axley et al., 2012; Ellingson et al., 2012; Saibu et al., 2011; http://www.prolibraries.com/anna/?select=session&sessionID=2131).

A. Etiology.
1. Accidental or traumatic separation of bloodlines.
2. Accidental dislodgement of needles from vascular access site.
3. Rupture of vascular access aneurysm or anastomosis.
4. Open central venous catheter limb or catheter dislodgement.
5. Dialyzer membrane rupture with failure of dialysate blood leak detector.
6. Failure to connect venous bloodline to the patient when discarding priming volume.
7. Undetected internal bleeding after anticoagulation (e.g., cardiac tamponade, GI, intracranial bleed) or inaccurate central venous catheter (CVC) placement.

B. Signs and symptoms.
1. Visualization of bleeding source.
2. Hypotension.
3. Increased heart rate.
4. Decrease in Hgb/Hct level.
5. Shock, seizures, and cardiovascular collapse.

C. Treatment.
1. Immediately stop blood pump and place a clamp on both sides of the separated bloodlines or catheter.
2. Apply pressure to any bleeding site. Apply tourniquet if unable to control bleeding.
3. Evaluate appropriateness of returning blood to the patient due to a ruptured dialyzer membrane.
4. Administer oxygen if blood loss is significant.
5. Administer volume expander if patient is hypotensive.
6. Monitor vital signs.
7. Obtain laboratory studies: Hgb/Hct.
8. Notify physician/APRN/PA.
9. Blood replacement as indicated.

D. Prevention.
1. Ensure all interlocking connections on bloodlines and access are secure throughout treatment.
2. Ensure continuous bloodline connections and vascular access visualization; do not leave patient unattended during the HD treatment.
3. Ensure access needles are securely taped according to facility procedure to avoid significant movement of needles in any direction. If a needle needs to be repositioned during treatment, replace existing tape with new tape to ensure needle security and tape adherence.
4. Ensure arterial and venous pressure monitors and dialysate blood leak detector are functioning properly.
5. Secure loosely looped bloodlines to the patient only during treatment. Do not secure to any other object.
6. Securely connect both the arterial and venous bloodlines to access lines at initiation of HD.
7. Use access clips to prevent needle dislodgement or catheter line separation if available.
8. Use moisture monitors or detection device for blood in the environment if available.
9. Appropriately cap and secure CVC when catheter use is completed.
10. Ensure complete stasis of access site prior to patient discharge.
11. Monitor patient throughout treatment for signs and symptoms of treatment and equipment-related complications.
12. Evaluate all patients for risk of venous dislodgement using the ANNA "Assessment of the Risk for a Serious Venous Needle Dislodgement

Incident" tool: ANNA, 2014, http://www.annanurse.org/resources/venous-needle-dislodgement
13. Use blood sensing devices at access site, if available.
14. *Safety alert.* Ensure the vascular access site is exposed and visible throughout the entire HD treatment and until the access needles are removed or the CVC is disconnected and securely closed (CMS, 2008, V407).

XII. Fever and chills/pyrogenic reaction (Nystrand, 2008; Roth & Jarvis, 2000; Schiffl, 2011; Schrauf, 2014; Ward & Ing, 2014, http://www.prolibraries.com/anna/?select=session&sessionID=3017).

A. Etiology.
1. Infection suspect with even small increases in temperature, 98° to 99°F, as average temperature for patient on HD is 96.8°F.
2. Introduction of pyrogens or endotoxins via dialysate, water, or reprocessed dialyzers; low-molecular-weight endotoxin fragments may be able to cross any dialyzer membrane.
3. Dialysate temperature higher than patient's temperature pretreatment can contribute to core body heating.

B. Signs and symptoms.
1. Patient feels cold after initiation of dialysis, often followed by involuntary shaking and sometimes fever.
2. Increase in body temperature.
3. Fever caused by pyrogenic or endotoxin reaction will most likely occur within the first 45 to 75 minutes of treatment, especially when the patient is afebrile prior to treatment.
4. Headache.
5. Hemodynamic instability.
6. Myalgia.
7. Nausea and vomiting.

C. Treatment.
1. Assess for signs and sources of infection such as vascular access, foot ulcer, decubiti, respiratory or urinary tract infections.
2. Obtain vital signs including temperature.
3. Notify physician/APRN/PA.
4. Obtain blood, inlet and outlet dialysate, and water cultures.
5. Obtain water and dialysate samples to test for Limulus amoebocyte lysate (LAL) assay to determine the presence of endotoxin. *Note:* LAL is an enzyme that is sensitive to the presence of endotoxin and a positive test is suggestive of endotoxin presence.

6. Discontinue HD without returning blood if a pyrogen or endotoxin reaction is suspected.
7. Administer antipyretics and antibiotics as ordered.
8. Assess and maintain proper dialysate temperature (34° to 36°C).

D. Prevention.
1. Appropriate water treatment.
2. Appropriate reuse procedures for dialyzers; follow facility policy and procedures/manufacturers' instructions.
3. Vigilant preparation of equipment and supplies to prevent contamination.
4. Aseptic treatment initiation to prevent contamination/infection.
5. Minimize the length of time supplies and extracorporeal system are prepared before treatment initiation.
   a. Multiple factors affect the possible introduction of contaminants into the extracorporeal system.
   b. The length of time that saline or blood can be safely recirculated is not defined and is elusive (Schrauf, 2014, http://www.prolibraries.com/anna/?select=session&sessionID=3017).
6. Protect patient from known and unknown infectious agents. Follow universal precautions and hand hygiene guidelines.
7. Appropriate handling of bicarbonate dialysate to avoid contamination.
8. Maintain a minimum UFR to prevent dialysate backflow into dialyzer.
9. Routine cleaning and disinfection of water treatment and concentration distribution systems.
10. Routine cleaning and disinfection of dialysate containers, particularly those used with bicarbonate dialysate.
11. Routine cleaning and disinfection of dialysis machines including the waste handling option (WHO) (if available on dialysis machine).
12. Isothermic dialysate.
13. Follow unit policies and procedures in preparing the dialyzer for treatment.
14. *Safety alert.* Maintain aseptic technique throughout dialyzer preparation and HD treatment.

XIII. Headache (Antoniazzi et al., 2003; IHS, 2013, http://www.ihs-classification.org/_downloads/mixed/International-Headache-Classification-III-ICHD-III-2013-Beta.pdf; Milinkovic et al., 2009; Sherman et al., 2014).

A. Etiology.
1. Occurs in as many as 70% of patients undergoing HD.
2. Common complaint during HD.
3. Cause is widely unknown.

4. International Headache Society (2013) diagnostic criteria for dialysis headache.
   a. Onset during HD.
   b. Worsens during the HD treatment or resolves within 72 hours after HD session.
   c. Has occurred during at least half of a prescribed dialysis treatment.
   d. Has occurred at least three times.
   e. Episodes do not recur after successful kidney transplantation or after HD is terminated.
5. May be due to mild DDS, caffeine withdrawal as caffeine level is reduced during dialysis, or biochemical changes in the body.
6. Magnesium deficiency is a rare occurrence but blood levels should be verified.
7. If headache is atypical or exceptionally severe, assess patient for neurological cause such as intracranial hemorrhage.
8. Hypervolemia or hypovolemia.
9. Hypertension.

B. Treatment.
1. Administer analgesic medication as ordered.
2. Adjust treatment parameters as indicated. A lower dialysate sodium concentration may be beneficial.

C. Prevention.
1. Ensure appropriate treatment parameters.
2. If serum magnesium levels are low, administer IV magnesium as ordered.

XIV. Hypotension (Bradshaw e t al., 2011; Charra, 2007; Damasiewicz & Polkinghorne, 2011; Henderson, 2012; House, 2011; NKF, 2006; Sherman et al., 2014; Tai et al., 2013).

A. Background.
1. It is estimated that hypotension occurs in 15% to 55% of all HD treatments.
2. Intradialytic hypotension (IDH) is associated with increased mortality and morbidity, decreased quality of life, and increased healthcare costs.
3. Low blood pressure impairs tissue perfusion and can compromise dialysis adequacy, contribute to loss of residual kidney function, and predispose patients to coronary and/or cerebral ischemia.
4. Low BP predialysis has been associated with higher risk of mortality and may be associated with cardiac failure, inadequate dialysis, hypervolemia, myocardial stunning, or other serious illnesses (NKF, 2006a, http://www2.kidney.org/professionals/KDOQI/guideline_upHD_PD_VA/hd_guide5.htm; Schreiber, 2003).
5. BP may increase with UF as the intravascular volume is reduced, improving cardiac contractility (see Figure 2.36 in Section D).

6 IDH is indicated by:
   a. A decrease in systolic blood pressure by equal to or greater than 20 mmHg or a decrease in mean arterial pressure (MAP) by 10 mmHg.
   b. If the predialysis systolic blood pressure is less than 100 mmHg, then intradialytic hypotension is defined as a decrease in systolic blood pressure by equal to or greater than 10 mmHg with associated symptoms.

B. Etiology.
BP = cardiac output (CO) x peripheral vascular resistance (PVR).
Cardiac output = stroke volume x heart rate.
Hypotension is a consequence of reduction in CO and/or PVR. Any minor decrease in PVR can precipitate a drop in blood pressure as the CO cannot increase to compensate during blood volume depletion. The inability to vasoconstrict the resistance in vessels is a significant cause of ultrafiltration induced hypotension. Causes include:
1. Posture changes: Autonomic neuropathy from diabetes or uremia blunts the normal PVR response to postural/orthostatic hypotension.
2. Hypoxemia and tissue ischemia cause a release of adenosine, a potent vasodilator.
3. Medications: antihypertensives or other vasodilator medications (narcotics, analgesics); beta-blockers decrease cardiac contractility and rate.
4. Decrease in PVR related to vasoactive substances that are administered or released by cells during dialysis; chemical inflammatory mediators from cells may induce potent vasodilatory effects.
5. Inaccuracies in the ultrafiltration (UF) rate or amount can result in volume depletion or overload. Decreased cardiac filling pressure and stroke volume can occur with either hypervolemia or hypovolemia.
   a. The rate of plasma volume change will be the difference between UF from the vascular compartment and the plasma refilling rate (PRR) from the interstitial compartment.
   b. The disparity in these rates and the precipitous fall in PRR supports the activation of the cardiodepressor (Bezold-Jarisch) reflex leading to a sudden loss of sympathetic tone and increased vascular bed capacitance (the ability to hold or contain).
   c. This reflex is initiated by cardiac stretch receptors that are maladaptively triggered by the hyperdynamic left ventricle becoming hypovolemic with UF.
   d. Autonomic neuropathy from diabetes or uremia may reduce the normal compensatory responses to a decrease in CO, attenuating the UF-induced contraction of the capacitance vessels and shift of volume from periphery to central circulation (DeJager-Krogh Phenomenon).
6. Incorrect end goal or target of dialysis body weight.
7. Reduced plasma osmolality: Low serum albumin, or low dialysate sodium relative to plasma sodium, can lead to movement of water into the intracellular compartment, reducing the extracellular compartment, hence fluid accessible for UF.
8. Core body heating stimulates vasodilation.
   a. Dialysate greater than 36° C; average temperature for patients on HD is 36° C (96.8° F).
   b. High UF rates generate heat and lead to heat accumulation, and eventual vasodilation.
9. Eating immediately prior to, during, or immediately after HD, can cause splanchnic vasodilatation; effects can last up to 2 hours.
10. Electrolyte imbalance can affect cardiac contractility and heart rate.
11. Acid-base imbalance can cause vasodilatation. Acetate dialysate may contribute to hypotension from vasodilatation if high blood concentrations are achieved during dialysis.
12. Anemia (Hct less than, 30% or Hgb less than 10 g/dL).
    a. Viscosity of blood affects PVR.
    b. Anemia leads to hypoxemia and tissue ischemia.
    c. Anemia can lead to decreased cardiac reserve related to chronic high output state.
13. Unstable cardiovascular status, arrhythmias, pericardial tamponade, myocardial infarction, and stiff hypertrophied heart compromise the heart's ability to maintain or increase CO in response to volume depletion.
14. Septicemia causes vasodilatation.
15. Dialyzer reaction, pulmonary leukostasis, hemolysis, and air embolism cause hypoxemia with resultant vasodilatation.
16. Carnitine deficiency alters cardiac and skeletal muscle function.
17. Hypotension perpetuates hypotension.
    a. Tissue ischemia causes the release of adenosine.
    b. Abrupt episodes support the activation of a cardiodepressor (Bezold-Jarisch) reflex, which causes a loss of sympathetic tone and PVR.

C. Signs and symptoms.
1. Anxiety.
2. Complaint of "not feeling well," feeling warm and fanning themselves may be early signs.
3. Cramps.
4. Decreased mental status, loss of consciousness.
5. Diaphoresis or cold clammy skin.

6. Dizziness upon standing.
7. Headache.
8. Pallor.
9. Posttreatment malaise and fatigue.
10. Nausea and vomiting.
11. Restlessness.
12. Arrhythmia, tachycardia, but may be blunted by calcium channel or beta blockers. Prolonged myocardial stunning and ischemia may lead to bradycardia or other arrhythmia.
13. Visual complaints.
14. Yawning, sighing.
15. Serious vascular complications include cerebral ischemia, atrophy, infarct, vision loss, vascular access thrombosis, nonocclusive mesenteric ischemia, cardiac ischemia, arrhythmias, infarct, decrease in residual kidney function, increased mortality.

D. Treatment.
1. Place patient in modified Trendelenburg position. Elevate legs 30 to 45 degrees, flexing at the hip, with the trunk remaining horizontal, and head level with trunk. *Note*: True Trendelenburg position may impair lung capacity and oxygenation, and result in more profound hypotension when the patient is gradually returned to the upright position. Compensatory mechanisms may be inadequate to support BP resulting from the extreme, true Trendelenburg position.
2. Reduce UFR to minimum (a minimum UFR prevents backflow of dialysate across the membrane).
3. Administer oxygen to prevent or treat tissue ischemia and improve myocardial function.
4. If necessary to reverse hypotension, administer suitable agents. If volume replacement is needed, the severity of symptoms will influence the volume.
   a. Normal saline (NS) replacement, if severe, can be used in bolus doses of 100 to 200 mL.
      Note: There are disadvantages to giving NS.
      (1) Fluid removal during HD will be less.
      (2) If given late in or after HD, the patient may experience postdialysis thirst resulting in increased interdialytic weight gain.
      (3) Rapid infusion of a large bolus may cause dysrhythmia or CHF.
   b. Osmotic agents, such as albumin, hypertonic saline, or hypertonic glucose solutions will facilitate movement of water from the interstitial and intracellular compartments into the vascular compartment. The use of mannitol is not supported due to continued fluid shifts after HD is completed and inadequate kidney function to clear the fluid, putting the patient at increased risk for hypervolemia, CHF, or pulmonary edema. Limitations of other osmotic agents include:
      (1) Unless cramps are also present, use of hypertonic solutions appears to offer no benefit over NS.
      (2) The KDOQI Guidelines (NKF, 2006a) discourages the increase of sodium balance during dialysis (e.g., includes sodium profiling) (http://www2.kidney.org/professionals/KDOQI/guideline_upHD_PD_VA/hd_guide5.htm).
      (3) Use above agents with caution.
      (4) Disadvantages.
         (a) Hyperosmolality of hypertonic saline.
            i. Increases postdialysis thirst.
            ii. A large portion is retained even when given 2 hours before the end of HD treatment.
            iii. 78% is retained when given 1 hour prior to the end of HD.
         (b) Hypertonic glucose solutions are better tolerated in patients without diabetes. One study demonstrated improved dialysis adequacy and blood pressure control with its use (Tayebi et al., 2013, http://www.inhc.ir/browse.php?a_code=A-10-327-5&slc_lang=en&sid=1).
   c. Administer oral fluids if less severe: water; black coffee, if allowed, will increase sympathetic tone.

E. Prevention.
1. Accurate predialysis and postdialysis weights.
2. As accurate an estimate of dry weight as possible.
3. Dry weight should be systematically reevaluated after each dialysis treatment as it may change under various conditions (e.g., intercurrent illness leading to loss of muscle mass and tissue weight, a patient newly dialyzed becoming less uremic and regains appetite, muscle and nonfluid weight changes). The plan of care changes should be documented to reflect efforts to attain/maintain dry weight (CMS, 2008).
4. Blood pressure and pulse before, during, and after HD; rapid pulse may indicate compensation.
5. NKF-KDOQI Clinical Practice Guidelines suggest use of a dialysis log to summarize relevant information (e.g., body weight, blood pressures, intradialytic events) to provide a longitudinal dynamic view of extracellular fluid volume and blood pressure changes (NKF, 2006b, http://www2.kidney.org/professionals/KDOQI/guideline_upHD_PD_VA/hd_guide5.htm).
6. Start HD with patient's feet one notch off the floor, elevated prophylactically. Instruct patient to sit up and stand slowly at end of HD treatment.

7. Assess for and treat hypoxemia prior to symptom occurrence.
8. Withhold antihypertensive medications immediately before and during dialysis per order.
   a. Reassess medication list frequently to look for possible side effects, interactions, and current need.
   b. Reductions in antihypertensive medication(s) may occur with fluid removal and achieving/maintaining ideal dry weight.
9. Dialyze with volumetrically controlled HD ultrafiltration systems, especially when using mid-flux or high-flux dialyzers.
10. Adjust and individualize the UFR to avoid intravascular volume depletion, myocardial stunning, hypotension, and other intradialytic morbidities. Net fluid loss ideally should not exceed 1 to 2 kg/week unless guided by hematocrit based blood volume monitoring (BVM) to observe PRR.

    Note: Use of multifrequency bioimpedence analysis is a relatively new technology for use on patients on hemodialysis. As of publication date of the *Core*, this has not been approved by the FDA, nor have enough studies been completed to verify efficacy in prevention of hypotension.

    a. UF profiling: varies the rate of fluid removal permitting the vascular space to refill. Periods of high UFR may not be tolerated and may cause myocardial stunning.
    b. Isolated ultrafiltration (no dialysate flow) also referred to as sequential ultrafiltration or pure UF.
       (1) Bypasses the dialysate solution to drain allowing UF only.
       (2) Removes iso-osmolar fluid from the systemic circulation via convection.
       (3) Removes excess fluid without changing blood solute concentrations.
       (4) Typical prescription is for 1 hour of isolated ultrafiltration prior to regularly prescribed HD time to avoid poor dialysis solute removal adequacy.
       (5) To avoid rebound hyperkalemia, it is suggested that isolated ultrafiltration be immediately followed by HD.
          (a) Intensive isolated ultrafiltration may lead to rebound hyperkalemia, perhaps from the exit of intracellular potassium into the extracellular fluid.
          (b) Although this complication is controversial, possible hyperkalemia can be avoided by immediate HD following isolated ultrafiltration.
       (6) The isolated ultrafiltration time is in addition to the prescribed HD treatment as it provides UF only, not dialysis.
          (7) High UFR with isolated UF may not be tolerated and may cause myocardial stunning.
    c. Hct-based blood volume monitoring noninvasively provides a measure of blood volume changes, Hct, and oxygen saturation.
       (1) Allows for the real-time calculation of plasma volume changes, UFR, and PRR disparity to proactively prevent intravascular volume depletion.
       (2) May promote optimization of extracellular fluid status.
       (3) Seems to reduce intra and post HD morbid complications.
       (4) May increase improvements in patient well-being.
       (5) Appears to provide an objective way of assigning ideal, true dry weight through plasma refill or "dry weight check" near end of treatment.
       (6) Provides numerical values for Hct and oxygen saturation for assessment of anemia/hypoxemia as potential causes of hypotension.
11. Sodium profiling if needed, due to reduced plasma osmolality.
    a. This technique increases dialysate sodium concentrations early in HD, followed by a progressive decrease (linear, step, or logarithmic) to a lower value at the end of HD.
    b. NKF-KDOQI Clinical Practice Guidelines state that increasing positive sodium balance by "sodium profiling" or using a high dialysate sodium concentration should be avoided to decrease thirst, fluid gains, and hypertension. Reviews showed uncertain benefit (NKF, 2006a, http://www2.kidney.org/professionals/KDOQI/guideline_upHD_PD_VA/hd_guide5.htm).
    c. The risk of intradialytic hypotension increases 13% for each 1 mEq fall in dialysate to serum sodium.
    d. The time-weighted average concentration determines the postdialysis serum sodium level. Base sodium recommended to be individualized to patient's sodium set-point.
12. Isothermic (cool) dialysate.
13. Encourage patients to eat a small, high-quality protein meal vs. large carbohydrate meal an hour before and after HD treatment. Discourage eating immediately prior to or during HD.
14. Assess laboratory values to identify and correct electrolyte/acid-base imbalances. The use of bicarbonate vs. acetate dialysate is recommended as the buffer of choice.

15. Maintain adequate Hgb/Hct levels. Transfuse blood products as needed.
16. Assess for and treat cardiovascular problems.
17. Correct identified carnitine deficiency.
18. Assess for and treat septicemia.
19. Follow procedures to avoid dialyzer reaction, hemolysis, and air embolism.
20. Administer an alpha-adrenergic agonist, such as midodrine, 15 to 30 minutes prior to HD. It may be repeated midway if needed to avoid hypotension in patients with autonomic neuropathy leading to impaired PVR or those with a tendency for hypotension. *Note*: Midodrine has a short half-life of 2 to 2½ hours.
21. Teach the patient to recognize and report early signs and symptoms of hypotension.
22. Instruct patients on taking blood pressure at home and parameters to assess prior to taking antihypertensive medication(s) post HD.
23. Encourage fluid restriction between HD treatments to 1 L plus urinary output.
    a. Ideal fluid gain is limited to 1 to 2 kg between treatments during the week for thrice weekly HD.
    b. Ideal fluid gain is limited to 1.5 to 3 kg during the weekend, or equal to or less than 3% of body weight.
24. Daily dietary sodium intake should be restricted to no more than 2.0 g of sodium; a more stringent daily sodium limit of 1 to 1.5 g is recommended for patients on HD who have hypertension.
25. Extend prescribed treatment time as needed to reduce the UFR.
26. Consider extra treatment vs. higher UFR to attain EDW.

XV. Hypertension (Zocali & Mallamaci, 2014).

A. Etiology.
   1. Controversial in literature; possible etiologies include:
      a. Temporary compensatory response to hypovolemia prior to BP drop in patients with active renin angiotension system (i.e., new to dialysis, have residual kidney function).
      b. Medications removed during the dialysis treatment. These patients may respond to more fluid removal, with eventual better BP control (NKF, 2006a, http://www2.kidney.org/professionals/KDOQI/guideline_upHD_PD_VA/hd_guide5.htm).
      c. Patient anxiety.

B. Treatment.
   1. Thorough assessment to determine cause.

2. Use BVM to determine accessibility of possible extra fluid to be removed.
3. Identification of cause/treatment of anxiety if identified.

XVI. Hypoxemia (Davenport, 2008; Kosmadakis & Medcalf, 2008; Manca-Di-Villahermosa et al., 2008; Zheng et al., 2009).

A. Etiology.
   1. Hemodialysis itself can provoke significant tissue hypoxemia and myocardial stunning, especially in patients with severe preexisting pulmonary or cardiac disease.
   2. Hypoventilation, especially when serum bicarbonate levels are high (equal to or greater than 35 mmol) and dialyzing against a bicarbonate dialysate (alkalosis).
   3. Anemia (Hct equal to or less than 30%; Hgb equal to or less than 10 g/dL).
   4. Bioincompatibility of the HD membrane.
   5. Chronic obstructive pulmonary disease (COPD).
   6. Congestive heart failure (CHF)/cardiovascular disease (CVD).
   7. Dialysate composition.
   8. Diffusion of oxygen through the dialyzer.
   9. Eating during HD.
   10. First use syndrome.
   11. Pulmonary edema.
   12. Pulmonary leukostasis.
   13. Pulmonary microembolization.
   14. Rebound of reprocessing agent.
   15. Sleep apnea occurs in as many as 70% of patients on HD related to uremic effects on the sleep center and throat mechanics.
   16. Warm dialysate (greater than 36°C).

B. Signs and symptoms (related to ensuing ischemia and/or vasodilation).
   1. Blurred vision.
   2. Chest pain.
   3. Confusion.
   4. Cramping.
   5. Cyanosis.
   6. Dizziness.
   7. Hypotension.
   8. Nausea and vomiting.
   9. Restlessness.
   10. Seizure.
   11. Shortness of breath.
   12. Tachycardia.
   13. Tachypnea.

C. Treatment.
   1. Supplemental oxygen.
   2. Nasal oxygen is usually sufficient.

3. Blood pressure support.
4. Reassess dialysate composition.

D. Prevention.
1. Consider supplemental oxygen proactively in the following situations.
   a. Anemia (Hct equal to or less than 30%; Hgb equal to or less than 10 g/dL).
   b. Arterial saturation less than 90%.
   c. Venous saturation less than 60%.
   d. Oxygen-carrying capacity below 19 to 20 mL/dL.
      (1) The normal range of overall oxygen-carrying capacity is 19 to 20 mL/dL.
      (2) This is calculated by multiplying 1.39 mL (the amount of oxygen each gram of hemoglobin carries) x hemoglobin x SaO_2 or SpO_2.
   e. Patients who frequently exhibit symptoms.
   f. Patients with a history of cardiac or respiratory disease.
   g. Pulse less than 60 or greater than 100 bpm.
   h. Respiratory rate greater than 24/minute.
   i. Sleep apnea.
   j. Systolic BP less than 100 mmHg.
   k. Unresolved edema.
2. Avoid weaning patient and/or decreasing oxygen during HD. If oxygen is applied during HD, continue oxygen posttreatment to promote plasma refill. Assess patient to establish that the patient is stable after oxygen is discontinued prior to discharge.
3. Have patient evaluated if sleep apnea is suspected.
4. Individualize bicarbonate dialysate based upon serum CO_2 and comorbidities, per physician/APRN/PA order.
5. Use thermal control for isothermic dialysis.
   a. Dialysate temperature significantly affects diffusion of oxygen, decreasing PaO_2.
   b. Most patients benefit from cool dialysate for prevention of hypoxia and report increased energy posttreatment.
6. Use dialyzer manufactured with biocompatible materials to reduce complement activation, especially for patients at high risk.
7. If dialyzers are reprocessed, follow facility's policies and procedures for removing and assessing for residual reprocessing agent and preventing sterilant rebound.
8. Discourage eating immediately prior to and during HD.
9. Maintain ideal dry weight to avoid CHF/pulmonary edema.
10. Maintain hematocrit to patient's individualized target per physician/APRN/PA orders/protocol.

XVII. Itching (Makari et al., 2013; Sherman et al., 2014).

A. Etiology and signs and symptoms.
1. Common problem in patients on HD; may be chronically present.
2. Can be precipitated or exacerbated by HD.
3. Can be precipitated or exacerbated by increase in patient temperature during HD.
4. Accumulation of substances not adequately removed by HD.
5. Hypercalcemia.
6. Hyperphosphatemia.
7. Hyperparathyroidism.
8. Inflammation.
9. Iron deficiency anemia.
10. Itching only during HD, especially if accompanied by additional minor allergic reaction(s), may indicate a low-grade sensitivity to the dialyzer or blood circuit components.
11. Liver disease: do not overlook viral or drug-induced hepatitis.
12. Neuropathy.

B. Treatment.
1. Acupuncture.
2. Medication as ordered (e.g., gabapentin).
3. Regular moisturizing and lubrication of skin using emollients.
4. Reduce serum calcium and phosphorous levels to the lower end of normal.
5. Symptomatic treatment with antihistamines.
6. Ultraviolet light therapy, especially UVB light.
7. Oral charcoal.
8. Nalfuralfine hydrochloride.
9. Switch from formaldehyde in dialyzer reprocessing to other disinfecting agents (DeOreo, 2014).
10. Isothermic dialysate.

C. Prevention.
1. Maintain serum calcium and phosphorous levels in normal range.
2. Routine moisturizing and lubrication of skin using emollients.
3. Use biocompatible membranes.
4. Wear light, loose clothing to keep body temperature cool.

XVIII. Membrane biocompatibility (Ahmad et al., 2014; Davenport, 2008; Heegard et al., 2013; Sherman et al., 2014; Ward, 2011).

A. Etiology.
1. Two types of reactions can occur: anaphylactic reactions (Type A) and a nonspecific reaction (Type B). Type A reactions can be severe while Type B reactions are milder and occur much less frequently than in the past.

2. Type A reactions.
   a. Allergy to the dialyzer membrane material; reaction may be amplified in patients taking angiotensin converting enzyme (ACE) inhibitors.
   b. Allergy to medications such as heparin and intravenous iron preparation.
   c. Bacterial or endotoxin contamination of water used for reprocessing or used to mix bicarbonate dialysate, especially when using a high flux dialyzer.
   d. Sensitivity to ethylene oxide (EO), a gas dialyzer sterilant.
   e. Occurs more readily in patients with mild to moderate eosinophilia.
3. Type B reactions are nonspecific and less severe.
   a. Complement activation has been implicated.
   b. May result from sensitivity to membrane material.
   c. Subclinical hemolysis should not be ruled out.

B. Signs and symptoms.
   1. Type A reaction.
      a. Occurs during the first 5 to 10 minutes (maximum 20) and progresses in severity.
      b. Initial feeling of uneasiness, warmth at the access site or throughout the body, a sense of impending doom; followed by agitation, chest tightness, back pain, and nausea.
      c. Can progress to shortness of breath, coughing, wheezing, urticaria, facial edema, flushing, anaphylaxis, cardiac arrest, and death.
      d. Milder case presents with itching, urticaria, cough, sneezing, watery eyes, or GI symptoms.
      e. BP can be high or low.
   2. Type B reaction.
      a. Occurs later in dialysis (20 to 40 minutes after initiation of treatment). Generally resolves after the first hour.
      b. Associated with back or chest pain.
      c. Hypotension in some instances.

C. Treatment.
   1. Type A reaction.
      a. Immediate termination of dialysis; do NOT return the patient's blood.
      b. Administer oxygen.
      c. Per physician/APRN/PA order or protocol, administer IV antihistamines, steroids, or epinephrine depending upon reaction severity.
      d. Cardiopulmonary support may be required for an anaphylactic reaction.
   2. Type B reaction.
      a. Treatment is supportive in nature. Oxygen for respiratory complaints and symptoms, antihistamines or analgesics for pain, treat angina promptly.

   b. Symptoms often resolve, and HD treatment does not usually need to be terminated.

D. Prevention.
   1. Type A reaction.
      a. Appropriate rinsing of dialyzers prior to treatment to remove ethylene oxide (ETO) sterilant, other sterilants, or other allergens.
      b. Use of dialyzer sterilized with electron beam, Gamma-radiation, or steam to avoid sterilant exposure and reactions.
      c. Administer antihistamines prior to treatment.
      d. Use reprocessed dialyzer or change to an alternate membrane and/or sterilant.
      e. Process reuse dialyzers prior to first use.
      f. Follow AAMI standards for water treatment.
      g. Change or stop heparin.
      h. Consideration should also be given to the possibility of a latex allergy.
   2. Type B reaction may result from sensitivity to membrane material.
      a. Possible benefit from dialyzer reuse program.
      b. Convert patient to a dialyzer with a more biocompatible membrane.
   3. Monitor patient throughout treatment for the onset of signs and symptoms of treatment and equipment-related complications.
   4. *Safety alert.*
      a. Patients should not be left unattended during HD treatment.
      b. Follow manufacturer's recommendations and facility's policies and procedures for dialyzer preparation to minimize opportunities for untoward membrane reactions.

XIX. **Methemoglobinemia**
(Carlson & Shapiro, 1970); NIH, 2011, http://dailymed.nlm.nih.gov/dailymed/lookup.cfm?setid=fde64824-2be5-4d85-8d57-5098ca6890bb; Davenport, 2006; Denshaw-Burke et al., 2013, http://emedicine.medscape.com/article/204178-overview#showall; FDA, 2011, http://www.fda.gov/drugs/drugsafety/ucm263190.htm; Fenves et al., 2000, http://onlinelibrary.wiley.com/doi/10.1046/j.1525-139x.2000.00094.x/abstract).

A. Definition: The presence of greater than 1% of Hgb having been oxidized to a ferric state.

B. Etiology.
   1. Abnormal preparation of dialysate composition due to:
      a. Elevated copper levels in treated water.
      b. Elevated nitrate levels in treated water.
      c. Elevated chloramine levels in treated water.

2. Diagnosis is by direct measurement of methemoglobin levels in blood.
3. *Safety alert.* It may take several hours for clinical symptoms to appear.

C. Signs and symptoms.
1. Cyanosis.
2. Dyspnea.
3. Headache.
4. Hemolysis.
5. Hypoxia.
6. Malaise.
7. Nausea/vomiting.
8. Palpitations.
9. Blood in bloodlines appear chocolate brown in color.

D. Treatment.
1. Discontinue treatment.
2. Monitor oxygen saturation and administer oxygen.
3. Notify physician/APRN/PA.
4. Treatment of choice is methylene blue IV in an acute care setting.
   a. If no or limited response to methylene blue, or patient is unable to be treated with methylene blue (glucose-6-phospate dehydrogenase (G6PD) deficiency), treatment may consist of:
      (1) Exchange transfusion.
      (2) Hyperbaric oxygen therapy.
   b. *Safety alert.*
      (1) Use caution when administering methylene blue; if given too rapidly, can worsen methemaglobinemia. Large IV doses can lead to nausea, headache, precordial and abdominal pain, profuse sweating, mental confusion (NIH, 2011, http://dailymed.nlm.nih.gov/dailymed/lookup.cfm?setid=fde64824-2be5-4d85-8d57-5098ca6890bb).
      (2) Patients taking serotonergic psychiatric medications may experience serious central nervous system toxicity resulting from a drug interaction with methylene blue (FDA, 2011, http://www.fda.gov/drugs/drugsafety/ucm263190.htm).

E. Prevention.
1. Follow AAMI recommendations for water treatment in hemodialysis.
2. Perform frequent chloramine testing of water treatment system.
3. Establish close relationship with water municipality to ensure notification occurs when chlorine is pulsed through water system and may overwhelm the carbon tank ability to remove chlorine.

XX. Muscle cramps (Raymond & Wazny, 2011; Sherman et al., 2014).

A. Etiology.
1. Excessive or rapid fluid removal.
2. Hypo-osmolality.
3. Hypotension.
4. Hypovolemia.
5. Tissue hypoxemia/ischemia.
6. Electrolyte disorders, imbalances/rapid shifts; low sodium, calcium, potassium, magnesium.
7. Any local irritating factor or metabolic abnormality of a muscle (e.g. severe cold, lack of blood flow, over-exercise).
8. Skeletal muscle structural changes.
9. Neuromuscular (motor system) diseases.
10. Peripheral vascular disease.
11. Polyneuropathy.
12. Postdialytic alkalemia.
13. Carnitine deficiency.

B. Signs and symptoms.
1. Painful cramps generally occurring in, but not limited to, the extremities or abdomen.
2. Muscle cramps usually occur late in HD.

C. Treatment.
1. Appropriate dialysate potassium and sodium concentration.
2. Thermal control (dialysate 34° to 36° C).
3. Correct anemia if hematocrit (Hct) is less than 30% or hemoglobin (Hgb) is less than 10 g/dL.
4. Treat hypoxemia (PaO_2 less than 90%; SvO_2 less than 60%; oxygen-carrying capacity below 19 to 20 mL/dL).
5. Reduce UFR to minimum.
6. Stretch affected muscle (e.g., dorsiflexion of foot).
7. Sequential compression devices.
8. Bolus dose of osmotic agents such as hypertonic saline or 50% glucose should be used with extreme caution. See caution statement under "Hypotension" regarding use of osmotic agents.
9. Volume expansion with normal saline.
10. Apply heat to site.
11. Treat identified carnitine deficiency with carnitine replacement.

D. Prevention.
1. Appropriate dietary control of fluid and electrolytes.
2. Adjust UFR to avoid intravascular volume depletion and myocardial stunning.
3. Individualize UFR based upon age, weight, and comorbidities.
4. Increase HD treatment time to reduce UFR.

5. Frequent assessment of correct postdialysis target body weight.
6. Evaluate appropriate dialysate sodium concentration.
7. Refrain from eating during HD.
8. Discourage sudden position changes, especially from recline to upright.
9. Isothermic dialysis.
10. Proactively identify and treat hypoxemia.
11. Correct anemia.
12. Stretching exercises before and during HD and at home may be beneficial.
13. Use Hct-based BVM to attain and maintain ideal body weight if available to assess PRR and if fluid is accessible for UF. Net fluid loss ideally should not exceed 1 to 2 kg/week unless guided by Hct based BVM to observe PRR.
14. Oxazepam or vitamin E may provide relief if given prophylactically.

Note: Use of multifrequency bioimpedence analysis is a relatively new technology for use on patients on hemodialysis. As of publication date of the *Core*, this has not been approved by the FDA nor have enough studies been completed to verify efficacy in prevention of hypotension.

XXI. Nausea and vomiting (Sherman et al., 2014).

A. Etiology.
1. Occurs in up to 10% of HD treatments.
2. Most cases are related to hypotension.
3. Can be an early symptom of dialysis disequilibrium syndrome.
4. Membrane incompatibility.
5. Contaminated or improperly mixed dialysate fluid.
6. Metabolic disturbance secondary to chronic kidney disease.
7. Medications.
8. GI: peptic ulcer, gallbladder, pancreas disease, pancreatitis, gastroparesis.
9. Pregnancy.

B. Signs and symptoms: nausea and vomiting.

C. Treatment.
1. Identify and treat appropriate cause.
2. Antiemetics, if needed, as ordered.
3. Consider use of alternative medications if related to medication administration.

D. Prevention.
1. Prevent hypotension.
2. Frequent reassessment of dry weight and ability to attain and maintain it.

3. Assess for root cause.
4. Antiemetics if needed.
5. Medications to control nausea and enhance gastric emptying.
6. Refer patient for further evaluation for recurring nausea and vomiting.
7. *Safety alert.*
   a. Encourage a small protein meal 1 hour before and 1 hour after HD. Avoid large carbohydrate meal.
   b. Discourage eating during HD or minimize intake if the patient must eat.
   c. Be aware of the risk of aspiration when the patient who is vomiting is also experiencing a decreased level of consciousness associated with hypotension.

XXII. Seizures (Brennan & Whitehouse, 2012; McIntyre, 2014).

A. Etiology.
1. Dialysis disequilibrium syndrome (DDS).
2. Dialysate composition errors.
3. Electrolyte/acid-base imbalances (e.g., hyponatremia or hypernatremia).
4. Hemodynamic instability including rapid blood pressure changes.
5. Hypoglycemia.
6. Hypotension.
7. Hypovolemia.
8. Hypoxemia.
9. Hypocalcemia.
10. Anaphylaxis.
11. Aluminum encephalopathy.
12. Intracranial bleeding hastened by heparin.
13. Removal of anticonvulsant medication by hemodialysis.
14. Severe hypertension.
15. Air embolism.
16. Too rapid infusion of blood.
17. Alcohol withdrawal.
18. Toxins; for example, starfruit ingestion has been documented to result in the following symptoms due to increased levels of oxalic acid in patients who are uremic.
   a. Symptoms typically occur 1 to 5 hours after ingestion.
   b. Persistent hiccups.
   c. Nausea/vomiting.
   d. Agitation.
   e. Insomnia.
   f. Mental confusion.
   g. Seizures.
19. *Safety alert.* Mental confusion and seizures have been associated with increased mortality.

B. Signs and symptoms.
  1. Change in level of consciousness.
  2. Twitching and jerking movements of extremities.

C. Treatment.
  1. Protect the patient and the access limb from harm.
  2. Treat hypotension and hypoglycemia if indicated.
  3. Administer oxygen.
  4. Treat DDS if indicated.
  5. Terminate treatment for severe seizures.
  6. Provide airway support.
  7. Obtain laboratory studies for glucose, calcium, and other electrolytes.

D. Prevention.
  1. Predialysis assessment of risk factors.
  2. Avoid large, rapid drops in BUN concentration during HD.
  3. Monitor blood pressure changes during HD.
  4. Minimize osmotic changes during HD.
  5. Administer anticonvulsant medication as ordered.
  6. Administer oxygen for patients with underlying cardiac or respiratory disease.
  7. Adjust UFR to avoid intravascular volume depletion, hypotension, and cerebral "stunning."
  8. Monitor the patient throughout treatment for the onset of signs and symptoms of treatment and equipment-related complications.
  9. Draw/monitor blood levels of anticonvulsant medications as ordered.
  10. Assess patient for adherence to prescribed anticonvulsants.
  11. *Safety alert.* The patient should not be left unattended during the HD treatment.

SECTION F
Dialyzer Reprocessing
Darlene Jalbert

I. Background information.

A. The blood and dialysate compartments of a hemodialyzer can be cleansed and sterilized or achieve a high level of disinfection to make it safe and effective for the patient to reuse the same dialyzer for multiple treatments.

B. Practiced safely in the United States since the 1960s and continues to be a common practice in many dialysis facilities today.
  1. In the beginning, reprocessing was done by hand, but is now most often done with automated equipment.

2. This practice became even more prevalent in the late 1980s due to Medicare setting a composite rate form of payment for dialysis facilities. Reprocessing was more cost effective.
3. Some dialysis providers are trending toward non-reuse due to improvement in single-use dialyzers and the rising cost of equipment, disinfectant, and labor for reprocessing (Morgan, 2008, http://www.renalbusiness.com/lib/download.ashx?d=1979).

C. Studies have shown reuse of hemodialyzers has an environmental impact because dialysis facilities generate less medical waste and thus reduce the cost and volume of their biohazard waste disposal (Medivators, 2007, http://medivators.com/international/resource/documents/msds/Renalin%20100%20English.pdf Morgan, 2008, http://www.renalbusiness.com/lib/download.ashx?d=1979).

D. Participating in reuse is voluntary.
  1. Benefits and risks associated with reuse must be fully disclosed to the patient.
  2. The patient must sign consent before being placed on reuse and annually thereafter.
  3. A physician's order for the patient participating in reuse must also be in the patient's medical record.

II. The Association for the Advancement of Medical Instrumentation (AAMI).

A. Founded in 1967 by a group of individuals from various professions such as engineers, physicians, nurses, and other industry professions.

B. The main goal: develop standards based on recommended practices for safe use of equipment and medical devices.

C. The Centers for Medicare and Medicaid Services (CMS) adopted these standards for the practice of dialyzer reprocessing and enforce them. (ANSI/AAMI, 2011; CMS, 2008, V301, http://www.cms.gov/Regulations-and-Guidance/Legislation/CFCsAndCoPs/downloads/ESRDfinalrule0415.pdf).

III. Clinical benefits of reuse for patients.

A. Reduce incidence of blood leak.
  1. A blood path integrity test is performed on each dialyzer during the reprocessing procedure for leaks by generating a transmembrane pressure (TMP) gradient across the membrane and observing for a pressure fall in either the blood or the dialysate compartment (DeOreo, 2014; MEI, 2014).
  2. Blood pathway integrity instills air or nitrogen into the blood side of the dialyzer or produces a

vacuum in the dialysate side. Only a minimal amount of air can leak through an intact wetted membrane (DeOreo, 2014).

B. Increase in dialyzer compatibility.
1. Reprocessing dialyzers allows the patient's blood to coat the fibers with the proteins from that patient's blood, making it more uniquely biocompatible for that specific patient, or more like the patient's own tissue.
2. The protein coating reduces the potential for "first use" reaction.
a. A "first use" reaction can occur when a patient's blood contacts a new dialyzer whose fibers are foreign to the patient's immune system.
b. Exposing the patient's blood to the reprocessed hemodialyzer reduces the potential for this reaction to occur.

C. Hypersensitivity to ethylene oxide (ETO).
1. Most dialyzers were historically sterilized by the manufacturer with a gas, ethylene oxide (ETO). Preprocessing and reprocessing of dialyzers reduced a patient's chance of a hypersensitive reaction to ETO exposure.
2. ETO is no longer used routinely and hence no longer a major concern in the United States because of the risk of a reaction to the gas.
3. Most dialyzers are now steam or gamma ray sterilized during manufacturing and prior to shipping.

IV. Potential risks to patients who participate in a dialyzer reuse program.

A. Chemical exposure.
1. Each reprocessed dialyzer is rendered sterile by introducing a germicide or high-level disinfectant into the dialyzer.
2. If the germicide is not rinsed out properly before the patient's next treatment, the patient may experience a chemical reaction from exposure to the sterilant.
3. Symptoms of chemical exposure that may be exhibited in the first 15 minutes of treatment include:
a. Burning in the access extremity.
b. Blurred vision.
c. Numbness in the lips.
d. Vision or hearing loss.
e. Death.

B. Loss of hemodialyzer clearance.
1. The membrane can change each time the dialyzer is reused or reprocessed, leading to:
a. Poor solute transport and poor ultrafiltration.

b. Patients will not receive their dialysis prescription as ordered (Bates et al., 2014; http://meiresearch.org/core_curriculum.php).
2. During reuse, the dialyzer fibers can become clogged with blood or other materials, reducing the effective surface area of the dialyzer.
3. A smaller surface area of lower flow rate due to clogged fibers can reduce the clearance, surface area, or UF rate of the dialyzer.

C. Bacterial/endotoxin contamination.
1. Bacteremia and pyrogen reactions due to endotoxins can result from an improperly processed dialyzer. Bacteria can enter the dialyzer from:
a. The water used to make dialysate.
b. Improper setup and contaminated blood lines.
c. Contaminated water used to flush the dialyzer during the preclean process.
2. Organisms may stay in the dialyzer from the dialysate side after a treatment and may multiply and enter the patient's bloodstream.
3. The hemodialyzer can absorb the endotoxins into the potting material in the headers (end caps) and casing. The endotoxin can then leach out during the treatment when blood contacts the dialyzer, resulting in bacteremia and/or pyrogenic reactions.
4. Conditions leading to potential contamination include:
a. The germicide prepared for disinfecting the dialyzer is outdated or improperly mixed.
b. The germicide has not dwelled or had required contact time in dialyzer.
c. The dialyzer is not stored properly.
d. The dialyzer is not properly filled or does not contain enough germicide (ANSI/AAMI, 2011, Preparation for dialysis and testing for chemical germicides and potentially toxic residues, 12.1, Visual Inspection, pg.142).
5. Symptoms of a pyrogenic reaction may be exhibited with:
a. Fever.
b. Chills.
c. Nausea and vomiting.
d. Low blood pressure.
e. Muscle pain (Bates et al., 2014, p. 231).
6. Symptoms of sepsis or bacteria in the blood.
a. Fever.
b. General malaise.
c. Positive blood cultures (Bates et al., 2014).

D. Water quality monitoring is essential and is required to protect patients from bacteria and endotoxin reactions (CMS, 2008, V317), http://www.cms.gov/Regulations-and-Guidance/Legislation/CFCsAndCoPs/downloads/ESRDfinalrule0415.pdf).

1. The AAMI standard for bacteria in the dialysis water must not exceed 200 colony forming units (CFU); the action level is 50 CFU.
2. Levels of endotoxin should be less than 2 endotoxin units/m (EU/mL) with an action level of 1 EU/mL (ANSI/AAMI, 2011; Layman-Amato, Curtis, & Payne, 2013, http://www.prolibraries .com/anna/?select=session&sessionID=2840).

V. Area design and process flow.

A. A reuse room is generally designed so that the flow process can occur from dirty to clean.

B. The room layout should consist of a:
1. Dirty, preclean sink and precleaning area.
2. The reprocessing area.
3. Data management area.
4. Clean sink.
5. The dialyzer storage area.

C. Clean and dirty dialyzers should be stored separately to prevent contaminating the clean dialyzers.

D. The reprocessing area should accommodate the work flow and maintain acceptable ambient concentrations of harmful substances and be kept clean and sanitary.

E. The reprocessing area may be part of the dialysis treatment area, if the equipment is properly vented and meets the requirements for environmental safety. (CMS, 2008, V322, http://www.cms.gov/Regulations-and-Guidance/Legislation/CFCsAndCoPs/download s/ESRDfinalrule0415.pdf).

VI. Dialyzer preprocessing.

A. A dry pack hemodialyzer labeled for reuse is filled with AAMI-quality water and the volume is measured.

B. Preprocessing the dialyzer establishes the baseline start volume for total cell volume (TCV) to determine the minimum volume requirement for subsequent uses. Dialyzers are discarded when this initial volume drops below 80% with subsequent uses.

C. The integrity of the membrane is tested for blood leaks.

D. Removing the dialyzer from its original sterile package requires that it be filled with germicide and disinfected before patient use and so indicated on the dialyzer label.

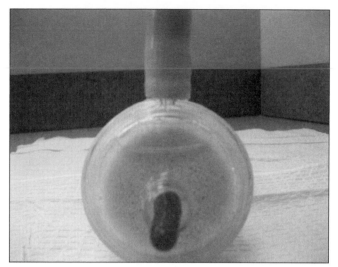

Figure 2.45. Dialyzer two-thirds full with sterilant.

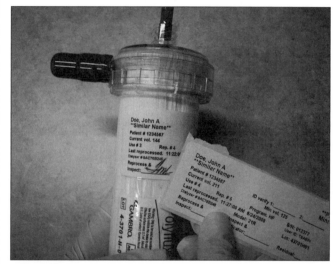

Figure 2.46. Legible labels.

E. Preprocessing is performed to decrease first-use syndrome (see Section E, XVIII, Membrane Biocompatability).

VII. Dialyzer preparation for use.

A. Pretreatment. The following checks should be made prior to priming the reprocessed dialyzer.
1. Verify the blood and dialysate port caps are intact and there are no leaks. A missing cap or leak will indicate the sterile barrier is broken.
2. Both dialyzer headers must be at least two-thirds full of germicide while holding the dialyzer horizontally with the dialysate port caps facing up (see Figure 2.45).
3. Dwell time of the germicide is verified on the label prior to priming and when verifying the prescription just prior to treatment initiation.

If the dwell time of the specified germicide is not met, there is a risk of bacterial and/or endotoxin contamination, and the hemodialyzer is rejected for further use.

4. Appearance of the dialyzer should be aesthetically acceptable.
   a. The outside of the dialyzer jacket should be free of blood, cracks, or leaks, and no more than a few dark clotted fibers evident on the inspection of the exterior of the hollow fibers.
   b. The headers (end caps) free of all but small peripheral clots or other deposits.
   c. The labels must be legible and the dialyzer should not be damaged (see Figure 2.46).
   d. *Safety alert.* Two staff members must verify the dialyzer is the correct dialyzer for the correct patient prior to priming.

5. The germicide should be verified for adequate presence prior to priming the dialyzer by performing a sterilant indicator test. The staff member(s) must document that the visual inspection was performed and that a positive presence test was obtained.

6. Reprocessed dialyzers must be labeled with the patient's first and last name; a medical record number; the number of uses, date, and last time of the last reuse; and the results of the tests done on the dialyzer.

7. *Safety alert.* Patients with the same or similar last names must have a warning or alert on the dialyzer.

8. All markings and labels should be legible and not conceal the blood path of the dialyzer.

B. Prime the dialyzer.
   1. Remove the germicide from the dialyzer prior to patient use.
      a. Flush or prime the dialyzer blood compartment with normal saline then flush/prime the dialysate compartment.
      b. Air must be removed from the arterial line prior to attaching it to the arterial port of the dialyzer to avoid introducing air into the dialyzer.
      c. Avoid introducing air into the extracorporeal circuit.
      d. Paracetic acid caveats.
         (1) Exposing the paracetic acid to the buffered dialysate can form gas bubbles. The bubbles can obstruct the dialyzer hollow fibers, preventing complete removed of the paracetic acid from the dialyzer. This can increase clotting of the fibers as well as interfere with complete removal of paracetic acid from the dialyzer.
         (2) The saline is generally recirculated through the extracorporeal circuit after a minimum

of 300 to 400 mL of NS has been flushed through the blood compartment.
      (3) Blood pump speed should be low enough to create minimal turbulence and enhance removal of air from the circuit.

2. *Safety alert.* A negative germicide residual test must be performed on the blood circuit immediately prior to patient use and must be verified by two individuals. One person verifying the information may be the patient, if appropriate.
   a. The residual test must be within the acceptable levels for the germicide being used immediately prior to initiating the HD treatment; this verifies there is no rebound of germicide in the extracorporeal circuit that would lead to germicidal patient exposure.
   b. Germicide rebound can occur if the dialysate or blood pump is stopped after the priming procedures are completed and prior to residual testing.
   c. Ensure the blood pump and dialysate flow are maintained to reduce the potential for rebound.
   d. If the blood pump stops during the recirculation process, additional time should be added to the recirculation time.
   e. Maintain a slight negative pressure in the dialysate compartment while the blood compartment is being recirculated with NS to reduce the potential of germicide rebound.
   f. Flush fresh NS through the extracorporeal circuit immediately prior to treatment initiation to ensure the patient is not exposed to any residual sterilant.

C. *Safety alert.* Dialyzer and patient identification.
   1. Prior to treatment initiation.
      a. Two patient-care staff members must verify the dialyzer is labeled with the patient's first and last name.
      b. Any other appropriate identifying information must correspond to the identifying information in the patient's permanent record.
      c. The patient is encouraged to validate the information on the dialyzer is his/hers.
   2. The persons verifying the patient identification must document their verification.

VIII. Treatment termination, dialyzer handling, and transportation posttreatment.

A. Treatment termination.
   1. NS is used to reinfuse the patient's blood at treatment termination.
   2. Avoid the introduction of air during reinfusion to preserve dialyzer patency as air predisposes the dialyzer hollow fibers to clotting. *Safety alert.* Do not air rinse the dialyzer!

3. Staff members should evaluate the dialyzer for clotted fibers and document the findings.
4. Excessive clotting may require that anticoagulation be adjusted prospectively.

B. Posttreatment.
 1. Proper capping and transport is important to reduce the opportunity for air to be introduced into the dialyzer.
 2. Remove one dialysate line at a time and immediately cap the port to prevent fluid from escaping from the dialyzer or air entering it.
 3. The dialysate compartment should remain filled with dialysate.

C. Dialyzer transport.
 1. The dialyzer should be transported to the reuse area in a clean, timely, and sanitary manner.
 2. Placing the capped dialyzer in a plastic bag for transportation to the reuse room prevents cross contamination or leakage of fluids into the environment.

IX. Precleaning-fiber flush, reverse ultrafiltration, and header cleaning.

A. Precleaning is the first step in reprocessing: the dialyzer is flushed with AAMI-quality water to remove residual blood from the blood compartment.

B. Precleaning may also involve the use of reverse ultrafiltration.
 1. A cap is placed on one of the dialysate ports and water is instilled into the dialyzer under a controlled amount of water pressure across the dialysate compartment.
 2. The amount of pressure is based on the dialyzer manufacturer's recommendations; the use of

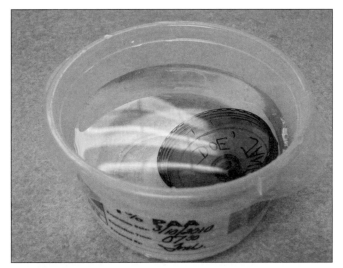

Figure 2.47. Header removal.

pressure higher than the recommendation can result in fiber breakage and cause blood leaks.

C. Some dialyzers have removable headers (end caps).
 1. The dialyzer header caps are removed and any clotted blood is removed from the header.
 2. A free flowing stream of AAMI-quality water must be used to clean the header, header caps, and O-rings: no foreign objects such as paper clips, 4x4's, or cloths should be used to clean the headers.
 3. The header caps are immersed in disinfectant prior to being replaced on the dialyzer. Figure 2.47 shows the header caps and O-rings separated and immersed completely in germicide.
 4. All parts, including headers, caps, and O-rings, should remain with the respective dialyzer to avoid exposure across patients (CMS, 2008, VCode 337; http://www.cms.gov/Regulations-and-Guidance/Legislation/CFCsAndCoPs/downloads/ESRDfinalrule0415.pdf).

X. Dialyzer reprocessing and performance measurements; performed after the dialyzer is rinsed and cleaned.

A. After the dialyzer is rinsed and cleaned, the dialyzer will be tested for total cell volume (TCV) of the dialyzer.
 1. The TCV must be at least 80% of the original TCV as a 20% decrease in TCV equates to a 10% decrease in small molecular clearance (CMS, 2008, VCode338; http://www.cms.gov/Regulations-and-Guidance/Legislation/CFCsAndCoPs/downloads/ESRDfinalrule0415.pdf).
 2. Many dialyzers fail to reach more than 15 reuses due to low fiber cell volume. This is usually caused by excessive clotting during dialysis.

B. A blood path integrity test is then performed by creating a TMP gradient across the membrane and observing for a pressure fail or leak.

C. Once the dialyzer is tested, the dialyzer is disinfected with germicide.
 1. The dialyzer is subsequently inspected for dialyzer leaks, cracks, or defects in the plastic housing.
 2. If the dialyzer passes testing and inspection, the dialyzer casing is wiped with germicide, labeled, and stored in a clean storage area.
 3. *Safety alert.* At any step during the process, one disinfectant must be rinsed before another is introduced unless mixing is shown to be safe and effective. For example, mixing formaldehyde and bleach, or paracetic acid and bleach, creates noxious vapors that are dangerous (http://medivators.com/international/resource/documents/msds/Renalin%20100%20English.pdf).

XI. Patient safety.

A. Dialyzer reuse is safe if done correctly. Done incorrectly, it can cause patient harm or death.
   1. Exposure to bacteria or endotoxin is a major risk to patients.
   2. The patient's temperature must be checked and recorded pretreatment and posttreatment to determine a baseline to facilitate assessment for untoward reactions to reprocessing.

B. The introduction of germicide into the patient's blood may cause the following symptoms.
   1. Burning in the access site.
   2. Blurred vision.
   3. Burning in the lips.
   4. Vision or hearing loss.
   5. Death.

C. All patients are monitored for inadequate dialysis with kinetic modeling at least monthly.

D. Matching the patient and dialyzer must be verified and documented every treatment by two persons prior to the patient being placed on the reprocessed dialyzer.

XII. Staff members' safety is an integral part of dialyzer reprocessing. Staff members' safety issues include blood, chemical, and respiratory exposure.

A. Dialyzer reprocessing exposes staff members to blood – contact that may result in exposure to blood borne pathogens.
   1. Pathogens of particular concern in a dialysis facility are hepatitis B, hepatitis C, human immunodeficiency virus (HIV), and Ebola Virus Disease (EVD).
   2. Blood exposure occurs any time blood comes in contact with a person's skin, eyes, and/or mucous membranes, which may result in the transmission of a bloodborne disease.
   3. *Safety alert.* Staff members should wear personal protective equipment (PPE) to include:
      a. Durable gloves and protective clothing when handling the dialyzer during initiation and termination of dialysis and during the reprocessing procedure.
      b. Eye protection should be worn when performing tasks that may result in spills or splashes.

B. A second hazard to reuse personnel and staff is the potential for injury from breathing vapors released by the chemicals used in reprocessing.
   1. Chemical fumes released during reprocessing can reach toxic levels if reprocessing chemicals are used improperly or in poorly ventilated reprocessing rooms.
   2. Exposure to chemical fumes may produce mucous membrane and respiratory irritation that can lead to more serious conditions such as bronchitis, pulmonary edema, and may even result in death (Bates et al., 2014).
   3. *Safety alert.* Air testing must be done regularly to verify the air is at safe levels. Ventilation should also be checked at specified intervals (ANSI/AAMI, 2011).

C. Personnel should follow the directions of the manufacturer's chemical Material Safety Data Sheet (MSDS) carefully for their protection to avoid chemical burns to the skin or eyes during all phases of dialyzer reprocessing (http://medivators.com/international/resource/documents/msds/Renalin%20100%20English.pdf).

XIII. Staff training.

A. All reuse technicians must participate in an in-depth reprocessing training program. The dialysis facility's Medical Director must establish a training course for individuals who are to perform the reprocessing procedures. This training course must be outlined in a written document that must outline the details of the training curriculum. The curriculum should include at least the following (ANSI/AAMI, 2011; CMS, 2008, V310) http://www.cms.gov/Regulations-and-Guidance/Legislation/CFCsAndCoPs/downloads/ESRDfinalrule0415.pdf):
   1. The dialysis facility's specific reprocessing procedure, including rationale for each step.
   2. Basic documentation requirements of the program.
   3. The operation and maintenance of the facility's specific equipment for reprocessing the hemodialyzers, and if applicable, the hemodialysis systems and components.
   4. Proper aseptic technique for the collection and handling of samples, and personnel safety and precautions for infectious hazards.
   5. The risks and hazards of multiple uses of hemodialyzers.
   6. The consequences of not performing tasks properly.
   7. Training that has been successfully completed will be documented in the employee's file.

XIV. Centralized reprocessing is the practice of reprocessing dialyzers from more than one facility; dialyzers are transported to one site for reprocessing and returned to the source units for reuse.

A. Advantages of centralized reprocessing.
   1. A small, focused staff.
   2. Closer supervision and controlled environment.
   3. Removes reuse from the chronic dialysis facility; therefore, fewer distractions during reprocessing.
   4. Most likely will use automated systems for reprocessing.

B. Disadvantages and risks.
   1. Transportation of used dialyzers.
   2. Maintenance of temperature control during transport.
   3. Power failure.
   4. If problems arise or are cited, it affects multiple units or dialysis facilities.

XV. Quality monitoring. Federal guidelines require dialysis facilities that participate in reprocessing have a continuous quality improvement (CQI) program to assess their reprocessing systems on an ongoing basis (ANSI/AAMI, 2011, 14.2 pg.145 vcode 376). Staff members have the responsibility to carry out critical scrutiny of all materials used, all practices, operation of reuse program, and patient outcomes of those who participate in the reuse program. Reviews of the reuse program processes must be documented and reviewed by the person who is responsible for the oversight of the reuse program and all policies and procedures related to reuse. Reviews of records, trend analysis, and conclusions that arise from the CQI practices should be reviewed regularly. Issues identified, based on the CQI reviews, should be addressed and solutions put in place that demonstrate that the solutions were effective. The medical director is responsible for frequency of reviews, endorsement of findings, and then the implementation of changes (http://www.cms.gov/Regulations-and-Guidance/Legislation/CFCsAndCoPs/downloads/ESRDfinalrule0415.pdf).

A. The reprocessing facility must demonstrate that their CQI program addresses reprocessing policies and procedures as written, and must include state and federal guidelines.

B. All policies and procedures must be reviewed at least yearly and whenever problems arise related to reprocessing equipment failures.

C. Quality management meetings should review and document review of all reuse practices.

D. If problems with reuse processes are identified, the problems should be reviewed and documented until solutions are in effect and have shown the actions taken were effective.

E. The Medical Director must determine the frequency of reviews.

F. The Medical Director must approve findings and be responsible where applicable for the recommended changes being implemented (ANSI/AAMI, 2011; Bates et al., 2014).

References

Agar, J. (2012). *Technology: What's coming.* Retrieved from http://www.nocturnaldialysis.org/technology_whats_coming.htm

Agency for Healthcare Research & Quality (AHRQ), Health Research & Educational Trust (HRET), End Stage Renal Disease (ESRD) Network 11, University of Michigan – Kidney Epidemiology Cost Center (UM-KECC). (2011). National opportunity to improve infection control in ESRD (NOTICE). *Infection control worksheet, Infection control checklists.* Retrieved from http://www.hret.org/quality/projects/resources/infection_control_checklist_11212011.pdf

Ahmad, S., Misra, M., Hoenich, N., & Daugirdas, J.T. (2014). Hemodialysis apparatus. In J.T. Daugirdas, P.G. Blake, & T.S. Ing (Eds.) *Handbook of dialysis* (5th ed., pp. 66-88), Philadelphia: Lippincott Williams & Wilkins

American Nephrology Nurses' Association. (n.d.) *Venous needle dislodgement project.* Pitman, NJ: Author. Retrieved from http://www.annanurse.org/resources/venous-needle-dislodgement

ANSI/AAMI. (2011). Association for the Advancement of Medical Instrumentation. *Reprocessing of Hemodialyzers.* Arlington, VA: Author.

Antoniazzi, A.L., Bigal, M.E., Bordini, C.A., & Speciali, J.G. (2003). Headache associated with dialysis: The international headache society criteria revisited. *Cephalalgia, 23*(2),146-149. doi:10.1177/0333102413485658. Retrieved from http://www.ihs-classification.org/_downloads/mixed/International-Headache-Classification-III-ICHD-III-2013-Beta.pdf

Ash, S. (2008). *Sorbent dialysis systems: An expert commentary.* Retrieved from www.medscape.com/viewarticle/576534_print

Ashton, D. (2014). Blood transfusion during hemodialysis: An evidence-based procedure. *Nephrology Nursing Journal, 41*(4), 424-428. Also available at http://www.prolibraries.com/anna/?select=session&sessionID=3058

Association for Professionals in Infection Control and Epidemiology (APIC). (2010). *Guide to the elimination of infections in hemodialysis.* Washington, D.C.: Author. Retrieved from http://www.apic.org/Resource_/EliminationGuideForm/7966d850-0c5a-48ae-9090-a1da00bcf988/File/APIC-Hemodialysis.pdf

Association for the Advancement of Medical Instrumentation (AAMI). (n.d.) *About the standards program.* Arlington, VA: Author. Retrieved from http://www.aami.org/standards/index.html

Association for the Advancement of Medical Instrumentation (AAMI). (2004). ANSI/AAMI RD 52, 2004. *Dialysate for hemodialysis.* Arlington, VA: Author.

Association for the Advancement of Medical Instrumentation (AAMI). (2014a). ANSI/AAMI 13959:2014. *Water for hemodialysis and related therapies.* Arlington VA: Author.

Association for the Advancement of Medical Instrumentation (AAMI). (2014b). ANSI/AAMI 26722:2014. *Water treatment equipment for hemodialysis applications and related therapies.* Arlington, VA: Author.

Association for the Advancement of Medical Instrumentation (AAMI). (2014c). ANSI/AAMI 11663:2014. *Quality of dialysis fluid for hemodialysis and related therapies.* Arlington, VA: Author.

Association for the Advancement of Medical Instrumentation (AAMI). (2014d). ANSI/AAMI 13958:2014. *Concentrates for hemodialysis and related therapies.* Arlington, VA: Author.

Association for the Advancement of Medical Instrumentation (AAMI). (2014e). ANSI/AAMI 23500:2014. *Guidance for the preparation and quality management of fluids for hemodialysis and related therapies.* Arlington, VA: Author.

Axley, A., Speranza-Reid, J., & Williams, H. (2012). Venous needle dislodgement in patients on hemodialysis. *Nephrology Nursing Journal, 39*(6), 435-445. http://www.prolibraries.com/anna/?select=session&sessionID=2131

Barth, C., Boer, W., Garzoni, D., Kuenzi, T., Ries, W., Schaefer, R., & Passlick-Deetjen, J. (2003). Characteristics of hypotenion-prone haemodialysis patients: Is there a critical relative blood volume? *Nephrology Dialysis Transplantation, 18,* 1353-1360.

Bates, J.W., Dahlin, J., Johnson, C.H., & Varughese, P. (2014). Dialyzer reprocessing. In *Core curriculum for the dialysis technician* (5th ed., pp. 219-236). Madison, WI: Medical Education Institute, Inc. Retrieved from http://meiresearch.org/core_curriculum.php

Baxter. (2009). *High-performance dialyzers for total patient care.* McGaw Park, IL. Retrieved from http://www.baxter.com/downloads/healthcare_professionals/products/AL09086_cellulosic_brochure_final.pdf

Bradshaw, W., Ockerby, C., & Bennett, P. (2011). Pre-emptively pausing ultrafiltration to minimise dialysis hypotension. *Renal Society of Australasia Journal, 7*(3), 130-134.

Bragg-Gresham, S.R., Levin, J.L., Twadowski, Z.J., Wizmann, V,, Saitor, A., & Port, F.K. (2006). Longer treatment time and slower ultrafiltration in hemodialysis: Association with reduced mortality in the DOPPS. *Kidney International, 69*(7), 1222-1228.

Brennan, M.R., & Whitehouse, F.W. (2012). Case study: Seizures and hypoglycemia. *Clinical Diabetes, 30*(1), 23-24.

Brown, M., Burrows, L., Pruett, T., & Burrows, T. (2015). Hemodialysis-induced myocardial stunning: A review. *Nephrology Nursing Journal, 42*(1), 59-66. Retrieved from http://www.prolibraries.com/anna/?select=session&sessionID=3140

Burton, J., Jefferies, H., Selby, N., & McIntyre, C. (2009). Hemodialysis induced repetitive myocardial injury results in global and segmental reduction in systolic cardiac function. *Clinical Journal of the American Society of Nephrology: CJASN, 4*(12), 1925-1931.

Carlson, D.J., & Shapiro, F.L. (1970). Methemoglobinemia from well water nitrates: A complication of home dialysis. *Annals of Internal Medicine, 73*(5), 757-759.

Carson, J.L. Grossman, B.J., Kleinman, S., Tinmouth, A.T., Marques, M.B., Fung, M.K., ... Djulbegovic, B. (2012). Red blood cell transfusion: A clinical practice guideline from the AABB. *Annals of Internal Medicine, 157*(1), 49-58.

Centers for Disease Control and Prevention (CDC). (2013a). *Infection training video and print resources for preventing bloodstream and other infections in outpatient hemodialysis patients.* Author. Retrieved from http://www.cdc.gov/dialysis/prevention-tools/training-video.html

Centers for Disease Control and Prevention (CDC). (2013b). *Infection prevention tools.* Author. Retrieved from http://www.cdc.gov/dialysis/prevention-tools/index.html

Centers for Disease Control and Prevention (CDC) (2013c). *Preventing bloodstream infections in ouptatient hemodialysis patients: Best practices for dialysis staff.* Author. Retrieved from https://www.youtube.com/watch?v=_0zhY0JMGCA&feature=youtu.be

Centers for Medicare & Medicaid Services (CMS). (2008a). *Conditions for coverage for end-stage renal disease facilities.* Final Rule, 73 Fed. Reg. 20481 (April 15, 2008) (42 CFR Parts 405, 410, 413 et al.). Retrieved from http://www.cms.gov/Regulations-and-Guidance/Legislation/CFCsAndCoPs/downloads/ESRDfinalrule0415.pdf

Centers for Medicare & Medicaid Services (CMS). (2008b). *Conditions for coverage for end-stage renal disease facilities: Interpretive guidance.* Retrieved from http://www.cms.gov/Medicare/Provider-Enrollment-and-Certification/SurveyCertificationGenInfo/downloads/SCletter09-01.pdf

Centers for Medicare and Medicaid Services (CMS). (2013). *End-stage renal disease (ESRD) quality initiative.* Retrieved from http://www.cms.gov/Medicare/End-Stage-Renal-Disease/ESRDQualityImproveInit/index.html

Charra, B. (2007). Fluid balance, dry weight, and blood pressure in dialysis. *Hemodialysis International, 11*(1), 21-31.

Cvach, M. (2012). Monitor alarm fatigue: An integrative review. *Biomedical Instrumentation & Technology, 48*(4), 39-50

Damasiewicz, M.J., & Polkinghorne, K.R. (2011). Intra-dialytic hypotension and blood volume and blood temperature monitoring. *Nephrology, 16*(1), 13-18. Retrieved from http://onlinelibrary.wiley.com/doi/10.1111/j.1440-1797.2010.01362.x/full#ss2

Daugirdas, J.T. (2014). Chronic hemodialysis prescription. In J.T. Daugirdas, P.G. Blake, & T.S. Ing (Eds.), *Handbook of dialysis* (5th ed., pp. 192-214). Philadelphia: Lippincott Williams & Wilkins.

Davenport, A. (2006). Intradialytic complications during hemodialysis. *Hemodialysis International, 10*(2), 162-167.

Davenport, A. (2008). The role of dialyzer membrane flux in bio-incompatibility. *Hemodialysis International, 12*(11), 29-33.

Davenport, A., Lai, K.N., Hertel, J., & Caruana, R.J. (2014). Anticoagulation. In J.T. Daugirdas, P.G. Blake, & T.S. Ing (Eds.), *Handbook of dialysis* (5th ed., pp. 252-267). Philadelphia: Lippincott Williams & Wilkins.

Denshaw-Burke, M., DelGiacco, E., Curran, A.L., Savior, D.C., & Kumar, M. (2013). *Methemoglobinemia. Medscape: Drugs and diseases.* Retrieved from http://emedicine.medscape.com/article/204178-overview#showall

DeOreo, P.B. (2014). Dialyzer reuse in J.T Daugirdas, P.G. Blake, & T.S. Ing (Eds.), *Handbook of dialysis* (5th ed., pp. 237-251). Philadelphia: Lippincott Williams & Wilkins.

DePalma, J.R., & Pittard, J.P. (2001). *Body water – body weight.* Hemodialysis, Inc. Retrieved from http://www.hemodialysis-inc.com/articles/bodywater.pdf

Diroll, A., & Hlebovy, D. (2003). Inverse relationship between blood volume and blood pressure. *Nephrology Nursing Journal, 30*(4), 460-461. Available at http://www.prolibraries.com/anna/?select=speaker&speakerID=39187&conferenceID=42

Donauer, J., Kölblin, D., Bek, M., Krause, A., & Böhler, J. (2000). Ultrafiltration profiling and measurement of relative blood volume as strategies to reduce hemodialysis-related side effects. *American Journal of Kidney Diseases, 36*(1), 115-123.

Dutka, P., & Harmon, E. (2007). Hemolysis: Crisis intervention.

Nephrology Nursing Journal, 34(2), 219- 220, 223. Retrieved from http://www.prolibraries.com/anna/?select=speaker&speakerID=3 8904&conferenceID=42

Ellingson, K.D., Palekar, R.S., Lucero, C.A., Kurkjian, K.M., Chai, S.J., Schlossberg, D.S., … Patel, P.R. (2012). Vascular access hemorrhages contribute to deaths among hemodialysis patients. *Kidney International, 82*(6), 686-692.

Eloot, S., DeWachter, D., & Verdonck, P. (2002). Computational flow modeling in hollow-fiber dialyzers. *Artificial Organs, 26*(7), 590.

Environmental Protection Agency (EPA). (2014). *Drinking water contaminants.* Author. Retrieved from http://water.epa.gov/drink/contaminants/index.cfm

Fenves, A.Z., Gipson, J.S., & Pancorvo, C. (2000). Chloramine-induced methemoglobinemia in a hemodialysis patient. *Seminars in Dialysis, 13*(5), 327-329. Retrieved from http://onlinelibrary.wiley.com/doi/10.1046/j.1525-139x.2000.00094.x/abstract

Fischer, K.G. (2007). Essentials of anticoagulation in hemodialysis. *Hemodialysis International, 11*(2), 178-189.

Fishbane, S., & Shah, H.H. (2014). Hematologic abnormalities. In J.T. Daugirdas, P.G. Blake, & T.S. Ing (Eds.), *Handbook of dialysis* (5th ed., pp. 592-614), Philadelphia: Lippincott Williams & Wilkins.

Food and Drug Administration (FDA). (2011). *FDA drug safety communication: Serious CCNS reactions possible when methylene blue is given to patients taking certain psychiatric medications.* Retrieved from http://www.fda.gov/drugs/drugsafety/ucm263190.htm

Ford, L., Ward, R., & Cheung, A. (2009). Choice of the hemodialysis membrane. In W.L. Henrich (Ed.), *Principles and practice of dialysis* (4th ed., pp. 1-11). Philadelphia: Lippincott Williams & Wilkins.

Fresenius Medical Care. (2011). *Polysulfone dialyzers technical specifications.* Waltham, MA: Author. Retrieved from http://fmcna-dialyzers.com/dialyzers-site/products.html

Fresenius Medical Care North America. (n.d.) *Crit-Line III monitor-user's manual.* Waltham, MA: Retrieved from www.fmcna.com/fmcna/OperatorsManuals/operators-manual.html

Fresenius Medical Care (2013). *Crit-Line® III user manual.* Kaysville, UT: Retrieved from http://www.fmcna.com/fmcna/idcplg?IdcService=GET_FILE&allowInterrupt=1&RevisionSelectionMethod=LatestReleased&Rendition=Primary&dDocName=PDF_300 0049033

Gambro. (2010). *Products/hemodialyis/dialyzers home page.* Retrieved from http://www.gambro.com/en/usa/Products/Hemodialysis/Dialyzers/Revaclear/?tab=other2Tab

Gomez, N.J. (2011). Nephrology nursing process of care – Hemodialysis. In N.J Gomez (Ed.), *Nephrology Nursing scope and standards of practice* (7th ed., pp. 123-144). Pitman, NJ: American Nephrology Nurses' Association.

Graves, G.D. (2001). Arterial and venous pressure monitoring during hemodialysis. *Nephrology Nursing Journal, 28*(1), 23-28. Retrieved from http://www.prolibraries.com/anna/?select=speaker&speakerID=39390

Hansen, S. (n.d.). *Dialysis procedures: Initiation, monitoring, discontinuing.* Retrieved from http://www.hdcn.com/symp/09nant/content/09nant_han/flash/09nant_han.pdf

Health Research & Educational Trust (HRET). (2010). *National opportunity to improve infection control in ESRD.* Chicago: Author. Retrieved from http://www.hret.org/quality/projects/improving-infection-coontrol-practices-ESRD-facilities.shtml

Heegard, K.D., Tilley, M.A., Stewart, I.J., Edgecombe, H.P., Lundy, J.B., Renz, E.M., & Chung, K.K. (2013). Anaphylactoid reaction during first hemofiltration with a PUREMAR polysulfone membrane. *The International Journal of Artificial Organs, 36*(5), 363-366.

Hema Metrics. (2006). *Inservice training manual section 2: Theory Crit-Line III TQA.* Retrieved from http://www.slideshare.net/ringer21/section-2-theory-critline-iii-tqa

Henderson, L.W. (2012). Symptomatic Intradialytic hypotension and mortality: An opinioned review. *Seminars in Dialysis, 25*(3), 320-324.

Herzog, C.A. (2004). Cardiac arrest in dialysis patients: Taking a small step. *Seminars in Dialysis, 17*(3), 184-185.

Hlebovy, D. (2006). Fluid management: Moving and removing fluid during hemodialysis. *Nephrology Nursing Journal, 33*(4), 441-446.

Hoenich, N.A., & Levin, N.W. (2007). Hemodialysis machines. *Biomedical Instrumentation & Technology, 41*(3), 215-218.

Hoenich, N., & Ronco, C. (2008). Selecting a dialyzer; technical and clinical considerations. In A.R Nissenson & R.N. Fine (Eds.), *Handbook of dialysis therapy* (4th ed., p. 274). Philadelphia: Saunders

Horkan, A.M. (2014). Alarm fatigue and patient safety. *Nephrology Nursing Journal, 41*(1), 83-85. Retrieved from http://www.prolibraries.com/anna/?select=session&sessionID=2975

House, A.A. (2011). Are there any contraindications to using midodrine for intradialytic hypotension? *Seminars in Dialysis, 24*(4), 402-403.

Jefferies, H.J., Voirk, B., Schiller, B., Moran, J., & McIntyre, C.W. (2011). Frequent hemodialysis schedules are associated with reduced levels of dialysis-induced cardia injurn (myocardial stunning). *Clinical Journal of the American Society of Nephrology.* doi:10.2215/CJN.05200610. Retrieved from http://cjasn.asnjournals.org/content/6/6/1326.full

Jepson, R., & Alonzo, E. (2009). Overheated dialysate: A case study and review. *Nephrology Nursing Journal, 36*(5), 551-553. Retrieved from http://www.prolibraries.com/anna/?select=session&sessionID=1014

The Joint Commission (2012). *Improving patient and worker safety: Opportunities for synergy, collaboration and innovation.* Author: Oak Brook Terrace, IL. Retrieved from http://www.jointcommission.org/assets/1/18/TJC-ImprovingPatientAndWorkerSafety-Monograph.pdf

Kalantari, K., Chang, J., Ronco, C., & Rosner, M. (2013). Assessment of intravascular volume status and volume responsiveness in critically ill patients. *Kidney International, 83*, 1017–1028; doi:10.1038/ki.2012.424. Retrieved from http://www.nature.com/ki/journal/v83/n6/abs/ki2012424a.html

Kallenbach, J.Z., Gutch, C.F., Stoner, M.G., & Corea, A.L. (Eds.). (2005). *Review of hemodialysis for nurses and dialysis technicians* (7th ed.). St Louis: Elsevier Mosby.

Katirci, Y. (2010). Accidental use of sodium hypochlorite instead of haemodialysis solution: A case report. *Hong Kong Journal of Emergency Medicine, 17* (5), 492-494.

Kidney Disease: Improving Global Outcomes (KDIGO). (2013). *Clinical practice guidelines.* Retrieved from http://kdigo.org/home/guidelines/

Kinnel, K. (2005). Should patients eat during hemodialysis treatments? *Nephrology Nursing Journal, 32*(5), 513-515. Retrieved from http://www.prolibraries.com/anna/?select=speaker&speakerID=39010&conferenceID=42

Kloner, R.A., Prayklnek, K., & Patel, B. (1989). Altered myocardial states: The stunned and hibernating myocardium. *The American Journal of Medicine, 86*(1), S1, 14-22. Retrieved from http://www.sciencedirect.com/science/article/pii/0002934389900053

Konner, K. (2005). History of vascular access. *Nephrology Dialysis Transplantation, 20*(12), 2629-2635. doi:10.1093/ndt/gfi168 Retrieved from http://ndt.oxfordjournals.org/content/20/12/2629.full

Kosmadakis, G.C., & Medcalf, J.F. (2008). Sleep disorders in dialysis patients. T*he International Journal of Artificial Organs, 31*(11), 919-927.

Koster, A., Fischer, K-G., Harder, S., & Mertzlufft, F. (2007). The direct thrombin inhibitor argatroban: A review of its use in patients with and without HIT. *Biologics, 1*(2), 105-112.

Lamiere, N., & Mehta, R. (2000). Acute dialysis complications. In N. Lamiere & R. Mehta (Eds.), *Complications of dialysis* (pp. 307-326). New York: Marcel Dekker, Inc.

Latham, C. (2006). Hemodialysis technology. In A. Molzahn & E. Butera, (Eds.), *Contemporary nephrology nursing: Principles and practice* (2nd ed., pp. 531-558). Pitman, NJ: American Nephrology Nurses' Association.

Layman-Amato, R.L., Curtis, J., & Payne, G.M. (2013). Water treatment for hemodialysis: An update. *Nephrology Nursing Journal, 40*(5), 383-404, 465. Also available at http://www.prolibraries.com/anna/?select=speaker&speakerID=5 9083&conferenceID=42

Makari, J., Cameron, K., & Battistella, M. (2013). Understanding pruritis in dialysis patients. *CANNT Journal, 23*(1), 19-23.

Manca-Di-Villahermosa, S., Tedesco, M., Lonzi, M. Della-Rovere, F.R., Innocenzi, A., Colarieti, G., ... Taccone-Gallucci, M. (2008). Acid-base balance and oxygen tension during dialysis in uremic patients with chronic obstructive pulmonary disease. *Artificial Organs, 32*(12), 973-977.

McIntyre, C.W. (2010). Haemodialysis-induced myocardial stunning in chronic kidney disease – A new aspect of cardiovascular disease. *Blood Purification, 29*(2),105-110. doi:10.1159/000245634. Epub 2010 Jan 8. Retrieved from http://www.karger.com/Article/Pdf/245634

McIntyre, C.W. (2014). Nervous system and sleep disorders. In J.T. Daugirdas, P.G Blake, & T.S. Ing (Eds.), *Handbook of dialysis* (5th ed., pp. 754-776). Philadelphia: Lippincott Williams & Wilkins.

Medical Education Institute (MEI). (2013). *Home Dialysis Central, Dialysis machine museum*. Retrieved from http://www.homedialysis.org/home-dialysis-basics/machines-and-supplies/dialysis-museum

Medivators. (2007). *Material safety data sheet 2001/58/EC RENALIN® 100 Cold Sterilant Minntech BV*. Sweden: Author. Retrieved from http://medivators.com/international/resource/documents/msds/R enalin%20100%20English.pdf

Milinkovic, M., Zidverc-Trajkovic, J., Sternic, N., Trbojevic-Stankovic, J., Maric, I. Milic, M., ... Stojimirovic, B. (2009). Hemodialysis headache. *Clinical Nephrology, 71*(2), 158-163.

Merriam-Webster. (2015). Retrieved from: http://www.merriam-webster.com/medical/dialysance

Misra, M. (2005). The basics of hemodialysis equipment. *Hemodialysis International, 9*(1),30-36.

Morgan. D. (2008). Save cash while being environmentally friendly. *Renal Business Today, 3*(9), 22-27. Retrieved from http://www.renalbusiness.com/lib/download.ashx?d=1979

Murray, P.T., Reddy, B.V., Grossman, E.J., Trevino, S., Ferrell, J., Tang, I., ... Swan, S.K. (2004). A prospective comparison of three argatroban treatment regimens during hemodialysis in end-stage renal disease. *Kidney International, 66*(6), 2446-2453.

National Institutes of Health (NIH). (2011). What are the signs and symptoms of angina? National Heart Lung and Blood Institute (NHLBI). Retrieved from http://www.nhlbi.nih.gov/health/health-topics/topics/angina/signs

National Institutes of Health (NIH). (2011). *Methylene blue injection. DailyMed*. Retrieved from http://dailymed.nlm.nih.gov/dailymed/lookup.cfm?setid=fde64824-2be5-4d85-8d57-5098ca6890bb

National Kidney Foundation (NKF). (1997). NKF-DOQI™ Clinical practice guidelines. *American Journal of Kidney Diseases*. New York: Author.

National Kidney Foundation (NKF). (2002). NKF-KDOQI Guidelines, *Clinical practice guidelines for bone metabolism and disease in chronic kidney disease, 2002*. Retrieved from http://www2.kidney.org/professionals/KDOQI/guidelines_bone/

National Kidney Foundation (NKF). (2005). *Kidney Disease Outcomes Quality Initiative (K/DOQI) clinical practice guidelines for cardiovascular disease in dialysis patients*. S1-S154. Retrieved from http://www2.kidney.org/professionals/KDOQI/guidelines_cvd/

National Kidney Foundation (NKF). (2006a). NKF-KDOQI guidelines, Clinical practice guidelines for hemodialysis adequacy, update 2006, Guideline 5: Control of volume and blood pressure. Retrieved from http://www2.kidney.org/professionals/KDOQI/guideline_upHD_PD_VA/hd_guide5.htm

National Kidney Foundation (NKF). (2006b). NKF-KDOQI guidelines, Clinical practice guidelines for hemodialysis adequacy, update 2006; Guideline 2: Methods for measuring and expressing the hemodialysis dose. Retrieved from http://www2.kidney.org/professionals/KDOQI/guideline_upHD_PD_VA/hd_guide2.htm

National Kidney Foundation (NKF). (2006c). NKF-KDOQI guidelines, *Clinical practice guidelines for hemodialysis adequacy, update 2006; Guideline 7: Quality improvement programs*. Retrieved from http://www2.kidney.org/professionals/KDOQI/guideline_upHD_PD_VA/hd_guide7.htm

National Kidney Foundation (NKF). (2006d). *NKF-KDOQI clinical practice guidelines for hemodialysis adequacy: Guideline 4. Minimally adequate hemodialysis*. Retrieved from http://www2.kidney.org/professionals/KDOQI/guideline_upHD_PD_VA/hd_guide4.htm

National Kidney Foundation (NKF). (2006e). *NKF-KDOQI guidelines. Clinical practice guidelines and clinical practice recommendations, 2006 Updates*. Retrieved from http://www2.kidney.org/professionals/KDOQI/guideline_upHD_PD_VA/

National Kidney Foundation (NKF). (2006f.) *Clinical practice guidelines for hemodialysis adequacy, update 2006. Guideline 3: Methods for postdialysis blood sampling*. Retrieved from http://www2.kidney.org/professionals/KDOQI/guideline_upHD_PD_VA/hd_guide3.htm

News Medical: The Medical News. (2013, February 11). *WetAlert wireless wetness detector from Fresenius Medical Care*. Retrieved from http://www.news-medical.net/news/20130211/WetAlert-wireless-wetness-detector-from-Fresenius-Medical-Care.aspx

Nicholls, A.J., Benz, R.L., & Pressman, M.R. (2007). Nervous system and sleep disorders. In J.T. Daugirdas, P.G. Blake, & T.S. Ing (Eds.), *Handbook of dialysis* (4th ed., pp. 700-713), Philadelphia: Lippincott Williams & Wilkins.

NxStage Medical, Inc. (2011). *Chronic hemodialysis with the NxStage® Pureflow™ SL*. Lawrence, MA: Author.

Nystrand, R. (2008). The microbial world and fluids in dialysis. *Biomedical Instrumentation & Technology, 42*(2), 150-159.

Palmer, B (2009). Dialysate composition in hemodialysis and peritoneal dialysis. In W.L. Henrich (Ed.), *Principles and practice of dialysis* (4th ed., pp. 25-39). Philadelphia: Lippincott Williams & Wilkins.

Parker, T.F., Hakim, R., Nissenson A.R., Krishnan, M., Bond, T.C., Chan, K., ... Glassock, R. (2013). Reducing rates of hospitalizations by objectively monitoring fluid removal. *Nephrology News & Issues, 27*(3), 30-36.

Patel, N., Dalal, P., & Panesar, M. (2008). Dialysis disequilibrium syndrome: A narrative review. *Seminars in Dialysis, 20*(3), 493-497.

Peacock, W.F. (2010). Use of bioimpedance vector analysis in critically ill and cardiorenal patients. *Contributions to Nephrology, 165,* 1257-1269.

Pedrini, L.A. (2011). Transmembrane pressure, ultrafiltration coefficient and the optimal infusion rate in haemodiafiltration. *Nephrology Dialysis Transplantation, 26*(4), 1445-1446. doi:10.1093/ndt/gfq795. Retrieved from http://ndt.oxfordjournals.org/content/early/2011/02/18/ndt.gfq795.full

Pittard, J.(2008). Safety monitors in hemodialysis. In A.R Nissenson & R.N. Fine (Eds.), *Handbook of dialysis therapy* (4th ed., pp. 188-223). Philadelphia: Saunders

Pun, P.H., Lehrich, R.W., Honeycutt, E.F., Herzog, C.A., & Middleton, J.P. (2011). Modifiable risk factors associated with sudden cardiac arrest within hemodialysis clinics. *Kidney International, 79*(2), 218-227.

Purcell, W., Manias, E., Williams, A., & Walker, R. (2004). Accurate dry weight assessment: Reducing the incidence hypertension and cardiac disease in patients on hemodialysis. *Nephrology Nursing Journal, 31*(6), 631-638.

Rahmani, S.H., Ahmadi, S., Vahdati, S.S., & Moghaddam, H.H. (2012). Venous thrombosis following intravenous injection of household bleach. *Human and Experimental Toxicology, 31*(6), 637-639.

Raymond, C.B., & Wazny, L.D. (2011). Treatment of leg cramps in patients with chronic kidney disease receiving hemodialysis. *CANNT Journal, 21*(3), 19-21.

Rob, P.M., Niederstadt, C., & Reusche, E. (2001). Dementia in patients undergoing long-term dialysis: Aetiology, differential diagnosis, epidemiology and management. *CNS Drugs, 15*(9), 691-699.

Roberts, R., Jeffrey, E.C., Carlisle, E.G., & Brierley, E.E. (2007). Prospective investigation of the incidence of falls, dizziness, and syncope in haemodialysis patients. *International Urology and Nephrology, 39*(1), 275–279.

Rocco, C., Levin, N., Brendolan, A., Nalesso, F., Cruz, D., Ocampo, C., … Ricci, Z. (2006). Flow distribution analysis by helical scanning in polysulfone hemodialyzers: Effects of fiber structure and design on flow patterns and solute clearance. *Hemodialysis International, 10*(4), 380.

Rodriguez, H.J., Domenici, R., Diroll, A., & Goykhman, I. (2005). Assessment of dry weight by monitoring changes in blood volume using Crit-Line. *Kidney International, 68,* 854-861.

Roth, V.R., & Jarvis, W.R. (2000). Outbreaks of infection and/or pyrogenic reactions in dialysis patients. *Seminars in Dialysis, 13*(2), 92-96.

Saibu, R., Mitchell, P., Alleyne, J., Blackman, J., DeConcilio, K., Joseph, A., & Salifu, M.O. (2011). Dialysis line separation: Maximizing patient safety through education and visibility of access site for patients on hemodialysis. *Nephrology Nursing Journal, 38*(6), 515-519, 526.

Santos, S.F.F., & Peixoto, A.J. (2008). Revisiting the dialysate sodium prescription as a tool for better blood pressure and interdialysic weight gain management in hemodialysis patients. *Clinical Journal American Society of Nephrology, 3,* 522-530.

Schiffl, H. (2011). High-flux dialyzers, backfiltration, and dialysis fluid quality. *Seminars in Dialysis, 24*(1), 1-4.

Schrauf, C.M. (2014). Factors affecting the safety of infusing recirculated saline or blood in hemodialysis. *Nephrology Nursing Journal, 41*(2), 213-216. Retrieved from http://www.prolibraries.com/anna/?select=session&sessionID=3017

Schreiber, M.J. (2003). *Intradialytic complications.* Paper presented at the RCG Sixth Annual Medical Conference, Tucson, AZ.

Schroeder, K.L., Sallustio, J.E., & Ross, E.A. (2004). Continuous haematocrit monitoring during intradialytic hypotension: Precipitous decline in plasma refill rates. *Nephrology Dialysis Transplant, 19*(3), 652-656. Retrieved from http://ndt.oxfordjournals.org/content/19/3/652.short

Schulman, G. (2008). Clinical application of high efficiency dislysis. In A.R Nissenson & R.N. Fine (Eds.), *Handbook of dialysis therapy* (4th ed., pp .481-497). Philadelphia: Saunders.

Selby, N.M., & McIntyre, C.W. (2007). The acute cardiac effects of dialysis. *Seminars in Dialysis, 20*(3), 220-228.

Shaz, B.H., & Hillyer, C.D. (2011). Transfusion therapy. In H.M. Lazarus, & A.H. Schmaier (Eds.), *Concise guide to hematology* (pp 332-343). Oxford, UK: Wiley-Blackwell. doi:10.1002/9781444345254.ch25

Sherman, R.A., Daugirdas, J.T., & Ing, T.S. (2014). Complications of dialysis. In J.T. Daugirdas, P.G. Blake, & T.S. Ing (Eds.), *Handbook of dialysis* (5th ed., pp. 215-236). Philadelphia: Lippincott Williams & Wilkins.

Shoji, T., Tsubakihara, Y., Fujii, M., & Imai, E. (2004). Hemodialysis-associated hypotension as an independent factor for two-year mortality in hemodialysis patients. *Kidney International, 66,* 1212-1220.

Sodemann, K., & Polascheggm, H.D. (2001). *Monitoring of mixed venous oxygen saturation by Critline III as a parameter of continuous cardiac output.* ASN/ISN World Congress of Nephrology: Abstract #553720.

Spiegal, P., Michelis, M., Panagopoulos, G., DeVita, M.V., & Schwimmer, J.A. (2005). Reducing hospital utilization by hemodialysis patients. *Dialysis and Transplantation, 34*(3), 131-136.

Sweet, S.J., McCarthy, S., Steingart, R., & Callahan, T. (1996). Hemolytic reactions mechanically induced by kinked hemodialysis lines. *American Journal of Kidney Diseases, 27*(2), 262-266. Retrieved from http://www.sciencedirect.com/science/article/pii/S0272638696905508

Tai, D.J., Conley, J., Ravani, P., Hemmelgarn, B.R., & MacRae, J.M. (2013). Hemodialysis prescription education decreases intradialytic hypotension. *Journal of Nephrology, 26*(2), 315-322.

Tanhehco, Y.C., & Berns, J.S. (2012). Red blood cell transfusion risks in patients with end-stage renal disease. *Seminars in Dialysis, 25*(5), 539-544.

Tayebi, A., Shasti, S., Tadrisi, S., Sadeghi Shermeh, M., & Einollahi B. (2013). The effect of infusion hypertonic glucose on dialysis adequacy in non diabetic hemodialysis patients. *Iranian Journal of Critical Care Nursing, 5*(4), 188-195. Retrieved from http://www.inhc.ir/browse.php?a_code=A-10-327-5&slc_lang=en&sid=1

Tsai, M-H., Chang, W-N., Lui, C-C., Chuung, K-J., Hsu, K-T., Huang, C-R., … Chuang, Y-C. (2005). Status epilepticus induced by star fruit intoxication in patients with chronic renal failure. *Seizure, 14*(7), 521-525.

Twardowski, Z. (2000). Safety of high venous and arterial line pressures during hemodialysis. *Seminars in Dialysis, 13*(5), 336.

Voroneanu, L., & Covic, A. (2009). Arrhythmias in hemodialysis patients. *Journal of Nephrology, 22*(6), 716-725.

Ward, R. (2008). Single–patient hemodialysis machines, safety monitors in hemodialysis, clinical application of high-efficiency hemodialyzers. In A.R Nissenson & R.N. Fine (Eds.), *Handbook of dialysis therapy* (4th ed., pp. 159-167). Philadelphia: Saunders.

Ward, R.A. (2011). Do clinical outcomes in chronic hemodialysis depend on the choice of a dialyzer? *Seminars in Dialysis, 24*(1), 65-71.

Weiner, D.E., & Saranak, M.J. (2014). Cardiovascular disease. In J.T. Daugirdas, P.G. Blake, & T.S. Ing (Eds.), *Handbook of dialysis* (5th ed., pp. 713-735). Philadelphia: Lippincott Williams & Wilkins.

Zheng, Z.L., Hwang, Y-H., Kim, S.K., Kim, S., Son, M.J., Ro, H., … Yang, J. (2009). Genetic polymorphisms of hypoxia-inducible factor-1 alpha and cardiovascular disease in hemodialysis patients. *Nephron, 113*(2), 104-111.

Zocali, C., & Mallamaci, F. (2014). Hypertension. In J.T. Daugirdas, P.G Blake, & T.S. Ing (Eds.), *Handbook of dialysis* (5th ed., pp. 578-591). Philadelphia: Lippincott Williams & Wilkins.

Vascular Access for Hemodialysis

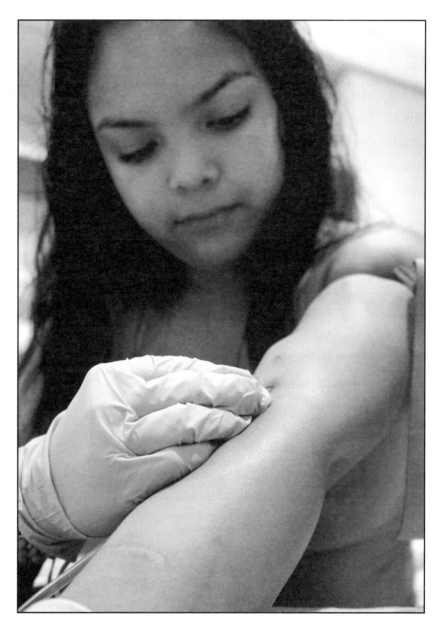

Chapter Editor
Kim Deaver, MSN, RN, CNN

Authors
Kim Deaver, MSN, RN, CNN
Caroline S. Counts, MSN, RN, CNN

CHAPTER **3**

Vascular Access for Hemodialysis

This offering for **1.8 contact hours** is provided by the American Nephrology Nurses' Association (ANNA).

American Nephrology Nurses' Association is accredited as a provider of continuing nursing education by the American Nurses Credentialing Center Commission on Accreditation.

ANNA is a provider approved by the California Board of Registered Nursing, provider number CEP 00910.

This CNE offering meets the continuing nursing education requirements for certification and recertification by the Nephrology Nursing Certification Commission (NNCC).

To be awarded contact hours for this activity, read this chapter in its entirety. Then complete the CNE evaluation found at **www.annanurse.org/corecne** and submit it; or print it, complete it, and mail it in. Contact hours are not awarded until the evaluation for the activity is complete.

Example of reference for Chapter 3 in APA format.

Deaver, K., & Counts, C. (2015). Vascular access for hemodialysis. In C.S. Counts (Ed.), *Core curriculum for nephrology nursing: Module 3. Treatment options for patients with chronic kidney failure* (6th ed., pp. 167-226). Pitman, NJ: American Nephrology Nurses' Association.

Interpreted: Section author(s). (2015). Title of chapter: Title of section. In ...

Cover photo by Robin Davis, BS, CCLS, Child Life Specialist, Texas Children's Hospital.

Special thanks to Chris Chmielewski and Sandra Schwaner for their contributions to this chapter.

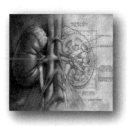

CHAPTER 3

Vascular Access for Hemodialysis

Purpose

This chapter will provide a comprehensive overview of the various types of vascular access used for hemodialysis and information related to each type. The material covers a wide array of topics related to the time before the need for dialysis through the dialysis treatment. The vascular access (1) provides an established pathway through which the blood can leave the body, enter the dialysis circuit, and return to the body after exiting the dialysis circuit, and (2) requires observation and care by both the nursing staff and the patient to prevent or limit potential complications.

Objectives

Upon completion of this chapter, the learner will be able to:
1. Describe the advantages and disadvantages of various types of vascular access.
2. Identify potential complications and appropriate interventions connected with each type of vascular access.
3. Describe the nursing care required to maintain a vascular access and to sustain its longevity and successful functioning.
4. Provide adequate and appropriate education to patients and their significant others.
5. Participate in continuous quality improvement (CQI) activities and other programs designed to protect and maintain the vascular access.

Introduction

Resources used to develop this chapter are grounded in recommendations and evidence-based practice. In particular, the chapter references the National Kidney Foundation's (NKF) KDOQI 2006 Clinical Practice Guidelines and Clinical Practice Recommendations regarding vascular access, the Fistula First Breakthrough Initiative (FFBI) started by the Centers for Medicare & Medicaid Services (CMS) – both of which are endorsed by the American Nephrology Nurses' Association (ANNA, 2013) – and other published materials. It must be noted that hardcore clinical research is missing and will be difficult, if not impossible, to accomplish given the nature of the topic.

In addition, per the 2006 KDOQI disclaimer, those guidelines are not meant to define the standards of care. Organizations and facilities must establish their own policies and procedures for their staffs to follow. Healthcare professionals must assess each patient as an individual in determining the specific needs of that person. The material in this chapter can help and should be used to guide, teach, and educate the nursing staff and, subsequently, the patients.

The success and longevity of the vascular access is in part dependent upon knowledgeable and skilled staff members coupled with the routine surveillance and maintenance of the access. The desired patient outcomes

from the published nephrology nursing process of care for vascular access by ANNA (2011, p. 123) are:
1. The patient's vascular access will provide a blood flow rate adequate to achieve the dialysis prescription.
2. The patient's vascular access will have a long use life and be free of complications.
3. The patient and patient's family will demonstrate knowledge regarding his/her vascular access.

A vascular access is necessary for hemodialysis therapy. The development of the vascular access has evolved over decades (see blue box on next page). The first long-term access to be used for hemodialysis was developed in the early 1960s. Today there are basically three types of vascular access, and each is presented in this chapter.

The type of access the patient has depends upon many variables including vessel size and diameter, anatomic and physiologic limitations, surgical preference and skill, and the patient's personal choice. The personal preference for an access is associated with the knowledge and education provided by the medical and nursing staff to the patient and his/her support system. The type of vascular access in use is directly related to the rate of blood flow through the dialysis machine and the patient's quality outcomes.

Significant Dates in the History of the Vascular Access

1960   Scribner and Quinton developed the first permanent access for chronic hemodialytic therapy. It consisted of Teflon tubes, one placed in an artery and one in a vein, which exited through the skin and were joined by a Teflon loop by means of swedge locks. On March 9, 1960, patient Clyde Shields became the first patient to receive this "permanent" access for dialysis. (The shunt had a life expectancy of 7 to 10 months.)

1961   Shaldon described a technique for cannulation of femoral veins.

1962   Siliconized rubber used for external shunt loop and Teflon used for vessel tips. A curved loop connected the two cannulas forming the shunt, which was specifically made for each patient. Siliconized rubber segments had steps and bends formed in them to make them more comfortable for patients, and to extend the life of the shunt by bringing it back up to the limb and away from the joint (reverse-winged shunt).

1966   Brescia and Cimino developed the internal arteriovenous fistula (AVF) for repeated venipunctures for maintenance hemodialysis.

1966   Ramirez developed the straight-winged shunt for better stabilization and easier declotting.

1966   Buselmeier shunt developed.

1969   The first of several modified AVFs were being used for dialysis, including the saphenous vein bridge graft. It used the saphenous vein harvested from a leg; it was implanted in an arm and connected an artery at one end to a vein at the other end.

1972   Allen-Brown shunt developed.

1974   Bovine carotid artery biologic graft used for circulatory access. This was the beginning of the arteriovenous graft (AVG).

1975   GORE-TEX® graft, a self-sealing synthetic product, became commercially available for use as an access for hemodialysis.

1977   Umbilical cord vein used for AV graft.

1977   Expanded polytetrafluoroethylene (ePTFE) AVG was used as an AV conduit for hemodialysis; still in use today.

1979   Uldall developed a catheter that allowed repeated cannulation of subclavian vein for temporary access for hemodialysis; introduced the concept of subclavian vein as temporary access to avoid destruction of peripheral vessels that later may be needed for creation of permanent vascular access. This led to the development of subclavian and jugular vein catheters that could be used as permanent circulatory access for hemodialysis when peripheral vasculature was inadequate to support creation and patency of either an AV fistula or an AV graft.

1980   Button needle-free vascular access for hemodialysis developed; not to be confused with the buttonhole cannulation technique in use today. The devices were expensive and plagued with problems related to infection and thrombosis.

1980   Interventional radiology procedures for the treatment of underlying anatomic stenotic lesions emerged.

1980   Urokinase® used for thrombolysis of AV access, especially catheters.

1983   The tunneled, cuffed catheter for long-term hemodialysis access introduced.

1990s   New fistula techniques emerged, such as the middle arm fistula, reverse flow fistulas, and basilica vein transpositions. All were intended to make better use of the limited available access sites.

1997   National Kidney Foundation Dialysis Outcome Quality Initiative (NKF-DOQI) Clinical Practice Guidelines were published. The guidelines identified the need for quality improvement and maintenance programs for vascular access.

1998   Trials began for subcutaneous port/catheter devices for hemodialysis – the LifeSite® (Vasca, Inc.) The device was implanted subcutaneously and used central venous vessels. Increased reports of infections, complications, and patient deaths resulted in the company ceasing operations other than providing support for patients who still had the device.

1999   Clinical Performance Measures (CPMs) based on the NKF-DOQI guidelines were introduced.

1999   Centers dedicated to vascular access were established with many using interventional nephrologists.

2001   The DOQI guidelines were revised and renamed the Kidney Disease Outcomes Quality Initiative (KDOQI). The most significant change in these Vascular Access guidelines was in the section on Monitoring and Surveillance.

2003   The National Vascular Access Improvement Initiative (NVAII) began because the AVF growth and the catheter reduction goals in the KDOQI guidelines were not being met. It soon came to be known as the Fistula First Program. In March 2005, this program was elevated by CMS to breakthrough initiative status and is now known as the Fistula First Breakthrough Initiative (FFBI).

2006   The NKF-KDOQI guidelines for Vascular Access were revised with major format changes. There are now eight clinical practice guidelines (CPGs) and a section for clinical practice recommendations (CPRs) with specific recommendations for pediatrics. The CPGs are evidence-based. The CPRs are supported by a combination of weaker evidence and expert opinion. Four topics were intensively reviewed and revised for this iteration and all others updated. While the goal for long-term catheter reduction (< 10%) is unchanged, the goal for AVFs, incident and prevalent, is now 65% (NKF-KDOQI, 2006, CPG 8). It is to be noted that the NKF-KDOQI guidelines are not standards of care.

2008   The HeRO™ vascular access implant was introduced. This device has components of an AVG and a tube-like outflow component. One anastomosis is on the arterial (inflow) end and the venous end has a titanium connector that attaches the graft to the tube-like outflow component.

2008   On October 3, 2008, the Centers for Medicaid and Medicare (CMS) Conditions for Coverage for End-Stage Renal Disease (ESRD) Programs Interpretive Guidance became rule. The Survey and Certification Program certifies ESRD facilities for inclusion in the Medicare Program by validating that the care and services of each facility meet specified safety and quality standards, called "Conditions for Coverage." The Survey and Certification Program provides initial certification of each dialysis facility and ongoing monitoring to ensure that these facilities continue to meet these basic requirements (CMS, 2014; access at http://www.cms.gov). The interpretive guidelines include areas for Dialysis Access. The interpretive guidelines are included with surveyor training and core surveys at ESRD facilities. Website: http://www.cms.gov/Medicare/Provider-Enrollment-and-Certification/GuidanceforLawsAndRegulations/downloads/esrdpgmguidance.pdf

I. Anatomy of the vascular access for hemodialysis (Vachharajani, 2010; Ball, 2009).

A. A basic comprehension of the anatomy of the blood vessels used to create a vascular access is helpful in understanding the complexity and required proper care of that access (see Figure 3.1).

B. The venous system in the upper extremity includes both superficial and deep veins. It is the superficial system that is most important for access creation.

C. The radiocephalic AVF at the wrist is the first choice hemodialysis access and uses the forearm segment of the cephalic vein.

D. It should be noted that each patient must be looked at as an individual, each with many variables – such as comorbid conditions, age, gender – as the person is being assessed for a vascular access. There will always be some patients who are not good candidates for an AVF.

E. The reader is referred to *Atlas of Dialysis Vascular Access* by Tushar J. Vachharajani, MD, FASN, FACP. It contains a wealth of information regarding the vascular access in pictorial information. It is simple

and straightforward and includes tunneled catheters, AVFs, and AVGs. It is intended to be used by everyone on the healthcare team. It can be found on the End-Stage Renal Disease (ESRD) Network Coordinating Center's (NCC) website at http://www.esrdncc.org/index/lifeline-for-a-lifetime.

II. Patient evaluation (Banerjee, 2009; Gomez, 2011; NKF-KDOQI, 2006, CPG1).

A. Placement of a vascular access for hemodialysis begins with the crucial steps of assessment, evaluation, and preservation.
1. The process should begin when the patient has a glomerular filtration rate (GFR) less than 30 mL/min/1.72 m^2 (CKD stage 4).
2. Early referral for permanent dialysis access allows sufficient time for access maturation.
3. Preservation of the veins of the forearm and upper-arm begins with:
   a. Using veins on the dorsal surface of the hand for intravenous (IV) cannulation.
   b. Avoiding the use of forearm and upper-arm veins for venipuncture. If they must be used, rotation of sites is recommended.
   c. Not using forearm and upper-arm veins for the placement of IV catheters, subclavian catheters, or peripherally inserted central catheter lines (PICCs).
   d. Educating the patient and his/her family regarding the importance of preserving these veins.
4. The recommended timeline.
   a. An arteriovenous fistula (AVF) should be placed 6 months prior to the anticipated need for dialysis.
   b. If a fistula is not possible, an arteriovenous graft (AVG) should be inserted at least 3 to 6 weeks ahead of the anticipated need for dialysis.
5. Nurses play a crucial role in educating, explaining, and reassuring patients during the process of vascular access creation and management.

B. The evaluation of the patient prior to access placement.
1. The evaluation process helps to optimize access survival while minimizing potential complications.
2. Evaluations should include:
   a. History and physical examination.
   b. Duplex ultrasound of the upper extremity blood vessels to show how blood moves through the arteries and veins.
      (1) Vessel or vascular mapping done > 6 months prior to surgery should be repeated to ensure accuracy.

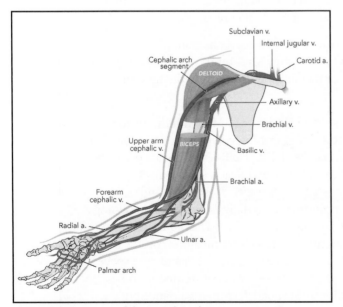

Figure 3.1. Anatomy of the vessels in the upper extremity.

Source: Vachharajani, T.J. (2010). *Atlas of dialysis vascular access.* Wake Forest University School of Medicine, North Carolina. Used with permission.

(2) Conditions in the vasculature change over time.
c. Central vein evaluation if the patient is known to have had a previous catheter or pacemaker.
(1) Duplex Doppler ultrasound (DDU).
(2) Magnetic imaging/magnetic resonance angiography (MRA) to show any problems with the blood vessels including blood flow and the condition of the blood vessel walls.

III. Selection and placement of the vascular access.

A. Choices in vascular access are shown in Figure 3.2 (CDC, 2014a; NKF-KDOQI 2006, CPG2).
1. The arteriovenous fistula (AVF) is created by surgically connecting a native artery to a native vein and allowing the vein to "arterialize." It is considered the gold standard of vascular access.
2. The arteriovenous graft (AVG) is a surgically created connection between an artery and a vein using an implanted material. The prosthetic AVG is made of synthetic or biologic material and provides a permanent vascular access for hemodialysis.
3. Central venous catheters (CVC) also provide a means of vascular access for hemodialysis. As compared to the AVF or the AVG, the catheters are associated with a higher rate of morbidity and mortality and should be avoided when possible.
a. A nontunneled catheter is a type of CVC that is held in place at the site of insertion. It travels directly from the entry site through a vein and terminates close to the heart or one of the great

vessels. It is intended to be used as a temporary catheter for short-term use.
b. A tunneled cuffed catheter is a CVC that travels a distance under the skin from the point of insertion before entering a vein. It terminates at or close to the heart or one of the great vessels.

B. The placement of the vascular access in order of preference in descending order.
1. The preferred fistula.
a. A wrist (radiocephalic) primary fistula.
b. An elbow (brachiocephalic) primary fistula.
c. A transposed brachial-basilic vein fistula.
2. The acceptable graft whether made of synthetic or biologic material.
a. A forearm loop graft which is preferable to a straight configuration.
b. An upper-arm graft.
c. A chestwall ("necklace") graft or lower extremity fistula or graft.

Note. All upper-arm sites should be exhausted.

d. The majority of past experience has been with the use of PTFE grafts. However, there are others, such as the polyurethane (PU) and biologic (bovine) grafts, which have similar outcomes.

Note. The access should be placed distally and in the upper extremities whenever possible.

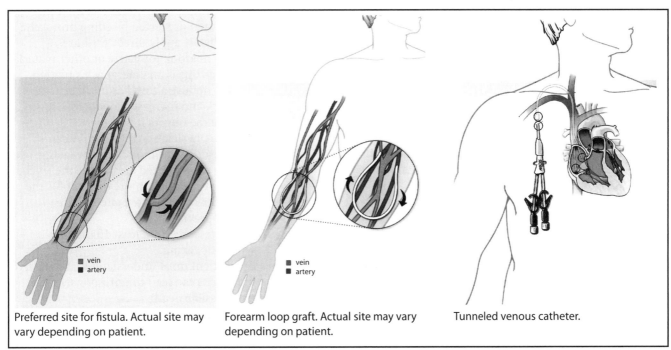

Preferred site for fistula. Actual site may vary depending on patient.

■ vein
■ artery

Forearm loop graft. Actual site may vary depending on patient.

■ vein
■ artery

Tunneled venous catheter.

Figure 3.2. Choices of vascular access. Used with permission from Arrow International, Inc.

3. The short-term catheter.
   a. Used for acute dialysis only.
   b. Used for a limited duration in hospitalized patients – less than 1 week.
   c. Noncuffed femoral catheters are for bed-bound patients only.
4. The unavoidable long-term catheter.
   a. The right internal jugular (IJ) is the preferred insertion site.
   b. Other possible sites include right external jugular vein, the left internal and external jugular veins, subclavian veins, femoral veins, and translumbar and transhepatic access to the inferior vena cava (IVC). The subclavian catheter is reserved for those instances when no other upper-arm or chest-wall options are available.
   c. Ultrasound should be used in the placement of catheters.
   d. The position of the tip of the catheter should be verified radiologically.
   e. When used, a plan for a permanent access should be in place.
   f. Catheters capable of rapid flow rates are preferable.
   g. The choice of catheter should be based on experience, technical detail, goals for use, and cost.
   h. Catheters should not be inserted on the same side as a maturing AV access if possible.

Note. Femoral catheters should be avoided in the patient who is or will be a transplant candidate.

IV. Education regarding the vascular access.

A. Patient education related to a vascular access (ANNA, 2011; Ball, 2013; CPG4; NIDDK, 2008; NKF, 2006).
   1. All patients with a vascular access should learn how to:
      a. Compress a bleeding access since a majority of fatal access bleeds and ruptures occur at home.
      b. Keep the access clean at all times.
      c. Wash the skin over the access with soap and water every day and before dialysis.
      d. Recognize signs and symptoms of infection.
      e. Select proper methods for exercising the fistula arm with some resistance to blood flow.
      f. Palpate for the thrill/pulse daily and after any episodes of hypotension, dizziness, or lightheadedness.
      g. Listen for the bruit with the ear opposite the access if they cannot palpate for any reason.

   2. All patients with a vascular access should know to:
      a. Avoid carrying heavy items draped over the access arm or wearing occlusive clothing.
      b. Avoid sleeping on the access arm.
      c. Avoid wearing tight jewelry or clothing on the access arm.
      d. Avoid injury to the access, such as bumps or cuts.
      e. Not allow the access site to be used for anything but dialysis treatments.
      f. Not allow blood pressure readings, blood draws, or injections on the access side.
      g. Ensure the staff checks the access prior to each treatment.
      h. Insist that staff rotate the needle sites each treatment if applicable.
      i. Ensure that the staff is using proper techniques in preparing the skin before cannulation and wearing masks for all access connections.
      j. Report any signs or symptoms of infection or absence of bruit/thrill to dialysis personnel immediately.
      k. Be willing to discuss with the nephrologist, advanced practice registered nurse (APRN), physician's assistant (PA), and/or surgeon any questions or concerns regarding the vascular access – this is a very important concept as some patients are hesitant to speak up.

   3. Preparation for an emergency response to bleeding begins with practice in the unit.
      a. It is important that the patient hold the access site postdialysis if able. This will help to elicit an automatic response should bleeding occur outside of the unit.
      b. Ask the patient, "What would you do if the access ruptured or started bleeding profusely?"
         (1) Immediately apply direct pressure.
            (a) Do not look for gauze or other material since this is an emergency situation.
            (b) Do not use a towel as it can act as a wick and increase blood loss.
            (c) Use the fingers if necessary.
            (d) The physician, APRN, or PA can prescribe antibiotic therapy later.
         (2) Elevate the ruptured area above the level of the heart making it more difficult for the blood flow to reach the affected area against gravity.
         (3) Hold pressure for at least 10 minutes without peeking.
         (4) The patient must understand that excessive blood loss can lead to unresponsiveness and possible death.
         (5) If bleeding stops, observe the site for 1 to 2 hours for any recurrence.
         (6) If bleeding does not stop, call 911.

(7) If it is a true rupture with uncontrolled bleeding, call 911 and apply a tourniquet at the arterial anastomosis to stop the flow of blood into the access.

Note. The use of a tourniquet is controversial. The patient may lose valuable time looking for the tourniquet. Additionally, the use of a tourniquet could possibly lead to the loss of the limb. Therefore, it is suggested that a careful evaluation of the patient be performed to assess if the correct use of a tourniquet is likely. Nonetheless, it is probably wise to educate patients who live alone, who have an aneurysm or false-aneurysm, or who have high blood flows through the access, to apply a tourniquet.

---

    c. Reinforcement of practice should be performed on a regular basis.
    d. The staff can evaluate learning through a return demonstration.
    e. If the patient is unable to perform, the patient should be reeducated.
    f. Family members and significant others should also know how to handle this emergency situation.
    g. It is extremely important to document all steps taken in the patient's medical record.
  3. Resources for patient education specific to the vascular access.
    a. *Vascular Access: A Lifeline for Dialysis* http://kidneyschool.org/pdfs/KSModule8.pdf
    b. *Vascular Access for Hemodialysis* http://kidney.niddk.nih.gov/kudiseases/pubs/vascularaccess/index.aspx
    c. *Hemodialysis Access: What You Need to Know* http://www.kidney.org/atoz/pdf/va.pdf

---

Note: Between the years 2000 and 2006, 1,654 patients on hemodialysis died from fatal vascular access hemorrhages (FVAHs), and this is likely an underestimation. Risk factors for FVAH include:
- Having an AVG – over half of the access ruptures occurred in grafts.
- Residing at home, in a nursing home, or an assisted living facility – approximately 75% of the deaths occurred in one of these locations.
- Experiencing access-related complications within 6 months before the FVAH.
- Hypertension.

How many of these incidents could have been prevented? Education and observation for infection, stenosis, aneurysms, and pseudoaneurysms are critically important.

B. Education of healthcare personnel outside of the dialysis facility (Ball, 2013; Rushing, 2010).

  1. When the patient is hospitalized or in a nursing home, extended care facility, etc., it is important that the staff members at those facilities know how to care for the patient's access.
  2. The staff should know to:
    a. Remove any restrictive clothing or jewelry from the arm.
    b. Place a nonrestrictive armband on the patient or a sign over the bed that says no blood pressure (BP) measurements, venipunctures, or injections on the affected limb.
    c. Perform hand hygiene before assessing or touching the access.
    d. Wear gloves if it is a new access with a wound.
    e. Position the arm so the access can be easily visualized.
    f. Assess for patency at least every 8 hours.
      (1) Palpate to feel the thrill.
      (2) Auscultate to detect the bruit.
    g. Assess circulation in the area distal to the access.
      (1) Palpate the pulse.
      (2) Observe capillary refill in the fingers.
      (3) Assess for numbness, tingling, altered sensation, coldness, and pallor.
    h. Notify the appropriate healthcare provider if clotting is suspected.
    i. Assess the access for signs and symptoms of infection: redness, warmth, tenderness, purulent drainage, open sores, swelling.
    j. After dialysis, monitor the access for bleeding or hemorrhage.
    k. Take appropriate emergency measures if bleeding occurs.
      (1) A significant number of bleeding episodes occur in nursing homes or assisted-living facilities.
      (2) Apply direct pressure and elevate the bleeding/ruptured area.
      (3) Hold pressure for at least 10 minutes before reevaluating.
      (4) Once bleeding has stopped, observe the patient for 1 to 2 hours for any recurrence.
      (5) If bleeding does not stop, call 911.
    l. Monitor any aneurysms that may be present.
    m. Avoid trauma or excessive pressure when moving the patient or assisting with ambulation.
    n. Document assessment findings, any interventions and the patient's response, any patient education, and level of understanding.

C. Education of healthcare personnel in the dialysis facility would include the material in this chapter. See Table 3.1 for a list of topics.

Table 3.1

Dialysis Caregiver Education Topics

- ❑ Vascular anatomy relevant to access creation/placement
- ❑ Vascular mapping for access creation
- ❑ Vascular access types
- ❑ Fistula creation vs. graft placement surgical decision
- ❑ Access placement surgeries
- ❑ Care of the newly created access
- ❑ Access assessment techniques
  - ○ Physical exam
  - ○ Arm elevation
  - ○ Fistula augmentation
  - ○ Interpretation of machine and lab data
  - ○ Intra-access blood flow volume measurement
- ❑ Fistula maturation – evaluating cannulation readiness
- ❑ Special considerations for initial fistula cannulation
- ❑ Cannulation techniques – site rotation vs. buttonhole
- ❑ Common fistula/graft complications
  - ○ Stenosis
  - ○ Thrombosis
  - ○ Aneurysm/pseudoaneurysm
  - ○ Infection
- ❑ Indications of access dysfunction and need for evaluation
- ❑ Endovascular procedures and treatment of fistula/graft complications
  - ○ Angiogram
  - ○ Angioplasty with or without stent placement
  - ○ Thrombectomy
  - ○ Embolization/ligation of draining veins
- ❑ Hemodialysis catheter insertion
- ❑ Catheter complications
  - ○ Malposition
  - ○ Infection
  - ○ Thrombosis
  - ○ Fibrin sheath
  - ○ Cuff extrusion
- ❑ Endovascular procedures and treatment of catheter complications
  - ○ Catheter exchange
  - ○ Fibrin sheath disruption

Courtesy of Christina Beale, RN, CNN.

SECTION B
The Arteriovenous Fistula (AVF)

I. Overview of the arteriovenous fistula (AVF).

A. Definition: a surgically created direct connection between an artery and a nearby vein allowing the high pressure arterial blood to flow into the vein causing engorgement, enlargement, and wall thickening (Ball, 2005; CDC, 2014a; NKF-KDOQI, 2006, CPG 1 &2; SVU, 2009).
   1. This process is known as *arterialization* or maturation of the vein. It provides a vessel that has adequate flow for hemodialysis and is sufficiently strong to allow effective cannulation.
   2. The number of sites is limited and requires proper handling and care during dialysis.
   3. The outflow vessel should be naturally superficial or surgically superficialized.
   4. The artery and the site of the anastomosis should never be cannulated.
   5. A variety of surgical anastomotic techniques and configurations can be used to create the fistula (see Figure 3.3).

B. Surgical classifications and process.
   1. Anatomic locations. The sites for creation of an AVF are limited only by the patient's suitable vasculature and the skill and creativity of the clinicians creating and caring for it. The surgical placement in order of priority includes:
      a. A wrist (radial-cephalic) primary fistula (see Figure 3.4).
      b. An elbow (brachial-cephalic) primary fistula.
      c. An upper-arm (brachial-basilic) fistula with vein transposition.
   2. Surgical techniques.
      a. The traditional AVF (such as the radial-cephalic or brachial-cephalic) is created with just the construction of the AV anastomosis – a one-step procedure, sometimes known as a primary fistula.
      b. With the increased impetus to give priority to AVF creation, more innovative surgical techniques are being used to superficialize the outflow vein.
         (1) Transposition of the vein or surgical removal of the tissue between the skin and the vein.
         (2) This technique involves surgically dissecting out and tunneling in a superficial, accessible area of limb.
         (3) AVFs with vein transposition are frequently created with two separate

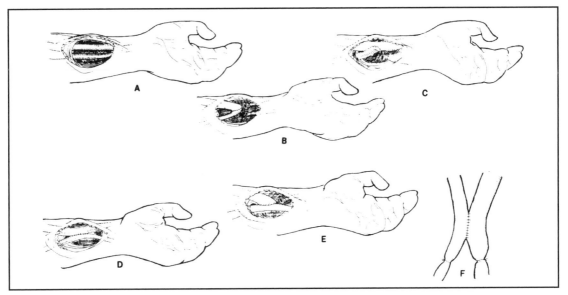

Figure 3.3. Examples of various configurations for AV fistula anastomoses: (a) normal artery-vein relationship, (b) end-to-end anastomosis, (c) end-vein to side-artery anastomosis, (d) side-to-side anastomosis, (e) side-vein to end-artery anastomosis, (f) side-to-side converted to end-to-end anastomosis.

procedures to allow for arterialization of the vein prior to superficialization.

(4) Examples of transposition: forearm radial-basilic fistula with vein transposition, upper-arm brachial-basilic fistula with vein transposition, and saphenous vein transposition fistula.

3. The timing of creating an AVF.

a. A fistula should be placed at least 6 months prior to the anticipated start of hemodialysis treatments. This timing allows for access evaluation and additional time for revision to ensure that a working, fully functional fistula is available at initiation of dialysis.

b. Patients should be considered for construction of an AV fistula whenever there is a failure of an access being used for dialysis.

c. In patients performing peritoneal dialysis who manifest signs of modality failure, an individualized consideration to create a backup fistula should be made.

4. When assessing a patient for fistula placement, the physical exam should include:

a. Examining the skin for scarring.

b. Checking the arterial blood supply in all extremities noting:
   (1) Character of peripheral pulses.
   (2) Color of digits.
   (3) Temperature of hands and feet.
   (4) Presence of lesions.
   (5) Deficits in function.

c. Performing the Allen test (see Table 3.2).

d. Listening to apical pulse for rate and rhythm.

e. Measuring bilateral upper-arm blood pressures to detect differences in arterial flow.

f. Examining venous drainage in all extremities.
   (1) Compare both arms for:
       (a) Presence and degree of edema.
       (b) Differences in size (evidence of venous and/or lymphatic obstruction).
       (c) Patency of veins noting compressibility and mobility of superficial veins in arms.

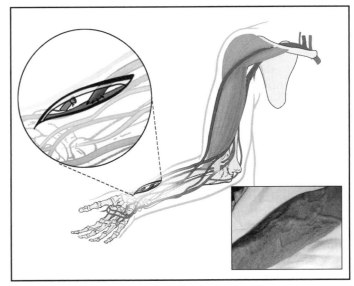

Figure 3.4. A normal radiocephalic fistula. The anastomosis is proximal to the wrist.

Source: Vachharajani, T.J. (2010). *Atlas of dialysis vascular access*. Wake Forest University School of Medicine, North Carolina. Used with permission.

Table 3.2

Allen Test

1. Patient clenches the fist of one hand to produce pallor in the hand.
2. Clinician occludes arterial flow by compressing both radial and ulnar arteries.
3. Patient opens clenched fist.
4. Clinician releases pressure on the ulnar artery and counts the seconds required for color to return to the hand. More than 3 seconds indicates decreased ulnar arterial supply to the hand if the radial artery is used for the vascular access.
5. Repeat the procedure, but release pressure on radial artery this time to assess radial arterial flow to hand.
6. Repeat procedure with opposite hand.

   (d) Note degree of change in superficial vessels with application of a tourniquet.
   (2) Compare both legs for:
      (a) Presence and degree of edema.
      (b) Difference in size (evidence of lymphatic and/or venous obstruction).
      (c) Presence of varicosities.
   (3) Look for swelling and presence of collateral veins in the chest wall and neck indicating central venous obstruction.
5. Potential diagnostic evaluations.
   a. Duplex ultrasound mapping of the upper extremity arteries and veins is recommended for all patients.
      (1) Determines the diameter, length, and suitability of the superficial veins for access placement.
      (2) Interference to adequate mapping can be the result of IV lines, bandages, patient positioning (the arm should not be above the level of the heart), or open wounds.
   b. Central vein evaluation in patients known to have:
      (1) A previous catheter, pacemaker, and/or internal defibrillator.
      (2) Edema or unilateral enlargement in the extremity of choice.
      (3) Collateral veins above the planned access site.
      (4) Evidence of any surgery or trauma to the neck, chest, breast, or arm involving the planned access vessels.
   c. Central venography can be accomplished with dilute contrast, CO_2, magnetic resonance imaging (MRI), and duplex ultrasound to avoid nephrotoxicity and preserve residual kidney function.

Note. Gadolinium-based contrast agents for MRI should not be used in patients with CKD stage 4 or 5 due to risk of nephrogenic systemic fibrosis (NSF).

C. Advantages of the AVF (Dhingra et al., 2001; Huber et al., 2003; Pisoni et al., 2002; Sofocleous, 2013; Vachharajani, 2010; Vachharajani et al., 2014).
   1. After creation and maturation of the native fistula, the average problem-free patency period is approximately 3 years.
   2. With interventions to treat underlying stenosis and thrombosis, the long-term secondary patency rate is 7 years for the forearm fistula and 3 to 5 years in the upper-arm fistula.
   3. Have the lowest rate of thrombosis and require the fewest interventions, providing longer survival of the access.
   4. Have lower rates of infection than grafts (which, in turn, are less prone to infection than percutaneous catheters).
   5. Cost of implantation and access maintenance are the lowest long-term.
   6. Are associated with increased patient survival and lower hospitalization rates.
   7. Avoid the complications associated with the venous anastomosis in AVGs.
   8. Avoid the potential for allergic response to synthetic materials.
   9. Outflow veins are autogenous tissue that seal and heal after cannulation. Synthetic grafts only seal by means of a fibrin plug.
   10. Can use the buttonhole cannulation technique.

D. Disadvantages of the AVF (Vachharajani, 2010).
   1. The vein may fail to enlarge or increase wall thickness (i.e., fail to mature). This may be caused by inadequate inflow or the presence of collateral or accessory veins that divert both volume and pressure from the intended outflow vein.
   2. The fistula has a comparatively long maturation time. Following surgery weeks to months must elapse before the AVF can be used. If maturation has not taken place prior to the need for dialysis, an alternative method of vascular access must be used until the fistula develops.
   3. In some individuals, the vein may be more difficult to cannulate.
   4. AVF creation and cannulation require different skill sets than for AVGs. Proficiency in one type of access does not assure proficiency in the other.
   5. A thrombosed AVF may be more difficult to restore the flow as compared to other types of access.
   6. The enlarged vein may be visible and be perceived as cosmetically unattractive by some individuals, especially when located in the forearm.

7. A hypertrophied outflow vein may significantly increase cardiac output (in turn increasing cardiopulmonary recirculation) and myocardial load. It may cause steal syndrome in the patient with compromised peripheral vasculature.

E. The Fistula First Breakthrough Initiative (FFBI) (Compton, 2005; Jackson & Litchfield, 2006; *Nephrology News & Issues*, 2014; USRDS Annual Report; http://esrdncc.org/ffcl).

1. In April 2004, a national initiative was launched by CMS to address the long-standing problems with vascular access and to increase the use of the AV fistula.
   a. CMS gave the program a "Breakthrough Initiative" status.
   b. The program is a top-level priority.
   c. In 2007, the use of an AVF as the primary access for patients on dialysis was 50%. In 1998, that number was 27%. In 2012, 79% of patients were using either an AVF or AVG without the presence of a catheter.
   d. The use of a catheter as the only mode of vascular access has remained stable since the 1990s. In 2007, 28% of prevalent patients had catheters.
   e. Overall, in 2011, just 35% of patients who were starting on dialysis had a maturing fistula or were using one as their primary access. In 2012, the number was 36.8%.
   f. Unfortunately, the use of catheters at the start of dialysis has remained high and unchanged at 81% when including patients with maturing AVFs or AVGs.
2. The FFBI is a coalition with representatives from CMS, the End-Stage Renal Disease (ESRD) Networks, patients, the renal community, and other stakeholders.
3. The mission of the FFBI is to improve the survival and quality of life of patients on hemodialysis by supporting the fistula as the optimal vascular access while at the same time reducing the use of the central venous catheter.
4. In 2014, the initiative became managed by the ESRD Network Coordinating Center (NCC).
   a. It provides support and coordination at the national level for the Medicare ESRD Network Program under a contract with CMS.
   b. http://www.esrdncc.org/index/lifeline-for-a-lifetime
5. The FFBI developed *13 Change Concepts for Increasing AV Fistulas* that can provide a road map to implement the NKF-KDOQI vascular access recommendations if followed. These changes include:
   a. **Change Concept 1**. Routine Continuous

Quality Improvement (CQI) review of vascular access (VA) is conducted.
   (1) Designate a staff member in the dialysis facility (RN if feasible) who will be responsible for VA CQI.
   (2) Assemble a multidisciplinary VA CQI team in the facility or hospital.
   (3) Minimally: the medical director and an RN (VA CQI Coordinator).
   (4) Ideally the team includes representatives of all key disciplines including access surgeons and interventionalists.
   (5) Investigate and track all non-AVF access placements and AVF failures.
   b. **Change Concept 2**. Timely referrals to nephrologist are made.
   (1) Primary care providers (PCPs) use ESRD/CKD referral criteria to ensure timely referral of patients to nephrologists.
   (2) Establish meaningful criteria for PCPs who may not perform GFR or creatinine clearance testing.
   (3) Nephrologist documents AVF plan for all patients expected to require kidney replacement therapy (KRT).
   (4) Designated nephrology staff person educates the patient and family to protect vessels, when possible using bracelet as reminder.
   c. **Change Concept 3**. Early referral to the surgeon for "AVF only" evaluation and timely placement.
   (1) Nephrologist/skilled nurse perform appropriate evaluation and physical exam prior to a referral for surgery.
   (2) Referral by the nephrologist for the patient to undergo vessel mapping where feasible, prior to surgical referral.
   (3) Nephrologist refers patients to surgeons for "AVF only" evaluation, no later than stage 4 CKD (GFR < 30). Surgery scheduled with sufficient lead time for AVF maturation.
   (4) Nephrologist defines AVF expectations to surgeon, including vessel mapping (if not already performed).
   (5) If timely placement of AVF does not occur, nephrologist ensures that patient receives AVF evaluation and placement at the time of initial hospitalization for temporary access (e.g., catheter).
   d. **Change Concept 4**. Surgeon selection is based on best outcomes, willingness, and ability to provide access services.
   (1) Nephrologists communicate standards and expectations to surgeons performing access, e.g., NKF-KDOQI minimal

standards for AVF placement, and training in current techniques for AVFs.

(2) Nephrologists refer to surgeons who are willing and able to meet the standards and expectations.

(3) Surgeons are continuously evaluated on frequency, quality, and patency of access placements. Data collection ideally is initiated and reported at the dialysis center as part of ongoing CQI process, and can be aggregated at the Network level.

e. **Change Concept 5.** Full range of surgical approaches to AV fistula evaluation and placement.

(1) Surgeons use current techniques for AVF placement including vein transposition.

(2) Surgeons ensure mapping is performed for any patient not clearly suitable for AVF based only on physical exam.

(3) Surgeons work with nephrologists to plan for and place secondary AVFs in suitable patients with AV grafts.

f. **Change Concept 6.** Secondary AV fistula placement in patients with AV grafts.

(1) Nephrologists evaluate every patient with an AV graft for possible secondary AV fistula conversion, including mapping as indicated, and document the plan in the patient's record.

(2) Dialysis facility staff and/or rounding nephrologists examine the outflow vein of all patients with grafts ("sleeves up") during dialysis treatments (minimum frequency, monthly). Identify patients who may be suitable for elective secondary AVF conversion in upper arm and inform nephrologist of suitable outflow vein.

(3) Nephrologists refer to surgeon for placement of secondary AVF before failure of the graft.

g. **Change Concept 7.** AV fistula placement in patients with catheters where indicated.

(1) Regardless of prior access (e.g., AV graft), nephrologists and surgeons evaluate all catheter patients as soon as possible for an AVF, including mapping as indicated.

(2) Facility implements protocol to track all catheter patients for early removal of catheter.

h. **Change Concept 8.** AV fistula cannulation training.

(1) Facility uses best cannulators and best teaching tools (e.g., videos) to teach AVF cannulation to all appropriate dialysis staff.

(2) Dialysis staff use specific protocols for initial dialysis treatments with new AVFs and assign the most skilled staff to such patients.

(3) Facility offers option of self-cannulation to patients who are interested and able.

i. **Change Concept 9.** Monitoring and maintenance to ensure adequate access function.

(1) Nephrologists and surgeons conduct postoperative physical evaluation of AVFs in 4 weeks to detect early signs of failure and refer for intervention as indicated.

(2) Facilities adopt standard procedures for monitoring, surveillance, and timely referral for the failing AVF.

(3) Nephrologists, interventional radiologists, and surgeons adopt standard criteria, and a plan for each patient, to determine the appropriate extent of intervention on an existing access before considering placing a new access.

j. **Change Concept 10.** Education for caregivers and patients.

(1) Routine facility staff in-servicing and education programs that focus on the vascular access.

(2) Continuing education for all caregivers to include periodic in-services by nephrologists, surgeons, and interventionalists.

(3) Facilities educate patients to improve quality of care and outcomes (e.g., prepping puncture sites, applying pressure at needle sites, etc.).

k. **Change Concept 11.** Outcomes feedback to guide practice.

(1) Networks work with dialysis providers to give specific feedback to all decision makers on incident and prevalent rates of AVF, AVG, and catheter use.

(2) Review data monthly or quarterly in facility staff meetings. Present and evaluate data trended over time for incident and prevalent rates of AVF, AVG, and catheter use.

l. **Change Concept 12.** Modify hospital systems to detect CKD and promote AV fistula planning and placement.

(1) Hospitals develop a comprehensive plan for early identification of patients with kidney disease.

(2) The goal is to allow for interdepartmental coordination for protective measures programs to prevent nephrotoxicity or other causes of further kidney damage, to allow for vessel preservation, patient and family support, and vascular access planning and/or placement.

m. **Change Concept 13.** Support patient efforts to live the best possible quality of life through self-management.

(1) Patient achieves optimum treatment outcomes and health status through collaborative knowledge-building related to CKD progression and treatment and through effective application of self-management interventions, such as self-monitoring and decision-making.

(2) Healthcare clinicians use techniques and strategies for the education of those who participate in vascular access education and management that are designed to encourage, enhance, and support patient self-management. This includes motivational interviewing, health coaching, and other patient empowerment strategies and techniques.

F. Assessment of the Fistula – Look, Listen, Feel (ANNA, 2011; Ball, 2005; Banerjee, 2009; Vachharajani, 2010).

Note. A series of educational videos for professionals is available on the Fistula First website and/or the ESRD Network Coordinating Center (NCC). They include:

http://esrdncc.org/navigating-your-esrd-journey/lifeline-for-a-lifetime/ – This tool reviews the assessment of the fistula. Among other vital information, the sounds of a bruit can be heard.

https://www.youtube.com/watch?v=m1-C61AOY3Q
In this video Tushar Vachharajani, MD, FASN, FACP, shows the full exam for a lower arm AVF (24 minutes).

http://esrdncc.org/navigating-your-esrd-journey/lifeline-for-a-lifetime/access-monitoring/professional-resources-for-access-monitoring/
In this video Dr. Gerald Beathard demonstrates an exam of upper-arm AVF (8 minutes).

Several other videos can be accessed from the site.
• AVF Cannulation Training videos
• Provider Educational videos
• Surgical Training videos
• AV Fistula Bruit Normal
• AV Fistula with Stenosis
• Abnormal AV Fistula Whistle
• Normal AV Graft
• AV Graft with Stenosis
• Abnormal AV Graft Whistle

1. Inspection – look.
   a. Compare the access extremity with the other extremity noting any obvious differences.
   b. Assess the access extremity for swelling, the presence of collateral veins, change in color or temperature, tortuosity of the fistula, decreased

sensation, limitation of movement, and/or capillary refill in the nail beds.

Note. A pink color should return to the nail beds in less than 2 seconds after pressure is removed.

   c. Assess the fistula itself for redness, warmth, drainage from previous needle sites, ecchymosis, hematoma formation, a rash or break in the skin, aneurysm or pseudoaneurysm, or stenosis.
      (1) A skin rash can be an allergic reaction to the soap or cleansing solution used to clean the access, the antibiotic ointment if used, or tape used for securing the needles in place.
      (2) Allergies should be well documented in the patient's medical record.

Note. When the arm is raised above the head, the outflow vein should collapse either partially or fully. If it does not, it is a sign of venous stenosis.

2. Auscultate – listen.
   a. The bruit is a continuous "whooshing" sound caused by the turbulence at the anastomosis.
      (1) The sounds should blend into each other and not have separate systolic and diastolic components.
      (2) A high-pitched bruit might be a sign of an underlying stenosis.
   b. Note any change in the sound or character of the blood flowing through the fistula.
3. Palpate – feel.
   a. Enables one to determine that blood is flowing through the fistula.
   b. The thrill is the sensation that is felt over the fistula.
      (1) Described as a continuous vibration or purring.
      (2) It is the result of the turbulence created as the blood flow from the high-pressured arterial system merges with the blood flow in the low-pressured venous system.
      (3) A pulsatile thrill may indicate stenosis.
         (a) Pulsatility occurs when the pulse overtakes the gentle thrill.
         (b) The vibration can no longer be felt; a pulse is felt.

Note. It is important to assess the entire access. If only the anastomosis is checked, indications of dysfunction occurring within the body of the fistula can be missed. It is also important to assess the character of the bruit and thrill and not just their presence.

II. Overview of potential problems and complications with the AVF.

A. Infection (ANNA, 2011; Ball, 2005; CDC, 2014a; CMS, 2008; Deaver, 2010; Kaplowitz et al., 1988; NKF-KDOQI, 2006, CPG 5; Schanzer, 2002).

Note. Of all the types of vascular access, the primary AVF is at least risk for infection.

1. Causes.
   a. *Staphylococcus aureus* is the leading cause of infections. It is known that patients on dialysis have more staph on their skin and in their nares than the general public.
   b. Poor patient hygiene.
   c. Inadequate skin preparation prior to cannulation.
   d. Not using aseptic technique for cannulation.
   e. Seeding from another infected site in the body.
   f. Introduction of microorganisms can also be related to:
      (1) Aneurysms. The thin walls make it easier for bacteria to be introduced into the vessel if the area is not avoided.
      (2) Clots formed near or within the aneurysm or at the site of an infiltration provide a site to which bacteria can attach.
2. Signs and symptoms.
   a. Inflammation.
   b. Pain.
   c. Skin break with drainage along the course of the vessel.
   d. Fever.
3. Potential interventions and treatments.

Note. Cannulation of an access with an infected segment should be done only with a physician's, APRN's, or PA's order if dialysis is extremely urgent. The infected area must be avoided.

   a. Healthcare providers, including physicians, nurses, and technicians, can prevent many infections by following basic infection prevention recommendations.
   b. Assessing the AVF every treatment is critical and is considered a primary intervention.
   c. Report findings to the vascular access team.
   d. Obtain culture of any exudates per protocol or as ordered.
   e. Administer IV broad spectrum or organism sensitive antibiotics as ordered. Infections of a primary fistula should be treated as subacute bacterial endocarditis within 6 weeks of antibiotic therapy.
   f. The surgical takedown of an AVF may become

necessary if there is evidence of septic emboli.
   g. A surveillance system must be in place that identifies at least the date of infection onset, infection site, full identification of the infecting organism(s), and antimicrobial susceptibility results.
      (1) Requires participation of the interdisciplinary team.
      (2) Necessary because of the high correlation to morbidity and mortality.

Note. Infection occurring within 3 weeks of surgery is generally considered perioperative infection and is usually prevented by prophylactic antibiotics at the time of surgery.

B. Venous stenosis (Ball, 2005; Kumar et al., 2007; NKF-KDOQI, 2006, CPG 4 & 5; Schanzer, 2005; Solocleous, 2013; Vachharajani, 2010; White, 2006).
   1. Definition: venous stenosis is an abnormal narrowing of the lumen of the vessel as a result of injury to the wall, causing intimal hyperplasia. The result is disturbances in flow dynamics and changes in pressures within the vessel.
      a. The bruit changes to a choppy, distinctly separate sound.
      b. At the site of the stenosis, the bruit may be higher pitched because of the narrowing, or it may be louder than at the anastomosis.
      c. The pulse will become a harsher, water hammer feel.
   2. Related problems.
      a. Venous hypertension: engorgement of vessels distal to anastomosis when resistance to flow is greater in proximal veins due to venous stenosis.
      b. Sore thumb syndrome: engorgement of thumb veins with sometimes painful throbbing or pulsating of distal veins and edema of thumb that may extend to entire hand; cyanotic nail bed with potential for serous oozing if obstruction of venous capillary drainage continues.
      c. Increased venous return can cause arm, breast, neck, chest, and facial swelling if stenosis develops in the central vessels. Blue or purple veins become visible in the upper arm and chest wall in the area close to the central stenosis.
   3. Related abnormalities.
      a. Reduction in blood flow rate and potential clotting of the fistula.
         (1) Average blood flow rate through an AVF = 500 to 800 mL/min.
         (2) A blood flow rate of 200 mL/min is needed to maintain patency.
      b. Increase in static venous pressures.
      c. Access recirculation leading to inadequate dialysis.

    d. Unexplained reduction in KT/V.

    e. Abnormal physical findings such as those described above.

    f. Other clues indicating stenosis.

      (1) Inability to maintain prescribed blood flow rate.

      (2) Increasing venous pressures.

      (3) Clotting of the extracorporeal circuit not related to anticoagulation issues.

      (4) Difficulty cannulation or having blood squirt out around needles during cannulation.

      (5) Increased bleeding times postdialysis due to the increased pressure.

4. Any abnormal findings or problems should be reported to the vascular access team.

5. Potential interventions and treatment,

    a. Noninvasive technique to assess a fistula.

      (1) Have patient hold the arm down while pumping the fist, allowing the fistula to engorge.

      (2) Have patient raise the arm straight up while keeping the fist clenched.

      (3) With no stenosis the fistula will drain and flatten out.

      (4) With stenosis, the fistula will not drain completely and will remain engorged and will feel firm when palpated rather than soft and compressible.

    b. Doppler ultrasound or fistulogram/venogram to measure flow and detect stenosis.

    c. Balloon angioplasty is the preferred treatment for hemodynamically significant stenosis.

      (1) Angioplasty by its very nature can injure the endothelium and underlying smooth muscle in the access because of the force behind it.

      (2) Can be beneficial or inadvertently harmful.

    d. Stent placement is useful in patients who have central venous stenosis, limited residual access sites, surgically inaccessible lesions, and/or contraindications to surgery.

      (1) Self-expanding stents are preferable because of their flexibility and radial force.

      (2) Indicated as a last resort when the stenosis persists after angioplasty.

      (3) Cannulation through a stent is an off-label use of the device and should never be done without a physician's, APRN's, or PA's order.

    e. Surgical revision may be indicated.

    f. For venous hypertension, elevate the arm above the level of the heart.

C. Central venous stenosis (CVS) (Kotoda et al., 2011; NKF-KDOQI, 2006, CPG 5; Vachharajani, 2010).

CVS is a serious complication for patients on hemodialysis and one that requires more research to understand its causes, prevention, and treatment.

1. Causes or contributing factors.

    a. History of multiple central venous catheters; however, CVS may develop without a history of central venous catheter placement.

      (1) Majority of stenotic lesions have been found in the subclavian vein.

      (2) Another common site is the junction of the subclavian and cephalic veins.

      (3) Possibly related to catheter insertion technique or catheter movement leading to endothelial damage, hyperplasia, and fibrosis.

    b. Mechanical compression of the central venous system by surrounding structures may play a role such as the position and size of muscles, ligaments, and bones.

    c. The arterialized high flow in the central veins coming from the access leads to changes in flow dynamics and results in abnormal shear stress, turbulence, and platelet aggregation.

    d. Other potential culprits include indwelling intracardiac wires or PICCs.

    e. Some occur without an identifiable cause.

2. Signs and symptoms (see Figure 3.5).

    a. Considerable to massive swelling in the upper extremity (access arm).

    b. Extensive network of collateral veins over the shoulder and chest develop.

    c. Pain and discomfort that increases during the dialysis session.

3. Potential interventions and treatments.

    a. Prevention of CVS through the avoidance of central venous catheters for dialysis, especially subclavian inserted catheters.

    b. Early detection and treatment of CVS reduces the rate of thrombosis and increases the likelihood of preserving the extremity for future access.

    c. Transluminal angioplasty with possible stent placement.

    d. Surgical treatment is very complex and has been associated with substantial morbidity and should be reserved for extreme situations.

D. Thrombosis (Jindal et al., 2006; NKF-KDOQI, 2006, CPG 4 & 5).

1. Causes.

    a. Stenosis of main outflow vein without collateral circulation.

    b. Significant hypotension due to volume depletion.

    c. Hypercoagulable states.

    d. Prolonged occlusive compression from a pressure dressing, clamps, tight clothing, or

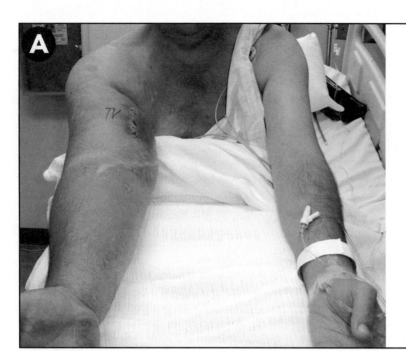

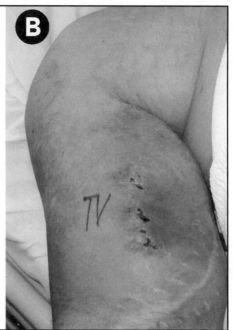

A. Massively swollen right upper extremity from completely occluded right subclavian vein. The transposed vasilic vein arteriovenous fistula is patent.

B. Extensive network of collateral veins over the right shoulder and chest area.

Figure 3.5. Central vein stenosis.

Source: Vachharajani, T.J. (2010). *Atlas of dialysis vascular access.* Wake Forest University School of Medicine, North Carolina. Used with permission.

jewelry. Anything that leaves an impression is considered too tight.
  e. Supporting heavy objects such as a basket handle or a sleeping head.

> **Note.** Lifting heavy objects with the hands once the suture line is well healed > 10 days postoperatively will not damage the AVF.

2. Signs and symptoms of impending thrombosis.
   a. The vein is distended and does not soften when the arm is elevated overhead.
   b. Significantly decreased intra-access blood flow (400 to 500 mL/min for AVF).
   c. Increased static venous pressures and standardized dynamic venous pressures.
   d. Changes in the quality of the bruit.
   e. Pulsation rather than thrill.
   f. Difficulty cannulating or pain with cannulation.
   g. Evacuation of clots.
      (1) Even with the needle properly inserted into the center of the vessel.
      (2) Without previous traumatic cannulation and/or infiltration.
   h. Increased viscosity of intra-access flow as evidenced by:
      (1) Difficulty maintaining extracorporeal blood flow at prescribed rate without an increase in the venous pressure and a decrease in the arterial pressure.
      (2) Access recirculation causing unexplained

decrease in Kt/V and URR. This is a late sign.
      (3) Late stage recirculation (black blood syndrome) develops when the same blood is being recirculated through the dialyzer and becomes deoxygenated as well as hemoconcentrated. This is a very late sign and constitutes an emergency requiring same day intervention.

> **Note.** Recirculation can be verified by introducing saline into the venous bloodline; if the blood in the arterial bloodline lightens in color, recirculation is confirmed.

   i. The final signs of thrombosis in AVF are the absence of the thrill and the bruit along the access vessel.
      (1) There may be a strong pulse in the artery at the inflow anastomosis.
      (2) Do not cannulate vessel to confirm. Needle holes in a thrombosed access complicate thrombectomy or prevent lytic administration.
3. Report any abnormal findings or problems to the vascular access team.
4. Potential interventions and treatments.
   a. Urgent referral to an interventionalist or surgeon to:
      (1) Prevent thrombosis formation by detecting and treating stenosis.

(2) Potentially perform a thrombectomy by lysing with a thrombolytic such as tPA (tissue plasminogen activator) to soften or resolve clot.
  (a) This is frequently used before mechanical thrombectomy.
  (b) Should be followed by correction of causative stenosis if indicated with angioplasty or surgical revision.
(3) Thrombectomy.
  (a) The thrombus may spread into side branches of the vessel making it more difficult to declot.
  (b) While thrombectomy should be attempted as early as possible after clot formation, the procedure can still be successful even after several days.
  (c) A major goal is to prevent the need for a temporary access.
b. Access monitoring and surveillance postprocedure to assure normal flow and pressure parameters.
c. Anticoagulation therapy for patients with proven hypercoagulable states.
d. Targeted ultrafiltration to patient tolerance.
e. Patient and staff education about prevention of:
  (1) Prolonged occlusive pressure.
  (2) Hypovolemic hypotension.

E. Aneurysm/pseudoaneurysm (NKF-KDOQI, 2006, CPG 5) (see Table 3.3).
  1. Potential contributing factors.
    a. Cannulating the AVF in the same area, also known as "one-site-itis," weakens the vessel wall (see Figure 3.6).
    b. Outflow stenosis/occlusion.
    c. Persistent hypertension.
  2. Signs (see Figure 3.6).
    a. Vessel enlargement in the specific area of constant needle insertion sites.
    b. Dilatation of the weakened vessel wall.
  3. Potential complications.
    a. Recirculation and poor clearance.
    b. Rupture and loss of blood – a potential life-threatening situation.
    c. Cosmetic concern for some patients.
  4. Diagnosis.
    a. Physical assessment of area for cannulation.
    b. Possible changes in bruit – louder than normal turbulence.
  5. Potential interventions and treatments.
    a. Assessing the AVF every treatment is critical and is considered a primary intervention; look for shiny skin and changes in pigmentation over the affected area.

Table 3.3

Aneurysm or Pseudoaneurysm?

What is the difference between an aneurysm and a pseudoaneurysm?

■ An aneurysm is an abnormal blood-filled dilation of a blood vessel wall (most commonly in arteries) resulting from disease or repeated injury of the vessel wall.

■ A pseudoaneurysm is a vascular abnormality that resembles an aneurysm, but the outpouching is not limited by a true vessel wall, but rather by external fibrous tissue.

Adapted from the glossary (NKF, 2006).

Note. Cannulation into an aneurysm or pseudoaneurysm must be avoided. Never cannulate in an area that has thin, shiny skin where the vessel appears to be ready to rupture.

---

  b. Report findings to the vascular access team.
  c. Education of the staff (or patient) who inserts the needles to either rotate sites (rope ladder) or use the same-site/buttonhole technique.
  d. Surgical referral when indicated.
  e. Based on severity of aneurysm, emergent surgery may be warranted.

F. Nonmaturing outflow vein and early failure (Ball, 2005; Banerjee, 2005; Dinwiddie, 2002; NKF-KDOQI, 2006, CPG 2, 4 & 5).
  1. Maturation is the dilatation and thickening of the vein wall in response to the increased flow and pressure of the arterial blood. Maturation is dependent upon three anatomical variants.
    a. Cardiac output.
    b. Arterial inflow.
    c. Venous outflow.

Note. Maturation is evidenced by the presence of the bruit and thrill. Fistulae may take weeks to months to mature.

---

  2. Definition of *failure to mature* – an AVF that either never physically develops enough to be cannulated for dialysis or fails to produce enough blood flow for adequate dialysis in a reasonable treatment time.
    a. Considered an early failure.
    b. Occurs within the 3-month period following the fistula's creation.
  3. Primary nondevelopment of the outflow vein may be caused by insufficient vasculature resulting from poor arterial flow and/or small vein size.

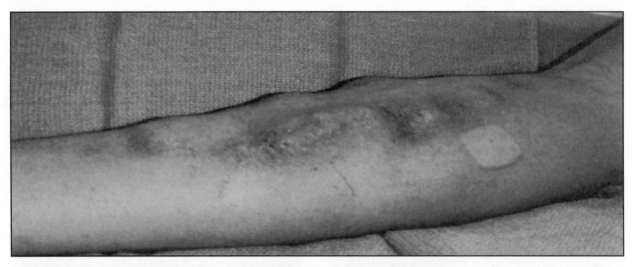

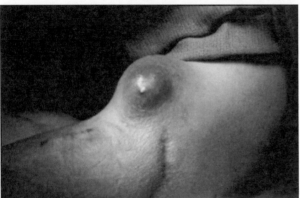
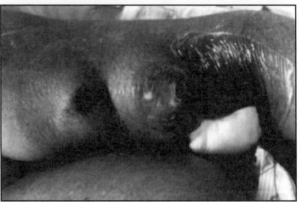

Figure 3.6. Emergent situations associated with aneurysms.
Pictured above are possible consequences of poor rotation of cannulation sites which can lead to an imminent danger of bleeding from the aneurysm. Surgical intervention in a timely manner is crucial. In addition, education regarding methods to control bleeding from the access and proper cannulation techniques should be provided to the patient and the staff.

The aneurysm pictured below would warrant urgent surgical intervention to prevent rupture and massive blood loss leading to possible death. Nursing assessment skills are important in monitoring a patient's access. In addition, the nurse must educate and mentor individuals in proper cannulation technique.

Photos courtesy of W.G. Schenk, University of Virginia Professor of Surgery. Used with permission.

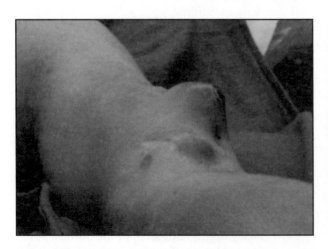
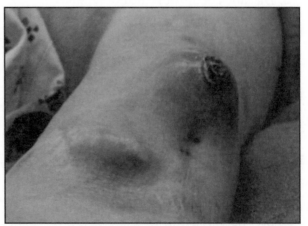

4. Signs.
   a. Minimal increase in vein size and the bruit is limited to the area of the anastomosis.
   b. Absence of palpable thrill and bruit by auscultation along the outflow vein.
   c. Persistent swelling of the hand.
   d. High negative pressure prior to the blood pump that results in:
      (1) Collapse of the blood pump segment.
      (2) Reduction of the actual blood flow rate by as much as 15% of the machine reading.
      (3) Hemolysis.
5. Potential interventions and treatments.
   a. Early identification and timely intervention are critical.
   b. Report any abnormal findings or problems to the vascular access team.
   c. Requires the evaluation of the AVF for early detection of access dysfunction – should be within 6 weeks after placement.
   d. Surgical revision of the fistula if possible.
   e. Maturation of the fistula may be enhanced by selective obliteration of major venous side branches provided there is no downstream stenosis.
   f. Exercising the fistula hand and arm may assist in the development of the fistula.
      (1) Builds muscle mass and increases circulation in the extremity.
      (2) May make the veins more prominent.

Note. Exercising the fistula hand and arm will not fix the cause of the failure to mature. The healthcare provider must be cognizant of this fact when patients are instructed to use this technique. If the fistula fails to mature, patients can perceive this as a personal failure for which they are responsible.

---

6. Appropriate interventions for access dysfunction may prolong the survival of the fistula.

G. Accessory veins (Vachharajani, 2010).
   1. Arterial flow through multiple outflow veins prevents the arterialization of a single outflow vein and, therefore, the development of a functional fistula.
   2. The thrill and bruit are present but appropriate vein development is absent.
   3. Report any abnormal findings or problems to the vascular access team.
   4. To detect the presence of an accessory vein.
      a. Occlude the main outflow vein with finger pressure sequentially along the vein.
      b. Note the character of the flow with the occlusion.
      c. If there is no accessory vein, the flow will become an augmented pulse.
      d. If an accessory vein is present between the anastomosis and the occlusion point, the thrill will continue.
   5. Treatment for accessory veins is surgical ligation or percutaneous coil ablation (coils are injected into the veins and expand to block and clot the veins).

Note. Multiple collateral veins without the presence of significant stenosis and with increased distal blood flow can cause "red hand" syndrome from venous stasis. The hand and possibly the arm appear swollen and red.

H. Steal syndrome is ischemia of the extremity distal to the arterial anastomosis (Leon & Asif, 2007; Malik et al., 2008; Suding & Wilson, 2007; Tordoir et al., 2004; Vachharajani, 2010).
   1. Cause: diversion of significant volume of blood away from the peripheral circulation.
   2. Occurs more frequently in patients who:
      a. Are elderly.
      b. Have peripheral vascular disease.
      c. Have diabetes.
      d. Have a history of multiple access surgeries in same extremity.
   3. Signs and symptoms may increase during dialysis.
      a. Pain distal to anastomosis.
      b. Cold, pale hand.
      c. Impaired hand movement and strength.
      d. Paresthesia: numbness, tingling (pins and needles).
      e. Poor capillary refill of affected nail beds (> 2 seconds).
      f. Potential progression to ulcerated, necrotic fingertips.
   4. Diagnosis.
      a. Based on physical examination.
      b. Confirmed with ultrasound to measure arterial flow to fingertips (plethysmyography/PPGs).
   5. Potential interventions and treatments.
      a. Report any abnormal findings or problems to the vascular access team.
      b. Surgical reperfusion of the hand using the DRIL (distal revascularization-interval ligation) procedure while maintaining flow through the fistula.
      c. Banding of inflow to the AVF to reduce flow.
      d. Severe ischemia not amenable to surgical revision may require urgent ligation of the access.
      e. Symptoms of mild ischemia may be improved by wearing a glove, keeping the hand dependent as much as possible, exercising, and/or massaging.

I. High output cardiac failure (MacRae et al., 2006; Mehta & Dubrey, 2008; Stern & Klemmer, 2011; Utescue et al., 2009).

1. Background information.
   a. Associating heart failure with the formation of an AVF started a few years after the use of this surgical technique began. Nonetheless, the fistula is still considered the access of choice.
   b. The AVF creates a high flow, low resistance vascular system. A large proportion of arterial blood from the left-sided circulation is shunted to the right-sided circulation via the fistula. The increase in preload can result in increased cardiac output. Over time the demands of the increased workload can lead to left ventricular hypertrophy and exacerbation of coronary ischemia.
   c. The condition can be aggravated by preexisting anemia and/or cardiovascular disease.
   d. Typically the AVF is quite large and located in the upper arm and more proximal to the heart.
   e. The high blood flow rate through the fistula can be a disadvantage to the peripheral circulation and can lead to tissue hypoxemia followed by a compensatory increase in cardiac output.
2. Signs and symptoms can include:
   a. Tachycardia.
   b. Elevated pulse pressure.
   c. Nicoladoni-Branham sign.
      (1) Compression of the artery proximal to the AVF results in a reflex bradycardia.
      (2) When the artery supplying the fistula is compressed, there is an increase in peripheral vascular resistance and afterload.
      (3) Secondary to the increased afterload, there is a reflex bradycardia.
   d. Tachypnea.
   e. Shortness of breath at rest or on exertion.
   f. Pulmonary crackles/rales.
   g. Pleural effusion.
   h. Cyanosis of lips and nail beds.
   i. Exercise intolerance.
   j. Fatigue.
   k. Fluid retention/edema.
   l. Jugular vein distension (if patent).
   m. Confusion.
3. Potential complications.
   a. Pulmonary edema.
   b. Angina.
   c. Cardiac dysrhythmias.
4. Diagnosis:
   a. Chest x-ray to assess cardiomegaly, pulmonary congestion, and pleural fluid accumulation.
   b. Blood gas to estimate oxygen consumption/ delivery ratio and an approximation of cardiac output and organ perfusion.
   c. Echocardiogram can reveal either a high or low left ventricular ejection fraction.
5. Potential interventions and treatments.

   a. Report any abnormal findings or problems to the vascular access team.
   b. Surgical reduction of the blood flow through the AVF with a banding procedure, plication of the fistula (reduce entire fistula size), or surgical ligation.
   c. Correction of anemia.
   d. Review cardiac pharmacotherapy.

Note. To reduce interdialytic symptoms, the AVF and outflow vein can be wrapped with an elastic bandage to reduce cardiac output. This requires an order from a physician, APRN, or PA. The nurse or patient must be able to comfortably slide an index finger under the bandage to be sure the fistula is not occluded.

III. Preparing the fistula for dialysis.

A. Applicable principles (Ball, 2005, CDC, 2002, 2014b; 2014c; CMS, 2008, V113; NKDOQI, 2006, CPG 3).
   1. The life of the fistula may be prolonged and morbidity improved through:
      a. The use of aseptic technique during cannulation. The CDC explains aseptic technique as taking great care to not contaminate the fistula site before or during the cannulation or decannulation procedures.
      b. The AVF being mature and ready for cannulation when first used.
         (1) Decreases the risk of infiltration.
         (2) Means the fistula is able to deliver the prescribed blood flow rate for adequate dialysis.
      c. The characteristics of the Rule of 6s should be used to insure the fistula is mature (see Table 3.4). This requires imaging studies, such as ultrasound, to measure flow, diameter, and depth.

Table 3.4

Rule of 6s for AVF Maturation

- The AVF should be expertly assessed within 6 weeks of creation for maturation.
- Flow through the vessel should exceed 600 mL per min.
- The vessel should be greater than 6 mm in diameter.
- The vessel should be less than 6 mm from the skin surface.
- A straight segment that is 6 cm in length.

Source: NKF KDOQI, 2006, CPG 3; Vachharajani et al., 2014.

(1) Flow > 600 cc/minute.

(2) Diameter at least 0.6 cm.

(3) No more than 0.6 cm deep with discernable margins.

d. Fistula hand-arm exercises should be performed.

Note. If a fistula fails to mature by 6 weeks, a fistulogram or other imaging study should be obtained to determine the cause of the problem.

---

2. Recommended skin preparation prior to dialysis.

a. Hand hygiene performed by staff and patients is the cornerstone of infection prevention.

(1) Wash hands with soap and water.

Note. Soap and water must be used if the hands are visibly soiled, meaning visible dirt or contamination with proteinaceous material such as blood or other body fluid.

---

(2) May use a waterless, alcohol-based antiseptic hand rub; usually contains 60% to 95% alcohol content.

(a) Vigorously rub hands together for 15 seconds.

(b) Cover all surfaces of the hands and fingers.

(c) Continue until hands are dry.

(3) It is important to wash hands even when gloves are to be worn and again after the gloves are removed.

b. The sites for cannulation should be determined prior to skin preparation. The prep should be repeated if the skin is touched by the staff or patient.

c. The access site should be washed using an antibacterial soap or scrub and water. Patients must be educated regarding the necessity of this step. Some patients may have washed before they left home and be reluctant to wash again.

d. The skin should be cleansed with the appropriate antimicrobial product in use by the facility using the manufacturer's instructions for use, especially the required contact time for efficacy.

(1) This is one of the most important aspects of cannulation.

(2) The proper cleansing technique (e.g., circular motion, back and forth motion, etc.) should be used for the antimicrobial product being applied. (See manufacturer's recommendations.)

e. The importance of dialysis precautions and aseptic technique cannot be overemphasized.

B. Cannulating the AVF for hemodialysis (Banerjee, 2009; Ball, 2005; Brouwer, 1995; Kumar et al., 2007; NKF-KDOQI, 2006, CPG 3 & Table 3; Vacharajani, 2010; Van Waeleghem et al., 2008).

1. Required dialysis precautions and facility policies and procedures must be followed.

2. Needle selection.

a. For the first cannulation, needle selection is critical; usually a 17G with a back-eye is used for initial attempts.

Note. The cannulator in the facility who is recognized for expert skills should be the person assigned to insert the initial needles. This is a skills-based determination and should not be based solely on licensure, certification, or seniority. It may be helpful to perform the cannulation during a nonturnover period to allow more time for the procedure to take place in a more relaxed atmosphere. Staff should be cognizant of the anxiety and pain that accompanies needle insertion (see Table 3.5).

---

b. The appropriate needle size can be selected by visualizing and feeling the AVF; follow the facility's policies and procedures.

c. As an alternate method, place a 17G and 16G (leaving the protective cap in place to prevent

---

Table 3.5

Needle Phobia

A phobia is an abnormal fearful response to a danger that is either imagined or is irrationally exaggerated. One subtype of specific phobias is blood-injection-injury; it was first recognized in the Diagnostic and Statistical Manual of Mental Disorders (DSM) in 1994. It has been estimated that up to 10% of the population is affected. The fear of needles is termed "belonephobia." (Fear of pointed objects is aichmophobia; fear of injections is trypanophobia.)

The etiology of a needle phobia is embedded in an inherited vasovagal reflex of shock and/or a learned behavior. The phobia can develop during childhood and eventually disappear; if not, treatment may be required.

Symptoms can range from rapid heartbeat, shortness of breath, trembling, feelings of panic, to dread, horror, or terror. Needle phobia is highly associated with avoidance behavior. When a patient who has this disturbing fear avoids a dialysis treatment, or habitually delays the dialysis treatment by coming in late, profound consequences can result.

Staff members must recognize this fear and be compassionate, offer reassurance, and show respect. The treatment of needle phobia can include cognitive behavioral therapy, medications, or both.

Source: American Psychiatric Association; Hamilton, 1995; Harvard Health Publication; Sokolowski, Giovannitti, & Boynes, 2010.

injury) needle over the chosen cannulation site to determine the appropriate size needle.

(1) Compare the vein size with the needle size with and without a tourniquet applied.

(2) If the needle is larger than the vein with the tourniquet on, it is too large and is likely to cause infiltration.

(3) Use the needle size that is equal to or smaller than the vein when the tourniquet was not applied.

(4) Blood flow delivered by a 17G needle is limited.

(5) Prepump arterial pressure monitoring is recommended.

    (a) This pressure should not exceed -250 mmHg.

    (b) Excessive negative pressure can result in hemolysis.

3. Anesthetics for needle insertion.

a. Intradermal lidocaine.

(1) Used immediately prior to needle insertion.

(2) Causes a bee-like stinging sensation and may be more painful than the needle.

(3) Risk of accidental intravenous infusion.

b. Topical anesthetic cream.

(1) Correct contact time is important for the drug to be effective.

(2) Needs to be applied by the patient prior to coming to the facility.

    (a) Maximum depth of 3 mm requires 60 minutes of contact.

    (b) Maximum depth of 5 mm requires 120 minutes of contact.

    (c) After application, the patient covers the site with plastic wrap to protect clothing and to ensure that the drug does not get wiped off prematurely.

    (d) There has been some concern that the cream is not sterile and may provide a medium for bacterial growth.

c. Patient preference per facility policy.

4. Needle insertion with a mature fistula (see Table 3.6).

a. Needle placement.

(1) A mature fistula is usually cannulated using a 15-gauge fistula needle.

(2) The arterial needle can be inserted in the direction of the blood flow in the fistula (antegrade) or against the direction of the blood flow (retrograde) (see Figure 3.7).

(3) The venous needle should always be inserted in the same direction as the blood flow.

b. The NKF-KDOQI Guideline 3 recommends the use of wet needles for cannulation.

(1) Use 8 mL of normal saline (NS) in a 10 mL syringe.

Table 3.6

Vascular Access Terminology for Physical Examination

■ **Proximal**: that portion of the access used for "arterial needle." In both a graft and AVF, this is the part of the access vessel that is closest to the arterial anastomosis.

■ **Distal**: that portion of the access that is used for the "venous needle" and leads to the draining veins of the central venous system.

Adapted from the glossary (NKF, 2006).

---

(2) Do not prime the needle until immediately prior to use.

(3) Used to confirm proper needle placement prior to starting the dialysis treatment.

c. After the skin has been prepped, apply a tourniquet.

(1) Increases the venous pressure.

(2) Enlarges and stabilizes the vein.

(3) Makes cannulation easier.

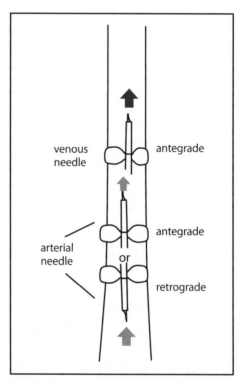

Figure 3.7. Direction of needles. Venous needle always points toward the venous return, while the arterial needle may point in either direction. Blue arrow shows venous needle. Gray arrows show arterial.

Source: Brouwer, D. (1995). Cannulation camp: Basic needle cannulation training for dialysis staff. *Dialysis and Transplantation, 24*(11), 606-612. Used with permission of John Wiley & Sons, Inc.

Note: Using a tourniquet for a fistula is a must. If a tourniquet is not needed for cannulation, the possibility of an outflow stenosis should be considered. If a tourniquet is needed during the treatment to obtain and maintain the prescribed blood pump speed, investigate the possibility of an inflow stenosis. The use of a tourniquet for this purpose is not an acceptable practice.

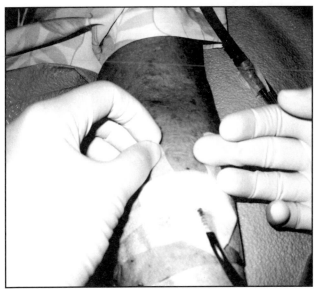

Figure 3.8. Needle taping.
Courtesy of Janet Holland and the FFBI.

d. The three-point method provides accuracy and may assist in limiting any pain.
  (1) The thumb and forefinger of the nonneedle hand are placed lightly on either side of the vessel.
    (a) Helps prevent the vessel from rolling.
    (b) Serves as a guide when threading the needle down the center of the vessel.
  (2) The pinky or ring finger of the needle hand pulls the skin taut.
    (a) Enables the needle to slide into the skin and vessel with less resistance.
    (b) Increases surface tension and lessens the surface area contacting the cutting edge of the needle.
    (c) Compresses the nerve endings that may interrupt the pain-to-brain sensation for approximately 20 seconds.
e. Grasp the butterfly needles by the wings.
  (1) Prime the needle with NS until all air is purged. Clamp the needle.
  (2) Remove the protective cap and immediately proceed with cannulating the AVF.
f. A 25-degree angle with the bevel up is used for needle insertion in an easily palpable vessel.
  (1) A less steep angle increases the risk of dragging the cutting edge of the needle on the vessel's surface.
  (2) Steeper angles increase the risk of perforating the back-wall of the vessel.
  (3) Having the bevel up facilitates entrance through the skin, subcutaneous tissue, and the vessel wall.
g. When the needle is advanced, blood flashback should be visible; the clamp may need to be opened.
  (1) Remove the tourniquet.
  (2) Aspirate back 1 to 5 mL with the 10 mL syringe; flush the needle and clamp.
  (3) The syringe must aspirate and flush easily. Observe for signs and symptoms of infiltration.

Note: Using dry needles for cannulation poses the risk of blood exposure to the staff, the patient, and other patients if the blood sprays or spills when the line is unclamped and the cap is removed to purge the line of air. In addition, proper needle placement cannot be confirmed prior to initiating dialysis.

h. Do not flip or rotate the needle as it may traumatize the intima of the vessel or cause infiltration.
i. Once in place, secure the needle with tape (see Figure 3.8).
  (1) Tape the needle at the same angle of insertion to prevent moving the tip of the needle from the desired position within the lumen of the vessel.
  (2) It may be helpful if facilities/units have a consistent procedure for taping needles and bloodlines. Using the same technique will make it easier for the staff to spot potential or impending needle dislodgement as the patients are being monitored.
  (3) The chevron technique (U-shaped) for taping needles is widely recommended.
j. The vascular access and needles must be visible at all times during the treatment.
k. Needle removal at the end of treatment is just as important as needle insertion to protect the access from damage and to facilitate proper hemostasis.
  (1) Remove the needle in the same angle as used for insertion.
  (2) Never apply pressure before the needle is completely out.

(a) This prevents the cutting edge of the needle from pressing into the intima.

(b) Dragging the cutting edge along the vessel can also traumitize the intima.

(3) There are two holes created by each needle – one through the skin and the other through the vessel wall.

(a) Appropriate compression to both holes must be applied using two fingers to hold the site.

(b) If both sites are not properly compressed, bruising, hematoma formation, and/or breakthrough bleeding (usually in the waiting room) can result.

(c) The access can become at-risk for difficult cannulation, limitation of potential needle sites, and access failure secondary to increased pressure or stenosis formation.

(4) To encourage hemostasis, the sites should be held by the staff or preferably by the patient, if able, for a minimum of 10 minutes without releasing.

(5) Excessive bleeding postdialysis (generally > 20 minutes, but should be patient specific) may indicate:

(a) Increase pressure indicative of an unsuspected outflow stenosis.

(b) Effects of anticoagulation from a medication, such as warfarin.

(6) Ensure a thrill can be felt in the access. If not, reduce the digital pressure.

5. Prior to discharge from the facility bleeding should be controlled, the needle sites should be bandaged per facility policies and procedures, the access should be assessed, and needed patient education should be completed, including removing the bandage within 24 hours and what to do should bleeding occur.

C. Cannulation site techniques (Atkar & MacRae, 2013; Ball, 2005, 2006, 2010; Ball et al., 2007; Ball & Mott, 2010; Birchenough et al., 2010; Evans, 2012; Kim & Kim, 2012; Mott & Moore, 2011; NKF-KDOQI, 2006, CPG 3; Pergolotti et al., 2011).

1. The rope ladder technique.

a. This technique has been the standard since 1966 and refers to rotating the cannulation sites.

(1) New sites are chosen every dialysis treatment allowing healing between sessions.

(a) In reality, certain sites are favored because "they work."

(b) This practice is discouraged because it leads to weakness in the vessel wall.

(2) The entire length of the AVF is used.

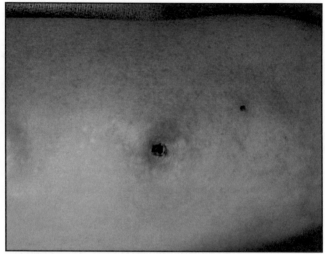

Figure 3.9. Alteration in scab size due to manipulation (center), normal size scab (on right).

Source: Ball, L. (2010).The buttonhole technique: Strategies to reduce infections. *Nephrology Nursing Journal, 37*(5), 473-478. Photo by Tony Samaha, MD. Used with permission.

(3) The needles are kept 1.5 to 2 inches apart and 1.5 inches from the anastomoses.

b. Rotating sites prevents aneurysm formation and intimal hyperplasia.

c. Potential problems with the technique.

(1) Cannulation sites can be limited if the AVF is short or curvy.

(2) Cannulation with sharp needles can be painful.

(3) Reduction in patient satisfaction is a possibility if pain and difficult cannulation become issues.

(4) The patient's quality of life may be affected if anxiety begins to play a role.

2. The buttonhole technique. See Figure 3.9 to see a healthy, mature buttonhole.

a. Refers to inserting the needle into the same site, at the same angle and depth and direction for each cannulation to create a scar tissue tunnel or track leading through the vein wall (see Figure 3.10).

b. During the creation process, sharp needles are used and do not come with sterile picks. The needles should never be used for scab removal. It is critical that the cannulator use a separate sterile device, e.g., tweezers, for each site for this purpose.

(1) The process of creating the buttonhole begins with a physical assessment of the AVF.

(2) The cannulation sites must be selected carefully. Consideration should be given to:

(a) Straight areas.

(b) Needle orientation.

(c) Ability of the patient to self-cannulate

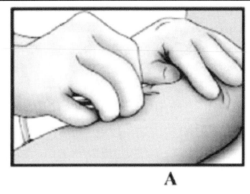

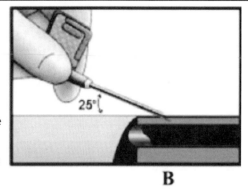

Arterial and venous sites may not develop at the same rate. Once a scar tissue tunnel track is well formed, the blunt bevel needles should be used. If standard sharp needles are used beyond the creation of the buttonhole sites, the scar tissue tunnel can be cut. More pressure and more needle manipulation will be required to advance the blunt needle down the tunnel track. This can lead to bleeding or oozing from the needle site during hemodialysis. The sharp needle can also puncture the vessel at a new site or cause an infiltration. The quick transition to the blunt needle will preserve the integrity of the buttonhole site and prevent complications.

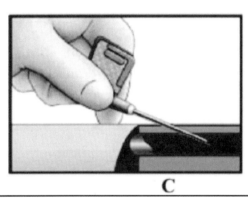

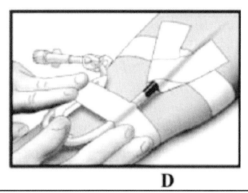

Figure 3.10. Starting a buttonhole.
© NxStage Medical, Inc. Used with permission by NxStage Medical, Inc.

(will require a steeper angle of cannulation).
    (d) Presence of aneurysms (to be avoided).
    (e) Enough area to allow a minimum of 2 inches between the tips of the needles.
(3) Requires a single cannulator until the sites are well established. This is a critical concept to the success of buttonhole development.
    (a) The time required to establish the buttonhole must be individualized.
    (b) It can take 3 weeks or more for the track to form.
    (c) If the patient has diabetes, track formation can take longer.
    (d) Moving too quickly can result in a conical track instead of a tube-shaped track, bleeding difficulties, and a higher infection rate.
(4) Once the track of scar tissue is formed from the entry site at the skin to the underlying vessel, further cannulation can be accomplished by using specialized blunt needles (see Figure 3.11).
    (a) Avoid the term "dull."
    (b) Blunt needles reduce the risk of vessel damage.

    (c) Only gentle pressure is needed to cannulate with a blunt needle. Applying force can damage the vessel wall or the track and result in infiltration or hematoma formation.
c. Potential advantages.
    (1) Fewer missed sticks and infiltrations.
    (2) Decreased aneurysm formation as compared to poor rope ladder techniques.
    (3) Decreased hematoma formation when forceful cannulation is avoided.
    (4) Less anxiety for the patient.
    (5) Ideal for patients dialyzing at home.
    (6) Some patients report less pain while others report no reduction in pain.
        (a) Pain is a subjective experience that can only be assessed by the individual.
        (b) This may result in inconsistencies in reported pain reduction outcomes.
    (7) Shortened hemostasis time.
    (8) Decreased staff stress.
        (a) Improved ease of cannulation.
        (b) The technique takes less time since there is no need to identify new sites and fewer complications.
d. Potential issues.
    (1) The staff.
        (a) It is difficult to schedule one staff

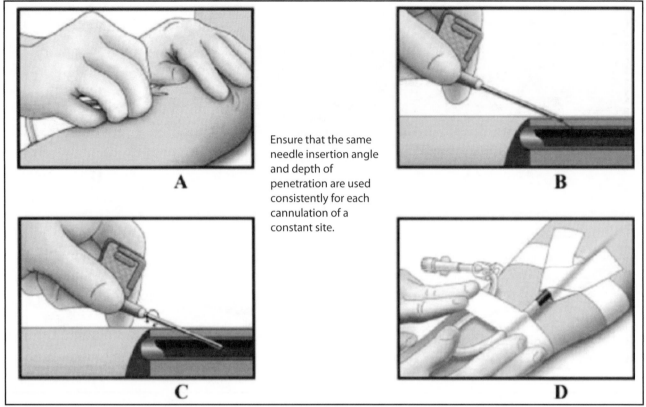

Ensure that the same needle insertion angle and depth of penetration are used consistently for each cannulation of a constant site.

Figure 3.11. Cannulating a buttonhole.

© NxStage Medical, Inc. Used with permission by NxStage Medical, Inc.

member to be present for each dialysis treatment to accommodate the process of track formation.

(b) In some units, if the original cannulator cannot be present, other staff members do not use the buttonhole sites for dialysis.

(c) Following the transition to the blunt needles, the single cannulator is no longer required. Subsequent staff should use only the blunt needles and must follow the direction and angle of the established track. The track is what it is and cannulation needs to be done exactly as it was done by the original cannulator to prevent damage to the site.

(2) Physical barriers that make the buttonhole technique challenging.

(a) Scar tissue from previous difficult cannulations, lidocaine use, keloid formation, or old AVFs will make make needle insertion difficult as the vessel moves beneath the fingers of the cannulator.

(b) Excessive amounts of subcutaneous tissue, adipose tissue, or excessive skin resulting from weight loss or loss of muscle mass make the tissue unstable or less firm.

(3) Increased risk of infection at the exit site and the tunnel and septic complications via the bloodstream.

(a) Inconsistent and improper techniques during cannulation can lead to serious infections such as septicemia, septic arthritis, or pericarditis. Meticulous skin preparation of the buttonhole sites is essential before and after dialysis.

(b) Strict adherence to the cannulation procedure is extremely important.

(c) Incorporating the use of antimicrobial ointment to the exit sites may be beneficial.

(d) The scabs covering the buttonhole puncture sites must be completely removed. *Staphylococcus aureus* can become imbedded in the scab and lead to infection.

(e) Having scabs that are larger than the needle hole indicates that the tunnel has been manipulated. For example, it was entered at multiple angles, was created at an overly steep angle, or someone was searching for the tunnel.

(4) Indented buttonhole sites – "hubbing."
  (a) The needle hub exerts a constant pressure on the skin at the point of entrance that does not rotate. With repeated cannulations, the mouth of buttonhole enlarges. With further use and deterioration a concave area develops.
  (b) The hub of the needle becomes buried in the entrance to the tunnel and becomes invisible.
  (c) Potential issues: inability to remove scab or clean the entrance completely, trauma to the entrance can increase, and/or breakdown of the epithelial lining of the tunnel.
  (d) Prevention: leave approximately 1/16th inch of the needle exposed preventing the hub from coming into contact with the skin.
  (e) Relocation of the buttonhole may be indicated.
e. Cannulation.
  (1) Assess fistula as previously described.
  (2) The patient (or staff if patient unable) must wash the access with antimicrobial soap just before dialysis. Overall hygiene is extremely important and must be emphasized.
  (3) Disinfect the cannulation sites per facility policy and procedure and manufacturer's recommendations.
  (4) Remove the scabs using a separate sterile device for each buttonhole site to insure precise needle insertion into the tunnel.
    (a) Moistening the scabs may ease the procedure and lessen any pain.
    (b) Care must be taken to not traumatize the sites as this can increase the chance of infection.
    (c) Care must also be taken not to fragment the scab making it necessary to remove the remaining pieces.
    (d) See Table 3.8 to see various methods for scab removal that were found in the literature.
  (5) Perform a second disinfection of the cannulation sites per facility policy and procedure and manufacturer's recommendations.
  (6) Continue with cannulation using aseptic technique. The tunnel and the entrance to the vessel must be aligned. If they are not, it could be due to:
    (a) The cannulator trying to manipulate the needle through the tunnel. A point of resistance will be felt. Do not push

on the tunnel as it will get displaced from the vessel's entrance.
    (b) Excessive fluid intake or previous inadequate fluid removal leading to the blood vessels stretching and shifting the vessel wall out of alignment with the tunnel.
    (c) The cannulator not using the exact procedure as when the tunnel was created; for example, using a tourniquet or not.
  (7) To realign the tunnel and the vessel's opening.
    (a) Position the blunt needle up to the point of resistance.
    (b) Lift the tunnel slightly until the opening is found.
    (c) If this does not work, the needle should be removed, the site bandaged, and a sharp needle inserted elsewhere preserving the buttonhole for future use. Avoid the area 3/4 inch in front of the buttonhole site.
    (d) Do not insert a sharp needle into the buttonhole. While it will work, it will also create the potential for aneurysm formation, especially if done frequently.

D. Needles that infiltrate (KDOQI, 2006, CPG 3; Rosenthal, 2014; Vachharajani, 2010).
  1. Definition (see Figure 3.12).
    a. The inadvertent administration of fluid into the tissue surrounding the fistula; occurs when the needle is no longer in the fistula.
    b. Can be secondary to improper cannulation technique.
    c. Can occur before dialysis, during dialysis when the blood pump is running, or after dialysis with needle removal.
  2. Symptoms: edema, taut or stretched skin, pain.
  3. Prevention.
    a. Monitor closely for signs and symptoms of infiltration. A quick response to a needle infiltration can help minimize damage to the access.
    b. Use caution when taping needles. Avoid lifting up on the needle after it is in the vein. An improper needle flip or taping procedure can cause an infiltration.
    c. Closely monitor the arterial and venous pressures during the treatment and observe the access site frequently.
    d. Proper needle removal prevents postdialysis infiltrations.
      (1) Apply the gauze dressing over the needle site, but do not apply pressure.

Table 3.7

Methods for Scab Removal for the Buttonhole Technique

Below are methods for scab removal when using the buttonhole technique for needle insertion that were described in the literature. It must be remembered that whichever technique is used, the entire scab must be removed, the mouth of the tunnel must be protected from trauma, and infection control is imperative. Per CDC guidelines, a separate sterile device should be used for each site.

Potential utensils and techniques are included in the discussion below.

1. Aseptic tweezers.
2. Sterile pick supplied by some manufacturers with the needle package.
3. Soak the site with a moist towel prior to scab removal; followed with soaking the site with an antiseptic solution; stretch the skin around the scab; and then, remove the scab with a blunt needle.
4. Stretching the skin around the buttonhole may aid in loosening the scab.
5. Gentle wiping is preferred over scrubbing as it can cause irritation to the area.
6. Cover the scab for 5 minutes with an alcohol pad; then remove the scab with a sterile needle.
7. Cover the scab and presoak with a two 2x2s saturated with tap water and antibacterial soap. May need to soak for up to 20 minutes.
8. Cover the scab with two 2x2s soaked with normal saline that is drawn out of the saline bag used to prime the system. Allow to soak as the patient's pre-assessment is completed. Use the thumb and forefinger to grasp the 2x2 and pull the scab off insuring that the entire scab is removed. (Alcohol based gel could be used instead of normal saline.)
9. Send the patient home with some alcohol pads and roll of tape. Have the patient tape an alcohol pad over the scab prior to coming to the facility for dialysis.
10. Use of a facial sponge or shower scrubber.
    a. The sponge/scrubber is never used by another person or for another purpose.
    b. After use the item is washed with antimicrobial soap, rinsed under hot tap water, squeezed to remove excess water, allowed to air dry, and stored in a sealable container that is cleaned with a diluted bleach solution weekly.
    c. Prior to coming to the facility for treatment, the patient completes the following procedure: immerse the sponge/scrubber in hot water for a minimum of 30 to 45 seconds prior to use; apply antibacterial soap to the buttonhole site and move the scrubber in a circular motion; use moderate pressure over the site until the scab comes off. The small slit will be covered with thin, new dermis that can be seen with close inspection. This is the entrance to the buttonhole track.
    d. When the patient is at the facility, the site is disinfected and cannulated following the facility's policies and procedures.
11. Note: Sterile needles should not be used because of the risk of cutting the skin and fragmenting the scab.

Source: Ball, 2006; Ball & Mott, 2010; Deaver, 2010; Doss et al., 2008; Mott & Moore, 201

(2) Carefully remove the needle at approximately the same angle as it was inserted. This prevents dragging the needle across the patient's skin. Using too steep of an angle during needle removal may cause the needle's cutting edge to puncture the vein wall.

(3) Do not apply pressure to the puncture site until the needle has been completely removed.

4. Potential interventions and treatments.
   a. If the infiltration occurs after the administration of heparin, care must be taken to properly clot the needle tract and not the fistula. In some cases, the decision to leave the needle in place and cannulate another site may be appropriate.
   b. The immediate application of ice can help decrease the pain and size of the infiltration and may decrease bleeding time. Use a thin towel to prevent frostbite. Follow the facility's policy and procedures.
   c. If the fistula is infiltrated, it is best to rest the fistula for at least one treatment.
      (1) If this is not possible, the next cannulation should be above the site of the infiltration.
      (2) If the patient still has a catheter in place, restart use of the fistula with one needle and advance to two needles, larger needle size, and greater BFRs as the access allows.
      (3) Imaging studies could be considered.

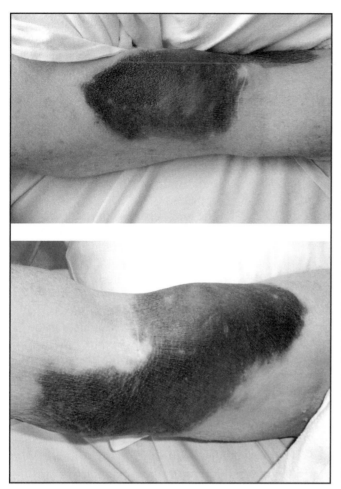

Figure 3.12. Massive infiltration due to improper cannulation technique.

Source: Vachharajani, T.J. (2010). *Atlas of dialysis vascular access*. Wake Forest University School of Medicine, North Carolina. Used with permission.

SECTION C
The Arteriovenous Graft (AVG)

I. Overview of the AVG.

A. Definition and characteristics (Kumar et al., 2007; NKF-KDOQI, 2006, CPG 1 & 2; CDC, 2014a).
   1. A surgically created connection between an artery and a vein using an implanted material (typically synthetic or, less frequently, biologic) to provide a permanent vascular access for hemodialysis.
   2. Needles are inserted into the graft to remove and return blood during hemodialysis.

Note. Needles are never inserted into the anastomoses.

---

   3. The average graft diameter is 6 mm, although some grafts have a diameter of 8 mm.
   4. A mature graft is one in which the edema and

erythema have resolved and the course of the graft is easy to palpate. This helps to prevent inaccurate needle placement or laceration during needle insertion.
   5. The maximum flow rate through the graft is reached in a matter of days to weeks.

B. Surgical classifications and process (Houle, 2004; Kumar et al., 2007; NKF-KDOQI, 2006, CPG 2; Vachharajani; 2010).
   1. Patients are candidates for grafts if they do not have adequate native vessels suitable for an AVF or have a failed fistula that is in the same location of the planned graft. An AVG is the second best option for hemodialysis.
   2. Types of grafts.
      a. Synthetic grafts are usually made of expanded polytetrafluoroethylene (ePTFE/Teflon®) and may be tapered for the arterial anastomosis or contain ringed segments to prevent kinking at the apex of the loop. Tapering and external reinforcement have not been shown to significantly improve the outcomes for the AVG.
      b. The composite/polyurethane graft has a temporary advantage over ePTFE. Because of its self-sealing property, it can be cannulated within hours of placement.
         (1) Use of this graft may avoid the need for a temporary catheter.
         (2) More skill is required for insertion to prevent kinking and twisting in the tunnel.
         (3) Preferably 24 hours can pass before it is used to allow the swelling to decrease and make the AVG easier to palpate.
      c. Biologic grafts are sometimes autogenous veins or cryopreserved human veins but most frequently are from treated bovine vessels. The latter have been shown to provide functional access for patients who have failed PTFE.
   3. Anatomic locations, configurations, and placement priority.
      a. A forearm loop graft is preferable to a straight configuration and is the most common AVG (See Figure 3.13).
      b. An upper-arm graft is usually a straight connection between the brachial artery and the basilic or axillary vein.
      c. Chest wall or "necklace" prosthetic graft or lower-extremity graft; used after all arm sites have been exhausted.
      d. "Femoral placement of access has been associated with proximal venous stenosis, which may be problematic later in patients receiving kidney transplantation" (NKF-KDOQI, 2006). Generally, a thigh AVG is a last resort.

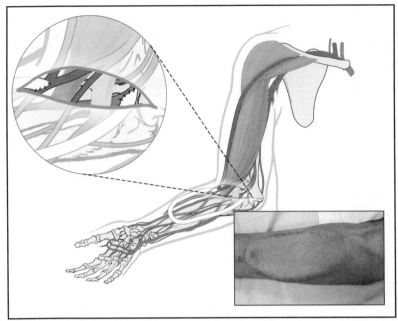

Figure 3.13. Forearm loop AV graft.

Source: Vachharajani, T.J. (2010). *Atlas of dialysis vascular access.* Wake Forest University School of Medicine, North Carolina. Used with permission.

1. The graft has a higher rate of stenosis and thrombosis as compared to the AVF.
2. The AVG has a higher rate of infections as compared to the AVF.
3. With a graft, there is a higher mortality rate as compared to the AVF.
4. The AVG has a shorter length of patency as compared to the AVF.
   a. Grafts last 1 to 2 years before indications of failure or thrombosis appear.
   b. The long-term patency rate with treatment of stenosis and thrombosis remains at 2 years for the AVG.
5. The sites where needles were inserted seal but do not heal.
6. There is potential for allergic reaction to the material that the graft is made out of.
7. Potential for steal syndrome exists in patients with compromised peripheral vasculature.

C. Advantages of the AVG (Ball, 2010; Kumar et al., 2007; NKF-KDOQI, 2006, CPG 2;).
   1. The AVG has a large surface area available for needle insertion.
   2. Technically a graft is easier to cannulate as compared to a new fistula.
   3. The time from surgical insertion to maturation is short.
      a. For the ePTFE graft, it is recommended to wait 1 to 3 weeks prior to cannulation.
      b. This time allows for healing and the incorporation of the surrounding tissue into the graft. This minimizes the amount of blood that might leak into the tissues after needles are removed.
      c. Preferably the AVG is not used for 3 to 6 weeks to allow healing of the incision and resolution of pain and swelling.
      d. Some grafts have self-sealing properties that allow them to be safely used earlier.
   4. The AVG can be placed in many areas of the body, including the upper surface of the thighs and the anterior chest wall.
   5. It can be placed in a variety of shapes to facilitate placement and cannulation.
   6. The AVG is easier for the surgeon to handle, implant, and connect the vascular anastomoses.
   7. The graft is comparatively easier to repair either surgically or by going through a small incision made into the vascular system.

D. Disadvantages of the AVG (Kumar, 2007; NKF-KDOQI, 2006, CPG 2; Sofocleous, 2013; Vachharajani, 2010).

E. Assessment of the Graft – Look, Listen, Feel (ANNA, 2011; Ball, 2005; Banerjee, 2009; NKF-KDOQI, 2006, CPG 4; Vachharajani, 2010).

Note. The reader is referred to the Assessment of the Fistula as much of the information is the same.

   1. Inspection – look.
      a. The patient with a forearm graft should have routine "sleeves up" examinations of that upper arm. If it has a well-developed cephalic vein, it may be able to be converted into a secondary fistula at a later time if and when needed.
      b. Compare the access extremity with the other extremity noting any obvious differences.
      c. Assess the access extremity for swelling, presence of collateral veins, change in color or temperature, decreased sensation, limitation of movement, and/or capillary refill in the nail beds.
      d. Assess the graft for redness, warmth, drainage from previous needle sites, ecchymosis, hematoma formation, rash, break in the skin, pseudoaneurysm, or stenosis.
   2. Auscultate – listen.
      a. Note any change in the sound or character of the blood flowing through the graft.
      b. The bruit is the "whooshing" sound; a high-pitched bruit might be a sign of an underlying stenosis.
   3. Palpate – feel.
      a. Enables one to determine that blood is flowing through the graft.

b. The thrill is the sensation that is felt over the graft.

II. Overview of potential problems and complications of the AVG.

A. Infection (ANNA, 2011; Ball, 2005; CDC, 2014a; CMS, 2008, April 15; Deaver, 2010; Kaplowitz et al., 1988; NKF-KDOQI, 2006, CPG 5; Schanzer, 2002).
   1. Potential causes.
      a. *Staphylococcus aureus* is the leading cause. It is known that patients on dialysis have more staph on their skin and in their nares than the general public.
      b. Poor patient hygiene.
      c. Inadequate skin preparation before cannulation.
      d. Not using aseptic technique for cannulation.
      e. Seeding from another infected site in the body.
      f. Bacteria can also be introduced from:
         (1) Pseudoaneurysms/aneurysms. The walls are thin and allow bacteria to be more easily introduced into the vessel if the area is not avoided.
         (2) Clot formation near or within the aneurysm or at the site of an infiltration. Clots provide a site to which bacteria can attach.

Note. Retained graft material can cause a subclinical infection. It might manifest itself as resistance to erythropoiesis-stimulating agents (ESAs) along with evidence of an inflammatory response. An abandoned and nonfunctioning graft is often the culprit and needs to be removed to stop the response.

   2. Signs and symptoms.
      a. Inflammation.
      b. Pain.
      c. Skin break with drainage along the course of the graft.
      d. Fever.
   3. Potential interventions and treatments.
      a. Healthcare providers, including physicians, nurses, and technicians, can prevent many infections by following basic infection prevention recommendations.
      b. Assessing the AVG every treatment is a critical step and can be considered a primary intervention.

Note. Cannulation of an access with an infected segment should be done only with a physician's, APRN's, or PA's order if dialysis is extremely urgent. The infected area must be avoided.

c. Report any abnormal findings or problems to the vascular access team.
d. Obtain culture of any exudates per protocol or as ordered.
e. Administer parenteral broad spectrum or organism sensitive antibiotics as ordered.
   (1) The initial antibiotic therapy should cover both gram negative and gram positive microorganisms.
   (2) Culture results should specify which subsequent antibiotics are appropriate.
   (3) Incision and drainage might be helpful.
f. Surgical resection and removal of the affected portion or all of graft may be needed.
g. A surveillance system must be in place that identifies at least the date of infection onset, infection site, full identification of the infecting organism(s), and antimicrobial susceptibility results.
   (1) Requires participation of the interdisciplinary team.
   (2) Necessary because of the high correlation to morbidity and mortality.

Note. Infection occurring within 3 weeks of surgery is generally considered perioperative infection and is usually prevented by prophylactic antibiotics at the time of surgery.

B. Stenosis and edema in the extremity (Ball, 2005; Kumar et al., 2007; NKF-KDOQI, 2006, CPG 4 & 5; Schanzer, 2005; Solocleous, 2013; Vachharajani, 2010; White, 2006).
   1. Causes.
      a. Begins with hyperplasia of the venous intima at or downstream from the anastomosis between the graft and the vein.
      b. The hyperplasia is probably caused by turbulence at the anastomosis and compliance mismatch between the graft and the vein.
      c. The stenosis leads to obstruction and eventually thrombosis. Approximately 90% of clotted grafts are associated with stenosis.
         (1) The blood flow in the graft is decreased.
            (a) The average blood flow rate through an AVG is 1,000 mL per minute; that rate can be up to 3,000 mL per minute.
            (b) A blood flow rate of 600 mL to 800 mL per minute is needed to maintain patency.
         (2) The intragraft pressure is increased.
         (3) The lower blood flow may reduce the efficiency of the hemodialysis treatment.
      d. The most common lesions in AVGs; occur most often in the venous end of the graft – an outflow stenosis.

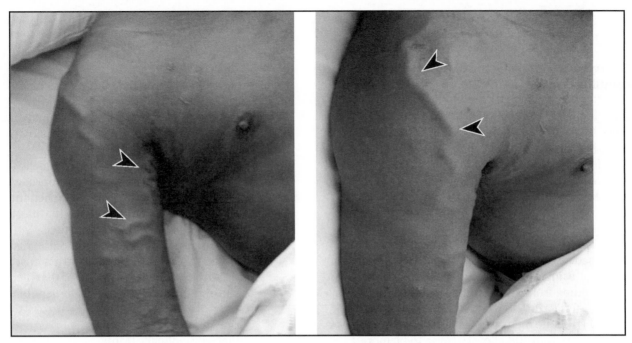

Figure 3.14. Central venous stenosis. The collateral veins can be seen on the patient's shoulder and chest (arrowheads).
Source: Vachharajani, T.J. (2010). *Atlas of dialysis vascular access.* Wake Forest University School of Medicine, North Carolina. Used with permission.

e. It is estimated that 20–25% of lesions occur in the artery or the arterial anastomosis and affect blood flow into the graft.

f. Lesions that are considered hemodynamically significant reduce the vessel's diameter by at least 50%.

2. Potential interventions and treatments.

a. If the graft was recently inserted and edema is present, the arm should be kept elevated above the level of the heart whenever the patient is sitting or lying down.

b. Report any abnormal findings or problems to the vascular access team.

c. If the swelling persists beyond 2 to 3 weeks, imaging to detect pathologic stenosis is indicated.

(1) If present, angioplasty will be needed for correction.

(2) A stent may need to be inserted if the stenosis returns after angioplasty (known as recoiling).

d. Preemptive treatment of stenosis may prevent clotting.

C. Central venous stenosis (CVS) (Gottmann et al., 2012; Kotoda et al., 2011; NKF-KDOQI, 2006, CPG 6; Vachharajani, 2010). CVS is a serious complication for patients on hemodialysis and one that requires more research to understand its causes, prevention, and treatment (see Figure 3.14).

1. Causes or contributing factors.

a. History of multiple central venous catheters but may develop without a history of central venous catheter placement.

(1) Majority of stenotic lesions have been found in the subclavian vein.

(2) Another common site is the junction of the subclavian and cephalic veins.

(3) Possibly related to catheter insertion technique or catheter movement, leading to endothelial damage, hyperplasia, and fibrosis.

b. Mechanical compression of the central venous system by surrounding structures may play a role, such as the position and size of muscles, ligaments, and bones.

c. The arterialized high flow in the central veins coming from the access leads to changes in flow dynamics and results in abnormal shear stress, turbulence, and platelet aggregation.

d. Other potential culprits: indwelling intracardiac wires or PICCs.

e. Some occur without an identifiable cause.

2. Signs and symptoms.

a. Massive swelling in the upper extremity (in the same arm with the access).

b. An extensive network of collateral veins over the shoulder and chest develop.

c. Pain and discomfort that increases during the dialysis session.

3. Potential interventions and treatments.

a. Prevention of CVS through the avoidance of central venous catheters for dialysis, especially catheters inserted into the subclavian.

b. Report any abnormal findings or problems to the vascular access team.

c. Early detection and treatment of CVS reduces the rate of thrombosis and increases the likelihood of preserving the extremity for future access.

d. Transluminal angioplasty with possible stent placement.

e. Surgical treatment is very complex and has been associated with substantial morbidity and should be reserved for extreme situations.

D. Thrombosis (Jindal et al., 2006; NKF-KDOQI, 2006, CPG 4&5).

1. Causes.
   a. Stenosis at the anastomoses, within the graft, in the outflow vein or the central veins.
      (1) Though the venous anastomosis is the most common site of stenosis, inflow stenosis at the arterial end can be as high as 20–25%.
      (2) Stenosis is the cause of 90% of the clotted grafts.
   b. Significant hypotension due to volume depletion.
   c. Hypercoagulable states.
   d. Prolonged occlusive compression from a pressure dressing, clamps, tight clothing or jewelry. Anything that leaves an impression is considered too tight.
   e. Supporting heavy objects such as a basket handle or a sleeping head.

Note. Lifting heavy objects with the hands once the suture line is well healed > 10 days postoperatively will not damage the AVG.

---

2. Signs and symptoms of impending thrombosis.
   a. Significantly decreased intra-access blood flow (< 600 mL/min for AVG).
   b. Increased static venous pressures proximal to the stenosis. This can lead to extended time to control bleeding postdialysis and to the appearance of new pseudoaneurysms.
   c. Increased standardized dynamic venous pressures.
   d. Changes in the quality of the bruit.
   e. Pulsation rather than thrill.
   f. Difficulty cannulating the graft or pain with cannulation.
   g. Abnormal coagulation studies that indicate a hypercoagulable state.
   h. Evacuation of clots even when the needle is properly inserted into the center of the vessel.
   i. Increased viscosity of intra-access flow as evidenced by:
      (1) Difficulty maintaining extracorporeal blood flow at the prescribed rate without

an increase in the venous pressure and a decrease in the arterial pressure.
      (2) Access recirculation causing unexplained decrease in Kt/V and URR. This is a late sign.
      (3) Late stage recirculation (black blood syndrome) develops when the same blood is being recirculated through the dialyzer and becomes deoxygenated as well as hemoconcentrated. This is a very late sign and constitutes an emergency requiring same day intervention.

Note. Recirculation can be verified by introducing saline into the venous bloodline; if the blood in the arterial bloodline lightens in color, recirculation is confirmed.

---

   j. The final signs of thrombosis in an AVG are the absence of thrill and bruit along the access vessel.
      (1) There may be a strong pulse in the artery at the inflow anastomosis.
      (2) Do not cannulate the graft to confirm. Needle holes in a thrombosed access complicate thrombectomy and complicate or prevent lytic administration.

3. Report any abnormal findings or problems to the vascular access team.

4. Potential interventions and treatments.
   a. Urgent referral to an interventionalist or surgeon to:
      (1) Prevent thrombosis by detecting and treating stenosis.
      (2) Potentially perform a thrombectomy by lysing with a thrombolytic such as tPA (tissue plasminogen activator) to soften or resolve clot.
         (a) This is frequently used before mechanical thrombectomy.
         (b) Should be followed by correction of causative stenosis if indicated with angioplasty or surgical revision.
         (c) Graft survival will be longer after elective angioplasty than with an urgent thrombectomy.
      (3) Thrombectomy.
         (a) While thrombectomy should be attempted as early as possible after clot formation, the procedure can still be successful even after several days.
         (b) A major goal is to prevent the need for a temporary access.
   b. Access monitoring and surveillance postprocedure to assure normal flow and pressure parameters.

c. Anticoagulation in proven hypercoagulable states.

d. Targeted ultrafiltration to patient tolerance.

e. Patient and staff education about prevention of:
  (1) Prolonged occlusive pressure.
  (2) Hypovolemic hypotension.

E. Graft deterioration and pseudoaneurysm (NKF-KDOQI, 2006, CPG 5).

1. Cause: repeatedly inserting the needles in the same area of a graft leads to bleeding into the incorporating tissue; this forms the pseudoaneurysm which is not uncommon (see Figure 3.15).

  a. As the pseudoaneurysm expands, it can cause stretching of the overlying subcutaneous tissue.

  b. Combined with the scar tissue that results from multiple cannulations, the microcirculation can become compromised.

  c. This causes tissue breakdown and puts the patient at risk for bleeding and/or graft rupture.

  d. Chronic outflow stenosis or obstruction contributes to aneurysm formation.

2. Signs.

  a. A sudden appearance of an irregular, pulsatile mass on the surface of the graft.

  b. An increase in the size of the pseudoaneurysm resulting from increased pressure in the vessel.

  c. A shiny appearance secondary to the thinning of the skin overlying the vessel.

  d. Poor healing of needle sites.

  e. A pseudoaneurysm tends to develop clots and can lead to clotting of the graft.

3. Potential interventions and treatments.

  a. Rotate the needle puncture sites to prevent this complication.

  b. Report any abnormal findings or problems to the vascular access team.

  c. Never cannulate a pseudoaneurysm. Doing so can cause further vessel deterioration and can make it more difficult to locate the center of the underlying vessel flow.

  d. A rapidly progressing pseudoaneurysm is one that is more than twice the diameter of the graft. It requires surgical repair or placement of a covered stent.

  e. Skin deterioration also requires surgical repair. The patient is put at risk for infection and access rupture that is a life-threatening emergency.

Note. Cannulation through a stent is an off-label use of the device and should never be done without a physician's, APRN's, or PA's order.

F. Steal syndrome is ischemia of the extremity distal to the arterial anastomosis. It is usually seen early after

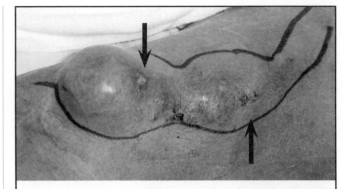
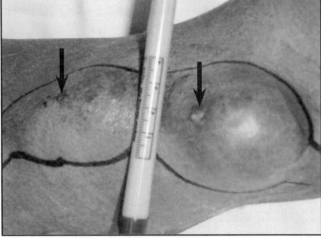

Figure 3.15. Pseudoaneurysm. The AVG in the upper extremity has a lumen diameter of 0.6 cm. The current KDOQI recommendation is to refer patients for surgical evaluation if the diameter is 1.5 to 2 times the normal.

Source: Vacharajani, T.J. (2010). *Atlas of dialysis vascular access.* Wake Forest University School of Medicine, North Carolina. Used with permission.

---

the placement of an AVG (Leon & Asif, 2007; Malik et al., 2008; Suding & Wilson, 2007; Tordoir et al., 2004; Vacharajani, 2010).

1. Cause: diversion of significant volume of blood away from the peripheral circulation.

2. Occurs more frequently in patients who:
  a. Are elderly.
  b. Have peripheral vascular disease.
  c. Have diabetes.
  d. Have a history of multiple access surgeries in same extremity.

3. Signs and symptoms may increase during dialysis.
  a. Pain distal to anastomosis.
  b. Cold, pale hand.
  c. Impaired hand movement and strength.
  d. Paresthesias: numbness, tingling (pins and needles).
  e. Poor capillary refill of affected nail beds (> 2 seconds).
  f. Potential progression to ulcerated, necrotic fingertips.

4. Diagnosis.
   a. Based on physical examination.
   b. Confirmed with ultrasound to measure arterial flow to fingertips (plethysmyography/PPGs).
5. Potential interventions and treatments.
   a. Report any abnormal findings or problems to the vascular access team.
   b. Surgical reperfusion of the hand using the DRIL (distal revascularization-interval ligation) procedure while maintaining flow through the graft or fistula.
   c. Banding of inflow to the graft to reduce flow.
   d. Severe ischemia not amenable to surgical revision may require urgent ligation of the access.
   e. Symptoms of mild ischemia may be improved by wearing of a glove, keeping the hand dependent as much as possible, exercising, and/or massaging.

G. Traumatic fistula formation.
   1. Cause. A needle passes through the graft during cannulation and creates an abnormal fistula or open track between the graft and an underlying artery. Blood from the artery shunts into the vessel and disturbs the existing flow pattern.
   2. Signs.
      a. Abnormal presence of a strong pulsation in area of graft not previously observed. May be more pronounced than at the arterial anastomosis.
      b. A sudden increase in venous pressure not present during the previous dialysis session is possible.
   3. A referral is needed to an interventionalist for evaluation and/or to a surgeon for possible repair.

III. Preparing the graft for dialysis.

A. Applicable principles (Ball, 2005, CDC, 2002, 2014b; CMS V113, 2008a; NKF-KDOQI, 2006, CPG 3).
   1. The life of the graft may be prolonged and morbidity improved through:
      a. The use of aseptic technique during cannulation. The CDC explains aseptic technique as taking great care to not contaminate the graft site before or during the cannulation or decannulation procedures.
      b. The AVG being mature and ready for cannulation when first used.
         (1) Decreases the risk of infiltration.
         (2) A mature graft is one in which the edema and erythema have resolved and the course of the graft is easy to palpate.
            (a) Helps to prevent inaccurate needle placement.

         (b) Helps to prevent laceration during needle insertion.
   2. Recommended skin preparation prior to dialysis.
      a. Hand hygiene performed by staff and patients is the cornerstone of infection prevention.
         (1) Wash hands with soap and water.

___

Note. Soap and water must be used if the hands are visibly soiled, meaning there is visible dirt or contamination with proteinaceous material such as blood or other body fluid.

___

         (2) May use a waterless, alcohol-based, antiseptic hand rub; usually contains 60–95% alcohol content.
            (a) Vigorously rub hands together for 15 seconds.
            (b) Cover all surfaces of the hands and fingers.
            (c) Continue until hands are dry.
         (3) It is important to wash hands even when gloves are to be worn and after they are removed.
      b. The sites for cannulation should be determined before skin preparation. The prep should be repeated if the skin is touched by the staff or patient.
      c. The access site should be washed using an antibacterial soap or scrub and water. Patients must be educated regarding the necessity of this step. Some patients may have washed before they left home and be reluctant to wash again.
      d. The skin should be cleansed with the appropriate antimicrobial product in use by the facility using the manufacturer's instructions for use – especially the required contact time for efficacy.
         (1) This is one of the most important aspects of cannulation.
         (2) The proper cleansing technique should be used for the antimicrobial product being applied. (See manufacturer's recommendations.)
      e. The importance of dialysis precautions and aseptic technique cannot be over emphasized.

B. Cannulating the AVG for hemodialysis (Atkar & McCrae, 2013; Ball, 2005, 2006, 2010; Ball & Mott, 2010; Ball et al., 2007; Banerjee, 2009; Birchenough et al., 2010; Brouwer, 1995; Evans, 2012; Kim & Kim, 2012; NKF-KDOQI, 2006, CPG 3 & Table 4; Mott & Moore, 2011; Pergolotti et al., 2011; Vachharajani, 2010; Van Waeleghem et al., 2008).
   1. Required dialysis precautions and facility policies and procedures must be followed.

2. In the beginning, the cannulator in the facility who is recognized for expert skills should be the person assigned to insert the initial needles. This is a skills-based determination and should not be based solely on licensure, certification, or seniority. It may be helpful to perform the cannulation during a nonturnover time to allow more time for the procedure in a more relaxed atmosphere. Staff should be cognizant of the anxiety and pain that accompanies needle insertion (refer to Table 3.5).

3. Select the appropriate needle size by visualizing and feeling the AVG.

4. Anesthetics for needle insertion.
   a. Intradermal lidocaine.
      (1) Used immediately prior to needle insertion.
      (2) Causes a bee-like stinging sensation and may be more painful than the needle.
      (3) Risk of accidental intravenous infusion.
   b. Topical anesthetic cream.
      (1) Correct contact time is important for the drug to be effective.
      (2) Needs to be applied by the patient prior to coming to the facility.
         (a) Maximum depth of 3 mm requires 60 minutes of contact.
         (b) Maximum depth of 5 mm requires 120 minutes of contact.
         (c) After application, the patient covers the site with plastic wrap to protect clothing and to ensure that it does not get wiped off prematurely.
   c. Patient preference per facility policy.

5. Needle insertion with a graft.
   a. The rope ladder technique refers to rotating the cannulation sites.
      (1) New sites are chosen every dialysis treatment allowing healing between sessions.
         (a) Too often, certain sites are favored because "they work."
         (b) This practice must be avoided because it leads to weakness in the graft wall.
      (2) Rotating sites prevents pseudoaneurysm formation.
      (3) Potential issues with the rope ladder technique.
         (a) Cannulation with sharp needles can be painful.
         (b) With the associated pain, the patient's satisfaction with care may be reduced.
         (c) The patient's quality of life may be affected if anxiety develops.
   b. Needle placement.
      (1) A tourniquet is not used with an AVG.
      (2) The needles are kept 1.5 to 2.0 inches apart and 1.5 inches from the anastomoses.

      (3) The arterial needle is inserted in the direction of the blood flow into the graft.
      (4) The venous needle should always be inserted in the same direction as the blood flow out of the graft.
      (5) When cannulating a loop graft, a diagram or a specific written description from the surgeon is recommended.
         (a) In most cases, carefully occluding for a brief moment the loop of the graft with a finger will reveal a pulsation that indicates the arterial side of the graft and the direction of the blood flow.
         (b) Reverse needle placement can increase recirculation 20% and lead to inadequate dialysis.
   c. NKF-KDOQI Guideline 3 recommends the use of wet needles for cannulation.
      (1) Use 8 mL of normal saline (NS) in a 10 mL syringe.
      (2) Do not prime the needle until immediately prior to use.
      (3) Used to confirm proper needle placement prior to starting the dialysis treatment.
   d. Pull the skin taut in the opposite direction of needle insertion.
      (1) Avoid excessive pressure to the site to stabilize and prevent the graft from flattening out.
      (2) Compresses the nerve endings that may interrupt the pain-to-brain sensation for approximately 20 seconds.
      (3) Increases surface tension and lessens the surface area contacting the cutting edge of the needle.
      (4) Helps prevent the vessel from rolling.
   e. Grasp the butterfly needles by the wings.
      (1) Prime the needle with NS until all air is purged. Clamp the needle.
      (2) Remove the protective cap and immediately proceed with cannulating the AVG.
   f. A 45-degree angle with the bevel up is used for needle insertion.
      (1) Less steep angles increase the risk of dragging the cutting edge of the needle on the graft's surface.
      (2) Steeper angles increase the risk of perforating the back wall of the graft.
      (3) Having the bevel up facilitates entrance through the skin, subcutaneous tissue, and the graft wall.
   g. When the needle has penetrated, there are basically two methods described by the NKF-KDOQI Guidelines (2006) for advancing the needle.
      (1) Advance the needle slowly with the cutting

edge facing up and do not rotate the needle.
  (a) Any manipulation of the needle may traumatize the wall of the graft.
  (b) This is the preferred method.
 (2) If the AVG is deep and hard to feel, immediately rotate the needle 180° and advance slowly. The bevel/cutting edge of the needle will be facing the bottom of the graft.
  (a) The rotation prevents the top of the intima from being traumatized and averts the tip of the needle from going into the back of the graft.
  (b) Only used when the graft's back wall location is hard to ascertain.
 (3) As the needle is advanced, blood flashback should be visible; the clamp may need to be opened.
  (a) Aspirate back 1 to 5 mL with the 10 mL syringe; flush the needle and clamp.
  (b) The syringe must aspirate and flush easily. Observe for signs and symptoms of infiltration.

Note. Using dry needles for cannulation poses the risk of blood exposure to the staff, the patient, and other patients if the blood sprays or spills when the line is unclamped and the cap is removed to purge the line of air. In addition, proper needle placement cannot be confirmed prior to initiating dialysis.

 h. Once in place, secure the needle with tape.
  (1) Tape the needle at the same angle of insertion to prevent moving the tip of the needle from the desired position within the lumen of the graft.
  (2) It may be helpful if facilities/units have a consistent procedure for taping needles and bloodlines. This can make it easier for the staff to spot potential or impending needle dislodgement as patients are being monitored.
  (3) The chevron technique (U-shaped) for taping needles is widely recommended (refer to Figure 3.8).
 i. The vascular access and needles must be visible at all times during the treatment.
 j. Needle removal at the end of treatment is just as important as needle insertion to protect the access from damage and to facilitate proper hemostasis.
  (1) Remove the needle in the same or similar angle as used for insertion.

 (2) Never apply pressure before the needle is completely out.
  (a) This prevents the cutting edge of the needle from pressing into the graft.
  (b) Dragging the cutting edge along the vessel can also traumitize the graft.
 (3) There are two holes created by each needle – one through the skin and the other through the graft wall.
  (a) Appropriate compression to both holes must be applied using two fingers to hold the site.
  (b) If both sites are not properly compressed, bruising, hematoma formation, and/or break through bleeding (usually in the waiting room) can result.
  (c) The access can become at risk for difficult cannulation, limitation of potential needle sites, and access failure secondary to increased pressure or stenosis formation.
 (4) To encourage hemostasis, the sites should be held by the staff or by the patient, if able, for a minimum of 10 minutes without releasing.
 (5) Excessive bleeding postdialysis (generally considered > 20 minutes but should be individualized) may indicate:
  (a) Increased pressure indicative of an unsuspected outflow stenosis.
  (b) Effects of anticoagulation from a medication, such as warfarin.
 (6) Ensure a thrill can be felt in the access. If not, reduce the digital pressure.
6. Prior to discharge from the facility.
 a. Bleeding should be controlled.
 b. The needle sites should be bandaged per facility policies and procedures.
 c. The access should be assessed.
 d. Needed patient education should be completed and documented, including removing the bandage within 24 hours and what to do should bleeding occur.

C. Needles that infiltrate (NKF-KDOQI, 2006, CPG 3; Rosenthal, 2014; Vachharajani, 2010).
 1. Definition (refer to Figure 3.12).
  a. The inadvertent administration of fluid into the tissue surrounding the graft; occurs when the needle is no longer in the graft.
  b. Can be secondary to improper cannulation technique.
  c. Can occur before dialysis, during dialysis when the blood pump is running, or after dialysis with needle removal.

d. Symptoms: edema, taut or stretched skin, pain.
2. Prevention.
   a. Closely monitor the arterial and venous pressures during treatment.
   b. Monitor closely for signs and symptoms of infiltration. A quick response to a needle infiltration can help minimize damage to the access.
   c. Use caution when taping needles. Avoid lifting up on the needle after it is in the vein.
   d. Proper needle removal prevents postdialysis infiltrations.
3. Potential interventions and treatments.
   a. If the infiltration occurs after the administration of heparin, care must be taken to properly clot the needle tract and not the graft. In some cases, the decision to leave the needle in place and cannulate another site may be appropriate.
   b. The immediate application of ice can help decrease the pain and size of the infiltration and may decrease bleeding time. Use a thin towel to prevent frostbite. Follow the facility's policy and procedures.
   c. If the graft is infiltrated, the next cannulation should avoid the site of the infiltration.

SECTION D
Central Venous Catheters (CVC)

I. Overview of the hemodialysis CVC.

A. Definition (NKF-KDOQI, 2006, CPG 7; CDC, 2014a).
   1. The CVC (see Figure 3.16).
      a. A synthetic, relatively large tube available in varying diameters that is placed into a high-flowing central vein
      b. The catheter either has two side-by-side chambers or lumens (called a dual lumen catheter) or two single lumen catheters (called twin catheters); needed because hemodialysis removes and returns blood at the same time.
         (1) The end of the catheter that enters the patient's bloodstream is the "tip" and has holes for blood to enter or exit.
         (2) The hub refers to the threaded end of the CVC that connects the CVC to the bloodlines during treatment or to a cap when the CVC is not in use.
         (3) The cap is a device that screws on to and occludes the hub.
         (4) The limb is the catheter portion that extends from the patient's body to the hub; also known as the "tail."

   (5) The exit site is where the catheter comes out through the skin.
2. Catheters are essential tools for providing urgent and, in some cases, long-term vascular access.
3. The associated morbidity and mortality that accompany the CVC could be greatly reduced through preventive measures and early treatment of complications.

B. General principles and classifications of the CVC (CDC, 2014a; Dutka & Brickel, 2010; NKF-KDOQI, 2006, CPG 2; Vachharajani, 2010).
   1. While the use of a CVC is not preferred, its use may be indicated when the patient:
      a. Is not a suitable candidate for an AVF or AVG as determined by documented vessel mapping; for example, the patient who has:
         (1) Peripheral vascular disease.
         (2) A limited life expectancy.
      b. Has a plan in place to undergo surgery for placement of an AVF or AVG.
      c. Has a maturing AVF or AVG in place.
      d. Is waiting for a scheduled live donor transplant although this is controversial.
   2. Catheters need to be made of rigid or semirigid material, or be structurally reinforced to prevent collapse of the lumen.
   3. Catheter lengths vary with the size of the patient and the site of placement.

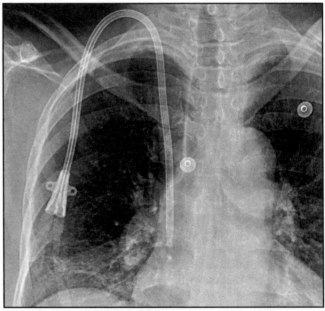

Figure 3.16. Central venous catheter right IJ. The catheter is placed in the right internal jugular vein with a smooth curve in the subcutaneous tunnel. The tip of the catheter is in the right atrium to achieve adequate blood flow during hemodialysis.
Source: Vachharajani, T.J. (2010). *Atlas of dialysis vascular access*. Wake Forest University School of Medicine, North Carolina. Used with permission.

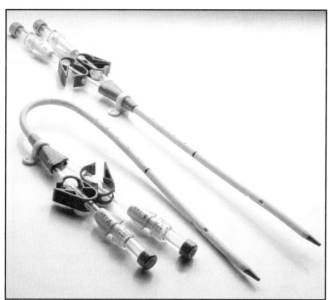

Figure 3.17. Nontunneled, noncuffed acute catheters for short-term use.
Used with permission from Arrow International, Inc.

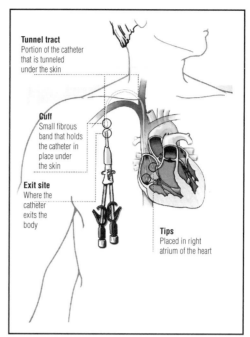

Tunnel tract
Portion of the catheter that is tunneled under the skin

Cuff
Small fibrous band that holds the catheter in place under the skin

Exit site
Where the catheter exits the body

Tips
Placed in right atrium of the heart

Figure 3.18. A tunneled, cuffed dialysis catheter for long-term use.
Used with permission from Arrow International, Inc.

4. Nontunneled, noncuffed catheters (NCC) (see Figure 3.17).
   a. Definition: a CVC that is fixed in place at the point of insertion, goes directly from the point of entry, and terminates close to the heart or one of the great vessels. It lacks a subcutaneous cuff and does not offer a barrier to infection.
   b. BEFORE starting dialysis, the location of the tip should be confirmed by chest x-ray or fluoroscopically at time of placement.
   c. It is intended for short-term use; that is, 3 to 5 dialysis treatments within 1 week.
   d. The patient should not be discharged from hospital with an NCC because of the risk of infection, accidental removal, hemorrhage, air embolism, and patient discomfort. Patient safety must come first.
5. Tunneled, cuffed catheters (TCC).
   a. Definition of the TCC: a CVC that travels a distance under the skin from the point of insertion before entering a vein and terminates at or close to the heart or one of the great vessels (see Figure 3.18).
      (1) A fibrous cuff is positioned subcutaneously about 1 cm from exit site inside the tunnel.
      (2) It is designed to incorporate the tunnel tissue to create a barrier to microorganisms.
      (3) The fibrous cuff also prevents catheter dislodgment.
      (4) When the catheter is inserted, it is sutured into place to allow for "integration" of the cuff with the tissue.

      (a) The process takes approximately 14 to 21 days.
      (b) Once this is complete, the sutures should be removed to prevent inflammation/infection.
   b. Anatomic locations.

Note. Catheters should not be placed on the same side as a slowly maturing long-term access.

---

      (1) Catheters are always inserted into veins.
      (2) The right internal (or external) jugular (RIJ) vein is the preferred site because it offers a more direct route to the right atrium than the left-sided great veins. Catheter insertion and maintenance in the RIJ is associated with a lower risk of complications compared to other potential catheter insertion sites (refer to Figure 3.16).
      (3) Using the left internal jugular (LIJ) vein for catheter placement may be associated with poorer blood flow rates and higher rates of stenosis and thrombosis than the RIJ due to the increased length.
      (4) Femoral placement is associated with the highest infection rates, and the catheter tip must be in the inferior vena cava to avoid regional recirculation (see Figure 3.19).
         (a) Placement of a femoral catheter in a transplant candidate should be avoided.

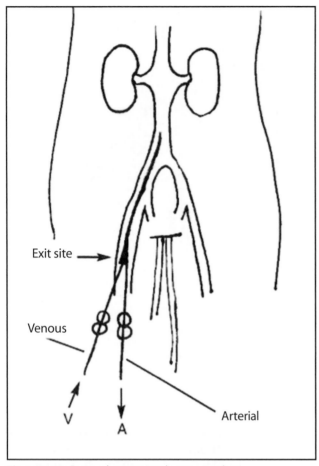

Exit site →

Venous

V   A   **Arterial**

Figure 3.19. Femoral vein central venous catheter.

Table 3.8

How to Differentiate Between an Internal Jugular Vein and a Subclavian Catheter Placement

Inspection

■ Where is the exit site — above or below the clavicle?

■ Can you see the outline of the catheter in a tunnel?

■ Can you see the tunneled catheter crossing the clavicle?

Palpation

■ With a gloved hand, feel the skin above the exit site. Can you feel the catheter in a tunnel?

■ Trace the tunnel till you can no longer feel the catheter. If it crosses the clavicle, it's jugular. If not, it's probably subclavian.

c. To determine whether the catheter is inserted into the internal jugular (IJ) or the subclavian (SC) vein, see Table 3.8.

C. Advantages of catheters (Dhingra et al., 2001; Haddad et al., 2012; NKF-KDOQI, 2006, CPG 2; Oliver et al., 2004; Pastan et al., 2003).
   1. Catheters are universally applicable – anyone can have one.
   2. They can be inserted into multiple sites relatively easily.
   3. They require no maturation time and can be used immediately after the tip position is confirmed by fluoroscopy or chest x-ray.
   4. Catheters cause no changes in the cardiac output or myocardial load.
   5. Not only can they provide an immediate access for dialysis, but also can remain in place over a period of months permitting time for a fistula to mature.

D. Disadvantages of catheters (Haddad et al., 2012; NKF-KDOQI, 2006, CPG 2; Oliver et al., 2004; Pastan et al.,2003).
   1. Infection rate leads to an increase in mortality and morbidity rates.
      a. Higher hospital admission rate associated with sepsis.
      b. Vegetation of heart valves associated with bacteria.
      c. Patients with catheters have a relative risk (RR) of death greater than patients with a fistula (RR = 2.3 for patients with diabetes and 1.83 for those without).
   2. Risk of permanent central venous stenosis or occlusion.

      (b) There is potential to damage the blood vessels needed for the transplant.
      (c) Stenosis of the iliac vein to which the transplanted kidney's vein is anastomosed must be avoided.
   (5) Subclavian veins must be strictly avoided due to risk of stenosis.
      (a) Using either vein can permanently exclude the possibility of a long-term upper-arm fistula or graft.
      (b) The subclavian veins should be used only when all access sites are exhausted in the ipsilateral (same side) arm.
      (c) In addition, subclavian placement puts the patient at greater risk for pneumothorax and/or hemothorax during insertion.
   (6) When all the above sites are exhausted, catheters may be inserted into the inferior vena cava using the translumbar or transhepatic approach.
   (7) In chest and neck placements, the exit site is usually a few centimeters below the clavicle.

E. Assessment (Gomez, 2011; Vachharajani, 2010).
   1. Verify the catheter tip's position before first use either by fluoroscopy or chest x-ray.
   2. Assess the exit site prior to every dialysis for signs of infection and/or skin irritation.
   3. Inspect the exit site for evidence of catheter migration, as evidenced by a visible cuff if it is a cuffed catheter.
   4. Verify the absence of respiratory distress, cardiac arrhythmia, and/or facial or neck edema.
   5. Check the catheter for integrity of the caps, hubs, tail, and dressing.
   6. Notify the physician, APRN, PA, or vascular access team of any assessment findings that will require an intervention.

F. Understanding patient's resistance to a permanent hemodialysis or peritoneal access (Axley & Rosenblum, 2012; Brouwer, 2005).
   1. Potential reasons for refusing a permanent access.
      a. Having had a previous negative experience with surgery (can include a specific surgeon).
      b. Experiencing a previous fistula or graft that did not work.
      c. Fearing the pain associated with needles and cannulation, including:
         (1) Fearing blood or bleeding.
         (2) Not trusting the staff.
         (3) Not wanting to hold the needle sites.
      d. Considering oneself too old for surgery.
      e. Awaiting a kidney transplant.
      f. Having been told that a CVC was appropriate for long-term use.
      g. Perceiving that initiating and terminating dialysis treatments is faster with a catheter.
      h. Sensing a better body image without a visible AVF or AVG.
      i. Having been told or believing that kidney function will return.
      j. Knowing other patients who had experienced problems with an AVF or AVG.
   2. Potential strategies and interventions.
      a. Listen carefully to the patient. Any strategy or intervention should be individualized.
      b. Unless the CVC is the only access option, avoid calling a tunneled cuff catheter a "permanent" catheter or "permcath" as it is misleading to the patient. Instilling the term "bridge" catheter from the very beginning may be helpful.
      c. Through continuous quality improvement activities, gather outcome data on vascular access results and timeliness on individual surgeons; share results with referring nephrologists, APRNs, or PAs.
      d. Facilitate patients sharing their positive experiences with their accesses.
      e. Provide appropriate patient education, including:
         (1) That PD is an option (if appropriate).
         (2) That age is not always a factor with the success of an access.
         (3) That CVCs come with higher rates of morbidity, hospitalizations, infections, and mortality.
         (4) Possible timelines while awaiting transplant.
      f. Limit cannulations of new or difficult accesses to the expert cannulators.
      g. Support patients with needle phobias.
      h. Discuss pain medication appropriate for cannulations with the physician, APRN, or PA.
      i. Explore coping mechanisms, such as visualization, breathing techniques, or music therapy. Involve the social worker as indicated.
      j. Confer with the nephrologist, APRN, or PA regarding patient's concerns and needs.

II. Overview of potential problems and complications.

A. Immediate issues (Haddad et al., 2012; NKF-KDOQI, 2006, CPG 2 & 7).

Note. All catheters should be placed using imaging such as fluoroscopy or ultrasound to assure correct tip placement and to minimize complications. Problems can be lessened and effectively managed by an experienced operator who possesses increased awareness and better technique.

   1. Immediate intraoperative and postoperative complications occur in less than 5% of patients.
   2. Potential complications.
      a. Bleeding.
      b. Catheter malposition or kink.
      c. Vein perforation.
      d. Damage to the carotid or femoral artery including puncture, dissection, or occlusion.
      e. Thrombosis.
      f. Cardiac arrhythmias.
      g. Reaction to medications.
      h. Pneumothorax.
      i. Hemothorax.
      j. Tissue perforation including the brachial plexus, trachea, superior vena cava, or myocardium.
      k. Poor flow from a malpositioned tip.
   3. Use of conditions and practices like those of an operating room must be used for placement of a catheter to prevent infection.

B. Infection (Bonkain et al., 2013; CDC, 2014d; Dutka & Brickel, 2010; Haddad et al., 2012; McAfee et al., 2010; NKF-KDOQI, 2006, CPG 7; Vachharajani, 2010).

Note.   All indwelling vascular catheters are colonized by microorganisms within 24 hours of insertion. "Biofilm" forms on the inside and outside of the catheter's surface and plays a significant role in the colonization process. The biofilm is formed by a combination of host factors and microbial products (slime). It has a critical role in the development of antibiotic resistance and intractable infections. Systemic antibiotics do not penetrate the biofilm.

---

1. Potential causes.
   a. Not using aseptic technique and appropriate cleansing procedures for accessing the catheter.
   b. Poor patient hygiene.
   c. Inadequate skin cleansing at dressing change.
2. Signs and symptoms.
   a. Inflammation and pain around the exit site and in tunnel.
   b. Drainage at exit site or from tunnel.
   c. Erosion of skin over the catheter.
   d. Fever and/or chills.
3. Definitions.
   a. An exit-site infection is localized to the area around the exit site. It does not extend beyond the cuff in the TCC. The exudate culture is confirmed to be positive (see Figure 3.20).
      (1) It is treated with topical and/or oral antibiotics.
      (2) It usually does not require catheter exchange or the insertion of a new catheter at a different site.
      (3) Exit-site erythema with crusting can also be a sign of an allergic response to the topical ointment or tape.
      (4) An exit-site infection can spread through the subcutaneous tunnel and cause more serious consequences.
   b. A tunnel infection occurs when the tract superior to the cuff is inflamed and painful. There may be drainage through the exit site that is culture positive (see Figure 3.21).
      (1) It is a more serious event.
      (2) It requires prompt catheter removal as well as treatment with antibiotics.
      (3) Catheter exchange with creation of a new tunnel may be an alternative if access options are limited.
   c. Catheter related bacteremia (CRB) is defined by positive blood cultures with or without the accompanying symptom of fever.

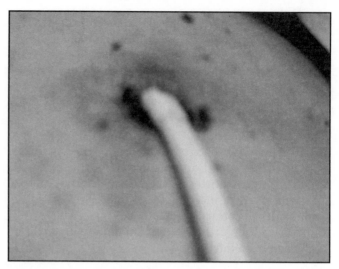

Figure 3.20. Exit site infection. Exit site erythema with crusting is suggestive of infection or allergic reaction to topical ointment or tape. The exit site should be evaluated before every dialysis treatment for early signs of infection. An exit site infection can spread through the subcutaneous tunnel and cause bacteremia, sepsis, and worsening morbidity and mortality.
Source: Vachharajani, T.J. (2010). *Atlas of dialysis vascular access.* Wake Forest University School of Medicine, North Carolina. Used with permission.

      (1) Definite bloodstream infection.
         (a) The same bacteria are identified from the catheter tip and from a peripheral or catheter blood sample.
         (b) There is no other apparent source of infection.
      (2) Probable bloodstream infection.
         (a) Either blood cultures confirm infection and cultures of the catheter tip do not, or cultures of the catheter tip confirm infection but blood cultures do not.
         (b) Fever is reduced after antibiotic therapy with or without catheter removal.
         (c) There is no other apparent source of infection.
      (3) Possible bloodstream infection.
         (a) Reduction in fever after antibiotic treatment or after the removal of the catheter.
         (b) There is no laboratory confirmation of bloodstream infection.
         (c) There is no other apparent source of infection.
4. Metastatic infections are serious life-threatening complications of CRB and require aggressive, long-term antibiotic therapy. Can include:
   a. Infective endocarditis.
   b. Osteomyelitis.
   c. Septic arthritis.
   d. Spinal abscess.

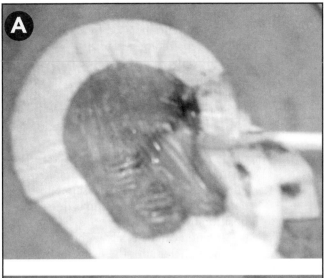

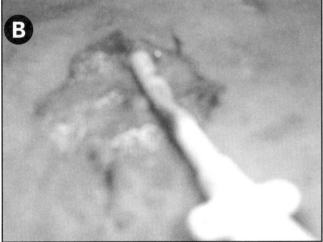

Figure 3.21. Tunnel infection. A. Purulent fluid collection under the dressing suggestive of infection. B. Purulent secretion, erythema over the tunnel and skin changes secondary to infection in the subcuaneous tunnel. The catether must be removed promptly for effective antibiotic therapy and morbidity reduction.

Source: Vachharajani, T.J. (2010). *Atlas of dialysis vascular access.* Wake Forest University School of Medicine, North Carolina. Used with permission.

5. Catheter related infections are not uncommon and are responsible for significant morbidity and mortality. Prevention is a key ingredient.
   a. The CDC's approaches to prevent bloodstream infections in a dialysis unit that are specific to, or can be applied to, a catheter include:
      (1) Observing hand hygiene monthly and sharing the results with the staff.
      (2) Observing catheter care quarterly, assessing aseptic technique when connecting or disconnecting catheters and during dressing changes, and sharing results with the staff.
      (3) Providing continuing education for the staff including the need for strict adherence

to guidelines, infection control, access care, and aseptic technique.
      (4) Evaluating the staff's competency skills (such as catheter care and accessing) every 6 to 12 months and upon hire.
   b. Staff members often have competing demands and time limitations which can lead to not following current guideline recommendations.
   c. The use of neutral-valve closed-system connectors may be useful in preventing CRB and catheter dysfunction.
      (1) The connectors easily interlock onto the catheter hubs and provide an unobstructed blood flow.
      (2) The connectors are flushed with normal saline and used for three consecutive hemodialysis treatments and are then changed out.
      (3) Provide a mechanically closed positive-pressure barrier.
6. Potential interventions and treatments.
   a. Begins with prevention.
      (1) Both staff and patients must be vigilant to potential breaks in infection control techniques.
      (2) Patients must be taught that poor personal hygiene is known to increase their risk for infection.
      (3) Patients with type 2 diabetes are at increased risk for nasal staphylococcal carriage.
   b. Intravenous broad spectrum or organism sensitive antibiotics for all infections except localized exit site where topical and/or oral antibiotics may be used.
   c. Catheter exchange within 72 hours of initiating antibiotic therapy with follow-up cultures 1 week after antibiotic therapy.
   d. Antibiotic lock therapy may be used instead of catheter exchange in cases where the patient is clinically stable and/or the catheter is reinfected with the same organism and catheter sites are limited.

C. Central venous stenosis (CVS) (Brouwer, 2005; Gottmann et al., 2012; Haddad et al., 2012; NKF-KDOQI, 2006, CPG 2 & 7).

Note. CVS has been previously described under the fistula and graft sections.

1. Causes.
   a. Catheters are known to cause CVS related to:
      (1) Site of insertion; this is particularly true of the subclavian vein catheters.
      (2) Number and duration of catheter uses.

(3) Occurrence of infection.
b. Catheter insertion and long-term placement can cause endothelial injury, inflammation, stenosis, and occlusion of any vein.
2. Superior vena cava syndrome.
   a. When CVS occurs in the superior vena cava, it has life-threatening implications and constitutes an emergency to be reported to the physician, APRN, or PA.
   b. It can have slow or rapid onset.
   c. It can prevent the future construction of any vascular access.
3. Signs and symptoms.
   a. Swelling of the chest/breast, arms, neck, and face with periorbital edema.
   b. Visible collateral veins on chest wall and jugular vein distension (if patent).
   c. Central nervous system (CNS) disturbances such as vision changes, dizziness, confusion, and/or pain.
   d. Dyspnea (difficulty breathing) and/or dysphagia (difficulty swallowing).
4. Potential interventions and treatments.
   a. Notify the physician, APRN, PA or vascular access team.
   b. Removal of any obstruction including an indwelling catheter.
   c. Lysing of thrombus with a thrombolytic infusion.
   d. Angioplasty of identified stenosis. Stents could be placed for recoiling stenosis.

D. Catheter dysfunction (Dutka & Brickel, 2010; Haddad et al., 2012; Niyyar & Lok, 2013; NKF-KDOQI, 2006, CPG 7; Vachharajani, 2010).
1. Definition.
   a. A catheter is considered dysfunctional when the attainable blood flow rate is < 300 mL/min at a prepump arterial pressure more negative than -250 mmHg.
   b. There are exceptions for pediatric patients and small adults. For these categories, dysfunction is defined as a significant reduction in baseline flows.
2. Consequences of catheter dysfunction.
   a. Increases in morbidity and mortality.
   b. Increase in economic expenditures.
   c. Effects on the patient's quality of life.
3. Mechanical problems.
   a. Potential causes.
      (1) Poor placement technique.
      (2) A kink in the catheter (see Figure 3.22).
      (3) Partial withdrawal with or without exposure of the cuff.
         (a) A catheter with an exposed cuff can be easily pulled out (see Figure 3.23).
         (b) An exposed cuff also suggests that the

tip is no longer in the correct position.
         (c) It should not be used for dialysis until it is repaired or replaced.
         (d) This catheter can be replaced over a guide wire.
      (4) Cracked hub or broken clamps.
      (5) Patient positioning.
      (6) Thrombosis or fibrin sheath formation (see Figure 3.24).
   b. Potential interventions and treatments.
      (1) Insure that the machine is calibrated.
      (2) Flush the CVC with normal saline to determine if the dysfunction is due to position or clot.
         (a) If blood can be easily withdrawn from the catheter after the flush, malposition of the tip is likely.
         (b) If after flushing, a brisk blood return is not attainable, the catheter is likely occluded by a fibrin sheath or clot.
      (3) Line reversal is attempted to increase the blood flow rate as a temporary fix. This intervention is discouraged due to the potential for:
         (a) Recirculation (86% chance) decreasing the effectiveness of the dialysis treatment.
         (b) Leaving a thrombus without treatment.
      (4) Definitive treatment is catheter exchange.

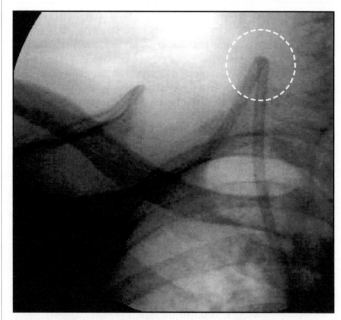

Figure 3.22. Kinked catheter. The catheter in the subcutaneous tunnel is acutely kinked causing mechanical obstruction to the blood flow.
Source: Vachharajani, T.J. (2010). *Atlas of dialysis vascular access.* Wake Forest University School of Medicine, North Carolina. Used with permission.

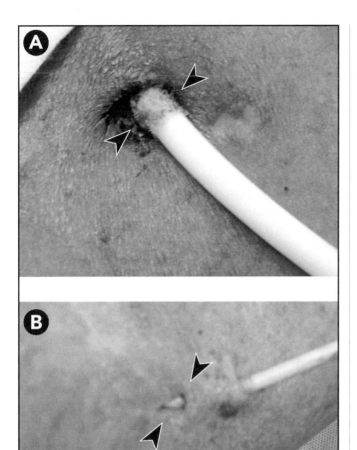

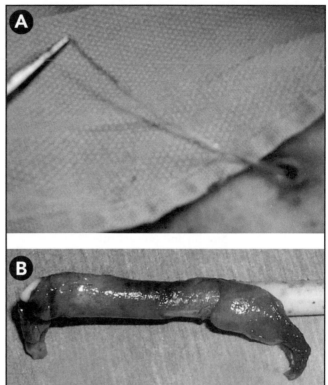

Figure 3.24. Fibrin sheath. An intact fibrin sheath pulled out along with the catheter. A fibrin sheath is a flimsy fibroepithelial tissue that extends from the cuff (A) to the tip of the catheter (B).

Source: Vachharajani, T.J. (2010). *Atlas of dialysis vascular access.* Wake Forest University School of Medicine, North Carolina. Used with permission.

Figure 3.23. Exposed cuff. A catheter with an exposed cuff can be easily pulled out and can lead to the loss of a vital access site. The exposed cuff would also suggest that the tip is no longer in the proper location and delivery of blood through this catheter may not be adequate.

Source: Vachharajani, T.J. (2010). *Atlas of dialysis vascular access.* Wake Forest University School of Medicine, North Carolina. Used with permission.

4. Thrombosis.

Note. An occluding thrombus can become the surface for bacterial proliferation and infection. Likewise, a catheter infection increases the risk of the catheter clotting.

a. Causes.
   (1) Endothelial trauma that occurs with the initial insertion leads to endothelial vessel wall damage.
   (2) The coagulation and inflammatory cascades are chronically activated.
   (3) Changes in the blood flow within the lumen of the catheter between dialysis treatments fuels a continuum of thrombus and fibrin sheath formation.
       (a) A fibrin sheath is composed of flimsy fibro-epithelial tissue.

   (b) It can extend from the cuff to beyond the tip of the catheter.
   (c) The sheath acts like a one-way valve and prevents adequate and free pulling of blood through the catheter.
   (d) The sheath can be disrupted with angioplasty or stripped with a snare device.
b. Types of thrombus.
   (1) Fibrin.
       (a) The fibrin sheath (sleeve) previously discussed. The fibrin adheres to the external surface of the catheter, and the thrombus is trapped between the sheath and the catheter tip.
       (b) The fibrin tail (or flap) which is also known as the ball-valve effect. The fibrin adheres to end of the catheter.
   (2) The intraluminal thrombus within the lumen of the catheter; can be a partial or a complete occlusion.
   (3) The mural thrombus along the wall of the catheter.
c. Warning signs of an impending thrombus.
   (1) Decreased blood flow.
   (2) Increases in the venous pressure.

(3) Decreases in the arterial pressure.
d. Potential interventions and treatments.
  (1) Trending catheter flows is the best predictor of impending failure.
  (2) Catheter "locks" per facility policy.
    (a) An anticoagulant is used to prevent embolic events and their recurrence.
    (b) A thrombolytic is used to break up or dissolve a clot.
       i. High cost with limited effectiveness.
       ii. Only works on clots contained within the lumen.
       iii. Does not work on fibrin sheaths.
    (c) An antibiotic is used to penetrate the biofilm and prevent infection.
  (3) Referral for imaging to check the catheter's position and the possible need for its replacement.

III. Preparing the central venous catheter for dialysis.

A. Applicable principles (CDC, n.d.; CDC, 2014b; NKDOQI, 2006, CPG 3 & Table 6).
1. The life of the catheter may be prolonged and morbidity improved through the use of aseptic technique including:
   a. Performing correct hand hygiene.
   b. Patients and staff wearing masks to prevent airborne contamination; masks should be worn whenever the catheter lumens or exit site are exposed.

Note. "Although data supporting the use of masks during catheter accessing/de-accessing to prevent vascular access infections is lacking, this practice is recommended for patients and staff in the 2000 KDOQI guidelines and is included in the Centers for Medicare and Medicaid Services (CMS) End-Stage Renal Disease Program Interpretive Guidance" (CDC, n.d., Central Venous Catheter Hub Cleaning Prior to Accessing, page 4).

   c. Using "no touch" technique to further reduce the risk for infection.
   d. Wearing disposable clean gloves to further reduce risk for infection.
   e. Allowing antiseptics to dry to obtain their maximal effect.
   f. Minimizing the time that the catheter lumens and exit site are exposed.
   g. Giving special attention to hub care as it can reduce the risk of catheter-related bacteremia.
2. Carefully following required dialysis precautions and facility policies and procedures is crucial.
3. The CDC published catheter connection and disconnection steps on their website: http://www.cdc.gov/dialysis/guidelines/index.html#CDC

B. Recommended practices for cleaning and dressing the CVC (CDC, n.d., 2011; NKF-KDOQI, 2006, CPG 3 & Table 6).
1. The skin around the catheter.
   a. Manufacturer's directions should be adhered to regarding the required contact time for efficacy.
   b. For the first-line skin antiseptic, the CDC recommends the alcohol-based chlorhexidine (greater than 0.5%) solution that is allowed to dry. If the patient cannot use chlorhexidine, use either:
     (1) Povidone-iodine, preferably with alcohol.
     (2) 70% alcohol sterile antiseptic pads that are labeled sterile.
2. The catheter hubs.
   a. The CDC recommends scrubbing the hubs with an appropriate antiseptic after the cap is removed and before accessing.
   b. There is insufficient evidence to recommend one antiseptic over the others. Choices include:
     (1) Greater than 0.5% chlorhexidine with alcohol.
     (2) 70% alcohol.
     (3) 10% povidone-iodine.
   c. The directions from the catheter's manufacturer should be followed regarding the choice of antiseptics as some contain ingredients that will interact with the catheter material.

Note. The CDC has online compatibility information for skin antiseptics and antimicrobial ointments with chronic hemodialysis catheters. Go to http://www.cdc.gov/dialysis/prevention-tools; under prevention tools, click on Hemodialysis Catheter Compatibility Information.

   d. If using an antiseptic that leaves a residue, such as chlorhexidine, avoid allowing large amounts of the solution to enter the lumen of the catheter. This avoids potential toxicities to the patient.
   e. For disinfecting the catheter, pads might be preferred over swabsticks because pads are malleable and allow for more vigorous cleaning of small spaces.
   f. If tape has been used on the caps between treatments, a residue can be left on the hub making disinfection more difficult.
   g. If blood residue is noted, it is important to remove it for the effects of chlorhexidine to be maximized.
   h. Disinfecting should be performed every time the catheter is accessed or disconnected for whatever reason.

i. The hubs should always be handled aseptically.
  (1) Once disinfected, the catheter hubs should not be allowed to come into contact with nonsterile surfaces.
  (2) When disinfecting the hubs, wear clean, nonsterile gloves.
3. Catheter dressings.
  a. The CDC recommends applying povidone-iodine ointment to the catheter exit site after catheter insertion and at each dialysis session. Other potential ointments include:
    (1) Bacitracin/gramicidin/polymyxin B ointment, but it is not currently available in the United States per the CDC website.
    (2) Bacitracin/neomycin/polymyxin B might have a similar benefit and is available in the United States. But studies have not thoroughly evaluated its effect for preventing bloodstream and exit site infections.
    (3) Single antibiotic ointments, e.g., mupirocin.
      (a) Concerns exist about the development of antimicrobial resistance.
      (b) Questions exist about their ability to cover a broad spectrum of potential pathogens; that is, both gram-negative and gram-positive bacteria.
  b. The use of a chlorhexidine-impregnated sponge dressing might be an alternative, for example, the Bio-patch®.
  c. The directions from the catheter's manufacturer should be followed regarding the choice of antibiotic ointment as some contain ingredients that will interact with the catheter material.
  d. The CDC does not have a preference between transparent, breathable dressings and gauze, although gauze is recommended if the exit site is oozing.

SECTION E
The Vascular Access Center

(Dobson et al., 2013; Favero, 2004; Jackson & Litchfield, 2006).

I. Definition.

A. The Vascular Access Center (VAC) is a facility that specializes in radiographic imaging and interventional procedures needed for vascular access care.
  1. It can be hospital based or office based.
  2. It is generally more cost effective if it is a freestanding facility.

B. A 4-year, retrospective cohort study conducted by Dobson et al. from 2006 to 2009, using Medicare claims data from the USRDS, demonstrated the following outcomes for patients treated in a freestanding, office-based center.
  1. There was an average Medicare per member per month payment (including dialysis and medications) that was $584 lower than those who received care in a hospital outpatient department. This amounts to an average annual Medicare savings of $7,008 per patient.
  2. There were 27,613 patients matched across each cohort, the total number of 55,226 representing about 10% of all patients with CKD stage 5 in the USRDS claims.
  3. Other significantly better outcomes included:
    a. A lower mortality rate (11.7%).
    b. Fewer related and unrelated hospitalizations.
    c. Fewer infections and septicemia-related hospitalizations.

C. Care is provided to the patient who has:
  1. Chronic kidney disease and not yet on dialysis.
  2. CKD stage 5 and requiring dialysis.

D. The VAC functions best when it is a part of an integrated vascular access management program.
  1. It does not replace the vascular access coordinator.
  2. While the VAC makes a positive contribution to the overall management of the vascular access, the maximum impact is seen when the other components are in place and strong.
  3. The center has a multidisciplinary team who are experts in hemodialysis access management.
  4. The VAC can increase the placement of fistulas in the persons awaiting dialysis by streamlining the referral process and providing the surgeon with vessel mapping.
  5. The center acts as a community resource for vascular access information and education.

E. The emphasis is on proactive care.

II. Operations and guidelines.

A. Applicable NKF-KDOQI guidelines, which the VAC can help meet.
  1. Placement of the access well in advance of the need for dialysis.
  2. Maximize the creation of the AVF over other types of access.
  3. Provide a system to detect potential problems with an existing access.
  4. Provide diagnostic testing to confirm the problem.

B. The Fistula First change package involves steps that could be carried out in a dedicated VAC.

1. Example: Change Concept 3 – early referral for "AVF only" evaluation and timely placement; vessel mapping can be done at the VAC prior to surgery.
2. Example: Change Concept 10 – education for caregivers and patients; can be carried out by the staff of the VAC.
   a. Provide continuing education activities for the staff.
   b. Supply written and verbal feedback on the findings and intervention required following a patient referral.
   c. Assist the patient in understanding the fistula and the current problem that is occurring.
3. Example: Change Concept 11 – outcome feedback to guide practice; data are sent back to the referring facility that can be used in ongoing improvement initiatives.

C. General areas of services.
1. Preoperative vessel mapping.
   a. Begins with a directed vascular history and physical examination.
   b. Improves the rate of fistula placement.
   c. Increases the rate of successful development of the fistula.
   d. Methods.
      (1) Venogram with contrast.
         (a) There is a potential for an acute worsening of kidney function or an allergic reaction, and there is a lack of arterial study.
         (b) The entire length and continuity of the venous drainage can be well visualized.
      (2) Ultrasonography.
         (a) Requires more operator expertise and more procedure time.
         (b) Yields quality information about the arteries and the veins.
      (3) A combination of venogram and ultrasound.
2. Fistula maturation procedures.
   a. Ultrasonography can assess the development of a young AVF.
   b. Research indicated that an experienced nurse at a dialysis facility well trained in AVF physical examination techniques can discern whether or not a fistula is developing well in 80% of the cases. The nurse is capable of recognizing when a referral needs to be made.
   c. Assessment of the maturation rate starts at the dialysis facility.
      (1) Referral to the VAC should be made if maturation appears to be lagging 8 weeks after surgery.
      (2) A fistulogram can be carried out to assess the entire vascular circuit and abnormalities

identified, for example, the presence of accessory veins or stenosis.
         (3) Potential treatments available at the VAC might include ligation and coil-obliteration of accessory veins or angioplasty.
3. Fistula and graft maintenance procedures.
   a. The dialysis facility staff is responsible for monitoring and trending the AVF/AVG for signs of dysfunction.
   b. The mature fistula can develop stenosis and/or clot; the VAC can carry out corrective angioplasty and thrombectomy if necessary.
4. Identification of opportunities for secondary AVFs.

SECTION F
Monitoring, Surveillance, and Diagnostic Testing – Detection of Access Dysfunction

(ANNA, 2013; CDC, 2014c; Gomez, 2011; NKF-KDOQI, 2006, CPG 4).

I.   Background information.

A. All patients who must start or who are already on hemodialysis require a vascular access. The vascular access must be maintained and kept functioning at an optimal level if the patient is to obtain at least adequate dialysis.
1. Long-standing problems are associated with the vascular access.
2. The effects on the patient's quality of life can be staggering.
3. The vascular access contributes highly to the morbidity and mortality of persons on dialysis.
4. The annual costs of placing, maintaining, treating complications, hospitalizations, and replacing the vascular access are enormous.

B. These costs caused CMS to implement guidelines to assure that patients' vascular accesses are addressed to ensure the best QOL outcomes.
1. CMS implemented guidelines for quality measures to be documented and recorded for quality purposes.
2. Quality measures help drive the implementation of improvements in patient care resulting in a better quality of life for patients and a decrease in the financial costs for organizations.
3. CMS uses the National Kidney Foundation's Kidney Disease Outcomes Quality Initiative guidelines for vascular access monitoring and surveillance as part of their requirements.
   a. CMS incorporates NKF-KDOQI guidelines

into their Interpretive Guidelines that are used when surveying facilities.

  b. The Fistula First Breakthrough Initiative also incorporates some of the guidelines into their change concepts.

 4. Facilities are allowed to implement and demonstrate best recommended practices for patients on hemodialysis.

C. Nephrology nurses have the primary responsibility to preserve the integrity of the vascular access by:

 1. Assuring the highest quality cannulation skills and techniques.

  a. Promoting expert cannulators.

  b. Developing formal cannulation protocols.

  c. Offering the patients the opportunity to self-cannulate.

 2. Identifying potential candidates for an AV fistula.

 3. Preventing access complications.

  a. Providing related education to staff and patients.

  b. Enforcing infection control policies and procedures.

  c. Assessing the vascular access.

  d. Conferring with the nephrologist, APRN, PA, or vascular access team regarding vascular access concerns or problems.

  e. Initiating consultations or request referrals as appropriate.

 4. Actively participating in the facility's access surveillance program and QAPI meetings.

II. Definition of terms in the NKF-KDOQI CPG 4 (page 273).

A. Monitoring – the examination and evaluation of the vascular access by means of physical examination to detect physical signs that suggest the presence of dysfunction.

B. Surveillance – the periodic evaluation of the vascular access by using tests that may involve special instrumentation and for which an abnormal test result suggests the presence of dysfunction.

C. Diagnostic testing – specialized testing that is prompted by some abnormality or other medical indication and that is undertaken to diagnose the cause of the vascular access dysfunction.

D. Access Surveillance Program – a program developed and implemented by an interdisciplinary group in the dialysis setting to assure that access dysfunction is detected early, so appropriate and timely interventions can be executed. This program should include a combination of routine (at least weekly) physical examinations of the access as well as some

form of objective monitoring such as static venous pressure or flow measurements (ANNA, 2013, p. 3).

III. Purpose of access surveillance.

A. A multidisciplinary team works proactively to ensure the patient is receiving an adequate dialysis dose by maintaining access function and patency.

B. Through monitoring and surveillance, the team may detect significant, but asymptomatic, stenosis that develops over variable lengths of time. If detected and corrected, episodes of underdialysis and thrombosis could be minimized or avoided.

C. Monitoring and surveillance can help in fostering the ability to salvage vascular access sites.

 1. Rather than urgent procedures or access replacement, planning, coordination of effort, and elective corrective intervention can prolong the quality and functioning of the access.

 2. There are several types of surveillance and monitoring methods used in the hemodialysis communities, including the inpatient areas. For example, sequential access flow through hemodialysis machines or transonics, sequential dynamic or static pressures, recirculation measurements, and physical examination.

D. The NKF-KDOQI guidelines state there is insufficient evidence to suggest one surveillance method over another. The choice at a particular facility is affected by many variables.

 1. Access type.

 2. Technology.

 3. Effect of operator.

 4. Cost, usually labor.

E. A regular monitoring/surveillance program is recommended to allow for tracking and implementation of issues that can affect patients' vascular accesses. This information should be included into Quality Assurance Program Initiative (QAPI).

 1. Vascular access is a very important part of the QAPI meeting where types of accesses are included as well as the infection rates.

 2. CMS requires dialysis facilities to enter information about vascular accesses into the CrownWeb database which, in turn, reports to CMS and the dialysis networks.

 3. Another reporting mechanism mandated to dialysis facilities is reporting to CDC's National Healthcare Safety Network (NHSN) all access types and infections.

  a. The reports give data for comparison that is discussed at the facility QAPI meetings.

b. The NHSN database reports to CMS and the dialysis networks.
   (1) Infection rates can be compared.
   (2) Low infection rates and best practices can be identified.
c. For further information, go to http://www.cdc.gov/nhsn/dialysis/

SECTION G
CMS ESRD Interpretive Guidelines Pertaining to the Vascular Access

I. Background Information.

A. The Centers for Medicare & Medicaid Services (CMS) Survey and Certification Program functions to:
   1. Certify ESRD facilities for inclusion in the Medicare Program by validating that the care and services of each facility meet specified safety and quality standards, called "Conditions for Coverage."
   2. Provide initial certification of each dialysis facility and ongoing monitoring to ensure that these facilities continue to meet these basic requirements.

B. Purposes of the ESRD survey process.
   1. Surveyors representing the CMS are able to identify deficient facility practices which have real potential for negatively impacting the safety and clinical outcomes for persons on dialysis.
   2. The impact of the survey may improve patient outcomes through individualizing the focus of each survey on the clinical areas where performance improvement is indicated in a facility based on that facility's specific data and information. The individual facility is identified by its single Medicare certification number.
   3. This survey process is intended to determine that the individual dialysis facility and the associated on-site staff are sufficiently qualified, knowledgeable, and equipped to provide safe and effective patient care in compliance with all applicable ESRD Conditions for Coverage.

C. Staff interviews.
   1. The staff interviews included in the survey must be with facility-based staff who routinely perform the care and duties in that area.
   2. The facility record reviews must be of those for that facility only.

II. The following V tag numbers that address the vascular access have been pulled from the ESRD Surveyor Training Interpretive Guidance manual. The entire manual can be found at http://www.cms.gov/Medicare/Provider-Enrollment-and-Certification/GuidanceforLawsAndRegulations/Dialysis.html

A. V-113 Infection control. Wear gloves/hand hygiene.
   1. Staff members should wear gloves while performing procedures which have the potential for exposure to blood, dialysate, and other potentially infectious substances. This includes procedures such as caring for patients' vascular accesses or catheters, setting up reprocessed dialyzers predialysis treatment, inserting or removing the vascular access needles, connecting the dialysis bloodlines to the vascular access needle lines or catheter lines, touching the dialysis bloodlines, dialyzer, or machine during or after a dialysis treatment, administering intravenous medications, handling bloodlines, dialyzers, dialysate tubing and machines postdialysis treatment, and cleaning and disinfecting the dialysis machine and chair postdialysis treatment.
   2. In addition, a new pair of clean gloves must be used each time for access site care, vascular access cannulation, administration of parenteral medications, or to perform invasive procedures.
   3. The intention is to ensure that clean gloves, which have not previously touched potentially contaminated surfaces, are in use whenever there is a risk for cross contamination to a patient's bloodstream to occur.

B. V-146 Infection control. Catheters, general.
   1. It is the intention of the Conditions for Coverage to incorporate relevant guidance from the CDC "Guidelines for the Prevention of Intravascular Catheter-Related Infections," MMWR August 9, 2002/Vol. 51/No. RR-10 into the requirements for facility infection control practices.
   2. Much of the material in this referenced guideline is general or relates to catheter selection, insertion, and use in acute or relatively short-term situations.
   3. The elements of this guidance which are most on point for hemodialysis facilities address the risks posed by intravascular catheters and the need for appropriate staff education, surveillance, vascular access care, and rigorous hand hygiene to reduce these risks.

C. V-147 Infection control. Staff education – catheters/catheter care.
   1. Healthcare worker education and training.
      a. Educate healthcare workers regarding the

appropriate infection control measures to prevent intravascular catheter-related infections.

b. Assess knowledge of and adherence to guidelines periodically for all persons who manage intravascular catheters.

c. Surveillance.

(1) Visually monitor the catheter sites of individual patients. If patients have tenderness at the insertion site, fever without obvious source, or other manifestations suggesting local or BSI (bloodstream infection), the dressing should be removed to allow through examination of the site.

(2) According to the CDC, intravascular catheters solve the problem of attaining vascular access quickly when there is insufficient time for development of a longer-term internal access: ideally a fistula, or secondarily a graft.

(a) Catheters also provide a solution of last resort when internal access site opportunities have been exhausted.

(b) However, despite their expedience, these catheters pose a threat of infection with the potential for immediate and long-term morbidity and mortality consequences for the patient.

(3) The use of catheters for hemodialysis is the most common factor contributing to bacteremia in patients on dialysis, and the relative risk for bacteremia in patients with dialysis catheters is seven times the risk for patients with primary arteriovenous fistulas. Staff must maintain aseptic technique for the care of all vascular accesses, including intravascular catheters.

(4) The CDC lists the two most common routes of catheter infection as:

(a) Migration of skin organisms through the insertion site and into the cutaneous catheter tract resulting in colonization of the catheter tip; and,

(b) Contamination of the hub, resulting in intraluminal colonization of the catheter.

i The initiation and termination of the dialysis process and manipu-lation and tension on the catheter provide frequent opportunity for such contamination.

ii Minimizing the use of intravascular catheters and protection of the insertion site and the catheter hub from contamination through

education and training about rigorous care is important in reducing catheter-related infections.

2. Catheter and catheter-site care including PICCs, hemodialysis, and pulmonary artery catheters in adult and pediatric patients.

a. Antibiotic lock solutions: Do not routinely use antibiotic lock solutions to prevent CRBSI (catheter-related bloodstream infections).

b. Catheter insertion sites should be routinely assessed by staff at each treatment.

(1) Most catheter sites are covered with either transparent dressings or gauze.

(2) Patients with catheters should be instructed to replace the dressing if a catheter site has sufficient bleeding or drainage to dampen or soil the dressing between treatments.

c. The CDC advises that prophylactic antibiotic lock solutions be reserved for use only in special circumstances, e.g., in units where the rate of catheter-related bloodstream infection (CRBSI) has not decreased despite optimal maximal adherence to aseptic technique.

d. Facility staff should follow guidance from the NKF-KDOQI Vascular Access Guideline (2006).

(1) "Airborne contaminants from both patients and staff are prevented best by the use of surgical masks when the catheter lumens or exit site are exposed. Wearing clean gloves and avoiding touching exposed surfaces further decreases the risk for infection. Aseptic technique includes minimizing the time that the catheter lumens or exit site are exposed."

(2) Manufacturers' directions should be adhered to for the types of antiseptics recommended for safe cleaning of the skin and catheter.

e. The facility should have an initial and ongoing training program for infection control practices, which includes information on the prevention of intravascular catheter-related infections. Facility policies should address the training and qualifications of staff that may access catheters, in accordance with any State licensure requirements, as well as the frequency for periodic practice audits to verify staff knowledge and adherence to infection control guidelines for intravascular catheters.

D. V-148 Infection control. Monitor catheter-related bloodstream infections (BSI) rates/surveillance.

1. Noncompliance with this requirement should be considered if there is lack of evidence of surveillance for catheter-related infections. A log or another tracking mechanism, such as the

Dialysis Module of the National Healthcare Safety Network (NHSN), should be used.

2. Both the surveillance log/database and the patient's individual medical records should contain detailed information on catheter infections and other adverse events such as, but not limited to, prolonged bleeding, stenosis/clotting, allergic reactions, pyrogenic reactions, cardiac arrests, hospitalizations, and deaths.

E. V-335 Reuse of hemodialyzers and bloodlines. Residual germicidal use.
   1. One of the symptoms of germicide infusion is severe pain and burning in the patient's vascular access.
   2. Patients may interpret pain in the vascular access at the onset of dialysis as pertaining to needle insertion pain.

F. V-405 Physical environment. The dialysis facility must:
   1. Maintain a comfortable temperature within the facility.
   2. Make reasonable accommodations for the patients who are not comfortable at this temperature.
   3. If patients choose to use a blanket or other covering, their vascular access site, bloodline connections, and face must be visible throughout the treatment. A head covering on a patient is acceptable, as are gloves.

G. V-406 Physical environment. The dialysis facility must make accommodations to provide for patient privacy.
   1. When patients are examined or treated and body exposure is required.
   2. For the use of a bedpan or commode during dialysis, initiating and discontinuing treatment when the vascular access is placed in an intimate area, for physical exams, and for sensitive communications.

H. V-407 Physical environment. Patients must be in view of staff during hemodialysis treatment to ensure patient safety (video surveillance will not meet this requirement).
   1. Each patient, including his/her face, vascular access site, and bloodline connections, must be able to be seen by a staff member throughout the dialysis treatment.
   2. Allowing patients to cover access sites and line connections provides an opportunity for accidental needle dislodgement or a line disconnection to go undetected. This dislodgement or disconnection could result in exsanguination and death in minutes.

I. V-454 Patients' Rights. Privacy and confidentiality in all aspects of treatment.
   1. Patients have the right to privacy during activities that expose private body parts while in the dialysis facility. This includes activities related to use of vascular access sites located in the groin or chest and physical examinations.
   2. Options for ways to comply with this requirement include the use of privacy screens, curtains, or blankets. Staff must be able to observe the patient's vascular access, bloodline connections, and face at all times. Refer to V407 under the Condition for Physical environment.

J. V-511 Patient assessment. Dialysis access type and maintenance. Evaluation of dialysis access type and maintenance (for example, arteriovenous fistulas, arteriovenous grafts, and peritoneal catheters).
   1. The efficacy of the HD patient's vascular access and the PD patient's peritoneal catheter correlates to the quality (adequacy) of their dialysis treatments and is of vital importance to their overall health status.
   2. Each HD patient should have an evaluation for the most appropriate type and location of vascular access and of the capacity of the vascular access to facilitate adequate dialysis treatments.
   3. Completion of this evaluation may include referrals to other entities, such as a radiologist or interventionist for vessel mapping or a vascular surgeon for access placement. Such referrals might take place as part of an assessment or as part of a plan of care, if the referral is to address an inadequate vascular access.

K. V-543 Patient plan of care. The plan of care must address, but not be limited to, the following.
   1. Dose of dialysis. The interdisciplinary team must provide the necessary care and services to manage the patient's volume status.
   2. Removal of too much fluid or removing it too fast in one dialysis treatment or going below the patient's target weight may cause hypotension, muscle cramping, and clotting of the vascular access.

L. V-544 Patient plan of care. Achieve and sustain the prescribed dose of dialysis to meet a hemodialysis Kt/V of at least 1.2 and a peritoneal dialysis weekly Kt/V of at least 1.7 or meet an alternative equivalent professionally accepted clinical practice standard for adequacy of dialysis.
   1. The patient's dialysis prescription (dialyzer, blood flow rate, dialysate flow rate, length of treatment time) and the efficacy of the vascular access affect the dose of dialysis delivered.
   2. If alarms stop the dialysis ultrafiltration "clock,"

the "remaining treatment time" or planned treatment time may need to be extended to fulfill the patient's dialysis prescription.

M. V-550 Patient plan of care. Vascular access – monitor/referrals.
   1. The interdisciplinary team must provide vascular access monitoring and appropriate, timely referrals to achieve and sustain vascular access.
      a. The patient on hemodialysis must be evaluated for the appropriate vascular access type, taking into consideration comorbid conditions, other risk factors, and whether the patient is a potential candidate for arteriovenous fistula placement.
      b. Based on the comprehensive assessment, the facility IDT must develop and implement a plan of care to facilitate each patient on hemodialysis receiving and maintaining the most appropriate and optimal vascular access identified for that patient.
   2. A well-functioning vascular access enables the patient on hemodialysis to receive efficient and adequate dialysis treatments, enhancing his/her quality of life.
      a. The determination of which type of vascular access is the most appropriate for the individual patient requires the integration and coordination between the facility IDT, including the patient/designee.
      b. It may include referrals for vessel mapping, surgical consult, Doppler studies, etc., enlisting the participation of other entities, such as primary care physicians, surgeons, interventional radiology, and surgical or vascular access centers for access placement and maintenance.
   3. To meet this requirement to "achieve and sustain" vascular access, the patient's medical record must include evidence of the evaluation and the basis for the decision for placement of the current vascular access.
      a. If the records from the surgeon are not available, the patient's physician, advanced practice registered nurse or physician assistant is expected to provide this information from communication with the surgeon.
      b. If the patient's vascular access is not an arteriovenous fistula, the record should indicate why the patient was determined to not be a candidate for a fistula.
      c. If a patient has been dialyzed with a central venous catheter in excess of 90 days, there should be an active plan in process for the placement of a more permanent vascular access or information in the record to demonstrate that a catheter is the most appropriate vascular access for that patient.

   d. Some patients may not be candidates for a fistula or graft; each patient has a right to make an informed choice.
      (1) Patients must be informed and educated about the benefits, risks, and hazards of each type of vascular access. Repeated education may be needed.
      (2) The IDT must involve the patient/designee in the plan for vascular access. The facility social worker should be involved and determine whether psychosocial considerations, such as body image, needle fear, or anxiety need to be addressed.
   4. Refer to the Measures Assessment Tool (MAT), which lists the current professionally accepted clinical standards and CMS CPMs for vascular access.
      a. The MAT incorporates measures and standards from the Department of Health and Human Services' Fistula First Breakthrough Initiative.
      b. This initiative has joint goals of increasing fistula use in patients on dialysis, while also decreasing the inappropriate use of catheters in these patients.

N. V-551 Patient plan of care. Vascular access – monitor/referrals. The patient's vascular access must be monitored to prevent access failure, including monitoring of arteriovenous grafts and fistulae for symptoms of stenosis.
   1. The facility must have an ongoing program for vascular access monitoring and surveillance for early detection of failure and to allow timely referral of patients for intervention when indications of significant stenosis are present.
   2. Patient education should address self-monitoring of the vascular access.
      a. "Monitoring" strategies may include physical examination of the vascular access, observance of changes in adequacy or in pressures measured during dialysis, and difficulties in cannulation or in achieving hemostasis.
      b. Precipitating events should also be noted, such as hypotension or hypovolemia.
   3. Surveillance strategies include device-based methods such as access flow measurements, direct or derived static venous pressure ratios, duplex ultrasound, etc.
   4. For patients with grafts and fistulas, the medical record should show evidence of periodic monitoring and surveillance of the vascular access for stenosis and signs of impending failure.
      a. The documentation of this may be on the dialysis treatment record, progress notes, or on a separate log.
      b. A member of the facility staff must review the vascular access monitoring/surveillance

documentation to identify adverse trends and take action if indicated.

O. V-562 Patient plan of care. Patient/family education and training.
1. The patient care plan must include, as applicable, education and training for patients and family members or caregivers or both, in aspects of the dialysis experience, dialysis management, infection prevention and personal care, home dialysis and self-care, quality of life, rehabilitation, transplantation, and the benefits and risks of various vascular access types. The dialysis facility must provide patients and their family members/caregivers with education and training in these listed areas, at a minimum.
2. The interdisciplinary team (IDT) must have the skills and expertise needed to educate patients on dialysis in these subjects, and to provide this education in a manner understood by the patient and family/caregiver.
3. Patients/designees must receive education regarding the types, risks, benefits, and care of their vascular access, personal hygiene related to dialysis access, infection prevention, dietary and fluid management, etc.
4. The patient's medical record must demonstrate the provision of patient education and training in all of the listed subject areas. There may be a single form or section of the medical record for information on patient education, or it may be located in various parts of the record, such as the progress notes of the members of the IDT.

P. V-582 Care at home.
1. The interdisciplinary team must oversee training of the patient on home dialysis, the designated caregiver, or self-dialysis patient before the initiation of home dialysis or self-dialysis (as defined in § 494.10) and when the home dialysis caregiver or home dialysis modality changes.
2. Home dialysis training must be provided and the patient and/or helper verified as competent to perform home dialysis before they are allowed to function independently.
   a. Although it is expected that most training for home dialysis would take place at the facility, home training may be provided in the patient's home to meet the individual needs of the patient and/or helper.
   b. Retraining must be provided whenever there is a change in home dialysis helper, treatment modality, or home dialysis equipment. Retraining may also be indicated if there are problems such as repeated episodes of peritonitis, vascular access infections, or a

failure to achieve expected outcomes, including goals for dialysis adequacy and anemia.

Q. V-585 Care at home. Be conducted for each home dialysis patient and address the specific needs of the patient.
1. The training must be individualized to the needs of each home dialysis patient.
2. Patients/helpers may be trained in small groups or individually, as long as the individual patient's needs are identified and addressed.
3. The information provided should be tailored to the patient's/helper's level of understanding. Each of the subject areas listed here should be addressed in the record of the training. Examples for clarification of the subject areas are as follows.
   a. The "full range" of home dialysis techniques would include:
      (1) Specific (step-by-step) instructions on how to use the patient's prescribed dialysis equipment (e.g., hemodialysis machine and water treatment components, peritoneal dialysis cycler).
      (2) Specific (step-by-step) instructions in home dialysis procedures (e.g., self-cannulation, peritoneal dialysis exchange) to facilitate adequate dialysis as prescribed by the physician.
   b. Report dialysis complications, including catheter, tunnel or exit site infection; peritonitis; catheter dislodgement; hypotension; hypokalemia; failure of sufficient dialysate to drain from the peritoneal space; protein malnutrition; etc.
   c. Patients on home hemodialysis must be taught to recognize, manage, and report such potential complications as vascular access problems (e.g., difficulty with cannulation, bleeding, and a change in bruit or thrill), infections, hypertension or hypotension, and hyperkalemia.
   d. Training for home patients to monitor their own health status should include the use of equipment to monitor heart rate, blood pressure, temperature, and weight; assessment of vascular or peritoneal dialysis access; recognizing adverse signs and symptoms; and when, how, and whom to contact if they experience problems with their health or treatment. Recording treatment and health status information for home dialysis patients includes documentation of the dialysis process, using hemodialysis or peritoneal dialysis specific treatment records.
   e. Training for infection control precautions should include, at a minimum, indications for the use of gloves, masks, and other personal

protective equipment, methods for hand hygiene, vascular access or peritoneal catheter care and dressing changes, cleaning and disinfecting dialysis equipment, and cleaning and disinfection procedures for spills and splashes of blood or effluent.

R. V-633 Vascular access.
1. The intent of QAPI in addressing vascular access is:
   a. To improve the rate of use and preservation of fistulas.
   b. To decrease the inappropriate use of catheters.
   c. To improve the care provided for all types of vascular access.
2. To identify opportunities for improvement and track progress in management of vascular access for its hemodialysis population, the IDT must use a standard that has achieved broadly accepted use in the ESRD community. Refer to the Measures Assessment Tool (MAT), which lists the current professionally accepted clinical practice standards and CMS CPMs for this and other areas.
3. Fistula survival may be affected by:
   a. Cannulation technique problems such as frequent infiltrations related to training issues or individual personnel difficulties.
   b. Episodes of hypotension or hypovolemia.
   c. Differences in surgical outcomes.
4. The QAPI program should include efforts to reduce the use of catheters and to reduce the incidence of infection related to catheter use. Requirements related to the care of catheters can be found under the Condition for Infection control, at V146, V147, and V148.

S. V-635 Infection control; with respect to this component the facility must:
1. Analyze and document the incidence of infection to identify trends and establish baseline information on infection incidence.
2. Develop recommendations and action plans to minimize infection transmission and promote immunization.
3. Take actions to reduce future incidents.
4. The intent of QAPI in addressing infection control is to minimize the number of patients and staff who are exposed to or acquire infectious diseases at the facility.
   a. The facility must record and follow up on all patient infections and serious adverse events.
      (1) The occurrence of these events should be recorded using a centralized log book or other tracking mechanism and regularly reviewed, with documentation of actions taken.

(2) Surveillance information available for review should include, but not be limited to, patient's vaccination status (hepatitis B, pneumococcal pneumonia, and influenza vaccines); viral hepatitis serologies and seroconversions for HBV(and HCV and ALT, if known); bacteremia episodes; pyrogenic reactions; vascular access infections; and vascular access loss due to infection.
   b. Surveillance information must include, at a minimum, the date of infection onset, site of infection, full identification of infecting organism(s), and antimicrobial susceptibility results.
      (1) Responsible staff must review the results of all routine and diagnostic testing (including culture and serology) upon receipt and ensure that the medical director periodically reviews recorded episodes of bacteremia, vascular access infections, soft tissue infections, and other communicable diseases to aid in tracking, trending, and prompt identification of potential environmental/staff practices issues or infection outbreaks among patients.
      (2) It is important to identify the method of transmission whenever possible as well as the immune status of affected and at-risk patients.

References

American Psychiatric Association (APA). (n.d.). *Phobias*. Retrieved from http://www.psychiatry.org/phobias

American Nephrology Nurses' Association. (2013). *Position statement: Vascular access for hemodialysis*. Pitman, NJ: Author.

Atkar, R.K., & MacRae, J.M. (2013). The buttonhole technique for fistula cannulation: Pros and cons. *Current Opinion Nephrology Hypertension, 22*, 629-636.

Axley, B., & Rosenblum, A. (2012). Learning why patients with central venous catheters resist permanent access placement. *Nephrology Nursing Journal, 39*(2), 99-103.

Ball, L.K. (2005). Improving arteriovenous fistula cannulation skills. *Nephrology Nursing Journal, 32*(6), 611-618.

Ball, L.K. (2006). The buttonhole technique for arteriovenous fistula cannulation. *Nephrology Nursing Journal, 33*(3), 299-304.

Ball, L.K. (2009). Forty years of vascular access. *Nephrology Nursing Journal, 36*(2), 119-123.

Ball, L.K. (2010). The buttonhole technique: Strategies to reduce infections. *Nephrology Nursing Journal, 37*(5), 473-477.

Ball, L.K. (2013). Fatal vascular access hemorrhage: Reducing the odds. *Nephrology Nursing Journal, 40*(4), 297-303.

Ball, L.K., & Mott, S. (2010). How do you prevent indented buttonhole sites? *Nephrology Nursing Journal, 37*(4), 427-431.

Ball, L.K., Treat, L., Riffle, V., Scherting, D., & Swift, L. (2007). A multi-center perspective of the buttonhole technique in the Pacific Northwest. *Nephrology Nursing Journal, 34*(2), 234-241.

Banerjee, S. (2009). Beyond needle placement: The role of the nephrology nurse in arteriovenous fistula management. *Nephrology Nursing Journal, 36*(6), 657-659.

Birchenough, E., Moore, C., Stevens, K., & Stewart, S. (2010). Buttonhole cannulation in adult patients on hemodialysis: An increased risk of infection? *Nephrology Nursing Journal, 37*(5), 491-498.

Bonkain, F., Racapé, J., Goncalvez, J., Moerman, M., Denis, O., Gammar, N., Gastaldello, K., & Nortier, J.L. (2013). Prevention of tunneled cuffed hemodialysis catheter-related dysfunction and bacteremia by a neutral-valve closed-system connector: A single-center randomized controlled trial. *American Journal of Kidney Disease, 61*(3), 459-465.

Brouwer, D.J. (1995). Cannulation camp: Basic needle cannulation training for dialysis staff. *Dialysis & Transplantation, 24*(11), 1-7.

Brouwer, D.J. (2005). Use of tunneled catheters must be minimized. *Nephrology Nursing Journal, 32*(6), 678-679.

Centers for Disease Control and Prevention (CDC). (n.d.). Central venous catheter hub cleaning prior to accessing Centers for Disease Control and Prevention (CDC) dialysis bloodstream infection (BSI) prevention collaborative protocol. Retrieved from http://www.cdc.gov/dialysis

Centers for Disease Control and Prevention (CDC). (2002).Guideline for hand hygiene in health-care settings. *Morbidity and mortality weekly report, 51*(RR-16), 1-22. Retrieved from http://www.cdc.gov/dialysis

Centers for Disease Control and Prevention (CDC). (2011). *Guideline for the prevention of intravascular catheter-related infections, 2011.* Retrieved from http://www.cdc.gov/dialysis

Centers for Disease Control and Prevention (CDC). (2014a). *Dialysis prevention process measures hand hygiene surveillance.* Retrieved from http://www.cdc.gov/dialysis

Centers for Disease Control and Prevention (CDC). (2014b). *Dialysis event protocol.* Retrieved from http://www.cdc.gov/dialysis

Centers for Disease Control and Prevention (CDC). (2014c). *Tracking infections in outpatient dialysis facilities.* Retrieved from http://www.cdc.gov/nhsn/dialysis/

Centers for Disease Control and Prevention (CDC). (2014d). *CDC approach to BSI prevention in dialysis facilities.* Retrieved from http://www.cdc.gov/dialysis

Centers for Medicare and Medicaid Services (CMS). (2008). *Survey & certification – Guidance to laws and regulations: Dialysis.* Retrieved from http://www.cms.gov/Medicare/Provider-Enrollment-and-Certification/GuidanceforLawsAndRegulations/Dialysis.html

Centers for Medicare and Medicaid Services (CMS). (2008, April 15). *Conditions of coverage for ESRD facilities: Final rule.* Retrieved from http://www.cms.gov/Regulations-and-Guidance/Legislation/CFCsAndCoPs/downloads/ESRDfinalrule0415.pdf

Centers for Medicare and Medicaid Services (CMS). (2014). *Survey & certification – Certification & compliance.* Retrieved from http://www.cms.gov/Medicare/Provider-Enrollment-and-Certification/CertificationandComplianc/index.html

Compton, A. (2005). National vascular access improvement initiative: "Fistula first." *Nephrology Nursing Journal, 32*(2), 221-222.

Deaver, K. (2010). Preventing infections in hemodialysis fistula and graft vascular accesses. *Nephrology Nursing Journal, 37*(5), 503-505.

Dhingra, R.K., Young, E.W., Hulbert-Shearon, T.E., Leavey, S.F., & Port, F.K. (2001). Type of vascular access and mortality in U.S. hemodialysis patients. *Kidney International, 60,* 1443-1451.

Dinwiddie, L.C. (2002). Interventions to promote fistula maturation. *Nephrology Nursing Journal, 29*(4), 377, 402.

Dobson, A., El-Gamil, A. M., Shimer, M.T., DaVanzo, J.E., Urbanes, A.Q., Beathard, G.A., & Foust Litchfield, T. (2013). Clinical and economic value of performing dialysis vascular access procedures in a freestanding office-based center as compared with the hospital outpatient department among medicare ESRD beneficiaries. *Seminars in Dialysis, 26*(5), 624-632. doi:10.1111/sdi.12120

Doss, S., Schiller, B., & Moran, J. (2008). Buttonhole cannulation – An unexpected outcome. *Nephrology Nursing Journal, 35*(4), 417-419.

Dutka, P., & Brickel, H. (2010). A practical review of the kidney dialysis outcomes quality initiative (KDOQI) guidelines for hemodialysis catheters and their potential impact on patient care. *Nephrology Nursing Journal, 37*(5), 531-535.

Evans, L.M. (2012). Buttonhole cannulation for haemodialysis: A nursing review. *Renal Society of Australasia Journal, 8*(3), 146-151.

Favero, H. (2004). Toward better vascular access management. *Nephrology Nursing Journal, 31*(1), 118.

Fistula First. (2009). *Thirteen change concepts for increasing AV fistulas.* Retrieved from http://esrdncc.org/ffcl/change-concepts

Gomez, N.J. (2011). Nephrology nursing process of care – Hemodialysis vascular access. In N.J Gomez (Ed.), *Nephrology nursing scope and standards of practice* (7th ed., pp. 123-128). Pitman, NJ: American Nephrology Nurses' Association.

Gottmann, U., Sadick, M., Kleinhuber, K., Benck, U., Huck, K., & Krämer, B.K. (2012). Central vein stenosis in a dialysis patient a case report. *Journal of Medical Case Reports, 6*(189), 1-4.

Haddad, N.J., Van Cleef, S., & Agarwal, A.K. (2012). Central venous catheters in dialysis: The good, the bad and the ugly. *The Open Urology & Nephrology Journal, 5*(Suppl. 1: M3), 12-18.

Hamilton, J.G. (1995). Needle phobia: A neglected diagnosis. *Journal of Family Practice, 41*(2), 169-175.

HealthCentral (n.d.). Needle phobia. *Harvard Health Publications.* Retrieved from http://www.healthcentral.com/anxiety/disorder-types-273889-5.html

Houle, K.H. (2004). Hemodialysis vascular access: Upper extremity graft versus anterior chest wall graft. *Nephrology Nursing Journal, 31*(6), 642-648.

Huber, T.S., Carter, J.S., Carter, R.L., & Seeger, J.M. (2003). Patency of autogenous and polytetrafluoroethylene upper extremity arteriovenous hemodialysis accesses: A systematic review. *Journal of Vascular Surgery, 38*(5), 1005-1011.

Jackson, J., & Litchfield, T. (2006). How a dedicated vascular access center can promote increased use of fistulas. *Nephrology Nursing Journal, 33*(2), 189-196.

Jindal, K., Chan, C.T., Deizel, C., Hirsch, D., Soroka, S.D., Tonelli, M., & Culleton, B.F. (2006). Chapter 4: Vascular access. *Journal of the American Society of Nephrology, 17*(S16-S23).

Kim, M-K., & Kim, H-S. (2012). Clinical effects of buttonhole cannulation method on hemodialysis patients. *Hemodialysis International, 17,* 294-299.

Kotoda, A., Akimoto, T, Kato, M., Kanazawa, H., Nakata, M., Sugase, T., … Kusano, E. (2011). Central venous stenosis among hemodialysis patients is often not associated with previous central venous catheters. *American Society of Artificial Society of Artificial Internal Organs (ASAIO) Journal, 57,* 439-443.

Leon, C., & Asif, A. (2007). Arteriovenous access and hand pain: The distal hypoperfusion ischemic syndrome. *Clinical Journal of the American Society of Nephrology, 2,* 175-183.

MacRae, J.M., Pandeya, S., Humen, D.P., Krivitski, N., & Lindsay, R.M. (2004). Arteriovenous fistula-associated high-output cardiac failure: A review of mechanisms. *American Journal of Kidney Diseases, 43*(5),17-22.

MacRae, J.M., Levin, A., & Belenkie, I. (2006).The cardiovascular effects of arteriovenous fistulas in chronic kidney disease: A cause for concern? *Seminars in Dialysis 19*(5), 349-352.

Malik, J., Tuka, V., Kasalova, Z., Chytilova, E., Slavikova, M., Clagett, P., … Gallieni, M. (2008). Understanding the dialysis access steal syndrome. A review of the etiologies, diagnosis, prevention and treatment strategies. *The Journal of Vascular Access, 9*(3), 155-166.

McAfee, N., Seidel, K. Watkins, S., & Flynn, J.T. (2010). A continuous quality improvement project to decrease hemodialysis catheter infections in pediatric patients: Use of a closed Luer-Lock access cap. *Nephrology Nursing Journal, 37*(5), 541-544.

Mehta, P.A., & Dubrey, S.W. (2008). High output heart failure. *Oxford Journals Medicine: An International Journal of Medicine, 102,* 235-241.

Mott, S., & Moore, H. (2011). Kinder, gentler methods for scab removal in buttonhole access. *Nephrology Nursing Journal, 38*(4), 439-443.

National Institute of Diabetes and Digestive and Kidney Diseases (NIDDK). (2008). *Vascular access for hemodialysis.* Retrieved from http://www.kidney.niddk.nih.gov

National Kidney Foundation (NKF). (2006). NKF Kidney Disease Outcomes Quality Initiative (KDOQI) clinical practice guidelines and clinical practice recommendations for 2006 Updates: Vascular access. *American Journal of Kidney Diseases, 48*(Suppl. 1), S231-S332. Retrieved from http://www2.kidney.org/professionals/KDOQI/guideline_upHD_PD_VA/

Nephrology News & Issues (2014, July 16). Fistula First offers new tools to improve outcomes, p. 23.

Niyyar, V.D., & Lok, C.E. (2013). Pros and cons of catheter lock solutions. *Current Opinion Nephrology Hypertension, 22*(6), 669-674.

Oliver, M.J., Rothwell, D.M., Fung, K., Hux, J.E., & Lok, C.E. (2004). Late creation of vascular access for hemodialysis and increased risk of sepsis. *Journal of the American Society of Nephrology, 15,* 1936-1942.

Paston, S., Soucie, J.M., & McClellan, W.M. (2002). Vascular access and increased risk of death among hemodialysis patients. *Kidney International, 62*(2), 620-626.

Pisoni, R.L., Young, E.W., Dykstra, D.M., Greenwood, R.N., Hecking, E., Gillespie, B., … Held, P.J. (2002). Vascular access use in Europe and the United States: Results from the DOPPS. *Kidney International, 61,* 305-316.

Pergolotti, A., Rich, E., & Lock, K. (2011). The effect of the buttonhole method vs. the traditional method of AV fistula cannulation on hemostasis, needle stick pain, preneedle stick anxiety, and presence of aneurysms in ambulatory patients on hemodialysis. *Nephrology Nursing Journal, 38*(4), 333-336.

Rosenthal, K. (ND). Infiltrations & extravasations. *Resource Nurse.* Retrieved from http://www.resourcenurse.com/feature_infiltration.html

Rushing, J. (2010). Caring for a patient's vascular access for hemodialysis. *Nursing Management, 41*(10), 47.

Schanzer, H. (2002). Overview of complications and after vascular access creation. In R.J. Gray & J.J. Sands (Eds.), *Dialysis access: A multidisciplinary approach* (pp. 93-97). Philadelphia: Lippincott Williams & Wilkins.

Society for Vascular Ultrasound (SVU). (2009). Upper extremity vein mapping for placement of a dialysis access. *Vascular Technology Professional Performance Guidelines.* Retrieved from http://www.svunet.org

Sofocleous, C.T. (2013). Dialysis fistulas. *Medscape Reference Drugs, Diseases, & Procedures.* Retrieved from http://emedicine.medscape.com/article/419393-overview

Sokolowski, C.J., Giovannitti, J.A., & Boynes, S.G. (2010). Needle phobia: Etiology, adverse consequences, and patient management. *Dental Clinics of North America, 54*(4), 731-744.

Stern, A.B., & Klemmer, P.I. (2011). High-ouput heart failure secondary to arteriovenous fistula. *Hemodialysis International.* Retrieved from http://www.ncbi.nlm.nih.gov/pubmed/21223485 doi:10.1111/j.1542-4758.2010.00518.x.

Suding, P.N., & Wilson, S.E. (2007). Strategies for management of ischemic steal syndrome. *Seminars in Vascular Surgery, 20*(3), 184-188.

Tordoir, J.H., Dammers, R., & van der Sande, F.M. (2004). Upper extremity ischemia and hemodialysis vascular access. *European Journal of Vascular and Endovascular Surgery, 27*(1), 1-5.

United States Renal Data System (USRDS). (2013). *Annual data report: Atlas of chronic kidney disease and end-stage renal disease in the United States.* Bethesda, MD: National Institutes of Health, National Institute of Diabetes and Digestive and Kidney Diseases.

United States Renal Data System (USRDS). (2014). *Annual data report: Atlas of chronic kidney disease and end-stage renal disease in the United States.* Bethesda, MD: National Institutes of Health, National Institute of Diabetes and Digestive and Kidney Diseases.

Utescu, M.S., LeBoeuf, A., Chbinou, N., Desmeules, S., Lebel, M., & Agharazii, M. (2009). The impact of arteriovenous fistulas on aortic stiffness in patients with chronic kidney disease. *Nephrology Dialysis Transplant, 24,* 3441-3446.

Vachharajani, T.J. (2010). *Atlas of dialysis vascular access.* Wake Forest University School of Medicine. Retrieved from http://fistulafirst.org/Home/VascularAccessAtlas.aspx

Vachharajani, T. J., Wu, S., Brouwer-Maier, D., & Asif, A. (2014). In J.T. Daugirdas, P.G. Blake, & T.S. Ing (Eds.), *Handbook of dialysis* (5th ed., pp. 99-120). Philadelphia: Lippincott Williams & Wilkins.

Van Waeleghem, J.P., Chamney, M., Lindley, E.J., & Pancirová, J. (2008). Venous needle dislodgement: How to minimise the risks. *Journal of Renal Care, 34*(4), 163-168.

White, R.B. (2006). Vascular access for hemodialysis. In A. Molzahn & E. Butera (Eds.), *Contemporary nephrology nursing: Principles and practice* (2nd ed., pp. 561-578). Pitman, NJ: American Nephrology Nurses' Association.

Yeuzlin, A., Agarwal, A. K., Salman, L., & Asif, A.K. (2014) In J.T. Daugirdas, P.G. Blake, & T.S. Ing (Eds.), *Handbook of dialysis* (5th ed., pp. 137-154). Philadelphia: Lippincott Williams & Wilkins.

CHAPTER **4**

Peritoneal Dialysis

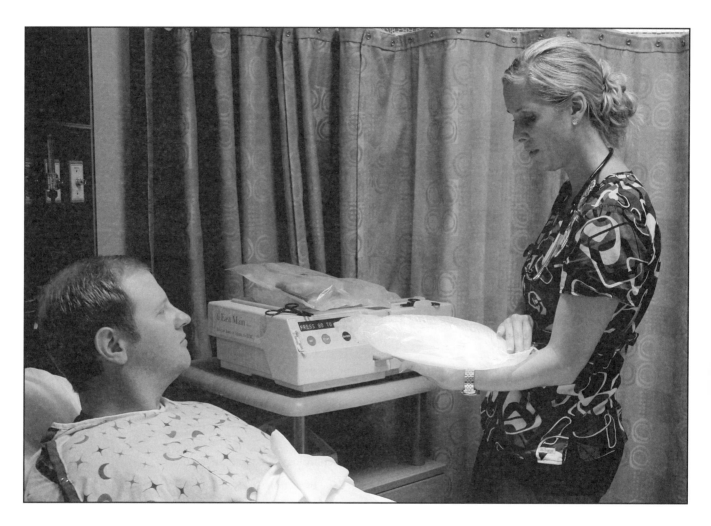

Chapter Editor
Lucy B. Todd, MSN, ACNP-BC, CNN

Authors
Lucy B. Todd, MSN, ACNP-BC, CNN
Lisa Ales, MSN, NP-C, FNP-BC, CNN
Cheryl L. Groenhoff, MSN, MBA, RN, CNN
Kim Lambertson, MSN, RN, CNN
Leonor P. Ponferrada, BSN, RN, CNN

CHAPTER **4**

Peritoneal Dialysis

This offering for **1.8 contact hours** is provided by the American Nephrology Nurses' Association (ANNA).

American Nephrology Nurses' Association is accredited as a provider of continuing nursing education by the American Nurses Credentialing Center Commission on Accreditation.

ANNA is a provider approved by the California Board of Registered Nursing, provider number CEP 00910.

This CNE offering meets the continuing nursing education requirements for certification and recertification by the Nephrology Nursing Certification Commission (NNCC).

To be awarded contact hours for this activity, read this chapter in its entirety. Then complete the CNE evaluation found at **www.annanurse.org/corecne** and submit it; or print it, complete it, and mail it in. Contact hours are not awarded until the evaluation for the activity is complete.

Example of reference for Chapter 4 in APA format. Use author of the section being cited. This example is based on Section A – Peritoneal Dialysis.

Lambertson, K. (2015). Peritoneal dialysis: Peritoneal dialysis access. In C.S. Counts (Ed.), *Core curriculum for nephrology nursing: Module 3. Treatment options for patients with chronic kidney failure* (6th ed., pp. 227-278). Pitman, NJ: American Nephrology Nurses' Association.

Interpreted: Section author(s). (2015). Title of chapter: Title of section. In …

Cover photo by Counts/Morganello.

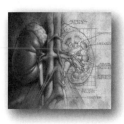

CHAPTER 4

Peritoneal Dialysis

Purpose

Peritoneal dialysis (PD) is experiencing a significant resurgence as a kidney replacement therapy modality. Many nurses now practicing in PD programs are relatively new to the therapy. This chapter was developed to meet the basic educational needs of all PD nurses, especially those with limited experience.

Objectives

Upon completion of this chapter, the learner will be able to:
1. Cite two absolute contraindications to PD therapy.
2. Discuss the factors that affect solute transport and total fluid removal in peritoneal dialysis.
3. Cite the current NKF Dialysis Outcomes Quality Initiative (KDOQI) Clinical Practice Guidelines recommendations for adequate PD.
4. Discuss strategies to preserve the peritoneal membrane.
5. Review the risk factors, diagnosis, treatment, and changes in dialysis prescription for the management of leaks, hernias, and genital edema.
6. Outline causes and interventions for hemoperitoneum, chyloperitoneum, peritonitis, and encapsulating peritoneal sclerosis.

Significant Dates in the History of Peritoneal Dialysis

1877   Wegner reported peritoneal lavage in animals.

1894   Starling and Tubby described absorption from the peritoneal cavity indicating that transport through the peritoneal membrane was bidirectional.

1923   Putnam published studies of peritoneal dialysis (PD) in dogs.

1923   Ganter reported the first use of peritoneal dialysis for uremia in a human. He used a needle for access in the first reported use of PD in humans.

1927   Heusser and Werder reported continuous flow PD in three patients with mercury poisoning. They used a needle for infusion and a rubber drain with multiple side perforations for drainage.

1934   Balazs and Rosenak performed continuous flow PD with two cannulae made of glass or fine wire with a bulbous tip and multiple holes.

1937   Wear, Sisk, and Trikle used two gall bladder trocars for acute PD. The drainage trocar had multiple side holes in the distal third.

1938   Wear reported what was thought to be the first patient treated with PD to recover from acute renal failure; Rhodes reported first attempt to use PD in chronic renal failure.

1946   Fine, Frank, and Seligman reported continuous flow dialysis for acute renal failure using combinations of stainless steel tubes, whistle tip, and mushroom-type catheters for inflow and outflow devices. This was the first report of rubber catheters inserted through a trocar. They also reported the use of heparin to minimize fibrin formation and adhesions.

1948	Rosenak and Oppenheimer developed the first "drain" specifically for PD. The intraperitoneal segment was spiral, stainless steel wire and a rounded tip and a plate for fixation to the abdominal wall. This was the first commercially available PD catheter.
1948	Odel, Ferris, and Power first used polyvinyl for the drain catheter. The tubing had multiple perforations to drain the dialysate. Both inflow and outflow tubes were weighted to keep the tips in the true pelvis. They argued against the use of inline bacterial filters, because they reduce flow rates and provide a potential site for multiplication of microorganisms.
1949	Derot and colleagues described a polyvinyl catheter inserted through a trocar.
1951	Grollman and colleagues reported a polyethylene plastic catheter, inserted through a trocar.
1959	Maxwell and colleagues used a "nonirritating" semi-rigid, nylon catheter with a rounded tip and numerous tiny side holes.
1959	Doolan et al. used a polyvinyl chloride catheter with grooves (20 per inch) designed to prevent omental wrapping.
1959	Sterile peritoneal dialysis solution became commercially available.
1962	Merrill and colleagues credit the availability of plastic catheters and commercial dialysis solution as instrumental in the wide acceptance of PD for treatment of renal failure in humans.
1962	Boen and colleagues implanted Teflon® or rubber tubes in the abdominal wall for reinsertion of the catheter in intermittent peritoneal dialysis. This was known as "Boen's button."
1962	Gutch and colleagues reported on the successful use of a less rigid, more comfortable polyvinyl catheter left in place for 110 days in a patient with chronic renal failure.
1963	Barry and colleagues from Walter Reed Hospital reported a new catheter with a balloon at the distal end. After placement in the peritoneal cavity, the balloon was filled with saline to extend it.
1963	McDonald developed a smaller trocar specifically for PD which significantly reduced leaks and bleeding.
1963	Palmer and Quinton developed a silicone rubber PD catheter with a coiled intraperitoneal segment: the prototype for current coiled catheters. The catheters were used for chronic renal failure and remained in place up to 2 years, but had problems associated with a tri-flange step located in the tunnel segment.
1964	Mallette and colleagues developed a conical shaped "button" implanted subcutaneously. The skin was punctured and a catheter inserted through the button for each treatment.
1964	Boen developed the first closed automated delivery system.
1965	Weston and Roberts designed an acute stylet catheter. This eliminated the need for general anesthesia, and it created a snug fit around the catheter, further reducing the incidence of leaks.
1966	Lasker developed an automated cycler.
1967	Tenckhoff designed the silicone double-cuff catheter. In 1968, Tenckhoff and Schechter published results with a silicone elastomer (Silastic®) catheter for chronic dialysis with two Dacron® polyester felt cuffs: one preperitoneal and one below the skin. The relatively short subcutaneous tunnel and straight intraperitoneal segment allowed implantation at the bedside. Tenckhoff and colleagues also developed a trocar for catheter insertion and described in detail a bedside insertion technique. The "Tenckhoff catheter" was commercially produced, was widely used, and remains the most commonly used catheter for PD access. It became the "gold standard" of peritoneal access and is the prototype for most modern catheters.
1972	Fully automated, reverse osmosis system developed.
1976	Popovich and Moncrief described continuous ambulatory peritoneal dialysis (CAPD) technique.

1976	The Toronto Western Hospital (TWH) catheter had three silicone discs placed on the intraperitoneal segment to reduce the incidence of catheter migration.
1978	The Food and Drug Administration (FDA) approved peritoneal dialysis solution in polyvinyl bags for use in the United States.
1980s	New CAPD systems, cycling machines, and catheter designs were developed; variations in dialysis prescriptions and regimens were prescribed.
1981	Diaz-Buxo et al. described continuous cycling peritoneal dialysis (CCPD).
1981	Ash and colleagues successfully placed Tenckhoff catheters using peritoneoscopy.
1985	Twardowski and colleagues developed a swan neck catheter with a bent or curved subcutaneous segment. The goal was to overcome the problems associated with catheter shape memory, when a straight silastic catheter is placed in a curved or arched tunnel (cuff extrusion and catheter malposition).
1988	Cruz reported development of a polyurethane "pail handle" catheter.
1990s	The emphasis on dialysis adequacy and nutrition increased with individualized dialysis prescriptions being used. There was increased use of cycler dialysis; > 30% of the patients on PD in the United States were using cyclers.
1991	Moncrief and Popovich reported a technique for catheter implantation leaving the external segment buried subcutaneously for 4 weeks to allow healing and tissue ingrowth into cuffs in a sterile environment. The external segment is eventually "exteriorized."
1992	Moncrief and colleagues reported a modified silastic, swan neck coiled catheter with the subcutaneous cuff lengthened to 2.5 cm. Both ends of the cuff were tapered and the catheter was implanted with the external segment buried as described above. This catheter, manufactured in North America, is distributed and used in many countries.
1992	A swan neck catheter with a long tunnel, third cuff, and presternal exit site on the chest was developed by Twardowski and colleagues in an effort to reduce exit-site complications and contamination. The presternal catheter is currently used in both adults and children.
2000s	Improved understanding of peritoneal biocompatibility led to the availability of new and more biocompatible peritoneal dialysis solutions. Approximately half of the PD population is using cyclers.
2010s	Use of urgent-start PD as an option for patients who urgently present with chronic kidney disease stage 5 without a plan for dialysis in place. The patients start on PD as an initial mode of therapy. At this point, more than half of the PD population is using cyclers.

Compiled by Leonor P. Ponferrada

SECTION A
Peritoneal Dialysis Access
Kim Lambertson

I. Peritoneal dialysis (PD) catheters.

A. Characteristics of the PD catheter.
   1. Background information.
      a. In the 1960s, Tenckhoff and Schecter designed a PD catheter that was less irritating to the peritoneal membrane and had cuffs to prevent leakage from the peritoneal cavity (Kathuria et al., 2009).
      b. The "Tenckhoff catheter" remains a broad term

to describe and discuss the generic PD catheter.
      c. Over the years, attempts have been made at designing different attributes to improve PD access. The attributes will be described below. Unfortunately, alternative designs to the original Tenckhoff design have failed to change PD catheter outcomes (Crabtree, 2006c).
      d. The most frequently used catheters in North America can be seen in Figure 4.1.
   2. Catheter materials.
      a. All catheters are made of silicone (Dell'Aquila et al., 2007).
      b. The Cruz catheter was made of polyurethane but is no longer produced.
   3. The extraperitoneal or subcutaneous segment.
      a. Straight.

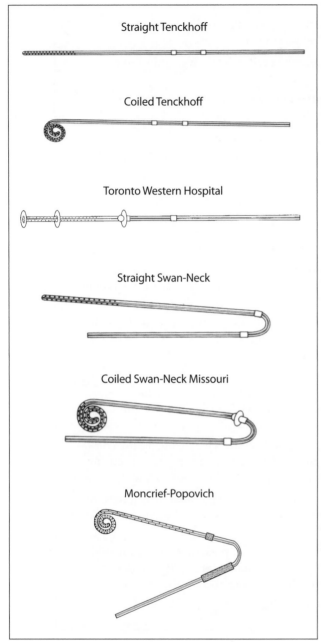

Straight Tenckhoff

Coiled Tenckhoff

Toronto Western Hospital

Straight Swan-Neck

Coiled Swan-Neck Missouri

Moncrief-Popovich

Figure 4.1. Chronic peritoneal dialysis catheters. From top: Double-cuff Tenckhoff catheter with straight intraperitoneal segment; double-cuff Tenckhoff catheter with coiled intraperitoneal segment; Toronto Western Hospital catheter with preperitoneal flange and bead and intraperitoneal discs; swan-neck catheter with straight intraperitoneal segment; swan-neck Missouri catheter with preperitoneal flange and bead and coiled intraperitoneal segment; Moncrief-Popovich catheter with wider tunnel angle and longer subcutaneous cuff.

b. Permanent, preformed, 150 to180-degree bend; commonly called a *swan neck*. The permanent bend allows for the insertion in a downward directed manner in both the rectus muscle and the exit site. This downward insertion is thought to prevent migration of the catheter outside of the pelvis (Dell'Aquila et al., 2007; Kathuria et al., 2009) (see Figure 4.2).

4. The cuff(s).
   a. Usually made of polyester (Dacron®). The purpose of the cuff(s) is to allow tissue ingrowth and prevent leaks and the migration of bacteria (Kathuria et al., 2009).
   b. A single cuff is placed in the rectus muscle (Dell'Aquila et al., 2007).
   c. In the case of a double cuff catheter, one cuff is placed in the rectus muscle and the other subcutaneously, approximately 2 to 4 cm from the exit site. All swan neck catheters are double cuffed (Crabtree 2006c; Kathuria et al., 2009).
   d. Missouri and Oreopoulous-Zellerman (also called the Toronto Western) catheters have a polyester disc that is implanted into the rectus muscle and a bead that is placed just inside the peritoneal cavity in place of a deep cuff. This style of catheter cannot be implanted laparoscopically (Covidien, 2011; Kathuria et al., 2009).
   e. The Moncreif-Popovich catheter has a longer subcutaneous cuff that is 2.5 cm compared to the standard 1 cm. This catheter was designed for embedding (Kathuria et al., 2009).

5. The intraperitoneal segment.
   a. Straight.
   b. Coiled to decrease inflow pain (Kathuria et al., 2009).
   c. The Oreopolous-Zellerman catheter has two silicone intraperitoneal discs to keep the catheter in the pelvis and prevent omental wrapping (Covidien, 2011).

6. The presternal catheter.
   a. The presternal catheter is a modification of a lower abdominal catheter that allows for an anterior chest exit site.
   b. Presternal catheters are two sections of catheter that are joined together internally with a titanium connector. The upper section has a preformed bend, two cuffs, and the external segment. The lower section may have a Missouri intraperitoneal design.
      (1) The ends of either piece of the presternal catheter can be cut in a length appropriate for the patient, allowing for the presternal or upper abdominal exit site.
      (2) All presternal catheters have a swan neck.
   c. The presternal catheter should not be placed over the sternum in the event the patient has to

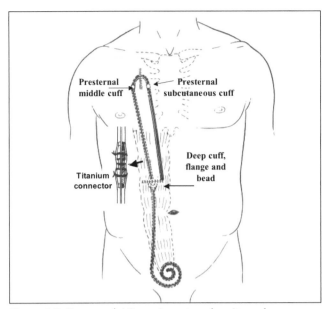

Figure 4.2. Swan-neck Missouri presternal peritoneal dialysis catheter.

Source: Twardowski, Z.J., Prowant, B.F., Pickett, B., Nichols, W.K., Nolph, K.D., & Khanna, R. (1996). Four-year experience with swan neck presternal peritoneal dialysis catheter. *American Journal of Kidney Diseases, 27*(1), 99-105. Used with permission.

have open heart surgery (Crabtree 2006c).
  d. Rationale for use of the presternal catheter.
    (1) There is less movement with the chest wall than abdominal location which facilitates healing and decreases trauma risk (Kathuria et al., 2009).
    (2) The presternal catheter configuration is helpful in patients with ostomies, incontinence, obese abdomens, or those who want to tub bathe (Crabtree, 2006c).
  7. Radiopaque strip.
    a. All catheters have a white or blue (in the case of catheters made by Merit Medical Systems, Inc.) stripe to assist with x-ray location.
    b. The radiopaque stripe also helps prevent or detect twists of the catheter during insertion (Kathuria et al., 2009).

B. Three catheter brands are available in the United States.
  1. Covidien – http://www.covidien.com/imageServer.aspx/doc215777.pdf?contentID=20743&contenttype=application/pdf
  2. Medcomp® – http://www.medcompnet.com/products/peritoneal/v-series.html#brochures
  3. Merit Medical Systems, Inc. – http://www.merit.com/products/default.aspx?code=pd

C. Catheter adapters.
  1. The catheter adapter is inserted into the external portion of the PD catheter. The adapter allows the patient to connect to PD solution administration sets. Adapters are made of titanium and plastics.
  2. The standard outer diameter of a PD catheter is 5 mm. The standard internal diameter is 2.6 mm with exception of the Flex-Neck® by Merit Medical Systems, Inc., which has an internal diameter of 3.5 mm (Dell'Aquila et al., 2007).
  3. The adapter has to correlate to the internal diameter of the catheter to prevent the adapter from falling out of the PD catheter.

II. PD catheter insertion.

A. Professionals responsible for placing the PD catheter.
  1. Surgeons place most of the PD catheters.
  2. Radiologists.
  3. Interventional nephrologists (Crabtree, 2010).

B. Placement techniques (see Table 4.1).
  1. Surgical dissection.
    a. Performed by a surgeon in an operating room and requires general anesthesia.
    b. There is no direct visualization of the abdominal cavity (Asif, 2004).
  2. Laparoscopic placement.
    a. Performed by a surgeon in the operating room and requires general anesthesia.

Table 4.1

How PD Catheters Are Placed

Placement Technique	Who Places and Where	Anesthesia
Surgical a. Dissection b. Laparoscope	Surgeon: Operating Room	General anesthesia
Percutaneous a. Blind insertion b. Guided by ultrasound, fluoroscopy c. Peritoneoscope	Interventional Radiologist or Nephrologist: Procedure Room, Interventional Room, Intensive Care Unit	Conscious sedation

b. Minimally invasive (Crabtree, 2010).
c. This method allows for the use of advanced laparoscopic techniques to proactively repair issues that may hinder proper catheter function.
d. Advanced laparoscopic techniques.
   (1) Rectus sheath tunneling is done to enter the abdominal cavity in such a manner that prevents catheter tip migration.
   (2) Omentopexy – tacking up redundant omentum so it does not interfere with catheter function. Omentopexy is an alternative to omentectomy (resection of the omentum); it is more time and cost effective and provides an equal or better outcome.
   (3) Resection of epiploic appendages, i.e., the removal of tabs of fat from the colon that can interfere with catheter function.
   (4) Adhesiolysis – the lysis of adhesions that cause dialysis solution to pocket within the peritoneal cavity.
   (5) Repair abdominal wall hernias (Crabtree, 2006c).
3. Percutaneous placement.
   a. Background information.
      (1) During percutaneous insertion, a needle is used to enter the peritoneal cavity.
      (2) A guide wire with a dilator and peel-away sheath are then advanced into the opening of the abdomen created by the needle.
      (3) The guide wire and dilator are removed.
      (4) The catheter is then put on a stylet and advanced into the peritoneal cavity through the sheath.
      (5) This technique is referred to as the Seldinger technique (Peppelenbosch, 2008).
   b. Percutaneous placement can be accomplished in three ways.
      (1) Blind percutaneous catheter insertion uses no imaging methods to visualize structures in the abdominal cavity. This method is not commonly used in the United States (Asif, 2004).
      (2) Ultrasound/fluoroscopic percutaneous catheter insertion uses ultrasound to guide the introduction of the needle into the abdomen, then fluoroscopy to assist with guide wire advancement. The use of ultrasound and fluoroscopy helps prevent the puncture of abdominal organs (Maya, 2008; Vaux et al., 2008).
      (3) The peritoneoscopic method uses a small laparoscopic port (2 mm) to guide the placement of the PD catheter. This allows for visualization of the abdominal structures and requires only small

incisions. This method is most commonly used by nephrologists (Asif, 2004).
   c. Advantages of percutaneous placement.
      (1) No general anesthesia; only conscious sedation (Maya, 2008).
      (2) Smaller incision into the peritoneal cavity (Vaux et al., 2008).
      (3) Frequently, referral for this method occurs in a more timely fashion than for surgical placement (Asif, 2004).
      (4) Percutaneous catheter placement can be done in a procedure room, an interventional room, or in the intensive care unit (Asif, 2004).
4. The embedding/Moncrief-Popovich technique allows for the placement of the PD catheter in advance need of dialysis. The catheter is placed by one of the methods previously described, but the external portion of the catheter is embedded subcutaneously in the patient's lower abdomen for 3 to 5 weeks or until dialysis is needed.
   a. Any type of catheter and surgical technique can be used when placing embedding catheters.
   b. When dialysis is needed, the catheter is externalized using local anesthesia in a clinic setting.
   c. Advantages of PD catheter embedding.
      (1) Efficient use of operating room and surgeon scheduling.
      (2) Reduction of the risk for urgent-start to hemodialysis with a central venous catheter.
      (3) The catheter is allowed to heal in a sterile environment although there is no data that shows reduced exit-site infections or risk of peritonitis.
      (4) Reduction in the costs of exit-site care and catheter flushing postoperatively (Crabtree, 2006c; Crabtree & Burchette 2013).
   d. One commonly asked question regarding embedded catheters is: *Does this practice cause catheter obstruction?* Crabtree and Burchette (2013) compared their study of 84 embedded catheter placements with the results of three other studies. In all four studies, more than 85% of catheters functioned immediately after externalization.

C. Preoperative catheter placement procedures.
   1. The PD catheter should be placed 2 weeks before starting PD. See Table 4.2 for information regarding dialysis after catheter placement.
      a. This period gives the catheter time for tissue ingrowth and prevents dialysate leaks.
      b. If dialysis needs to be started before the 2-week healing period is completed, PD can be commenced in the supine position with small fill volumes (Gokal et al., 1998).

Table 4.2

Dialysis After Catheter Placement

Traditional
Full-dose PD is started 2 weeks postimplantation to allow tissue ingrowth of catheter cuffs to prevent leaks.

Urgent-Start
Used when dialysis must start dialysis in less than 2 weeks but not before 48 hours (Ghaffari, 2012).
PD treatments are complete three times to six times per week over 5–12 hours in the outpatient PD unit with fill volumes of 500–1500 cc (Arramreddy et al., 2014).
This method of starting dialysis reduces the risk of infection compared to starting hemodialysis with a central venous catheter (CVC).
Several studies have demonstrated that urgent-start PD patients have outcomes similar to traditional start patients in regards to mechanical and infectious complications (Mahnensmith 2014).

2. For patients who do not receive routine nephrology care before reaching CKD stage 5, procedures should be in place to educate those patients about the option of PD. PD as an urgent-start modality has the advantage of decreasing the use of central venous catheters in HD (Arramreddy et al., 2014; Figueiredo et al., 2010).

3. Some programs do nasal cultures to assess for *Staphylococcus aureus* carriage and treat positive cultures with intranasal mupirocin. There is no data that shows if this is effective (Cho & Johnson, 2014; Li et al., 2010).

4. The abdominal wall should be assessed for hernias, and plans should be in place for repair at the time of catheter insertion (Gokal et al., 1998).

5. Exit-site planning and marking.
   a. The patient should be examined dressed and in the sitting and standing positions to evaluate exit-site placement.
      (1) If the belt line is above the umbilicus, the exit site should be below the belt line and facing downward. This can be accomplished using a catheter with a swan neck.
      (2) If the belt line is below the umbilicus, the exit site should be above the belt line and in a lateral position (Crabtree, 2006c).
   b. Stomas, bowel, and bladder incontinence, body habitus, and the desire for tub baths should be assessed when planning the exit site. In these patients, upper abdominal or presternal exit sites should be considered (Crabtree, 2006c).
   c. Penner and Crabtree (2013) reported on the

use of an extended catheter with an exit site on the patient's back. Using the back for an exit site may be helpful with patients who have altered mental status and are at risk for pulling or contaminating the catheter.
   d. The exit site should be visible to the patient and in an area of the abdomen that the patient can reach to perform exit-site care.
   e. Stencils are available from catheter manufacturers to ensure that the proper tunnel is created (Kathuria et al., 2009; Covidien and Merit Medical Systems, Inc. catalogs).
   f. The appropriate catheter configuration should be made available to the operating room (Crabtree, 2006c).

6. The morning of the insertion, the patient should shower, using chlorhexidine (Crabtree & Fishman, 2005).

7. The patient should have bowel preparation as a distended bowel can interfere with placement and function of the catheter (Campos et al., 2009).

8. The bladder should be empty. In patients with neurogenic bladders, a Foley catheter should be placed (Campos et al., 2009).

9. Hair should be clipped from the surgical site (Crabtree & Fishman, 2005).

10. Prophylactic intravenous antibiotics should be given at the time of catheter placement.
    a. First-generation cephalosporins are most commonly used.
    b. A randomized trial found that vancomycin is superior at preventing early peritonitis.
    c. The International Society for Peritoneal Dialysis (ISPD) recommends that each program examine the benefit of vancomycin versus the risk of resistant organisms (Li et al., 2010).

D. Intraoperative procedures.
   1. The catheter cuffs should be submerged in sterile saline.
      a. The cuffs should then be squeezed to eliminate air.
      b. This promotes better tissue ingrowth (Crabtree & Fishman, 2005; Kathuria et al., 2009).
   2. To prevent leaks and hernias, the insertion site should not be midline (Gokal et al., 1998).
   3. The deep cuff should be placed in the rectus muscle or the preperitoneal space, never in the peritoneal cavity (Gokal et al., 1998).
   4. The catheter tip should be placed between the visceral and parietal peritoneum and toward the pouch of Douglas (Gokal et al., 1998).
   5. Once the catheter tip is placed, the peritoneum is closed below the level of the catheter with a purse-string suture (Gokal et al., 1998).
   6. The subcutaneous tunnel should produce a lateral

or downward facing exit site. The direction depends on the configuration of the catheter (Crabtree, 2006c).
7. The exit site is made by exiting through the skin with a tunneling device rather than a scalpel.
   a. This technique will produce an exit site that is snug around the catheter and eliminates the need for sutures at the exit site.
   b. Sutures at the exit site increase the infection risk (Bender et al., 2006).
8. For catheters with a preformed bend, the superficial cuff should be 2 to 3 cm before the exit site; for straight catheters 4 cm (Crabtree, 2006c).
9. The function of the catheter should be evaluated by infusing 1 liter of normal saline.
   a. One liter should inflow in 5 minutes.
   b. The outflow should last 5 minutes (Crabtree & Fishman, 2005).
10. An adapter and transfer set should be connected to the catheter (Crabtree & Fishman, 2005).
11. The exit site should be covered with sterile gauze. Occlusive dressings should be avoided to eliminate the pooling of drainage in the sinus and exit site (Gokal et al., 1998).
12. To promote healing and reduce trauma, the catheter should be immobilized at all times (Bender et al., 2006).

E. Postimplantation care.
1. Exit=site care.
   a. The goal of immediate postoperative exit-site care is to prevent colonization and trauma to the exit site and tunnel (Gokal et al., 1998).
   b. For the first 2 to 3 weeks after catheter placement, dressings should be changed only weekly.
      (1) To eliminate contamination of the site.
      (2) To reduce trauma from catheter manipulation.
      (3) A dressing that becomes contaminated or wet should be changed more frequently (Gokal et al., 1998).
   c. During the postoperative period, dressing changes should be completed using aseptic technique with face masks, sterile gloves, and dressings (Bender et al., 2006).
   d. Nonocclusive dressings should be used during this period to allow any drainage to dry rather than pool at the sinus or exit site (Gokal et al., 1998).
   e. The patient should avoid submerging the exit site into water. This helps prevent the colonization of the new exit site from waterborne organisms (Gokal et al., 1998).
2. The catheter should be immobilized at all times to reduce trauma (Gokal et al., 1998).
3. Intraabdominal pressure should be minimized.

a. During the first 2 weeks after catheter insertion, if dialysis becomes necessary:
   (1) The patient should be in the supine position.
   (2) Low (500 to 1500 mL) dialysate volumes should be used (Gokal et al., 1998).
b. Other activities that increase intraabdominal pressure and should be avoided during healing include:
   (1) Coughing.
   (2) Straining with stool.
   (3) Bending over.
   (4) Squatting.
   (5) Stair climbing (Crabtree, 2006a).
4. Catheter flushing.
   a. There is no data that supports the routine flushing of the catheter until the start of PD.
   b. The practice of embedding catheters demonstrates that catheters not flushed until dialysis starts do not have higher rates of obstruction (Crabtree & Burchette, 2013; Gokal et al., 1998; McCormick et al., 2006).

F. Chronic exit-site care.
1. Goals of exit-site care.
   a. Prevent exit-site infections and assess the exit site (Prowant & Twardowski 1996).
   b. All healed exit sites will be colonized with bacteria. Appropriate exit-site care will reduce the colony-forming units and reduce the risk of infection (Bender et al., 2006).
2. Recommendations for chronic exit-site care. See Table 4.3.
   a. Begins when the exit site is healed.
      (1) Usually 2 to 3 weeks postimplantation (Prowant & Twardowski, 1996).
      (2) A healed exit site has no gapping, erythema, drainage, crusting, or tenderness (Bender et al., 2006).
      (3) Another way to assess for the need to start chronic exit-site care is by exit site classification. When the site can be classified as *good* or *equivocal*, chronic care can begin (Gokal et al., 1998).
   b. Cleansing.
      (1) There is no data on how frequently exit-site care should be done or what cleansing agent should be used.
         (a) Most clinics recommend daily care.
         (b) Exit-site care should be done if the site becomes wet or dirty (Cho & Johnson, 2014; Gokal et al., 1998).
      (2) Hand washing should be completed before touching the catheter or exit site (Piraino et al., 2011).
      (3) The site can be cleansed with liquid antibacterial soap or an antiseptic that is

Table 4.3

Key Elements of Chronic Exit-Site Care Recommendations

Thorough hand washing before touching catheter or exit site.
The exit site can be cleansed with liquid antibacterial soap or an antiseptic that is noncytotoxic (Piraino et al., 2011).
A clean washcloth and towel can be used for the healed exit site (Prowant & Twardowski, 1996).
A regimen for the prophylaxis of *S. aureus* at the exit site should be instituted (Piraino et al., 2011).
Nonsterile dressings can be used to cover the healed exit site (Prowant & Twardowski, 1996).
The catheter should be immobilized at all times to prevent trauma.
Submersion of the exit site into lakes, rivers, streams, bath tubs, and hot tubs should not be allowed due to high bacterial counts (Bender et al., 2006).

noncytotoxic (Piraino et al., 2011).

(a) To prevent contamination, soaps and antiseptics should not be transferred from one container to another (Prowant & Twardowski, 1996).

(b) Bacteria tend to grow in an environment with a pH of 6 to 8. Vinegar can be used for exit-site cleansing in conditions when water is contaminated or unavailable (see Table 4.4).

(4) A clean wash cloth and towel can be used for exit-site cleansing; sterile gauze is not

necessary (Prowant & Twardowski, 1996).

c. Prophylaxis for *S. aureus* at the exit site.

(1) The International Society for Peritoneal Dialysis (ISPD) recommends that PD units have a protocol for reducing S. aureus exit-site infections.

(a) The lack of *S. aureus* prophylaxis represents a significant danger to patients on PD.

(b) Once it has caused an exit-site infection, *S. aureus* is known to travel the subcutaneous tunnel and cause peritonitis.

(c) Once this occurs, catheter loss is common.

(2) Daily application of mupirocin cream around the exit site has been confirmed effective for reducing *S. aureus* exit-site infections and peritonitis.

(3) A large trial examining the use of intranasal mupirocin showed that regimen to be effective for reducing exit-site infections and peritonitis caused by *S. aureus*, but not other peritonitis causing organisms. *S. aureus* carriers were treated with 2% mupirocin nasal ointment three times daily for 7 days. They were recultured 7 days after the end of treatment, and then monthly to detect recolonization. Retreatment was used for recolonization (Perez-Fontan et al., 1993).

(4) Daily application of gentamicin has been shown to reduce *S. aureus* and *Pseudomonas aeruginosa* exit-site infections. An increased risk of fungal infections has been seen with the use of gentamicin (Piraino et al., 2011).

Table 4.4

Procedure for Vinegar Solution for Exit Site Care

A preparation of vinegar solution can be used when clean water is not accessible or when the exit site is inflamed or infected.		
To prepare solution	**For contaminated water, prevention of infection, or postinfection**	**For inflamed or infected exit site, perform the following twice daily**
• Combine 6 ounces (¾ cup) of boiled or bottled water, 4 ounces (½ cup) of white vinegar, and 1¾ teaspoons of table salt in a clean container. • Shake until salt is dissolved. • Pour solution into a clean spray bottle. • Discard unused solution after 7 days.	• Follow routine procedure for exit-site cleansing. • Rinse with tap water and pat dry. • Spray vinegar solution on exit site and pat dry.	• Follow routine procedure for exit-site cleansing. • Saturate a gauze pad with the vinegar solution. • Wrap around catheter or place over catheter exit site. • Leave in place for 20 minutes.

Source: Centers for Disease Control (CDC). (2005, September). *Infection control for peritoneal dialysis (PD) patients.* Retrieved from http://emergency.cdc.gov/disasters/pdf/icfordialysis.pdf

(5) There is concern that widespread resistance to mupirocin and gentamicin will develop. Several alternative agents have been studied, but results were insufficient for widespread recommendations (Cho & Johnson, 2014). The following agents were studied.

    (a) Medical honey was compared to intranasal mupriocin. The study could not recommend medical honey over intranasal mupriocin due to higher infection rates in patients with diabetes and high drop-out rates in patients who received treatment with medical honey versus intranasal mupirocin (Cho & Johnson, 2014).

    (b) Polysporin® triple ointment was compared to exit-site mupirocin. Polysporin® was found to be associated with higher rates of fungal exit-site infections and peritonitis (McQuillan et al., 2012).

    (c) A study comparing mupirocin to polyhexamethylene biguanide (PHMB) found that use of PHMB was associated with significantly higher exit-site infection rates (Findlay et al., 2013).

    (d) Creams are preferred to ointments. Ointments tend to hold moisture in at the exit site, as well as bacteria. They are contraindicated with Cruz catheters, although these are no longer being inserted.

d. Prevention of trauma.

(1) Discourage the removal of scabs and crusts as well as scratching the site.

(2) Discourage activities that cause tension, tugging, twisting, or pressure on the exit site.

(3) Avoid cleansing or topical agents that cause skin irritation.

(4) Avoid aggressive cleansing of the site.

(5) The catheter should be immobilized at all times (Prowant & Twardowski, 1996).

    (a) Many devices (belts, dressings) are available for this purpose.

    (b) Homedialysis.org is a website with information on such products.

e. Dressings.

(1) There is no data that shows the use of dressings over the exit site reduce infections.

(2) Nonsterile dressings can be used for chronic care to protect and keep the site clean.

(3) Sterile dressing should be used on infected sites (Prowant & Twardowski, 1996).

f. Swimming.

(1) Patients with healed exit sites may swim in the ocean or chlorinated swimming pools.

(2) Submersion in lakes, rivers, streams, bath tubs, and hot tubs should not be allowed.

(3) Exit-site care should be done after swimming (Bender et al., 2006).

3. Exit-site assessment (see Figures 4.3 and 4.4).

a. The site should be assessed by the patient during exit-site care.

b. The site should be assessed at each clinic visit.

(1) Assessment parameters.

    (a) Subjective.

        i. Tenderness or pain.

        ii. Recent trauma.

    (b) Tunnel.

        i. Palpate over exit-site cuff for induration.

        ii. Assess for inflammation along the tunnel.

    (c) External exit site.

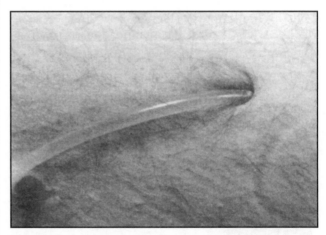

Figure 4.3. Healthy peritoneal dialysis catheter exit site.

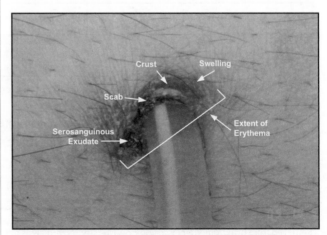

Figure 4.4. Infected peritoneal dialysis catheter exit site.

i. Observe for color and extent of discoloration.
ii. Edema.
(d) Scab and bleeding.
 i. May be the result of trauma.
 ii. Exuberant granulation tissue bleeds easily.
(e) Crusting.
 i. Crust is formed from dried, serous exudate.
 ii. A small, flaky crust is frequently found in an exit site.
 iii. Large, stubborn crusts often cover exuberant granulation tissue.
(f) Drainage.
 i. Assess the amount and characteristics of the drainage.
 ii. External drainage may not be present until after manipulation of the catheter and milking of the cuff or sinus track.
(g) Visible sinus.
 i. Assess how much of the visible sinus is covered by epithelium.
 ii. Describe the epithelium's appearance; for example:
  • Fragile, mucosal during healing after implantation.
  • Strong and mature in healthy exit sites.
  • Macerated (may be a sign of infection).
 iii. Assess how much of the visible sinus is covered by granulation tissue.
(h) Texture of granulation tissue.
 i. Plain, healthy granulation appears flat, firm, and dull.
 ii. Slightly exuberant granulation tissue protrudes slightly, appears shiny, and some vessels may be visible.
 iii. Exuberant granulation tissue or "proud flesh" is bulging, shiny, and moist; vessels are clearly visible.
 iv. Describe any drainage characteristics.
(2) Additional assessment parameters.
(a) Inspect the catheter tubing for damage.
(b) Check that adapter is fully inserted and fits tightly to transfer set.
(c) Note if cuff is visible in the sinus (Prowant et al., 2008).
c. Twardowski and Prowant (1996) devised a system for classifying the exit site into five categories.
(1) Perfect exit site.

(a) The exit site is a minimum of 6 months old.
(b) The visible sinus is covered with strong epithelial tissue.
(c) Erythema, drainage, and tenderness are absent.
(d) Small specks of crusting might be visible.
(2) Good exit site.
(a) Part of the sinus is covered with fragile epithelial or granulation tissue; mature epithelial tissue covers the remaining sinus.
(b) Erythema, drainage, and tenderness are absent.
(c) Crusts will be minimal and easily detached.
(3) Equivocal exit site.
(a) Epithelium is absent or covers only part of the sinus.
(b) Slightly exuberant or proud flesh may be present.
(c) Purulent drainage is present in the sinus or on the dressing. The drainage may be clear.
(d) Erythema is less than 13 mm around the diameter of the exit site.
(e) Pain and swelling are absent.
(4) Chronically infected.
(a) Epithelium is absent or covers only part of the sinus.
(b) Proud flesh or exuberant granulation tissues are present.
(c) Crusts are difficult to remove.
(d) Erythema is greater than 13 mm if the site is exacerbated.
(e) External drainage may be present.
(f) Site may be tender if the site is exacerbated.
(5) Acutely infected.
(a) Epithelium is regressed.
(b) Proud flesh is present.
(c) Erythema is greater than 13 mm.
(d) Purulent drainage, crusting, swelling, and tenderness are present (Kathuria et al., 2009).
4. Exit-site and tunnel infections (catheter infections).
a. Signs and symptoms.
(1) Purulent drainage at the exit site indicates infection. Erythema may or may not be present during catheter infection (Li et al., 2010).
(2) Tunnel infections are indicated by erythema, edema, and tenderness over the subcutaneous tunnel. Tunnel infection rarely occurs without the presence of an exit-site infection.

(3) *S. aureus* and *P. aeruginosa* are the most common causes of catheter infection. Since these two organisms frequently lead to peritonitis, treatment must be aggressive (Li et al., 2010).

b. Treatment.

(1) Once a catheter infection is noted, a culture and gram stain are completed.

(2) Initial therapy should be oral antibiotics that cover *S. aureus*. Once the culture results are available, treatment will be changed based on the antibiotic sensitivities.

　(a) Oral penicillinase-resistant penicillin is used for gram-positive organisms.

　(b) Vancomycin should only be used for methicillin-resistant *S. aureus* (MRSA) infections.

　(c) Oral fluoroquinolones are used for *P. aeruginosa*. For infections that are slow to resolve, a second antipseudomonal drug can be added.

　(d) Antibiotics should be continued until the exit site appears normal; this usually takes a minimum of 2 weeks (Li et al., 2010).

(3) Exit-site care may be intensified, and antibiotic cream may be used.

　(a) Sterile dressings should cover the infected exit site to absorb drainage and to help protect the exit site from other microorganisms.

　(b) The sterile dressing will help prevent trauma (Piraino et al., 2005).

(4) In addition to antibiotics, hypertonic saline soaks can be applied to the infected exit site up to two times daily for 15 minutes (see Table 4.5).

　(a) To make the hypertonic solution, add 1 tablespoon of salt to 500 cc of sterile water.

　(b) Soak gauze in the solution then place on exit site (Piraino et al., 2005).

(5) Exuberant granulation tissue may be cauterized with silver nitrate (Prowant & Twardowski, 1996).

(6) Sonography can be useful in evaluating the extent of tunnel infection and the response to antibiotic treatment (Li et al., 2010).

(7) Surgical treatment of catheter infections.

　(a) Tunnel and cuff revision: an incision in made around the exit site. The tunnel is then unroofed and the subcutaneous cuff is shaved off of the catheter. A new exit site is then created (Crabtree, 2006b).

　(b) Simultaneously, a new catheter is placed and the infected catheter is removed.

Table 4.5

Procedure for Hypertonic Saline Soaks for Inflamed or Infected PD Catheter Exit Sites

To prepare solution	To apply soaks
Add 1 tablespoon of salt to 1 pint (500 mL) of sterile water.	• Pour solution onto gauze. • Wrap saturated gauze around catheter/exit site. • Leave in place for 15 minutes once or twice a day.

Source: Piraino et al. (2005). Peritoneal dialysis-related infections recommendations: 2005 update. *Peritoneal Dialysis International, 25*(2), 107-131.

　(c) Both of these surgical treatments prevent the need for HD, but neither of the methods has been studied in large groups (Li et al., 2010).

G. Monitoring outcomes for the peritoneal access.

1. The ISPD recommends that outcomes be audited by the PD multidisciplinary team at least annually.

2. The following benchmarks are reached for catheter insertion.

a. Bowel perforation: < 1% of catheters placed.

b. Significant hemorrhage: < 1% of catheters placed.

c. Exit-site infection within 2 weeks of catheter insertion: < 5% of catheters placed.

d. Peritonitis within 2 weeks of catheter insertion: < 5% of catheters placed.

e. Catheter problems that require revision, replacement, or lead to transfer to HD: < 20% of catheters placed.

f. More than 80% of catheters should be functioning at 1 year (Figueiredo et al., 2010).

SECTION B
Peritoneal Dialysis Therapy
Cheryl L. Groenhoff, Lisa Ales, Lucy B. Todd

Note: When Level I or Level II evidence exists, treatment recommendations are identified as evidenced-based.

I. Contraindications to peritoneal dialysis.

A. Absolute contraindications.

1. Hypercatabolism: peritoneal dialysis is not able to adequately remove uremic metabolites.

2. Patent opening between the peritoneal and pleural cavities.

3. Inadequate transfer surface area because of adhesions and scarring from:
   a. Multiple surgeries.
   b. Previous peritonitis.
   c. Sclerosing peritonitis.

B. Relative contraindications.
   1. Chronic back pain.
   2. Chronic obstructive pulmonary disease (COPD).
   3. Severe diverticular disease.
   4. Abdominal disease or malignancy.
   5. Presence of a colostomy, ileostomy, nephrostromy, or ileal conduit.
   6. Patient unable or unwilling to do home dialysis and has no suitable partner(s).

II. Anatomy and physiology.

A. Description.
   1. The peritoneum is a serous membrane that covers the abdominal organs and lines the abdominal wall (see Figure 4.5).
   2. Approximately 60% of the peritoneum is visceral peritoneum, 30% is mesenterium and omentum, and 10% is parietal peritoneum.
   3. The peritoneum is composed of thin layers of connective tissue covered with mesothelium.

B. Size. The peritoneal membrane is 1 to 2 m² and approximates the body's surface area.

III. Nature.

A. The dialyzing membrane consists of the:
   1. Vascular wall.
   2. Interstitium.
   3. Mesothelium.
   4. Adjacent fluid films.

B. The peritoneal membrane is continuous and closed in males.

C. In females, the ovaries and fallopian tubes open into the peritoneal cavity.

D. The peritoneal cavity normally contains about 100 mL of fluid (transudate).

IV. Blood supply.

A. The parietal peritoneum receives blood from the arteries of the abdominal wall.

B. The blood from the parietal peritoneum and abdominal wall drains into the systemic circulation.

C. The visceral peritoneum receives blood from the mesenteric and celiac arteries.

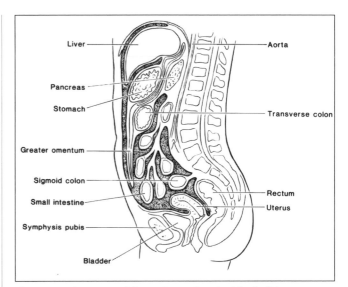

Figure 4.5. Anatomy of the peritoneal cavity (shaded) in an adult female.

D. Blood from the visceral peritoneum converges and enters the portal vein.

E. The aorta, inferior vena cava, and the mesenteric vascular network are retroperitoneal, so prolonged exposure to dialysis fluid of a different temperature may alter core body temperature.

V. Lymph drainage.

A. Lymph drainage from the peritoneal cavity occurs through a one-way system primarily involving specialized lymph openings found in the subdiaphragmatic peritoneum.

B. Intraperitoneal fluid is absorbed by convective flow. Fluid, solutes, and large molecules, such as proteins and blood cells, are all absorbed.

C. Lymph absorption is influenced by respiratory rate, intraabdominal pressure, and posture as intraabdominal pressure is lower in the supine position.

D. The average lymph absorption rate in patients on CAPD has been estimated to be between 1.0 and 1.5 mL/min, resulting in average daily lymph absorption of at least 1.5 to 2 L.

E. Lymph drainage is returned to the venous circulation primarily via the right lymph duct and the left thoracic duct.

F. Lymph drainage from the peritoneal cavity during peritoneal dialysis results in a net decrease in ultrafiltration and solute removal.

G. The lymphatics also contribute to the host defenses of the peritoneum through the absorption of foreign substances.

VI. Kinetics of peritoneal dialysis.

A. Diffusion.
   1. Diffusion across the peritoneal membrane into the dialysate is the primary mechanism of waste removal in PD, particularly for small solutes.
   2. Diffusion is defined as bidirectional movement of solutes across the peritoneal membrane from an area of higher solute concentration to an area of lower solute concentration.

B. Factors that influence solute transport.
   1. Peritoneal membrane permeability, which is affected by:
      a. Infection. Causes inflammation, which increases solute transfer.
      b. Medications. Depending upon the drug, solute transfer may either increase or decrease.
      c. Collagen and/or vascular diseases and membrane abnormalities.
   2. Peritoneal membrane size or available membrane area. This is also called *effective surface area* (may be reduced by scarring or adhesions).
   3. Concentration gradient. The higher the concentration gradient, the more rapid the solute exchange occurs.
   4. Solute characteristics.
      a. Size. Small molecules diffuse faster than larger molecules.
      b. Protein binding. Solutes that are protein bound have restricted transport.
      c. Water soluble substances are transferred more rapidly than lipid-soluble substances.
      d. Electrical charge. The peritoneal membrane has fixed negative charges.
   5. Peritoneal blood flow.
      a. Increased blood flow enhances clearances.
      b. However, dialysis occurs primarily in the microvasculature, so increasing blood flow is not very feasible.
   6. Dialysis solution volume. Larger exchange volumes increase total solute removal.
   7. Dialysis solution temperature.
      a. Solutions that are cooler than body temperature slow the rate of diffusion early in the exchange until the dialysate warms to body temperature.
      b. This has a greater effect in short dwell exchanges (as in acute dialysis or automated PD) than in long-dwell exchanges.

C. Routes of solute transport.
   1. Transcellular (across cell membranes).
   2. Extracellular (through cell junctions and gaps).

D. Factors that enhance diffusion.
   1. Increased dialysis solution flow.
      a. Dialysate flow is the total volume of solution used divided by total dwell time.
         (1) Example: in standard CAPD, 4 x 2 L = 8,000 mL divided by 1,440 (the number of minutes in 24 hours).
         (2) The dialysate flow is 5.56 mL/min.
      b. Increase exchange volume.
      c. Increase the number of exchanges.
   2. High concentration gradient. By increasing the volume and/or more frequent exchanges, the concentration gradient increases.
   3. Prewarmed dialysis solution.
   4. Ultrafiltration creates a solvent drag that pulls additional solute across the membrane.
      a. This is termed *convective transport,* and may be associated with sieving.
      b. Convective transport is the primary mechanism for middle and large molecule removal.
   5. Sieving means that solute transfer is lower than that of water transfer.
      a. The solute concentration in the ultrafiltrate is lower than that in the solution which was ultrafiltered.
      b. This occurs most often with sodium when the dwell is too short. Complaints of thirst are a diagnostic red flag that the dwells are too short.

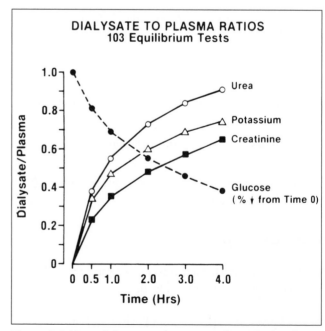

Figure 4.6. Mean dialysate to plasma ratios for multiple solutes related to dwell time; determined from 103 equilibration studies in 86 patients.

E. The rate of equilibration between the blood and dialysate occurs at a different rate for each solute as seen in Figure 4.6.
   1. Small molecular weight substances reach equilibrium more rapidly and are removed more efficiently than larger solutes.
   2. Sodium and potassium removal are most influenced by convective transport.

F. After an initial washout, the protein transport rate is almost constant.

G. Substances lost in the dialysate.
   1. Proteins.
   2. Amino acids.
   3. Water soluble vitamins.
   4. Electrolytes (e.g., sodium and potassium).
   5. Trace minerals.
   6. Some hormones (e.g., parathyroid hormone).
   7. Some drugs.

H. Substances absorbed from the dialysis solution into the systemic circulation include:
   1. Dextrose (100 to 200 g/day in CAPD with dextrose solutions).
   2. Icodextrin is absorbed by the lymphatic system when it is used as an osmotic agent.
   3. Lactate or bicarbonate.
   4. Calcium is absorbed from dialysis solutions containing 3.5 mEq/L calcium; however, most patients use 2.5 mEq/L solution.
   5. Amino acids are absorbed when present in dialysis solutions.
   6. Some drugs (e.g., insulin, antibiotics). Heparin is not absorbed.
   7. Removal and absorption rates vary among patients.

VII. Fluid removal.

A. Fluid removal in peritoneal dialysis is a two-step process.
   1. A two-step process.
      a. Water transport from the peritoneal capillaries to the interstitium.
      b. Transport across the peritoneal membrane into the peritoneal cavity.
   2. Both hydrostatic and colloid osmotic forces affect water transport.
   3. Transport of water across the walls of capillaries and venules is believed to occur through large and small pores and ultra-small pores (aquaporins).
   4. The aquaporins are transmembrane channels and only free water passes through.
      a. Aquaporins mediate 50% of UF during a hypertonic dwell.
      b. Movement of water through the aquaporins accounts for the sodium sieving.

B. Osmosis is the movement of water across the peritoneal membrane from an area of lower solute concentration to an area of higher solute concentration.

C. Factors that influence water removal in peritoneal dialysis.
   1. Peritoneal membrane permeability and surface area.
   2. Hydrostatic pressure gradient.
   3. Type and concentration of the osmotic pressure gradient.
      a. Dextrose is a crystalloid gradient.
      b. Icodextrin is a colloid or oncotic gradient.
   4. Dwell time.
      a. With dextrose, fluid is removed most rapidly early in the dwell when the osmotic gradient is greatest.
      b. During long-dwell exchanges with dextrose solutions, after several hours, fluid will be reabsorbed from the peritoneal cavity, decreasing the total drain volume.
   5. The amount of lymphatic absorption also affects the net volume of water removed.

D. Principles of fluid removal in PD.
   1. Dextrose is added to the dialysis solution to create an osmotic gradient.
   2. Icodextrin acts as a colloid osmotic agent.
   3. For dextrose solutions, the ultrafiltration rate is highest at the beginning of each exchange when the osmotic gradient is highest.
      a. Ultrafiltrate volume peaks at osmotic equilibrium when dialysate osmolality decreases (due to dilution and dextrose absorption) to the point where the rate of ultrafiltration is exceeded by the rate of lymphatic absorption.
      b. Reabsorption of water occurs if the dialysate is allowed to dwell past osmotic equilibrium.
      c. Use of dialysate solutions containing 1.5% (1.38 g/dL) dextrose will result in little or no fluid removal, especially with long-dwell exchanges.
      d. 2.5% (2.27 g/dL), 3.5% (3.18 g/dL), and 4.25% (3.86 g/dL) dextrose solutions are more hyperosmotic and are used to increase ultrafiltration and net fluid removal.
   4. Figure 4.7 illustrates how exchange volume and dextrose concentration affect ultrafiltration in long-dwell exchanges.
   5. For patients on continuous PD regimens, particularly those with high membrane permeability, shortening the exchange time (e.g., from 6 hours to 4 hours) will result in increased ultrafiltration volume.
   6. For patients on CAPD regimens who have a long overnight dwell, or patients on automated peritoneal dialysis (APD) with a long daytime

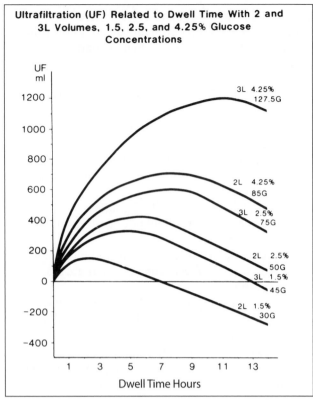

Figure 4.7. Ultrafiltration curves for 2-liter and 3-liter volumes, 2.5% and 4.25% dextrose dialysis solutions related to dwell time.

Source: Twardowski, Z.J., Khanna, R., & Nolph, K.D. (1986). Osmotic agents and ultrafiltration in peritoneal dialysis. *Nephron, 42*(2), 93-101.

dwell, icodextrin solutions will maintain the osmotic gradient throughout the long dwell.

7. Persistent use of hyperosmotic dialysis solutions may cause excessive fluid removal with the following results.
    a. Increased serum osmolality and/or hypovolemia.
    b. This leads to excessive thirst.
    c. This leads to increased fluid intake necessitating more ultrafiltration.
8. Rapid exchanges with dialysis solutions containing ≥ 4.25% dextrose.
    a. Can cause rapid water removal.
    b. This can result in an increased serum osmolality, hypernatremia, or hypovolemic shock.
    c. Historically, the use of solutions containing 7% dextrose was associated with dialysis disequilibrium. This is not standard practice.
9. Chronic use of hypertonic dialysis solutions.
    a. Results in greater exposure of the peritoneal membrane to glucose and glucose degradation products (GDPs), which may damage the membrane.
    b. Consequently, the use of 4.25% dextrose should not be part of the daily prescription.

VIII. Drug transport.

A. Effect of systemic drugs on dialysis kinetics.
    1. Systemic vasodilators may increase clearances somewhat by augmenting blood flow to adjacent capillary beds.
    2. Use of drugs that decrease abdominal blood flow will decrease clearances.

B. Effect of dialysis on drugs.
    1. Factors that affect solute clearances also affect clearance of systemic drugs. Drugs that have low molecular weights, which are poorly bound to protein and are water soluble, are more readily transported across the peritoneal membrane.
    2. Drugs administered intraperitoneally are transported into the systemic circulation.
    3. Drugs that are removed by peritoneal dialysis may need to be given in increased frequency or dosages.
    4. Drugs that are poorly removed by peritoneal dialysis and are normally excreted by the kidneys may need to be given in decreased dosages.
    5. The intraperitoneal route for drug administration, other than antibiotics for peritonitis, should be used with caution due to the potential for deleterious effects on the peritoneal membrane.

C. Intraperitoneal (IP) insulin administration.
    1. Insulin is absorbed from the peritoneal cavity and enters the systemic circulation via the hepatic portal system.
    2. Peak insulin levels are reached 20 to 30 minutes later than with endogenous insulin and are sustaned longer.
    3. Intraperitoneal insulin administration alone may be used to control serum glucose for patients on continuous forms of dialysis therapy. It is more difficult to calculate insulin dosage and control glucose for patients on continuous cycling peritoneal dialysis (CCPD) than on CAPD because most of the caloric load takes place during the day when there is only one long-dwell exchange.
    4. Intraperitoneal insulin may be used to provide supplemental insulin in intermittent peritoneal dialysis (IPD) or in acute dialysis with short exchanges.
    5. Regular insulin is added to the dialysis solution for each CAPD exchange.
    6. An increased dose of insulin is required due to:
        a. Insulin binds to the dialysis solution bags. Therefore, the amount of insulin needed is 2.5 to 5 times greater than subcutaneous dosing.
        b. Not all of the insulin is absorbed from the dialysis solution.
    7. Most clinics have abandoned IP insulin.

IX. Individual membrane characteristics.

A. Each individual's peritoneal membrane is unique. Therefore, rates of clearance and ultrafiltration differ among patients.

B. Objective evaluation of the peritoneal membrane permeability is useful in determining the most appropriate treatment modality and in prescribing the dialysis treatments.

C. The KDOQI guidelines outline three methods for the assessment of individual peritoneal membrane characteristics.
1. Peritoneal equilibration test (PET).
2. Standard peritoneal permeability analysis (SPA).
3. Peritoneal dialysis capacity (PDC).

D. All measurements of peritoneal transport characteristics should be obtained when the patient is clinically stable and at least 1 month after resolution of a peritonitis episode.

E. The peritoneal equilibration test (PET) is a standardized diagnostic test that measures the rate of solute removal and glucose absorption in individual patients.
1. Standardized PET procedure.
   a. The exchange prior to the PET exchange must have a long dwell (≥ 6 hours).
   b. Two liters of 2.5% dextrose dialysis solution is allowed to dwell in the peritoneal cavity for exactly 4 hours.
   c. Dialysate samples are collected at 0, 2, and 4 hours and analyzed for creatinine and glucose. This is a timed test so samples must be drawn at exact times.
   d. A blood sample is obtained at 2 hours for creatinine and glucose. These values are used in all calculations.
   e. The dialysate to plasma ratio for creatinine (D/P creatinine) is calculated for each sample time.
   f. The glucose over glucose at 0 dwell time (D/D0) is calculated for the 2-hour and 4-hour dwell times. There are several modeling programs that can be used for prescription predictors.
      (1) They require additional data such as obtaining an overnight specimen for BUN, creatinine, drain volume based on 2 L fill volume, and amount of total dwell time in minutes.
      (2) These data points are used for assumptions in the modeling program.
2. Faster and simpler PET procedures have been developed, but they are less reliable.
   a. A 4-hour PET with the initial drain and infusion done by the patient at home.
      (1) Patient compliance with instructions, documentation of infusion time, and accurate timing of drain are required.
      (2) There is only one 4-hour sample, so results may be more difficult to evaluate.
   b. In-center 1-hour and 2-hour PETs using extrapolated values have been described.
3. For additional information, an unabridged PET can be performed.
   a. Dialysate sampling is done at 0, 15, 30, 60, 120, and 240 minutes.
   b. Includes measurement of additional solutes (e.g., sodium, potassium, urea) (Twardowski et al., 1986).
4. Equilibration test results can be plotted on graphs representing equilibration curves from a large number of patients (see Figure 4.8).
5. The PET may be used to evaluate the patient's peritoneal membrane permeability at a single point in time, or serial studies may be used to evaluate whether changes in permeability have occurred.
6. The PET does not always provide good prediction of ultrafiltration volumes.
7. A PET using 4.25% dextrose is recommended to evaluate ultrafiltration failure.
   a. It is sometimes referred to as the "4–4–4 test."

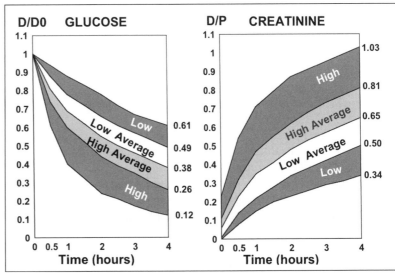

Figure 4.8. Peritoneal equilibration test curves for dialysate glucose to dialysis solution glucose at time 0 (D/D0) ratios (left) and corrected creatinine dialysate to plasma (D/P) ratios (right); determined from 103 equilibration studies in 86 patients.

b. Instill a fill volume of 2 L of 4.25% dextrose for 4 hours, and the patient should drain a net 400 mL of fluid, i.e., 2000 mL in and 2400 mL out.

c. Failure to achieve a minimum of 400 mL ultrafiltrate is diagnostic for UF failure.

8. Frequent errors in performing the PET.
   a. Short dwell time prior to the PET exchange. A long overnight dwell is necessary prior to the PET.
   b. Incomplete drain of prior exchange or of PET exchange.
      (1) Related to constipation.
      (2) Related to serum glucose greater than 300. The serum glucose must be less than 300 mg/dL.
      (3) Related to hypernatremia.
      (4) Related to catheter issues.
   c. Samples not drawn at designated times.
   d. Dialysate sample mixed with fresh dialysis solution due to improper sampling technique.
   e. Samples labeled incorrectly. Glucose numbers should go down in a linear manner, and creatinine numbers should go up in a linear manner.

9. Some assays use colorimetric methods to measure creatinine.
   a. These methods also read the unusually high glucose as creatinine.
   b. A correction factor (calculated for each laboratory) must be used to obtain accurate creatinine values.

10. The Standard Peritoneal Permeability Analysis (SPA) was developed to calculate mass transfer area coefficient (MTAC) of small and middle molecular-weight solutes and to determine residual volume and ultrafiltration kinetics. This technique is often used for research purposes.
    a. Dextrose 4.25% with dextran 70 solutions are used.
       (1) This results in less of an osmotic gradient for ultrafiltration.
       (2) There is better determination of the true diffusive MTAC characteristics of the membrane in a situation in which there is less ultrafiltration and associated convective removal of solutes.
    b. Similar to the PET, SPA uses a single dialysis exchange and direct measurements to characterize peritoneal transport properties.

11. The peritoneal dialysis capacity (PDC) test establishes the MTAC and, in addition, is better able to determine peritoneal fluid absorption rates and macromolecule permeability.
    a. Uses data from multiple dwells (typically 4 to 5) performed during a 24-hour period.
    b. Data are combined in a mathematical model to estimate peritoneal transport characteristics.

12. Interpretation of individual peritoneal membrane characteristics (based on PET).
    a. Patients with high permeability have high rates of solute transport and high rates of glucose absorption. Although clearances are good, ultrafiltration may be poor, particularly with long-dwell exchanges. These patients have many capillaries in the peritoneal membrane. They require short dwells to limit reabsorption and maximize UF.
       (1) Initial high transport associated with a low albumin is a predictor of increased risk of death. To achieve adequacy, care needs to be taken to increase fill volumes instead of exchanges to protect increased loss of protein in these patients.
       (2) Initial high transport not associated with low albumin, systemic inflammation, or atherosclerosis is not predictive of a poor prognosis.
    b. Patients with low permeability have low solute transport rates and slow rates of glucose absorption. Therefore, ultrafiltration is excellent, but clearances are low. These patients have few capillaries in the peritoneal membrane. They require long dwells to clear solutes.

13. Companies have developed computer software to help with the evaluation and interpretation of peritoneal membrane transport.
    a. PD Adequest®, developed by Baxter Healthcare Corporation (Deerfield, IL), is based on the D/P data from the standard PET.
    b. PatientOnLine®, developed by Fresenius Medical Care (Bad Homburg, Germany), uses the FT50 (equivalent to time D/P reaches 0.5) as the main parameter. Based on this value, all other parameters regarding small solute transport and ultrafiltration are calculated.

F. None of these tests (PET, SPA, PDC) has been shown to be clinically superior to the others, and KDOQI guidelines recommend that each center choose one of these tests and use it consistently to characterize peritoneal transport.

G. The PET is the simplest procedure to perform and has the most clinical experience related to its use.

H. Baseline peritoneal membrane transport characteristics should be established after initiating a daily PD therapy.
   1. The recommended time to perform the initial PET is at 4 to 6 weeks after initiation of PD.
   2. Allows ample time for healing, reducing inflammation of the peritoneal membrane, and achieving acceptable fluid balance.

I. Peritoneal membrane transport testing should be repeated when clinically indicated (e.g., loss of ultrafiltration or decrease in solute clearances).

X. Intraabdominal pressure during dialysis.

A. Peritoneal dialysis fluid can cause an increase in intraabdominal pressure proportionate to the volume of dialysis solution instilled.

B. Increased intraabdominal pressure is a risk factor for dialysate leaks, hernias, hemorrhoids, compromised pulmonary function, and vagal stimulation leading to bradycardia.

C. Factors that affect intraabdominal pressure.
1. The volume of dialysis solution. The intraabdominal pressure increases as the dialysis solution volume is increased.
2. The body's position. The intraabdominal pressure is lowest in the supine position and increases markedly in the sitting or upright positions.
3. Activity (see Figure 4.9).
a. Coughing and the valsalva maneuver induce extremely high intraabdominal pressures.

Table 4.6

Typical Electrolyte Concentration, pH, and Osmolality of Dialysis Solutions Commercially Available in the United States

	Standard Solution	Low Calcium Solutions	Icodextrin Solution
Sodium (mEq/L)	132.0	132.0	132.0
Calcium (mEq/L)	3.5	2.5	3.5
Magnesium (mEq/L)	0.5	0.5	0.5
Chloride (mEq/L)	96.0	95.0	96.0
Lactate (mEq/L)	40.0	40.0	40.0
pH	5.2–5.5	4.0–6.5	5.0–6.0
Osmolality (mOsm/L)			
1.5% Dextrose	346	344	
2.5% Dextrose	396	395	
3.5% Dextrose	447	445	
4.25% Dextrose	485	483	
Icodextrin			282–286

b. Jumping and weight lifting also cause very high intraabdominal pressures. Because of these high pressures, it may be recommended that patients perform some exercises without fluid in the peritoneal cavity.
c. Walking and riding a stationary bicycle are associated with lower intraabdominal pressures. Therefore, these are more appropriate exercise activities for patients on PD with intraperitoneal fluid.
4. Older and obese patients tend to have higher intraabdominal pressures.

D. Measurement of hydrostatic intraperitoneal pressure may be performed as an objective means of determining optimal fluid tolerance.

XI. Dialysis solution.

A. Composition.
1. The typical electrolyte concentration, pH, and osmolality of dialysis solutions commercially available in the United States are shown in Table 4.6.
2. Dialysis solution magnesium was lowered to 0.5 mEq/L.
a. This was done to ameliorate the high serum magnesium levels seen in patients on PD.
b. These lower magnesium-containing solutions should be used in patients with hypoparathyroidism (evidence-based).
3. Low calcium solutions are indicated for patients on PD with hypercalcemia (evidence-based);

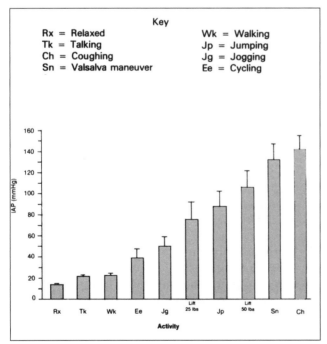

Figure 4.9. Mean ± SEM intraabdominal pressure in six upright men with 2 liters of dialysis solution in the peritoneal cavity during relaxation and various activities.

Source: Prowant, B., & Ryan, L. (1987). Intra-abdominal pressure in CAPD patients. *ANNA Journal, 14*(4), 253-257. Used with permission.

however, this is the standard formulation for most patients.

4. Sodium lactate is added as a buffer. Bicarbonate-based solutions are available in many countries.

5. Dextrose is added to increase the osmolality to enhance ultrafiltration.
   a. Most widely used osmotic agent.
   b. 1.5%, 2.5%, 3.5%, and 4.25% dextrose concentrations are available.
   c. Safe, effective, readily metabolized, and inexpensive.
   d. Exposure of the peritoneal membrane to high glucose concentrations and glucose degradation products (GDPs) may contribute to both structural and functional changes in the peritoneal membrane.

6. Amino acids in dialysis solutions also act as osmotic agents.
   a. Ultrafiltration is similar to 1.5% dextrose.
   b. Amino acid solutions are used for only one exchange per day with a long dwell to avoid uremic symptoms and metabolic acidosis.
   c. Short-term use of this solution has resulted in improvement of nitrogen balance in malnourished patients.
   d. Amino acid-containing solutions should be considered in malnourished patients as part of a strategy to improve nutritional status (evidence-based).

7. 7.5% icodextrin solution is an alternative nonglucose osmotic agent.
   a. This solution removes fluid by colloid osmotic pressure.
   b. It has a prolonged positive ultrafiltration effect because of the slow absorption via the lymphatics.
   c. Indications for clinicians may use the icodextrin solution for:
      (1) Patients with insufficient peritoneal ultrafiltration.
      (2) Patients with high/high average transport characteristics.
      (3) Those with insufficient ultrafiltration from the long-dwell exchanges in either CAPD or CCPD (evidence-based).
      (4) To avoid excessive exposure to glucose and GDPs.
      (5) Icodextrin is only used once a day for the longest dwell exchange (overnight in patients on CAPD; a long daytime exchange for patients on CCPD).
      (6) The icodextrin breaks down to maltose, primarily in the blood stream.
         (a) The maltose metabolizes to glucose intracellularly.
         (b) Its use is limited to only one exchange per day in the long dwell.

d. Allergic reactions have been reported in approximately 5% of patients.
   (1) Primarily, a skin rash develops within the first 3 weeks of use. Stop using the product.
   (2) A few patients have developed exfoliative dermatitis.
e. Maltose interferes with blood glucose monitoring results with test strips that use glucose dehydrogenase pyrroloquinoline-quinone (GDH PQQ)-based methods.
   (1) Falsely high glucose levels can result.
   (2) Blood glucose measurements must be done using a glucose-specific method to prevent maltose interference. Peripheral blood draws are not affected.
   (3) Go to http://www.glucosesafety.com to verify monitor status (Baxter Healthcare, Icodextrin package insert).

8. Outcomes.
   a. The use of icodextrin may help keep glucose exposure lower.
   b. There is no difference in peritonitis rates in patients using glucose as compared to those using icodextrin for the long dwell (evidenced-based).

B. Bicarbonate-buffered PD solutions are safe and well tolerated. Bicarbonate is a more physiologic buffer with a higher pH.
   1. Bicarbonate solutions come in double-chambered bags.
   2. Bicarbonate solutions may reduce infusion pain.
   3. Blood bicarbonate levels may increase and normalize with use of bicarbonate solutions.
   4. At the time of this writing, bicarbonate solutions were not available in the United States.
      a. High buffer-containing solutions should be used in patients with metabolic acidosis (evidence-based).
      b. Serum bicarbonate concentration should be monitored to avoid metabolic alkalosis.

C. Potassium.
   1. Omitted from dialysis solutions because patients with kidney failure require potassium removal.
   2. Acute dialysis with rapid exchanges may lower serum potassium to normal or below normal levels. Potassium chloride is then added to dialysis solutions per physician/APRN/PA's order.
   3. The goal is to maintain serum potassium levels within normal limits.

XII. The peritoneal dialysis process.

A. The exchange or cycle.
   1. An exchange or cycle is defined as the drainage, infusion, and dwell of dialysis solution, or drain-

fill-dwell. This cycle is repeated throughout the course of dialysis.

a. Infusion.
  (1) Dialysis solution flows into the peritoneal cavity by gravity with a manual system and with most cycling systems.
  (2) Other cyclers use a pump for solution infusion.
  (3) Infusion by gravity takes approximately 10 minutes for a 2 L volume if the catheter is patent and solution is elevated sufficiently above the level of the abdomen.

b. Factors that affect the rate of inflow by gravity include the height of the solution, the inner diameter of the catheter and tubing, the tubing length, catheter configuration, and intraabdominal pressure.
  (1) If the catheter and tubing diameters are equivalent, a straight Tenckhoff catheter has the fastest infusion time.
  (2) If the catheter and tubing diameters are equivalent, a coiled catheter has a longer infusion time because it is longer in total length and has more curves.
  (3) If the catheter and tubing diameters are equivalent, a swan neck, coiled catheter will have an even longer infusion time because of its greater length and additional curve.
  (4) These differences in flow rates are not clinically significant, especially in continuous PD.

2. Dwell. The dwell or equilibration period provides time for diffusion and osmosis to take place.
  a. A typical dwell time for acute intermittent peritoneal dialysis is 30 to 60 minutes.
  b. In CCPD, the cycler dwell time is approximately 1.5 to 2.0 hours.
    (1) A single daytime exchange may last as long as 12 to 16 hours.
    (2) Or, the daytime exchange may be drained after 4 to 6 hours and followed by a dry period or a second daytime exchange.
  c. CAPD daytime exchanges typically last 4 to 6 hours and the overnight exchange for 8 to 10 hours.

3. Drain.
  a. Dialysate typically drains from the peritoneal cavity by gravity.
  b. Some cyclers remove fluid by negative pressure.
  c. Drainage of 2 L plus UF takes about 20 minutes if the catheter is functioning optimally.
  d. Drain flow occurs through both the tip and side holes.
  e. Factors that affect the drain rate include the catheter position, internal or external pressure on the lines, intraabdominal pressure, catheter

configuration, the tubing diameter, tubing length, and the height or distance from the abdomen to the drain bag.
  (1) The dialysis solution drains rapidly and at a fairly constant rate during the first 7 to 10 minutes of the drain.
  (2) It then reaches a "breakpoint" where the drain flow slows dramatically.
  (3) At this point, most of the final drain volume, approximately 95%, has drained.
  (4) Prolonging the drain time further simply prolongs the period of time in which there is no dialysis taking place.
  (5) In "breakpoint APD."
    (a) The cycler is programmed to stop the drain at the breakpoint based on the patient's individual drain flow profile.
    (b) This increases clearances and reduces cycler alarms.

B. Warming methods.
  1. When exposed to high temperature for a period of time.
    a. Glucose in peritoneal dialysis solution degrades to toxic carbonyl compounds commonly known as glucose degradation products (GDPs).
    b. When there is extensive glucose degradation, the solution may have a light brown discoloration due to carmelization.
  2. Therefore, PD fluids should be warmed only to body temperature, and shortly before use.
  3. Regardless of the warming method used, the temperature of the solution must be monitored.
  4. The measured temperature should be approximately 37° C.
  5. The solution should be tepid to the touch.
  6. Dry heating is recommended.
    a. Heating cabinet or incubator.
      (1) Solutions should be warmed before use.
      (2) Solutions should not be left in the heater for an extended period of time.
    b. Heating pad.
    c. Microwave warming results in hot spots in the solution bag, especially in the medication port.
      (1) It can actually burn the peritoneal membrane.
      (2) It is for this reason that warming the solution bag in the microwave is not recommended.
    d. Home patients may place the dialysis solution on or near a heating source or in the sunshine.
    e. Water baths are not recommended for heating peritoneal dialysis solutions because they increase the risk of contamination to the system.

(1) Water is contaminated with microorganisms.

(2) Even though the dialysis solution container is dried when it is removed from the water bath, some moisture may remain and run down to the connection.

C. Shipping and storage of PD solutions.

1. When PD fluid is exposed to high temperatures during shipping or storage, the concentration of cytotoxic GDPs increases rapidly and doubles within a few hours.

   a. This can also occur with overheating or prolonged warming of dialysis solutions.

   b. This can happen regardless of the warming method used.

2. The concentration levels and cytotoxicity of GDPs gradually decrease when the PD fluid temperature is lowered to room temperature.

   a. They eventually return back to original levels.

   b. The process is slow and takes up to 40 days (Erixon et al., 2005).

XIII. Addition of medications.

A. It is recommended that medications be added immediately before the solution will be hung and used. For cyclers, it is recommended that medications be added to each individual bag.

B. Aseptic technique is critical.

C. Disinfect multiple-dose vials.

1. A 5-minute povidone-iodine soak is widely used.

2. Sodium hypochlorite preparations are also used (e.g., Amuchina®).

D. The injection port must be disinfected as the overwrap does not guarantee sterility of the bag exterior.

1. Alcavis 50 for 2 minutes is now a commonly used disinfectant method. Always consult package inserts and labeling for compatibility with system used. A darkening or shadow on the catheter has been seen near the exit site when Alcavis was used excessively on the catheter.

2. Aqueous-based providine iodine for 5 minutes is still in practice.

3. Chlorhexidine (Hibiclens®) is commonly used for 2 minutes predominantly in hospitals.

E. A ⅝-inch insulin needle will not consistently puncture the inner diaphragm of Baxter brand dialysis solution bags. A 1-inch needle is recommended.

F. Mix dialysis solution well after medication has been added.

Table 4.7

Evidence-Based Practice Guidelines for Peritoneal Dialysis, Level I and II Recommendations

■ Measurement of dialysis adequacy (KDOQI).

  • The first measurement should be performed within the first month after initiation of PD.

  • Adequacy studies should be repeated every 4 months.

  • If the patient has > 100 mL urine/day and renal clearances are used to determine the total weekly Kt/V_{urea}, a 24-hour urine collection for volume and clearances should be done every 2 months.

■ The **minimum** weekly total Kt/V_{urea} is 1.7 (KDOQI, EBPG).

■ The corrected creatinine clearance target for high and high average transporters is 60 L/week; for low and low average transporters, the target is 50 L/week (CARI, 2005).

■ The **minimum** target for net ultrafiltration in anuric patients on PD is 1.0 L/day (EBPG).

■ Subjective Global Nutritional Assessment (SGA) is a valid and clinically useful measure of protein-energy nutritional status in maintenance dialysis patients (KDOQI).

■ To preserve residual renal function, use angiotensin converting enzyme inhibitors (ACEs) or angiotensin receptor blockers (ARBs) in patients who require antihypertensive medications (KDOQI).

CARI = Caring for Australasians with Renal Impairment (2005)
EBPG = European Best Practice Guidelines (Dombros et al., 2005).
KDOQI = Kidney Disease Outcomes Quality Initiative (National Kidney Foundation, 2006)

G. Label solution container(s) with drug, dose, time, and initials. Do not use markers on the bag as the ink may penetrate it. Using labels can facilitate good communication and protect fluid sterility.

H. Record date and time of initial use on reusable medication vials.

I. Potassium chloride (KCl) comes in single dose vials without preservative. These vials should not be reused.

XIV. Peritoneal dialysis in the acute setting. See Module 4.

XV. Chronic peritoneal dialysis.

A. Evidence-based practice guidelines related to delivery of peritoneal dialysis therapy are summarized in Table 4.7.

B. Types of PD therapy.
1. Intermittent peritoneal dialysis (IPD). Treatments are performed periodically, at least several times during the week. The peritoneal cavity is empty or dry between treatments.
   a. Typically treatments are performed at night with a dry day.
   b. May be done during the day, similar to CAPD exchanges, but without an overnight exchange.
      (1) This is sometimes termed daily ambulatory peritoneal dialysis (DAPD).
      (2) Because of the shorter dialysis time, this therapy is only sufficient for patients with residual kidney function.
      (3) Because of the short dwell times, it is most appropriate for patients with high transport characteristics.
2. Continuous peritoneal dialysis, also known as CCPD. The patient dialyzes 24 hours, 7 days per week.
   a. There is always dialysis solution in the peritoneal cavity except for drain and fill.
   b. Nighttime exchanges last an average of 8 to 9 hours, with a last fill.
   c. There may be a possible additional day fill.
3. In CAPD, there are 3 to 4 daytime exchanges and a long overnight exchange.
C. Technique.
1. Intermittent flow is used for almost all chronic peritoneal dialysis.
2. Dialysis solution is first infused and then, after a dwell period, it is drained through the same catheter.
3. Each fluid exchange or cycle has three distinct modes.
   a. Inflow, dwell, and drain.
   b. Fill, dwell, and drain.
4. Intermittent flow should not be confused with intermittent dialysis. It simply describes the interruption of fluid flow through the catheter during the dwell period.
5. Tidal flow, not to be confused with tidal drain mode (defined below).
   a. After the initial volume of dialysis fluid is instilled into the peritoneal cavity, at the end of each exchange only a portion of the dialysate is drained and replaced with fresh fluid.
   b. This leaves the greater portion of dialyzing fluid in constant contact with the peritoneal membrane until the dialysate is completely drained at the end of the treatment.
      (1) A significant amount of solute removal continues during fill and drain times.
      (2) This increases the overall efficiency of the dialysis process.
      (3) Each tidal exchange has three distinct modes: inflow, dwell, and drain. However,

the initial fill and last drain have higher volumes as they are complete drains.
   c. An example of tidal dialysis is an initial fill volume of 2 L, drain volume of 1.2 L, and a tidal infusion volume of 1 L for subsequent exchanges, with a full final drain. This can help with drain pain in a patient new to PD.
6. Continuous flow is a type of intermittent PD. It is primarily a research technique aimed at enhancing dialysis efficiency.
   a. The patient has two catheters. Dialysis solution is continuously infused through one catheter and drained through the other.
   b. Theoretically, the constant infusion of new dialysis solution maintains a high concentration gradient facilitating diffusion, and a higher dextrose concentration enhancing ultrafiltration.
   c. Dialysate mixing must occur to prevent the stream of new dialysis solution from infusing through one catheter and draining right out the other.
7. Tidal drain.
   a. At the end of a CAPD or APD exchange, dialysate is drained for a set time or a set volume.
   b. The drain phase is interrupted before complete drainage is achieved.
   c. This shortens the standard drain time by eliminating the final phase where dialysate flows slowly and there is minimal additional drain volume.
   d. Thus, what would have been additional drain time becomes additional dialysis dwell time.
   e. Only at the end of the treatment is the dialysate drained completely.

XV. Method by which the peritoneal dialysis procedure is done.

A. The basic aims of any PD delivery system.
1. Security – to prevent bacterial contamination.
2. Simplicity – in terms of performing the procedure (both by staff and the patient).
3. Quality – in relation to the materials used (strong and resilient, biocompatible, disposable, recyclable).
4. Convenience – in terms of patient's preference, considering social background including employment, family, and patient's lifestyle.

B. Manual method.
1. Each fluid exchange is performed manually by the patient, partner, or nurse.
2. CAPD and DAPD are examples of PD using the manual method.

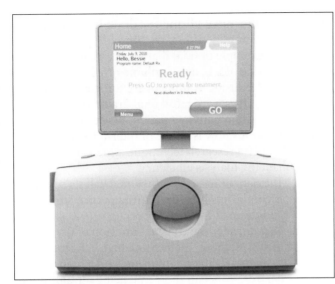

Figure 4.10. Amia cycler.
Courtesy of Baxter Healthcare.

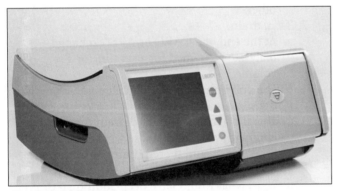

Figure 4.11. Liberty cycler.
Courtesy of Fresenius Medical Care.

C. Automated method (sometimes referred to as automated peritoneal dialysis [APD]).
   1. Exchanges or cycles are accomplished by a preset dialysis cycler.
   2. CCPD and NIPD are examples of PD treatments using an automated method.

XVI. Cycler.

A. Device used for automated peritoneal dialysis.
   1. Peritoneal dialysis cyclers require disposable tubing as well as prepared dialysis solution that must be attached and set up by the patient, assistant, or nurse using a specific procedure.
   2. Two types of cyclers are shown in Figures 4.10 and 4.11.

B. Warms dialysis solution.

C. Delivers dialysis solution to the patient and allows dialysate to remain in the peritoneal cavity for a preset period of time.

D. Controls are preset and determine inflow volume, dwell time, and outflow volume. The drain cycle can be controlled either by a predetermined volume or by time.

E. Generally monitors temperature, inflow and outflow rates, and inflow and outflow volumes.

F. Can be operated by the patient without assistance.

G. Requires mask, hand washing, and aseptic technique to add medications and perform connect/disconnect procedures.

H. Some cyclers can be disassembled and used for travel.

I. Some cyclers are equipped with memory chips that record details of each dialysis session.
   1. For example, Pro Card® for HomeChoice PRO system, Baxter Healthcare Corporation, Deerfield, IL; Newton IQ® and Liberty®, both by Fresenius Medical Care North America, Lexington, MA.
   2. The patient's treatment information can easily be downloaded, so nurses can review the patient's treatment history for a period of time.

XVII. Procedures.

A. An example of a procedure for initiating PD is shown in Table 4.8.

B. An example of a procedure for discontinuing PD is shown in Table 4.9.

C. An example of a procedure for changing the transfer set is shown in Table 4.10.

D. A study of transfer set procedures using both povidone-iodine and sodium hypochlorite reconfirmed that an external scrub or external scrub plus closed 5-minute soak does not completely disinfect the connection. Only procedures that incorporated a 5-minute open soak ensured disinfection of all surfaces (Kubey & Straka, 2005).

XVIII. The dialysis prescription.

A. The dialysis prescription should be individualized for each patient, taking into consideration:
   1. Peritoneal transport rate.
   2. Residual kidney function.
   3. Size (volume of urea distribution) or (total body surface area).
   4. Certain medical conditions.
   5. Personal preference.

Table 4.8

Example of a Procedure for Initiating PD

Using aseptic technique (wearing mask and sterile gloves):

1. Scrub the catheter-cap connection using a disinfectant.
2. Soak the catheter-cap connection in disinfectant.
3. Dry catheter-cap connection and remove cap.
4. Soak open catheter adapter in disinfectant.*
5. Connect sterile transfer set.
6. Connect dialysis solution system.
7. Drain any residual dialysate from the peritoneal cavity.
8. Flush PD system with dialysis solution.
9. Fill the peritoneal cavity with dialysis solution.

* Only procedures that incorporated a 5-minute open soak ensured disinfection of all surfaces (Kubey & Straka, 2005).

Table 4.9

Example of a Procedure for Discontinuing PD

Using aseptic technique (wearing mask and sterile gloves):

1. Scrub catheter-transfer set connection with disinfectant.
2. Soak catheter-transfer set connection in disinfectant.
3. Disconnect the transfer set from the catheter.
4. Soak open catheter adapter in disinfectant.*
5. Place cap on catheter adapter.

* Only procedures that incorporated a 5-minute open soak ensured disinfection of all surfaces (Kubey & Straka, 2005).

Table 4.10

Example of Rationale and a Procedure for Changing the Transfer Set

Key Steps	Rationale
Use aseptic technique	The inner lumen of the catheter and peritoneal cavity are sterile. Use of aseptic technique reduces the risk of contamination during the procedure.
Scrub	Physically removes dirt and debris from catheter and adapter.
Closed soak	Reduces bacteria present on the outside of the tubing, catheter, and adapter prior to disconnection.
Disconnect	Removes and discards old transfer set.
Open soak*	Reduces bacteria present on the adapter prior to connection of the new transfer set. (This will allow the disinfectant to come into contact with bacteria on the distal end of the adapter that may have been exposed when the connection was loose, but are not reached by the first soak if connection was later tightened.)
Connect new transfer set	Establishes a new, sterile transfer set for delivery of PD therapy.

* Only procedures that incorporated a 5-minute open soak ensured disinfection of all surfaces (Kubey & Straka, 2005).

B. Continuous PD therapies.
   1. Continuous ambulatory peritoneal dialysis (CAPD). This continuous dialysis therapy uses manual or manual-assisted methods.
      a. Schedule.
         (1) Dialysis solution is always present in the peritoneal cavity, except for brief interruptions to drain; then infuse fresh dialysis solution.
         (2) Dialysis takes place 24 hours, 7 days a week.
         (3) 4 to 5 exchanges per day.
      (4) Daytime exchanges usually last from 4 to 6 hours.
      (5) Overnight exchange usually lasts from 8 to 10 hours.
      (6) A typical pattern is to exchange the solution upon arising, at lunchtime, before or after dinner, and at bedtime.
      b. Indications.
         (1) Patients with average or low peritoneal membrane permeability.
         (2) Patients who want to avoid machines or confinement to bed.

c. Clearances are higher than those obtained with IPD because of the extremely long dwell times. Good control of fluid balance can be maintained.

2. Continuous cycling peritoneal dialysis (CCPD). This continuous therapy uses a cycler for automated overnight dialysis, with a long-dwell exchange during the day, or a single additional daytime exchange.

   a. Schedule.

     (1) 3 to 5 overnight cycles.

     (2) Overnight cycles last from 1.5 to 2 hours, or even 3 hours.

     (3) A single, long daytime exchange lasts 12 to 16 hours.

       (a) Use of hypertonic (4.25%) solution may prevent significant reabsorption, but is not recommended on a daily basis. An additional daytime exchange can be made as well.

       (b) Use of icodextrin should be considered for the long-dwell exchange (evidence-based).

   b. Indications for icodextrin.

     (1) High or high average peritoneal membrane transport characteristics to improve UF vs 4.25% (Baxter Healthcare, Icodextrin package insert).

       (a) Clearances are higher than those obtained with IPD.

       (b) Better control of fluid balance may be achieved.

       (c) Minimize glucose exposure.

     (2) Patients who choose CCPD.

       (a) Preference for uninterrupted days.

       (b) School or work schedules require uninterrupted days.

       (c) Those patients requiring the assistance of a partner for dialysis (e.g., children and older adults).

       (d) Teenagers to accommodate school.

3. Systems for continuous therapies.

   a. Common elements. Tubings are composed of polyvinyl, thermoplastic, silicone, or polypropylene materials with clamps to control fluid flow.

   b. The majority of the peritoneal dialysis systems are interlocking connector systems (e.g., Luer-Lok).

   c. Y-set tubing comes with a drain bag on one arm of the Y and the other arm is used to attach the new solution bag. The leg of the Y is connected to the patient's catheter or transfer set. This is commonly used to drain out solution when a patient goes part of the day dry.

   d. Double-bag systems are Y-sets manufactured with the dialysis solution bag already attached.

Double-bag or twin-bag systems are preferred for CAPD because they are more effective in preventing peritonitis (evidence-based). These are the systems most frequently used in North America and Europe. If a double-bag system is not available, any Y-set system is preferred to a spike system, because Y- and double-bag systems are more effective in preventing peritonitis (evidence-based).

4. Flush before fill concept.

   a. For both the Y and double-bag systems, approximately 100 mL dialysis solution is flushed from the new dialysis solution bag to the drain bag.

     (1) The patient then drains the dialysate from the peritoneal cavity.

     (2) This procedure is widely referred to as "flush-before-fill."

   b. In vitro studies have shown that the flushing procedure followed by a drain was effective in eliminating *Staphylococcus epidermidis* 5 minutes after contamination. *Staphylococcus aureus* and *Pseudomonas* species were reduced, but not consistently eliminated.

   c. Studies consistently demonstrated lower peritonitis rates using Y systems or Luer-Lok systems than standard spike, and the standard systems should not be used (evidence-based).

C. Intermittent peritoneal dialysis (IPD).

1. With IPD, any schedule that has a period off dialysis is considered intermittent.

   a. Typically, IPD uses a cycling device, although it can be done manually.

   b. IPD refers to peritoneal dialysis that is done for several hours, discontinued, and then repeated, either in a healthcare facility or at home.

   c. Exchange time on IPD is significantly shorter than in continuous dialysis.

   d. Therefore, it is ideal for patients with very high peritoneal transport characteristics or with significant residual kidney function.

2. Indications for IPD.

   a. Used during early use of a chronic catheter (catheter break-in period), as in urgent-start PD.

   b. When there are complications related to increased intraabdominal pressure (e.g., hernias and leaks). (*Reminder*: Intraabdominal pressure is lower in the supine position.)

   c. Used when patients are in hospitals and extended care facilities and staffing does not allow CAPD.

   d. Patients unable to achieve adequate ultrafiltration and solute clearances with CAPD (e.g., patients with high transport characteristics) (evidence-based).

   e. In patients with significant residual kidney

function, IPD may provide adequate clearances and fluid removal.

   f. Dialysis for acute kidney injury.

  3. Schedule. To achieve adequate clearances and fluid removal, chronic IPD is typically done 8 to 10 hours every night.

    a. This is sometimes called nightly intermittent peritoneal dialysis (NIPD).

    b. Additional time is required for patients without residual kidney function.

    c. Nightly tidal peritoneal dialysis (NTPD) is another variation of IPD. This therapy uses a cycler that delivers tidal volumes.

D. Tidal dialysis.

  1. In tidal dialysis, only a portion of the full exchange volume is drained and replaced for each exchange. For example, if a 2 L initial fill volume is used, the cycler could be set for a 1200 mL drain volume and 1000 mL tidal fill volume.

  2. Tidal volumes and dwell times must be individualized to achieve the most efficient clearances. Dwell times are shorter than in typical IPD (or CCPD).

  3. Tidal peritoneal dialysis requires special programming so that tidal volumes and cycles can be delivered.

  4. Indications for tidal dialysis.

    a. Need to increase dialysis efficiency and adequacy in a patient on cycler dialysis.

      (1) Weekly clearances are somewhat greater than for the equivalent time on NIPD.

      (2) This is due to the use of more fresh dialysis solution and greater diffusion time (due to decreased drain and fill times).

    b. Inflow or outflow pain (evidence-based).

    c. Slow drainage causing cycler alarms (evidenced-based).

  5. Tidal peritoneal dialysis may be more expensive because of the markedly higher volume of dialysis solution used.

E. Table 4.11 compares key elements of the three most widely used PD.

XIX. Achieving adequate peritoneal dialysis.

A. Residual kidney function (RKF) predicts survival and contributes significantly to peritoneal dialysis adequacy.

Table 4.11

Comparison of Chronic Peritoneal Dialysis Therapies

CAPD (continuous ambulatory peritoneal dialysis)	CCPD (continuous cycling peritoneal dialysis)	NIPD (nightly intermittent peritoneal dialysis)
4–5 manual exchanges during the day; may use assist device for extra nighttime exchange(s).	Automatic cycling of exchanges overnight with a long daytime dwell.	Automatic cycling of exchanges overnight.
Solution in peritoneal cavity continuously, except for drain and fill times.	Solution in peritoneal cavity continuously, except for drain and fill times.	Dialysate is drained completely at end of dialysis; no solution in the peritoneal cavity between dialyses.
Some techniques require portable equipment (e.g., an exchange assist device).	Requires cycler; typically uses 5 liter bags.	Requires cycler; typically uses 5-liter bags.
Closed system is opened for each exchange.	Closed system opened for setup and on/off procedures.	Closed system opened for setup and on/off procedures.
Requires 20–40 minutes/exchange.	Requires ~ 45 minutes for setup and on/off procedures.	Requires ~ 45 minutes for setup and on/off procedures.
Blood chemistries stable.	Small diurnal biochemical fluctuations.	Biochemical fluctuations.
Fluid balance stable.	Diurnal fluctuations in fluid balance.	Fluid balance fluctuations.
Daytime interruptions for exchanges; sleep uninterrupted.	Sleep may be disturbed; may require an additional daytime exchange.	Sleep may be disturbed; no interruption of daytime routine.

1. The Kidney Dialysis Outcomes Initiative (KDOQI) Guidelines for Peritoneal Dialysis Adequacy were revised in 2006 based upon results of two prospective randomized trials demonstrating the importance of residual kidney function versus the achievement of higher small solute clearances on survival in patients on PD. Additionally, a re-analysis of the Canada–United States (CANUSA) study, from which original guidelines were developed, revealed no survival benefit by increasing peritoneal small solute clearances (Bargman et al., 2001).
   a. Further examination of the CANUSA study showed that for each 5 L/week per 1.73 m^2 increment increase in the glomerular filtration rate (GFR), there was a 12% decrease in the relative risk of death (CANUSA, 1996).
      (1) The same association was not seen with peritoneal solute clearances.
      (2) Additionally, a 36% reduction in the relative risk of death was observed for every 250 mL incremental daily increase in urine volume (Bargman, et al., 2001).
   b. Results of the Adequacy of Peritoneal Dialysis in Mexico (Ademex Study) (Churchill, 2005).
      (1) This was a randomized clinical trial comparing the clinical outcomes of two groups of continuous ambulatory dialysis (CAPD) patients randomized to two distinct doses of PD.
      (2) The results were also considered in the revision of the most recent guidelines.
      (3) The Ademex study revealed no survival advantage between the control group of patients randomized to a Kt/V of 1.80 and the intervention group randomized to a Kt/V of 2.27.
   c. A similar interventional study conducted in Hong Kong examined the effect of Kt/V and patient survival in 320 anuric patients on CAPD.
      (1) Patients were randomized into three different Kt/V target groups.
      (2) The Hong Kong study demonstrated that increasing the Kt/V$_{urea}$ above 1.7 did not lead to improved survival (Lo et al., 2003).
2. Residual kidney function (RKF).
   a. An RKF of 1 mL/min contributes around 10 L to the total weekly creatinine clearance for a patient who has a body surface area (BSA) of 1.73 m^2.
   b. Conversely, each 1 mL/min of residual kidney urea clearance adds 0.25 to the total weekly Kt/V$_{urea}$ for a 70 kg male (Burkhart et al., 1996).
3. The current 2006 KDOQI guidelines now emphasize the importance of monitoring and preserving residual kidney function (evidenced-based).
4. The following strategies are recommended by KDOQI to preserve RKF.
   a. Preferential use of angiotensin-converting enzyme.
      (1) KDOQI recommends use of angiotensin-converting enzyme inhibitors (ACEs) or angiotensin receptor blockers (ARBs) in patients who require antihypertensive medications (evidenced-based).
      (2) Studies examining the effects of ACE inhibitors and ARBs in patients on PD indicate a slower decline in GFR and residual urine volume compared to patients not receiving ACE or ARB therapy (NKF, 2006a).
   b. Consideration of the use of ACE inhibitors or ARBs in normotensive patients with RKF (evidenced-based).
   c. Avoidance of nephrotoxic drugs (e.g., nonsteroidal antiinflammatory drugs [NSAIDs]), including COX-2 inhibitors and aminoglycoside antibiotics.
   d. Avoiding intravenous (IV) radiocontrast agents. Alternative diagnostic studies should be considered if feasible to avoid radiocontrast dyes or agents.
   e. Establish a protocol that outlines renal protective strategies when IV radiocontrast agents must be used. Recommended strategies include:
      (1) Use of the lowest dose of radiocontrast dye possible.
      (2) Administration of iso-osmolal nonionic radiocontrast.
      (3) Maintain adequate hydration.
      (4) Prophylactic administration of acetylcysteine.
   f. Patient education regarding preservation of residual kidney function.
   g. Avoiding excessive fluid removal, dehydration, and hypotension.

B. KDOQI Guidelines for Peritoneal Dialysis Adequacy – past and present.
   1. In 1997, the original Kidney Dialysis Outcomes Initiative (KDOQI) Guidelines for peritoneal dialysis adequacy were published. The origins of these early guidelines for peritoneal dialysis adequacy were primarily based on the Canada–United States (CANUSA) study that suggested higher solute clearance targets would improve patient outcomes.
      a. Initial results of the CANUSA study revealed:
         (1) For every 0.1 increase in the Kt/V$_{urea}$ per week, the relative mortality risk was

reduced by 5% (Bargman et al., 2001).

(2) For every 51 L/week/1.73 m² increase in creatinine clearance, the relative mortality risk was reduced by 7% (Bargman et al., 2001).

b. Residual kidney function was not separately examined as a risk factor impacting clinical outcomes as the clearance of small solutes from native kidneys was considered to be equal to small solute clearance by the peritoneal membrane. This was the major flaw in the paper.

c. Based upon these preliminary findings, the original KDOQI guideline recommendations (Churchill, 2005) were a Kt/V_{urea} of ≥ 2.0 for CAPD with incremental increases for CCPD and NIPD.

d. A total (dialysate + kidney) weekly target for corrected creatinine clearance was recommended according to peritoneal membrane transport status.

(1) High and high average transporters had a target of 60 L/week.

(2) Low and low average transporters had a target of 50 L/week of total corrected creatinine clearance (Churchill, 2005).

e. The ADEMEX study demonstrated increasing Kt/V_{urea} over 1.7 did not lead to improved survival (Paniagua et al., 2002).

f. Studies in Hong Kong found increasing Kt/V_{urea} over 1.7 did not lead to improved survival in anuric patients. There was a trend toward improved survival in patients with $Kt/V_{urea} > 2.0$, but was not statistically significant (Lo et al., 2003).

2. Current guidelines.

a. Current KDOQI guidelines recommend an absolute minimum Kt/V_{urea} of 1.7.

(1) This goal must be met by all patients on PD at all times.

(2) Regardless of type of PD therapy or prescription (evidence-based).

b. The same data used to determine Kt/V_{urea} can be used for calculations of urea generation rate, protein catabolic rate, and residual kidney function.

3. Creatinine clearance.

a. Creatinine clearance has been dropped from the KDOQI guidelines. A total weekly creatinine clearance of 60 L for high and high average transporters, and 50 L for low and low average transporters, is still recommended by the Australian guidelines (CARI, 2005).

b. The International Society for Peritoneal Dialysis (ISPD) 2006 Solute and Fluid Removal Guidelines recommend a target of 45 L per week of creatinine clearance in automated

peritoneal dialysis patients (Lo et al., 2006).

c. Creatinine clearance is calculated from 24-hour collections of both dialysate and urine, and is standardized using body surface area. Creatinine clearance can be easily and inexpensively measured from the same dialysate and urine collections and blood sample as the Kt/V_{urea}.

d. Creatinine diffuses more slowly than urea because of its higher molecular weight.

(1) Creatinine clearance can be used as a surrogate marker of clearance of molecules a bit larger than urea.

(2) Creatinine is both filtered in the glomerulus and secreted by the tubules and is more readily removed when patients have residual kidney function.

e. When both Kt/V_{urea} and creatinine clearance values are available and there is discordance between Kt/V_{urea} and creatinine clearance values, Kt/V_{urea} should be the determinant of adequacy.

f. The same data used to determine creatinine clearances can be used for estimation of lean body mass.

4. Frequency of adequacy testing as recommended by KDOQI guidelines.

a. The first measurement should be performed within the first month after initiation of PD. However, most clinicians wait at least a month after therapy initiation.

b. Adequacy studies should be repeated every 4 months thereafter.

c. If the patient has > 100 mL urine/day, and renal clearances are used to determine the total weekly Kt/V_{urea}, a 24-hour urine collection for volume and clearances should be done every 2 months.

d. Clinical experts recommend measurements be repeated if there is a change in residual kidney function, ultrafiltration, or a change in laboratory values that could signal a change in peritoneal membrane function.

e. Other clinical indications for measurement of dialysis adequacy can be seen in Table 4.12.

5. Evaluation of adequacy of peritoneal dialysis.

a. All patients should routinely have a careful clinical evaluation for adequacy of dialysis with special attention to signs of inadequate dialysis.

b. Elements of the evaluation.

(1) Appetite (e.g., presence of anorexia, dysgeusia, nausea, vomiting).

(2) Energy and activity levels.

(3) Muscle mass, strength, and endurance.

(4) Parathesias and asthenia.

(5) Quality of sleep.

(6) Nutritional status.

Table 4.12

Clinical Indications for Measurement of Peritoneal Dialysis Adequacy

- Documentation of delivered total solute clearance after a prescription change.
- Hypertension and volume-overload refractory to current therapy.
- Signs or symptoms of uremia.
- Changes in laboratory values (e.g., increasing serum creatinine, urea, or potassium).
- Failure to thrive on dialysis therapy.
- Evaluation of other undiagnosed clinical problems.

(7) Ability to achieve/maintain fluid balance and blood pressure control.

(8) Anemia and response to erythropoiesis-stimulating agents (ESAs).

6. Evaluation of fluid balance.
   a. The European guidelines recommend a minimum target for net ultrafiltration in patients with anuria and on PD, of 1.0 L/day (evidence-based) (Dombros et al., 2005).
   b. KDOQI guidelines do not recommend a minimum target for net ultrafiltration but do state that each facility should have a program to monitor fluid balance on a monthly basis, including blood pressure, PD drain volumes, and residual kidney function (evidence-based).
   c. KDOQI guidelines recommend the following strategies to optimize extracellular water and blood volume (evidence-based).
      (1) Restrict dietary sodium.
      (2) Restrict water intake.
      (3) Use diuretics in patients with residual kidney function.
      (4) Optimize peritoneal ultrafiltration and sodium removal.
         (a) Negative ultrafiltration during the long daytime dwell in APD, and nocturnal dwell in CAPD should be avoided.
         (b) Patients on APD may need shorter daytime dwells with a dry period to avoid peritoneal fluid reabsorption.
         (c) An alternative approach would be the use of icodextrin solution during the long dwell.
         (d) Patients on CAPD may need to be switched to APD.
   d. There should be ongoing assessment, monitoring, and evaluation of dry weight.

C. Techniques for measuring PD adequacy require 24-hour urine and dialysate collections.
   1. Urea kinetic modeling (Kt/V_{urea}).
      a. The formulas calculate the total clearance of urea (from 24-hour collections of both dialysate and urine) over a specified time, adjusted for the volume of body water estimated from sex, age, height, and weight. A formula and sample calculations are shown in Tables 4.13 and 4.14.
      b. The NKF-KDOQI guidelines recommend that urea distribution volume (the V in Kt/V_{urea}) should be estimated using either Watson and Watson or Hume-Weyers methods using ideal or standard weight rather than actual body weight.
      c. The volume should not be estimated as a percentage of total body water.
         (1) This method will overestimate V in obese patients, and underestimate V in underweight patients.
         (2) The volume has a large impact on the results of the Kt/V_{urea} equation.
         (3) Inaccurate estimated volumes can result in erroneous Kt/V_{urea} results in individual patients.
   2. Methods of collecting dialysate samples for adequacy testing.
      a. Batch method.
         (1) Collect all drain bags for 24 hours.
         (2) Weigh or measure dialysate in each bag to determine total volume.
         (3) Combine all dialysate in one container and mix well.
         (4) Take sample and send to laboratory for urea and creatinine.
      b. Aliquot method.
         (1) Collect all drain bags for 24 hours.
         (2) Weigh/measure each drain bag.
         (3) Record the total 24-hour volume.
         (4) Take at least 0.1% sample from each bag.
         (5) Combine all samples and mix well.
         (6) Send sample to laboratory for urea and creatinine.
   3. Problems with adequacy testing.
      a. 24-hour collections for adequacy assessment are typically done by the patient at home.
         (1) The dialysis done on the day of collection may not represent the dialysis that the patient routinely does.
         (2) In a case where the patient frequently skips an exchange, but does dialysis as ordered on the day of collection, the clearance indices will represent what the prescribed therapy could achieve, not the amount of dialysis the patient is actually receiving.
      b. The patient may make errors in performing the

Table 4.13

Urea Clearance and Kt/V$_{urea}$ Formulas for Continuous Peritoneal Dialysis

$K = D_{urea} \times D_{volume} / P_{urea} \times t$

K = Clearance
D = Dialysate
    urea in mg/dL
    volume in mL
P = Plasma
    urea in mg/dL
t = time in minutes

Kt/V = Clearance x time/volume (TBW)

TBW* = 2.45 – 0.0952** (age) + 0.107** (Ht.) + 0.336 (Wt.)

_____

*Total Body Water according to Watson formula for males.
**These numbers have been rounded in this example.

Table 4.14

Sample Kt/V$_{urea}$ Calculation

A 47-year-old Caucasian male, height 176 cm, weight 70 kg, is on CAPD with four 2 L exchanges per day.

Dialysate volume	10,000 mL
Dialysate urea nitrogen	53 mg/dL
Urine volume	950 mL
Urine urea nitrogen	408 mg/dL
Serum urea nitrogen	75 mg/dL

$K_{dialysis}$ = $\dfrac{53 \text{ mg/dL} \times 10,000 \text{ mL}}{75 \text{ mg/dL} \times 1440 \text{ minutes}}$
= 4.91 mL/min or 7.07 L/day*

K_{urine} = $\dfrac{408 \text{ mg/dL} \times 950 \text{ mL}}{75 \text{ mg/dL} \times 1440 \text{ minutes}}$
= 3.59 mL/min or 5.17 L/day*

$K_{combined}$ = 8.50 mL/min or 12.24 L/day

TBW = 2.45 – 0.0952 (47) + 0.107 (176 cm) + 0.336 (70 kg)
    = 40.33 L

Kt/V = 12.24/40.33 = .30/day or 2.1/week

_____

* In actual practice, only the final number would be rounded, and only to the least number of decimal places used in the entire calculation. Incorrect rounding results in error.

dialysis exactly as ordered, in saving a complete quantitative urine collection, or in bringing the collections or samples to the clinic or laboratory. Frequent errors include:
(1) Quantitative urine collection.
    (a) Not recording precise times the collection begins and ends.
    (b) Including the first voiding in the collection.
    (c) Failing to include all voidings or including partial voidings.
(2) Dialysate collection.
    (a) For continuous therapies, time is not exactly 24 hours.
        i. A longer time results in an increase in solute removal, somewhat overestimating clearances.
        ii. A shorter time results in less solute removal, thus underestimating clearances.
    (b) The patient adds an extra bag to the 24-hour collection, from the previous day or the following day.
    (c) The patient does not clamp bags securely when bringing them into clinic and dialysate is lost; the measured 24-hour volume is less than the actual volume.
    (d) Bags are not weighed or measured accurately when an aliquot is taken at home. The volume measurement is inaccurate.

D. Problems achieving targets.
    1. Unless a patient has residual kidney function, it is almost impossible to achieve recommended levels of creatinine clearance.
    2. Patients with low peritoneal membrane permeability will have a larger discrepancy between Kt/V$_{urea}$ and creatinine clearance than those with high membrane permeability. KDOQI guidelines state when there is discordance between Kt/V$_{urea}$ and creatinine clearance values, Kt/V$_{urea}$ should be the determinant of adequacy.

E. Patients at risk for inadequate dialysis.
    1. Patients with declining or no residual kidney function (RKF) require adjustments in the PD prescription to achieve an increase in small solute clearances and compensate for the loss of RKF clearance. KDOQI guidelines recommend a continuous PD prescription in patients with minimal RKF.
    2. Patients with low peritoneal membrane permeability.
    3. Large patients may have difficulty achieving

adequate dialysis. Larger patients may require the use of 3.0 L fill volumes.

4. Patients who are nonadherent must be assessed, including:
   a. Repeat counts of dialysis solution inventory.
   b. Monitor dialysis solution orders. Reviewing order history using Direct Access® (Baxter Healthcare Corporation, Deerfield, IL), an online Peritoneal Dialysis (PD) prescription management tool, or other online systems available from the PD supplies provider.
   c. Review data on computer memory cards from cycler machines.
   d. Review patient's home dialysis records.
   e. Clinical assessment for inadequate dialysis as outlined above.
5. Patients on intermittent dialysis.

F. Methods of increasing the dose of dialysis.
1. NKF-KDOQI guidelines state regardless of delivered dose, if a patient has signs and symptoms suggestive of inadequate dialysis, or if a patient is not thriving and has no other identifiable cause other than kidney failure, consideration should be given to increasing the dialysis dose. The guidelines list these reasons to consider when increasing the dose of dialysis (NKF-KDOQI, 2006b).
   a. Evidence of volume overload.
   b. Unexplained nausea or vomiting.
   c. Sleep disturbances.
   d. Restless leg syndrome.
   e. Pruritus.
   f. Uncontrolled hyperphosphatemia.
   g. Hyperkalemia.
   h. Metabolic acidosis unresponsive to oral bicarbonate therapy.
   i. Anemia refractory to or requiring large doses of ESAs.
   j. Uremic neuropathy.
   k. Uremic pericarditis.

2. CAPD.
   a. Increasing the exchange volume is a recommended first strategy to increasing clearance on CAPD for all membrane types.
      (1) An increase from 2.0 to 2.5 L per exchange increases clearances approximately 25%.
      (2) Some patients can tolerate 3 L exchanges.
   b. Increasing the number of exchanges will increase clearances on CAPD.
      (1) Increasing the number of exchanges per day on CAPD increases burden of therapy.
      (2) This can lead to poor adherence and poor quality of life.
3. CCPD.
   a. Increasing exchange volume. Larger exchange

volumes are sometimes better tolerated resting in the supine position because intraabdominal pressure is lower.
      (1) Night fill volumes can be increased over the course of a few weeks, increasing fill volumes in increments of 100 to 200 mL to enhance patient tolerance.
      (2) Increasing the exchange volume of four overnight cycles from 2.0 to 2.5 L increases clearances by 10–15%.
   b. Adding a second long-dwell daytime exchange.
      (1) This may increase Kt/V_{urea} another 20%.
      (2) Consider the use of icodextrin for the long 8–16-hour dwell to improve clearance of creatinine and urea nitrogen in high and high average transport types.
   c. Increasing the number of nocturnal cycles from 4 to 6 cycles typically results in a 10% increase in urea clearance.
   d. As the number of cycles increase, the dwell time for each cycle may decrease unless therapy time is increased on the cycler.
      (1) Shortened dwell times can reduce the urea concentration in each cycle.
      (2) For maximum increases in clearances, additional therapy time may need to be added.
4. Nightly intermittent peritoneal dialysis (NIPD).
   a. NIPD is indicated for patients with significant residual kidney function or high transport peritoneal membrane types.
      (1) NIPD may be an inadequate therapy for large patients and patients with low and low average transport types.
      (2) NIPD is not recommended in patients with anuria (Gahl & Jorres, 2000).
   b. Strategies to increase clearances on NIPD include:
      (1) Increasing exchange volume.
      (2) Increasing the number of exchanges.
      (3) Increasing the total time on the cycler.
      (4) Considering changing patient's therapy to a continuous (CCPD) vs. an intermittent PD prescription.
         (a) In a patient with minimal RKF, a continuous (24 hr/day) PD regimen rather than intermittent PD prescription should be used to maximize middle-molecule clearance.
         (b) This increases the Kt/V_{urea} up to 30%, depending on transport characteristics.
   c. The ISPD guidelines for solute and fluid removal (Lo et al., 2006) state that continuous around-the-clock dialysis is preferred to an intermittent schedule whenever possible (evidence-based).

XX. Nursing care of patients on chronic PD.

A. Chronic peritoneal dialysis is almost exclusively a home dialysis therapy. Home dialysis candidates must have an assessment of self-care abilities and suitability for home dialysis.
1. Assessment parameters for patient and/or family.
   a. Understanding of the diagnosis of CKD stage 5 disease and therapy options.
   b. Cultural orientation toward health and illness.
   c. Motivation for choosing home dialysis.
   d. Family support for patient's decision to dialyze at home.
   e. Past experiences with self-care.
   f. Level of independence in activities of daily living.
   g. Patient's roles and level of functioning prior to diagnosis.
   h. Any degree of disability given the complexity of the illness. The patient may be too ill to take the sole responsibility for dialysis. Even if a family member is willing to care for their loved one, assessment of partner burnout needs to be done routinely.
   i. Patient's physical abilities or handicaps.
      (1) Vision.
      (2) Muscular strength.
      (3) Fine motor coordination.
      (4) Cognitive impairment.
   j. Identify any family and community resources for assistance and support.
   k. Is a partner required to perform some or all of the assessments or procedures?
      (1) Is a partner available?
      (2) Is the partner willing and motivated?
      (3) Is there an alternative if the partner should be unable to perform dialysis?
   l. Patient and/or partner's decision-making abilities and adherence history.
   m. Physical characteristics of the home.
      (1) Access to electricity and drain for automated equipment.
      (2) Adequate space to store fluid and supplies.
      (3) Home size and number of inhabitants.
         (a) Is there an area that can be isolated for aseptic procedures?
         (b) Pets in the home are acceptable provided they are not in the room during dialysis, or in the bed at night when a cycler is used.
   n. Comorbid medical conditions. See contraindications.
   o. Mental status.
      (1) Mentally competent.
      (2) Has intact memory and sequencing skills.
      (3) Acceptance of diagnosis.
      (4) Any barriers to rehabilitation, real and perceived, including fears?
   p. Quality of life.
   q. Goals for vocational rehabilitation.
2. The National Kidney Foundation has published an outcome-driven nephrology social work assessment consisting of three components.
   a. Factors affecting adjustment to chronic kidney disease.
   b. Rehabilitation.
   c. Health-risk behavior assessment.

B. Patient education. (Also see Module 2, Chapter 3.)
1. The patient education process is a collaborative effort among the members of the peritoneal dialysis team, which includes at least a nurse, physician, dietitian, social worker, and the patient and family/significant other.
2. Goals of the patient education program.
   a. To provide the patient and family members the knowledge and skills to perform PD safely in their home environment.
   b. To maintain proper nutrition.
   c. To assist the patient and family in identifying the need for, and using, medical and community resources.
   d. To assist the patient and family in developing skills to cope with chronic kidney disease and achieve optimum quality of life and rehabilitation.
3. Patient education is most effective when principles of adult education are incorporated.
   a. Assess learning ability and readiness to learn.
   b. Be SMART about goals, objectives, and plan. SMART goals include:
      (1) Specific.
      (2) Measurable.
      (3) Attainable.
      (4) Realistic.
      (5) Timely.
   c. Differentiate what patient "needs to know" from "nice to know" to be successful and safe and prioritize this information.
   d. Use analogies to which patients can relate, i.e., semipermeable membrane is like a teabag.
      (1) This helps the patient, as an adult learner, link what they already know to the new information being taught.
      (2) The teabag analogy illustrates the semipermeable nature of the membrane: certain things can come through while others cannot.
   e. Always give objective evaluation and feedback.
4. Initial patient education should include:
   a. Description of the dialysis therapy and appropriate terminology.
   b. Principles of peritoneal dialysis – drain, fill, dwell.

c. Principles of asepsis and aseptic technique.
d. How to care for the peritoneal dialysis catheter and exit site.
e. How to monitor vital signs, especially the blood pressure and weight, and why these are important.
f. Fluid balance.
   (1) When to use 1.5%, 2.5%, and 4.25%.
   (2) Include why 4.25% should not be used daily.
   (3) Discuss how to recognize volume overload.
g. Discuss with the patient potential complications of peritoneal dialysis that are most likely to occur.
h. Problem solving, especially when to call the PD nurse or seek emergency assistance.
i. Medications.
j. Diet instruction.
   (1) Primarily with the dietitian.
   (2) Should include family members who cook and/or buy groceries.
k. Discuss appropriate activities and exercise, and ways to advance these as the catheter heals.
l. Maintenance of home dialysis records, including the need to bring in cycler-specific record devices as indicated.
m. Discuss the emergency communication system, or who to call when and for what issue. Most clinics teach patients to call the nurse first (Firanek, 2013).

5. Patient training after initial training.
   a. Explain the plan for follow-up.
      (1) Clinic visits.
      (2) Routine laboratory tests.
         (a) Urea and creatinine.
         (b) Potassium.
         (c) Calcium and phosphorus.
         (d) Hematocrit.
         (e) Serum albumin.
         (f) Kt/V_{urea} and creatinine clearance as markers of adequacy.
   b. How to order and inventory supplies.
      (1) Ensure there is adequate storage capacity in the home.
      (2) Many programs do not teach ordering during initial training, but wait until a week or two later when the patient returns to the clinic (Firanek, 2013).
   c. Emergency procedures.
      (1) Technical (performing dialysis procedures). This may be included in the initial training as well and reinforced later.
      (2) Medical emergencies (e.g., chest pain).
      (3) Natural disaster.
   d. Assess psychosocial issues and refer to social worker as indicated.
      (1) Coping with chronic kidney failure.

(2) Adjustment to dialysis therapy.
(3) Sexual concerns.
(4) Body image and alternative places for the PD catheter, such as presternal.
(5) Rehabilitation status.
   (a) Is the patient able, willing, and interested in working?
   (b) How will this impact the family, especially household finances?

6. Skills training.
   a. CAPD exchange procedure.
   b. Dialysis machine (cycler) procedures.
   c. Peritoneal dialysis catheter exit-site care.
   d. Procedure for adding medications to the dialysis solution if the patient is capable.
   e. Procedure for obtaining dialysate samples.
   f. Procedure for managing contamination of the PD system.
   g. Troubleshooting complications such as drain issues.
      (1) Constipation.
      (2) Fibrin formation.
      (3) Kinks.
      (4) Clamped lines.

C. Patient follow-up.
   1. It is equally important for both patients who are in transition from training to independence and those that have been established on home PD therapy to have follow-up and monitoring.
      a. Evaluate clinical status of home patients.
      b. Reinforce learning and provide positive feedback regarding self-care and home dialysis.
      c. Ongoing assessment of learning needs and continuing education when indicated.
         (1) Many programs have regular monthly education topics so that all patients receive reinforcement on common topics.
         (2) For example, exit-site care, hand washing, fluid selection, etc. (Firanek, 2013).
      d. Support adjustment to home dialysis and rehabilitation.
   2. Assessment parameters.
      a. Fluid balance.
      b. Blood pressure.
      c. Weight gains, dry weight.
      d. Exit site.
      e. Procedure technique.
      f. Dialysis adequacy.
      g. Nutrition.
      h. Laboratory results.
      i. Routine medications.
      j. Supply and inventory.
      k. Adherence to prescribed treatment.
   3. Encourage routine preventive health care (e.g., mammograms) and assist in referring or scheduling, if necessary.

4. Follow-up activities:
   a. Telephone calls.
   b. Routine clinic visits.
   c. Home visits.
   d. Additional clinic visits for specific problems (e.g., peritonitis, exit-site infection).
5. Education updates and reviews of technique procedure.
6. Individualized multidisciplinary care plan. In the United States, the Centers for Medicare and Medicaid Services (CMS) requires that the multidisciplinary follow-up includes at least with a physician, registered nurse, dietitian, and social worker.

D. Clinical management issues.
1. Nonadherence: In a study of adherence in patients on PD, "noncompliance," defined as performance of < 90% of dialysis exchanges and determined by repeated inventory of dialysis solution bags, was found in 30% of patients on PD in the first 6 months of PD, and in 13% of chronic patients on PD studied (Bernardini et al., 2000).
   a. Some patients who were initially noncompliant became compliant. Others were intermittently compliant. Only a small fraction were consistently noncompliant.
   b. Noncompliant patients experienced more hospital admissions and had more hospital days.
   c. Noncompliant patients had a measured Kt/V_{urea} 18% lower than compliant patients.
   d. Noncompliant patients were more likely to transfer to hemodialysis due to uremia.
   e. Noncompliant patients were more likely to die than compliant patients.
   f. Although there is a paucity of studies regarding improving adherence in PD, there is a large body of literature regarding adherence in healthcare settings.
2. Preserving peritoneal membrane function.
   a. A small proportion of patients continue to transfer to hemodialysis due to loss of peritoneal membrane function. These patients have signs and symptoms of inadequate dialysis and fluid overload despite attempts to optimize dialysis prescription.
   b. Changes in membrane function can be documented by repeat PET, SPA, or PDC tests.
   c. Strategies to preserve peritoneal membrane function include:
      (1) Prevent catheter-related infections.
      (2) Prophylactic antibiotics prior to catheter insertion (evidence-based).
      (3) Short course of antibiotic therapy for known contamination of the PD system.
      (4) Prophylactic antibiotic therapy for dental, gastrointestinal (e.g., colonoscopy with biopsy), and other invasive procedures.
      (5) Prevent exit-site trauma by effectively securing the catheter.
      (6) Prophylactic treatment for severe exit-site trauma.
      (7) Treat equivocal (infected) exit sites.
      (8) Use low glucose degradation products (GDP). Peritoneal membrane damage is caused by the transition of epithelial to mesenchymal cells. This is the result of high glucose exposure to the peritoneal membrane (Diaz-Buxo, 2007).
         (a) 1.5% rather than 2.5% rather than 4.25%
         (b) For the long dwell, use icodextrin since it is glucose free.
      (9) Use intraperitoneal heparin any time there is fibrin or blood in the dialysate.
      (10) If bleeding is severe, drain dialysate and perform short exchanges until bleeding subsides.
      (11) Avoid introduction of disinfectants into the peritoneal cavity.
      (12) Use intraperitoneal medications only when absolutely necessary.
      (13) Avoid use of overheated dialysis solutions.
      (14) Rotate stock of dialysis solution to avoid using old solutions.
3. Anemia management.
   a. Hemoglobin and hematocrit improve after starting PD related to both decrease in plasma volume and increase in red cell mass.
   b. Although some patients on PD achieve a normal hematocrit, most remain somewhat anemic.
   c. Erythropoiesis-stimulating agents (ESAs) (e.g., recombinant human erythropoietin and darbepoetin alfa) have been shown to be safe and effective in correcting anemia in patients on peritoneal dialysis.
   d. In addition to the correction of anemia, other benefits of ESAs include improvements in quality of life, cognitive abilities, exercise capacity, and overall well-being.
   e. Administration of ESAs.
      (1) Subcutaneous administration is preferred because an intravenous (IV) access is not readily available.
      (2) Most patients on PD are taught to self-administer ESAs.
      (3) Adherence with treatment regimens is an important factor in determining the efficacy of ESAs in patients on PD.
         (a) Risk factors for nonadherence are younger age, fewer comorbidities, and longer duration of therapy (Muirhead, 2005).

(b) Darbepoetin alfa, which is a hyper-glycosylated analog of epoetin alfa, is available for the treatment of anemia.
  i. It has a prolonged serum half-life.
  ii. This allows extended dosing intervals.
  iii. May prove beneficial in situations where patient adherence is a real concern.
(4) Patients on PD require iron supplementation to prevent iron deficiency and maintain iron stores. Targets for iron supplementation for this group of patients:
  (a) Transferrin saturation of > 20%.
  (b) Serum ferritin 200 to 500 ng/mL.
(5) The 2000 KDOQI guidelines for the treatment of anemia recommend an oral iron dose of ≥ 200 mg of elemental iron per day. Oral iron may not be sufficient to supply or replace iron needs since iron absorption is suboptimal.
(6) If oral iron fails, IV iron is recommended. For many patients treated with a home-based therapy, IV iron administration can present significant logistical problems.

E. Prevention of cardiovascular complications.
  1. Cardiovascular disease is the leading cause of death in this patient population.
  2. Good blood pressure control and fluid balance are critical in preventing left ventricular hypertrophy (LVH) and congestive heart failure. LVH may regress with good control of fluid.
    a. Many patients who start CAPD have a drop in blood pressure and improved blood pressure control and are able to discontinue some or all antihypertensive medications. The responsible mechanism is believed to be good control of salt and water balance.
    b. Some clinicians observe that blood pressure tends to go up again after 6 to 12 months, but this may be a function of dietary intake and fluid balance management.
  3. Some patients on low-sodium diets can become sodium depleted and will require liberalization of sodium intake.
  4. Patients with diabetic autonomic neuropathy and cardiac dysfunction can develop symptomatic orthostatic hypotension.
  5. Patients on CAPD have a more atherogenic lipoprotein profile than hemodialysis patients. Several studies have shown that patients on CAPD have fewer dysrhythmias than HD patients.

F. Malnutrition, inflammation, and atherosclerosis (MIA syndrome) is associated with high cardiovascular mortality and accounts for most of the premature deaths in patients on peritoneal dialysis. Proper nutritional support, enhanced dialysis prescriptions, and treatment of underlying inflammation may decrease morbidity and mortality associated with MIA.

G. Nutritional status.
  1. Protein energy malnutrition can be a major problem for patients on PD.
    a. Malnutrition may be present at the initiation of dialysis.
    b. Residual kidney function is significantly lower in patients with severe malnutrition.
    c. Older adults, patients with diabetes, and patients with renal vascular disease have a higher incidence of malnutrition.
    d. Factors that contribute to malnutrition.
      (1) Inadequate dialysis.
      (2) Comorbid illnesses.
      (3) Anorexia.
      (4) Losses of protein, amino acids, and other nutrients in the dialysate.
      (5) Endocrine abnormalities.
      (6) Activation of cellular catabolic pathways and displacement of other energy sources by glucose absorbed from the dialysate.
    e. Malnutrition is related to increased morbidity and mortality in patients on PD.
  2. Glucose.
    a. Glucose is absorbed from peritoneal dialysis solutions.
    b. Blood glucose and plasma insulin levels peak 45 to 90 minutes after infusing a hypertonic exchange. These levels remain high for a prolonged period.
    c. Isotonic solutions have minimal effects on blood glucose and insulin levels.
    d. The patients on CAPD have a tendency toward hyperglycemia with hyperinsulinemia. Some of these patients will develop overt diabetes mellitus.
    e. Clinical implications.
      (1) Constant glucose absorption can result in anorexia.
      (2) There will be an increase in total caloric load if dietary intake is not modified.
      (3) There may be a gradual increase in dry body weight.
    f. Monitoring and intervention. Monitor number of hypertonic exchanges, dietary patterns, serum glucose, and weight gain.
    g. Glucose absorption varies by membrane transport type and tonicity of dialysate used. Over an 8 hour 2 L dwell, expected glucose absorption of 4 calories/gram, would equal:
      (1) Low transporter: 1.5% = 20 g; 2.5% = 32 g; 4.25% = 48 g.

(2) Low average: 1.5% = 23 g; 2.5% = 40 g; 4.25% = 62 g.

(3) High average: 1.5% = 28 g; 2.5% = 47 g; 4.25% = 76 g.

(4) High transporter: 1.5% = 30 g; 2.5% = 50 g; 4.25% = 82 g (Gokal, 2002).

h. Avoid excessive use of hypertonic solutions by regulating sodium and fluid intake.

3. Weight control regimen.
   a. Avoid simple carbohydrates in diet.
   b. Increase activity and exercise.
   c. Restrict alcohol.
   d. Reduce excessive fat intake.
   e. Insulin administration as ordered for diabetic patients with careful monitoring of serum glucose.

4. Lipids.
   a. Patients on PD typically have an increase in serum cholesterol and triglyceride concentrations after starting dialysis therapy.
   b. They have more atherogenic serum lipid profiles than patients on hemodialysis.
      (1) 50% to 70% of patients on PD have elevated triglyceride concentrations.
      (2) Total cholesterol may also be high.
      (3) Increased LDL-cholesterol and VLDL-cholesterol fractions and decreased HDL-cholesterol.
      (4) Higher levels of apolipoprotein B.
   c. Intervention.
      (1) Restrict use of hypertonic dialysis solution.
      (2) Dietary modifications to reduce weight: reduce intake of saturated fats and carbohydrates.
      (3) Stop smoking.
      (4) Restrict alcohol.
      (5) Regular exercise program.
      (6) Lipid-lowering drugs.
   d. Attention to amount of glucose exposure, limiting it as feasible, may improve lipid profiles.

5. Proteins.
   a. Proteins and amino acids are lost in the dialysate (5 to 15 g/day).
   b. Total serum protein and albumin levels are often low.
   c. Abnormal plasma amino acid concentrations are similar to untreated uremia and those of patients on hemodialysis.
      (1) Decreased levels of essential amino acids.
      (2) Increased concentration of nonessential amino acids.
   d. Intervention for low protein and amino acids in conjunction with the dietitian.
      (1) Review individual dietary prescription.
      (2) Increase dietary intake of proteins.
      (3) 50% of protein intake should be of high

biologic value.
      (4) Nutritional supplements.
      (5) Amino acid supplements.
      (6) Education awareness days with the dietitian may be beneficial for patients and family members.
         (a) Cooking classes with recipe handouts that include nutritional content.
         (b) Field trips to supermarket with emphasis on how to read labels.
         (c) Protein smoothie classes that can accommodate almost everyone's dietary preferences.
   e. Amino acid supplementation via absorption from dialysis solution has been studied.
      (1) Amino acid solutions are used for only one exchange per day.
      (2) Use of amino acid solutions showed short-term improvement in protein nutrition and metabolic status.
      (3) BUN levels and dialysate protein losses increase.
      (4) A 3-year study in Hong Kong found that:
         (a) The use of amino acid solutions maintained a stable albumin and cholesterol and lowered triglycerides compared to the control group, which had decreasing albumin and cholesterol and stable or increasing triglycerides.
         (b) The group receiving amino acids did not have fewer hospitalizations or better survival.

6. Nutritional assessment.
   a. The NKF-KDOQI guidelines for maintenance patients on peritoneal dialysis, recommends routine monthly assessment of nutritional status including:
      (1) Serum albumin (or prealbumin) levels.
      (2) Estimation of dietary protein intake (such as protein equivalent of nitrogen appearance [PNA] calculated from urea kinetic modeling data).
   b. Other assessment parameters.
      (1) Subjective global assessment (SGA). A 7-point scale modified for patients on PD assesses weight change, anorexia, subcutaneous tissue, and muscle mass (evidence-based).
      (2) Serum creatinine and creatinine index are valid measures of protein-energy nutritional status.
      (3) Serum bicarbonate should be maintained above 22 mEq/L.
      (4) Anthropometric measurements.
      (5) Dual energy x-ray absorptiometry (DEXA).

(6) The NKF-KDOQI nutrition guidelines also recommend intensive nutritional counseling for every patient based on an individualized care plan.

H. Outcomes of peritoneal dialysis.
1. Residual kidney function.
2. Patients on PD maintain residual kidney function longer than patients on hemodialysis.
3. Even minimal residual kidney function contributes significantly to solute removal and dialysis adequacy.
4. Patients with no residual kidney function are at risk for poor outcomes.
   a. Inadequate dialysis.
   b. Increased morbidity.
   c. Transfer to hemodialysis.
   d. Increased mortality.

I. Morbidity (USRDS, 2014).
1. The United States Renal Data System (USRDS) data for 2014 shows overall all-cause hospital admission rate for patients on hemodialysis was 1.73/patient years and 1.61/patient years for patients on PD.
   a. This includes admissions for infection.
   b. Admissions for peritonitis have declined 37.5% since 1999 (USRDS, 2014).
2. HD compared with PD as an initial therapy doubles the risk of hospitalizations for septicemia (Nabeel et al., 2006).
3. The risk of bacteremia in patients on HD who start dialysis with a central venous catheter (CVC) is higher than the risk of peritonitis in patients who start on PD with a PD catheter during the first 3 months (Nabeel et al., 2006).
   a. This is an important point as the USRDS does not include data from the first 90 days.
   b. Healthy People (HP) 2010 goals called for an increase to 50% of those choosing HD to have a mature arteriovenous fistula (AVF) when starting dialysis.
   c. Despite this goal, according to the USRDS 2014 annual report, only 17% started HD with a mature fistula.
   d. USRDS reported that 81% of U.S. patients initiated dialysis with a central venous catheter (CVC), increasing the risk of death.
   e. To avoid this relative risk of death, many practices have incorporated treatment options even in the "urgent-start" unplanned access population (Casaretto et al., 2012; Ghaffari, 2012). A PD catheter is placed instead of a CVC when PD was chosen. The benefits include:
      (1) A temporary access becomes a permanent access, a one-stop-shop approach.

(2) Decreased risk of septicemia as stated by Nabeel and others (2006).
(3) Preservation of residual kidney function (RKF).
(4) Maintenance of employment.
(5) Decreased hospitalizations.
(6) Decreased cost to payer system, the median being:
   (a) $129,997 per year PD.
   (b) $173,507 per year HD.
   (c) $43,510 higher to maintain a patient on HD (Berger et al., 2009).

J. Patient dropout or transfer to another form of therapy.
1. This is still greater for PD therapies than for HD.
2. Infectious complications are still the main reason for changing modality.
3. Inadequate dialysis or fluid removal is the second most frequently cited reason for transfer.
   a. However, software tools can model patients for optimal prescription management.
   b. Provides a good indicator of needed changes in the PD prescription when the patient's RKF decreases.
4. PD catheter-related problems account for up to 15% of transfers.
5. Patient choice, malnutrition, and abdominal complications also contribute to dropout.

K. Transplantation.
1. PD before transplantation may be beneficial, as a lower incidence and severity of delayed recovery of kidney function after transplantation has been reported in patients on PD.
2. Transplant outcomes are similar in HD and CAPD for both adults and children.
3. Peritoneal dialysis can be used during delayed graft function after transplantation provided the peritoneal cavity remains intact during the transplant procedure.
4. The PD catheter can be left in for 3 to 4 months with a functioning graft. However, earlier removal after successful transplantation is advisable, because transplanted patients are at risk for catheter-related infections (Prowant et al., 2008).

L. Survival.
1. The USRDS (2014) database demonstrates that overall mortality rates continue to decline.
   a. The adjusted death rates fell by 9% from 1993 to 2002.
   b. The adjusted death rates fell by 26% from 2003 to 2012.
2. Mortality rates for patients on hemodialysis:
   a. Fell by 3% from 1993 to 2002.
   b. Fell by 25% from 2003 to 2012.

c. The net reduction since 1993 is 28%.
3. Mortality rates for patients on peritoneal dialysis:
   a. Fell by 15% from 1993 to 2002.
   b. Fell by 35% from 2003 to 2012.
   c. The net reduction since 1993 is 47%.
4. Mortality rates for patients receiving a kidney transplant:
   a. Fell by 27% from 1993 to 2002.
   b. Fell by 35% from 2003 to 2012.
   c. The net reduction since 1993 is 51%.
5. The 3-year survival probabilities for patients with CKD stage 5 after onset are as follows:
   a. Hemodialysis: 54%.
   b. Peritoneal dialysis: 65%.
6. The 5-year survival probabilities are as follows:
   a. Hemodialysis: 40%.
   b. Peritoneal dialysis: 49%.

Section C
Peritoneal Dialysis Complications
Kim Lambertson

I. Noninfectious complications of peritoneal dialysis.

A. Catheter obstruction.
   1. Etiology of inflow obstruction.
      a. External kinks or clamps.
      b. Kinks in the catheter in the subcutaneous tunnel.
      c. Clots/fibrin.
      d. Omental wrap (Gokal et al., 1998).
   2. Etiology of outflow obstruction.
      a. Intraluminal: Fibrin/clot (Gokal et al., 1998).
      b. Extraluminal.
         (1) Constipation, as the impacted stool can compress on the catheter lumen and also cause tip migration (McCormick & Bargman, 2007).
         (2) Omental entrapment.
         (3) Catheter tip migration or incorrect placement.
         (4) Entrapment in adhesions.
         (5) Occlusion from abdominal organs (Gokal et al., 1998).
   3. Interventions.
      a. Interventions should start with the least invasive measures (Gokal et al., 1998).
      b. Exam and evaluation.
      c. Check external tubing for kinks and clamps (Zorzanello et al., 2004).
      d. Flushing with saline or heparinized saline (Crabtree, 2006b; Miller et al., 2012).
      e. High-dose laxatives for constipation.

(1) 30 mL of 70% sorbitol solution every 2 hours.
(2) Stimulant laxatives (bisacodyl) and enemas should be avoided due to the risk of transmural migration of bacteria into the peritoneal cavity and risk of peritonitis (Crabtree, 2006b).
   f. Abdominal x-ray.
      (1) To assist with ruling out kinks and tip migration as well as evaluate the correction of constipation (Crabtree 2006b).
      (2) To rule out internal kinking of the catheter, both a flat plate and lateral view abdominal x-ray should be done (Zorzanello et al., 2004).
   g. Tissue plasminogen activator (tPA).
      (1) In a report by Zoranello et al. (2004), tPA was used in 29 cases of catheter obstruction. In 24 of the cases, catheter flow was restored.
      (2) The protocol used by Zorzanello et al. (2004):
         (a) 8 mg of tPA in 10 mL of sterile water was infused into the catheter.
         (b) The tPA was allowed to dwell for 1 hour; then the peritoneal cavity was drained.
   h. Fluoroscopy.
      (1) Is approximately 50% effective in restoring catheter function (Crabtree, 2006b; McCormick & Bargman, 2007; Miller et al., 2012) but has a lower complication rate than laparoscopic manipulation. Fluoroscopy does not require that the PD prescription be altered postprocedure (Miller et al., 2012).
      (2) Fluoroscopic manipulation is done after a sterile surgical field is prepared and the transfer set is taken off of the catheter. The procedure can be done with:
         (a) Guide wires.
         (b) Endoluminal brushes.
         (c) Fogarty balloons are useful with swan neck catheters as using a straight guide wire in such a tunnel can cause trauma (Crabtree, 2006b).
      (3) Fluoroscopy cannot be used in presternal catheters due to the length of the catheter (Crabtree, 2006b).
   i. Laparoscopic revision.
      (1) Rates of restoring catheter function with laparoscopic revision are reported to be 80% to 100% successful (Crabtree, 2006b; McCormick & Bargman, 2007; Miller et al., 2012).
      (2) Advanced laparoscopic techniques are used to eliminate catheter entrapment in

omentum, adhesions, or epiploic appendices. For further discussion of these techniques, see The Peritoneal Dialysis Access section.

   (3) The need for temporary hemodialysis after laparoscopic revision can be avoided by:
      (a) Use of small laparoscopic ports and watertight wound closure.
      (b) Use of low-volume supine dialysis (Crabtree 2006b).

B. Catheter cuff extrusion.
  1. The subcutaneous cuff becomes externalized.
  2. Causes.
    a. Incorrect placement of subcutaneous cuff (see section on Peritoneal Dialysis Access).
    b. Catheters have shape memory. A catheter with a straight subcutaneous segment that is bent during placement will eventually return to the straight shape.
    c. Trauma (pulling) of the catheter (Kathuria et al., 2009).
    d. Infection (Campos et al., 2009).
    e. Increased intraabdominal pressure.
    f. Implantation of the catheter into a site with edema (Kathuria et al., 2009).
  3. Treatment.
    a. If the cuff is not infected, it can be left alone (Kathuria et al., 2009).
    b. The cuff will frequently become infected.
      (1) Ultrasound of the tunnel can be used to determine the extent of infection (Li et al., 2010).
      (2) For localized infections, cuff shaving can be done. The scalpel blade is placed parallel to the surface of the cuff until all is removed. The scalpel blade should be replaced frequently so that heavy pressure is not applied, increasing the risk of catheter perforation (Crabtree, 2006b).
      (3) Systemic antibiotics are needed (Kathuria et al., 2009).

C. Abdominal pain not related to peritonitis.
  1. Etiologies.
    a. Low pH of the dialysis solution.
    b. Hypertonic dialysis solutions.
    c. Temperature of dialysate.
    d. Catheters with a straight intraperitoneal segment.
    e. Catheter malposition (Crabtree, 2006b).
    f. Infusion of air into the peritoneal cavity (Diaz-Buxo, 2006).
  2. Intervention.
    a. Many times the pain is transient and resolves without intervention.
    b. Slowing infusion rates.

    c. Ensuring appropriate temperature of dialysis solution (Crabtree, 2006b).
    d. Tidal peritoneal dialysis prescription (Kathuria et al., 2009).
    e. The use of catheters with a coiled intraperitoneal segment. The coiled tip is thought to decrease the "jet effect" of dialysate infusion (Crabtree, 2006b).
    f. Addition of 2 to 5 mEq/L of sodium bicarbonate to the dialysis solution for alkalinization (Kathuria et al., 2009).
    g. Addition of 2.5 mL/L of 1% lidocaine to the dialysate (Kathuria et al., 2009).
    h. Fluoroscopic catheter tip manipulation.
    i. Laparoscopic exploration (Crabtree, 2006b).

D. Pneumoperitoneum.
  1. Free air in the peritoneal cavity usually presents as air under the diaphragm.
  2. Air in the peritoneal cavity is usually the result of incorrect technique while completing PD exchanges. Pneumoperitoneum caused by infused air is benign; the air will be reabsorbed.
  3. Free air in an abdominal x-ray can also represent perforation. A patient assessment must be taken into account with x-ray results (Bargman, 2009).

E. Hernias.
  1. Umbilical hernias are the most common (Balda et al., 2014; Crabtree, 2006a).
  2. Risk factors for hernia.
    a. Older age.
    b. Female.
    c. Multiparous women.
    d. Previous hernia.
    e. Obesity.
    f. Polycystic kidney disease (Bargman, 2008).
    g. History of prior transplant (Balda et al., 2014).
  3. Studies have not found a correlation between larger fill volumes and hernia development (Balda et al 2014; Bleyer et al., 1998; Del Peso et al., 2003; Hussain et al., 1998).
  4. Signs and symptoms.
    a. Usually a lump or swelling on the abdomen.
    b. Genital edema (Bargman, 2009).
  5. Diagnosis.
    a. Scintigraphy. Isotope is added to the dialysate and administered to the patient. After ambulation, multiple images of the abdomen are taken (Crabtree, 2006a).
    b. Computerized tomographic (CT) scan. Nonionic contrast medium is added to 2 L of dialysate and administered to the patient. After the patient is ambulatory, images are taken (Crabtree, 2006a).
    c. Magnetic resonance imaging (MRI). The peritoneal dialysate is used as contrast to avoid

adding contrast to the dialysate and possible contamination (Prischl et al., 2002).
6. Potential complications.
   a. Bowel incarceration and strangulation.
   b. Rupture of hernia sac will cause edema of the abdominal wall and genitalia (Bargman, 2008).
7. Treatment.
   a. Surgical repair with mesh. The use of mesh is necessary because if the weakened tissues are sutured together, the hernia will recur due to the very thin and fragile tissue of the hernia sac and the increased intraperitoneal pressure associated with the dialysis fluid.
      (1) Mesh should not be placed in the peritoneal cavity.
      (2) Mesh does not increase the risk of peritonitis.
      (3) Prophylactic antibiotics should be given preoperatively (Crabtree, 2006a; Martinez-Mier et al., 2008).
   b. Postoperative care.
      (1) Decrease intraabdominal pressure.
         (a) Avoid coughing.
         (b) Avoid constipation and straining.
         (c) Avoid bending over.
         (d) Avoid squatting.
         (e) Avoid stair climbing (Crabtree, 2006a).
      (2) Dialysis.
         (a) There is no standardized recommendation for dialysis posthernia repair.
         (b) Low volume (1 to 1.5 L, supine dialysis for 2 weeks (Crabtree, 2006a; Martinez-Mier et al., 2008; Shah et al., 2006).
         (c) Due to the risk of peritonitis from enteric bacteria that translocate into the peritoneal cavity, it is recommended that patients with bowel ischemia or strangulation do hemodialysis postoperatively (Balda et al., 2013; Bargman 2008).

F. Leaks.
   1. Types of leaks.
      a. Early/pericatheter leaks.
         (1) Occur within 30 days of PD catheter placement.
         (2) Usually associated with catheter placement.
         (3) Associated with fluid leakage from the catheter exit site or surgical wound.
         (4) Because of an increased risk of tunnel infection and peritonitis due to the leaking of dialysis fluid into the tissues and subcutaneous tract, dialysis should be stopped and prophylactic antibiotics should be considered (Leblanc et al., 2001).

      (5) Temporary stop of PD.
      (6) Catheter replacement (Leblanc et al., 2001).
   b. Late leaks.
      (1) Occur 30 days after catheter placement.
      (2) Related to a mechanical tear in the peritoneal membrane that allows dialysis fluid to the tissues.
         (a) Abdominal wall.
         (b) Genitalia.
      (3) Signs and symptoms.
         (a) Swelling and edema of the abdominal wall.
         (b) Weight gain.
         (c) Peripheral edema.
         (d) Genital edema.
         (e) Decreasing dialysate drain volumes (Leblanc et al., 2001).
      (4) Diagnosis.
         (a) Peritoneography.
            i. Contrast medium is injected directly into the PD catheter using sterile technique.
            ii. Initial x-rays are taken in the supine position. Then the patient will roll from side to side and ambulate to coat the peritoneal cavity with contrast. Additional x-rays are in the supine, prone, and Trendelenburg positions (Scanziani et al., 2006).
         (b) CT with contrast dye (Leblanc et al., 2001).
         (c) Scintigraphy (Scanziani et al., 2006).
         (d) CT with contrast dye (Leblanc et al., 2001).
         (e) MRI with dialysate as contrast (Prischl et al., 2002).
      (5) Treatment.
         (a) Temporary stopping PD.
         (b) Supine, low volume PD.
         (c) Surgical repair (Leblanc et al., 2001).
   c. Pleural cavity leak (hydrothorax).
      (1) Usually occurs soon after dialysis is started and up to 88% are on the right side (Tapawan et al., 2011). The incidence of hydrothorax in the adult PD population ranges from 1.6% to 10% (Chavannes et al., 2014).
      (2) Etiology.
         (a) Congenital diaphragmatic defects.
         (b) Possibly a weakening in the diaphragmatic tissues caused by the high intraabdominal pressures associated with PD (Tapawan et al., 2011).
      (3) Signs and symptoms.
         (a) Symptoms will vary depending on the

severity of the leak; up to 25% of patients are asymptomatic.
  (b) Dyspnea.
  (c) Pulmonary function tests show reduced total lung capacity and vital capacity.
  (d) Diminished tactile fremitus on palpation.
  (e) Dullness or flatness upon percussion.
  (f) Diminished breath sounds.
  (g) Decreased effluent drain volume and ultrafiltration (Lew, 2010).
(4) Diagnosis.
  (a) Chest x-ray will show an effusion (Bargman, 2009; Chavannes et al., 2014).
  (b) Thoracocentesis can be used to both diagnose and relieve the symptoms of hydrothorax. Pleural fluid will be low in protein and high in glucose, and the presence of D-lactate from the dialysate will be noted.
    i. It should be noted that the glucose level will be dependent on size of the defect and the rate of glucose absorption by the mesothelium (Tapawan et al., 2011).
    ii. The assay necessary for detection of D-lactate may not be readily available (Tapawan et al., 2011).
  (c) Scintigraphy.
  (d) CT Scan.
  (e) MRI (Lew, 2010).
(5) Treatment.
  (a) Supine low volume PD.
  (b) Interruption of PD.
    i. PD should be held 4 to 6 weeks.
    ii This conservative measure is successful in 50% of cases (Lew 2010).
  (c) Pleurodesis. A chemical (such as tetracycline, talc, or autologous blood) is placed in the plueral cavity via a chest tube. The chemical will cause fibrosis that will close the communication between the pleural and peritoneal cavities.
    i. Pleurodesis has a success rate of approximately 48%.
    ii. It is recommended that PD be held until 10 days postpleurodesis (Tapawan, 2011).
  (d) Surgical repair with thoracotomy. Openings in the plueral cavity are sutured shut and possibly reinforced with Teflon patches (Chow et al., 2003).
  (e) Video-assisted thorascopic surgery (VATS) allows chemical pleurodesis

(talc) or mechanical pleurodesis (repair with Teflon patches or fibrin glue) with video assistance in a minimally invasive fashion. PD can be resumed in 3 to 4 weeks (Tapawan, 2011).

G. Genital edema.
  1. Dialysate leaks in to the labia majora, scrotum, or penis.
  2. Genital edema is seen less frequently in women than in men.
  3. The mechanism for the travel of fluid.
    a. Dialysate tracks through the plane from the catheter insertion site.
    b. A hernia sac tears and leaks fluid.
    c. Through a patent processus vaginalis.
  4. Diagnosis.
    a. CT.
    b. MRI.
    c. Scintigraphy.
  5. Treatment.
    a. Temporary rest from PD.
    b. Low volume, supine PD.
    c. Surgical repair of hernia or patent processus vaginalis (Bargman, 2009).

II. **Noninfectious causes of cloudy dialysate.** Most cloudy dialysate is caused by peritonitis. Three noninfectious causes of cloudy dialysate are outlined here.

A. Hemoperitoneum.
  1. A common complication of peritoneal dialysis that is usually benign and resolves spontaneously.
  2. The condition does not cause changes in the peritoneal membrane or increase risk of peritonitis.
  3. The condition can be unsettling for patients as just 2 mL of blood in a 2 L bag of dialysate will cause blood-tinged effluent (Lew, 2007).
  4. Gynecologic-related events are the most common causes (Lew, 2007).
    a. Menstruation.
    b. Ovulation.
    c. Pregnancy.
    d. Ovarian cysts.
  5. Other causes of hemoperitoneum.
    a. Trauma.
      (1) Coughing.
      (2) Heavy lifting (Balsera & Guest, 2013).
    b. Medical procedures.
      (1) Pericardiocentesis.
      (2) Radiation to the peritoneum.
      (3) Colonoscopy (Lew, 2007).
    c. Intraabdominal causes.
      (1) Liver or spleen rupture.
      (2) Liver tumors.

(3) Kidney and liver cysts (Lew, 2007).

(4) Retroperitoneal hematomas resulting from procedures such as cardiac catheterization (Guest, 2013).

(5) Rupture of aneurysm (Lew, 2007).

(6) Rectus sheath hematoma due to abdominal surgery or due to the combination of anticoagulant therapy and abdominal trauma (Balfa et al., 2014).

6. Interventions.
   a. Assess hemodynamic stability.
      (1) Follow trends in hemoglobin.
      (2) Monitor for coagulopathies (Balfa et al., 2014; Balsers & Guest, 2013).
   b. Rapid flushes with room temperature dialysate (Balsera & Guest, 2013).
   c. The addition of heparin in a dose of 500 units per liter of dialysate will prevent clotting and flow obstruction in the PD catheter (Lew, 2007).
   d. Persistent, worsening, or repeated hemoperitoneum can be evaluated with:
      (1) Ultrasound.
      (2) CT Scan.
      (3) MRI.
      (4) Surgically (Lew, 2007).

B. Chyloperitoneum.
   1. Presents as milky-white effluent (Bargman, 2009) as well as abdominal distention and pain after eating (Cheung & Khwaja, 2008).
   2. Chyloperitoneum is a rare complication of PD (Lee et al., 2005).
   3. Chylous effluent is the result of a communication between the peritoneal lymphatics that allows the movement of chylomicrons that are rich in triglycerides into the peritoneal cavity. The communication can be caused by conditions such as (Bargman, 2009):
      a. Injury during catheter placement.
      b. Neoplasm, especially lymphoma.
      c. Tuberculous peritonitis.
      d. Superior vena cava syndrome.
      e. Calcium channel blockers.
   4. Diagnosis.
      a. Triglyceride levels in the dialysis effluent are greater than the plasma (Bargman, 2009).
      b. Levels of triglycerides in the dialysate > 110 mg/dL (Lee et al., 2005).
      c. Presence of chylomicrons in the PD effluent (Jain et al., 2003).
   5. Treatment.
      a. Temporarily stopping PD (Bargman, 2009).
      b. A low-fat diet with medium-chain triglycerides (MCTs).
         (1) Long-chain triglycerides are converted into monoglycerides and free fatty acids then transported as chylomicrons into the intestinal lymph nodes.
         (2) MCTs are absorbed directly into the portal vein which reduces the production and flow of lymph (Cheung & Khwaja, 2008).
      c. Octreotide is an injectable somatostatin analogue (Lee et al., 2005).
         (1) The use of octreotide is based on the knowledge that somatostatin decreases intestinal fat absorption and lymphatic flow.
         (2) Octreotide has been used to treat postoperative chyloperitoneum in patients not on PD.
         (3) The dosage of octreotide has to be reduced by 50% in dialysis patients (Lee et al., 2005).

C. Eosinophilia.
   1. The patient may present with cloudy effluent and abdominal pain, usually occurring within the first few weeks of starting PD.
   2. Peritoneal effluent cell count with > 100 leukocytes per mm^3 and more than 10% eosinophils (Fourtounas et al., 2008).
   3. Peritoneal eosinophilia may or may not be associated with peripheral blood eosinophilia (Fourtounas et al., 2008).
   4. The condition is usually benign (Quinlan et al., 2010) and does not affect the peritoneal membrane (Ejaz, 1998).
   5. Causes and associations.
      a. Hypersensitivity to PD catheter and dialysis supplies.
      b. Intraperitoneal medications.
      c. Air in the peritoneal cavity.
      d. May be seen during peritonitis, especially fungal (Fourtounas et al., 2008).
   6. Treatment.
      a. Usually resolves spontaneously without treatment (Quinlan et al., 2010).
      b. Steroids (oral and IP) and antihistamines have been used to treat eosinophilia (Fourtounas et al., 2008; Quinlan et al., 2010).

III. Other complications of peritoneal dialysis.

A. Hypokalemia.
   1. Hypokalemia is defined as a serum potassium of < 3.5 mmol (Chuang et al., 2009).
   2. Hypokalemia affects approximately 30% of patients on PD (Bender, 2012; Chuang et al., 2009) and is more common in patients on PD than patients on HD (Delanaye et al., 2012).
   3. The dialysate for PD does not contain potassium because the daily oral intake of potassium in most patients would be greater than the amount removed by PD.

a. The daily consumption of potassium in patients on PD is approximately 50 to 60 mEq/day.

b. An 8-L/day CAPD prescription can remove approximately 40 mEq/day of potassium (Zanger, 2010).

4. Hypokalemia is associated with poor nutritional status and comorbidity (Chuang et al., 2009; Delanaye et al., 2012).

5. Patients on PD experience potassium loss through the bowel and increased intracellular uptake of potassium due to increased insulin levels because of the dextrose in dialysate (Bender, 2012).

6. Hypokalemia has been associated with increased risk of peritonitis. The state of hypokalemia slows bowel motility which allows bacterial overgrowth in the bowel and bacteria translocate into the peritoneal cavity (Chuang et al., 2009).

7. Interventions.
   a. Liberal oral potassium intake.
   b. Oral potassium supplements.
   c. Intraperitoneal (IP) potassium should only be used in the acute setting (Bender, 2012).
   d. Potassium 4.0 to 5 mm can be added to the dialysate (Korbet, 2007; Ponce et al., 2014).

B. Fluid management issues.
   1. The target weight for the patient on PD should be the weight at which the patient is euvolemic.
   2. Euvolemia can be defined as the state at which the patient is edema-free and free of symptoms of hypovolemia such as hypotension and cramping.
   3. The euvolemic state may be difficult for the patient and clinician to assess. For example, significant fluid overload may be present and the patient may still be edema-free (Mujais et al., 2000).
   4. On a monthly basis the following parameters should be assessed:
      a. Blood pressure. Optimal blood pressure (BP) for patients on PD is not known; most clinicians advocate for a BP < 140/90 (Bender, 2012).
      b. Volume status.
      c. Drain volume.
         (1) The 24-hour net ultrafiltration (UF) should be assessed.
         (2) Any long dwells that result in fluid absorption or a negative net should be assessed (Burkhart & Piraino, 2006).
         (3) In CAPD patients, dialysate bag overfill should be accounted for so as not to overassess UF (Davies, 2013).
      d. Residual kidney function. Per 2006 NKF-KDOQI Guidelines, the 24-hour urine volume should be measured for volume and solute removal every 2 months.
      e. Dietary salt and water intake. Salt and water intake can be evaluated by measuring the 24-hour urine volume and sodium and then calculating the difference between the volume and sodium over 1 day of dialysate effluent and solution. Overfill of the dialysate bag should be considered in this calculation.
      f. Clinical strategies for attaining euvolemia.
         (1) Reduce sodium and water intake.
         (2) Protect residual kidney function.
         (3) Augment urine volume with oral high-dose loop diuretics.
         (4) Increase peritoneal ultrafiltration.
            (a) Avoid dwells that cause fluid absorption.
            (b) Use of hypertonic dextrose.
            (c) Use of an alternative osmotic agent such as icodextrin (Burkhart & Piraino, 2006).

C. Heparin-induced thrombocytopenia (HIT).
   1. HIT most commonly occurs after intravenous administration of heparin.
   2. A case of HIT has been diagnosed in a PD patient receiving IP heparin.
   3. IP heparin does not cause systemic anticoagulation.
   4. It is thought that the mechanism for HIT with IP administration of heparin is absorption via the peritoneal lymphatic system (Kaplan et al., 2005).

D. Encapsulating peritoneal sclerosis (EPS).
   1. EPS is very rare with an incidence of 0.7% to 3.3%.
   2. Most of the cases of EPS have been reported in Japan and Europe. EPS is rare in the United States. Many suspect that fewer cases are seen in the United States because of lower use of PD and decreased time on PD therapy.
   3. The exact cause and risk factors for EPS are unknown. Currently it is thought that the membrane is damaged or sclerosed from long-term PD and receives a "double hit" that triggers EPS. Some of the triggers for EPS are thought to be peritonitis, hemoperitoneum, and stopping PD.
   4. Symptoms of EPS are typically vague gastrointestinal complaints such as loss of appetite, nausea, and vomiting. In the later stages of EPS, the symptoms of bowel obstruction can appear.
   5. The peritoneal equilibrium test shows increasing high transport and decreasing ultrafiltration.
   6. In the later stages of EPS, the bowel is "cocooned" by peritoneal thickening and calcification. Bowel obstructions are common.
   7. There is no data that shows the success of one treatment over the other. Currently, EPS is treated with nutritional support, corticosteroids, tamoxifen, and surgery (De Sousa et al., 2012).

E. Peritonitis.
1. Risk factors for peritonitis that may be modified have been outlined by Piraino et al. (2011).
   a. Technique errors.
   b. Hypoalbuminemia.
   c. Vitamin D deficiency.
   d. Hypokalemia.
   e. Prolonged use of antibiotics.
   f. Constipation.
   g. Exit site and tunnel infections.
   h. Exposure to animals.
2. Prevention.
   a. Proper hand-washing agents.
      (1) 70% alcohol-based hand rubs are considered most effective.
      (2) Alcohol-based agents are not effective for *Clostridium difficile* (Piraino et al., 2011).
   b. Exit-site care – see Section A for a detailed discussion on exit-site care.
   c. Patient training and home visits.
      (1) Detailed guidelines for patient training can be found at http://ispd.org
      (2) Home visits can assess adherence to training protocols.
      (3) Retraining should be considered after:
         (a) Hospitalization.
         (b) Peritonitis or catheter infection.
         (c) Changes in dexterity, vision, or mental acuity.
         (d) After initial training and at least yearly thereafter (Piraino et al., 2011).
      (4) Patients should be taught what contamination is and the proper response.
   d. Treatment of constipation. Bacteria can migrate over the bowel wall and into peritoneal cavity.
   e. Treatment of hypokalemia (see prior section on hypokalemia).
   f. Prophylactic antibiotics for procedures with the abdomen or pelvis or procedures that cause transient bacteremia such as dental work. Additionally, patients should empty the peritoneal cavity before procedures to the abdomen or pelvis (Piraino et al., 2011).
   g. Cycler cassettes should not be reused due to the high risk of peritonitis with water-borne organisms
   h. Antifungal prophylaxis when exposed to antibiotic therapy to prevent fungal peritonitis (Cho & Johnson, 2014).
3. Presentation.
   a. Cloudy fluid.
   b. Abdominal pain.
   c. Pain is usually generalized and associated with rebound (Li et al., 2010).
4. Procedures for suspected peritonitis.
   a. Peritonitis should always be ruled out in patients on PD with abdominal pain.
   b. The peritoneal cavity should be drained and the effluent inspected and sent for a cell count with differential, Gram stain, and culture. Often the Gram stain will be negative, but it should always be performed as a method to detect fungal peritonitis early in the course of peritonitis.
   c. An effluent cell count of > 100/µl with 50% polymorphonuclear neutrophilic cells indicates peritonitis.
   d. The number of cells in the effluent will depend on how long fluid has dwelled in the peritoneal cavity. In patients who have had a short dwell time, the percentage of neutrophils should be used for diagnosis. A neutrophil count > 50% indicates peritonitis.
   e. For patients with a dry abdomen who have abdominal pain, 1 liter of dialysate should be infused and dwelled for 1 to 2 hours, then examined and sent for a cell count with differential, Gram stain, and culture.
5. The exit site and tunnel should be examined and cultures taken of the drainage.
6. ISPD Guidelines for Treatment. These treatment guidelines have been outlined from the 2010 ISPD Guidelines.
   a. Antibiotics should be started as soon as cloudy effluent is seen. Do not delay treatment until results from the cell count and Gram stain are returned from the lab.
   b. Empiric therapy should cover both gram-positive and gram-negative organisms.
      (1) Center should select antibiotics based on local sensitivities.
      (2) Vancomycin or a cephalosporin can be used for gram-positive coverage.
      (3) A third-generation cephalosporin or aminoglycoside can be used for gram-negative coverage.
         (a) Intraperitoneal (IP) antibiotic administration is superior to intravenous dosing.
         (b) IP antibiotics can be given in each exchange (continuous dosing) or once daily (intermittent dosing). For intermittent dosing, the antibiotic solution should be allowed to dwell for 6 hours to allow for adequate absorption.
      (4) Once culture and sensitivities are known, antibiotics should be adjusted.
      (5) Within 48 hours of starting antibiotics, patients will show clinical improvement (decreasing pain and clearing of fluid).
   c. Catheter removal is recommended in certain situations to preserve the peritoneal membrane.

(1) Fungal peritonitis. Due to high mortality rates (25%), attempting treatment without catheter removal is discouraged.

(2) Refractory peritonitis. The catheter should be removed for peritonitis that fails to improve after 5 days of antibiotics.

(3) Relapsing peritonitis. This is when peritonitis reoccurs within 4 weeks of antibiotic completion with the same organism.

(4) Refractory catheter infections.

d. Catheter reinsertion.

(1) Simultaneous catheter reinsertion and removal can be used in the case of refractory exit-site infections and relapsing peritonitis. The patient should be covered with antibiotics.

(2) For refractory and fungal peritonitis, the appropriate time between catheter removal and reinsertion in unknown.

e. CQI/program monitoring for infectious complications. PD programs should monitor infection rates for exit site, tunnel infections, and peritonitis on at least a quarterly basis (Piraino et al., 2011).

(1) Overall rates can be examined as well as rates for each organism. Examining rates for each organism can help identify areas for improvement for the program.

(2) The ISPD recommends that a peritonitis rate of 0.36 episodes per patient year be reached.

(3) On a yearly basis, the program should examine the percentage of patients who are peritonitis-free. At least 80% of patients should remain peritonitis-free each year.

F. Trends, outcomes, and further investigation in peritoneal dialysis.

1. Catheter complications.

a. Approximately 20% to 35% of patients on PD transfer to HD due to catheter issues.

b. Patient survival in PD has improved, but technique survival has improved only slightly.

(1) More data is needed to show if specific catheters and insertion methods are better than others (Stylianou & Daphnis, 2014).

(2) The introduction of catheters that are more biocompatible and infection resistant could be helpful to PD therapy (Bieber et al., 2014).

2. Infectious complications.

a. Peritonitis causes approximately 20% of the technique failure in PD and 2% to 6% of deaths in patients on PD.

b. Over time, there has been a decrease in peritonitis rates in patients on PD. The decrease has been mostly seen with gram-positive peritonitis.

c. There is a great variability in reported peritonitis rates.

(1) Reported infection rates vary from 0.06 to 1.66 episodes/patient year.

(2) This bias may result from statistical bias, but it is also likely due to variation in practice and adherence to best demonstrated practices (Cho & Johnson, 2014).

d. More research is needed on topics related to the treatment of peritonitis.

(1) Interventions with modifiable risk factors reduce infections.

(2) Predialysis screening and treatment of *Staphlococcus aureus*.

(3) Agents used for exit-site cleansing.

(4) Continuous versus intermittent antibiotic dosing for peritonitis.

(5) Monitoring antibiotic levels during peritonitis treatment.

(6) Antibiotic prophylaxis for procedures (dental procedures, colonoscopy).

3. PD modality.

a. Over 70% of patients on PD in the United States are treated with APD.

b. A recent analysis comparing outcomes between CAPD and APD failed to show statistically significant differences between the two modalities in terms of loss of residual kidney function, peritonitis rates, fluid balance, technique, and patient survival or quality of life.

c. It is hypothesized that APD will grow in the United States due to increased use of PD, especially related to urgent-start PD.

d. Technical innovations with APD will also help with the transfer of data from the patient's home to the dialysis unit to increase safety and allow patients in remote areas more communication with providers (Bieber et al., 2014).

References

Arramreddy, R., Zheng, S., Saxena, A.B., Liebman, S.E., & Wong, L. (2014). Urgent-start peritoneal dialysis: A chance for a new beginning. *American Journal of Kidney Diseases, 63*(3), 390-395.

Asif, A. (2004). Peritoneal dialysis access-related procedures by nephrologists. *Seminars in Dialysis, 17*(5), 398-406.

Balafa, O., Koundouris, S., Mitsis, M., & Siamopoulos, K.C. (2014). An unusual case of hemoperitoneum: Spontaneous rectus sheath hematoma. *Peritoneal Dialysis International, 34*(1), 134-135.

Balda, S., Power, A., Papalois, V., & Brown, E. (2013). Impact of hernias on peritoneal dialysis technique survival and residual renal function. *Peritoneal Dialysis International, 33*(6), 629-634.

Balsera, C., & Guest, S. (2013). Hemoperitoneum in a peritoneal dialysis patient from retroperitoneal source. *Advances in Peritoneal Dialysis, 29,* 69-72.

Bargman, J.M. (2008). Hernias in peritoneal dialysis patients: Limiting occurrence and recurrence. *Peritoneal Dialysis International, 28*(4), 349-351.

Bargman, J.M. (2009). Noninfectious complications of peritoneal dialysis. In R. Khanna & R.T. Kredict (Eds.), *Nolph and Gokal's textbook of peritoneal dialysis* (3rd ed., pp. 571-609).New York: Springer.

Bargman, J., Thorpe, K., & Churchill, D. (2001). Relative contribution of residual renal function and peritoneal clearance to adequacy of dialysis: A reanalysis of the CANUSA study. *Journal of the American Society of Nephrology, 12,* 2158-2162.

Bender, F.H. (2012). Avoiding harm in peritoneal dialysis patients. *Advances in Chronic Kidney Disease, 19*(3), 171-178

Bender, F.H., Bernardini, J., & Piraino, B. (2006). Prevention of infectious complications in peritoneal dialysis: Best demonstrated practices, *Kidney International, 70,* S44-S54.

Berger, A., Edelsberg, J., Inglese, G.W., Bhattacharyya, S.K., & Oster, G. (2009). Cost comparison of peritoneal dialysis versus hemodialysis in end-stage renal disease. *American Journal of Managed Care, 15*(8), 509-518. Retrieved from http://www.ncbi.nlm.nih.gov/pubmed/19670954

Bernardini, J., Nagy, M., & Piraino, B. (2000). Pattern of noncompliance with dialysis exchanges in peritoneal dialysis patients. *American Journal of Kidney Diseases, 35*(6), 1104-1110.

Bieber, S.D., Burkart, J., Golper, T.A., Teitelbaum, I., & Mehrotra, R. (2014). Comparative outcomes between continuous ambulatory and automated peritoneal dialysis: A narrative review. *American Journal of Kidney Disease, 63*(6), 1027-1037.

Bleyer, A.J., Casey, M.J., Russell, G.B., Kandt, M., & Burkart, J.M., (1998). Peritoneal dialysate fill-volumes and hernia development in a cohort of peritoneal dialysis patients. *Advances in Peritoneal Dialysis, 14,* 102-104.

Burkhart, J.M., & Piraino, B. (2006). Clinical practice guidelines for peritoneal adequacy. *American Journal of Kidney Diseases, 48*(1), S99-S102.

Campos, R.P., Chula, D.C., & Riella, M.C. (2009). *Complications of the peritoneal access and their management.* Contributions in Nephrology, 163, 183-197.

CANADA-USA (CANUSA) Peritoneal Dialysis Study Group. (1996). Adequacy of dialysis and nutrition in continuous peritoneal dialysis: Association with clinical outcomes. *Journal of the American Society of Nephrology, 7*(2), 198-207.

The Kidney Health Australia – Caring for Australasians with Renal Impairment (KHA-CARI). (2005). *Dialysis adequacy (PD).* Retrieved from http://www.cari.org.au/Dialysis/dialysis_guidelines.html

Casaretto, A., Rosario, R., Kotzker, W., Rosario-Pagan, Y., Groenhoff, C., & Guest, S. (2012). Urgent-start peritoneal dialysis: Report from a U.S. private nephrology practice. *Advances in Peritoneal Dialysis, 28,* 102-105.

Centers for Disease Control (CDC). (2005, September). Infection control for peritoneal dialysis (PD) patients. Retrieved from http://emergency.cdc.gov/disasters/pdf/icfordialysis.pdf

Centers for Medicare & Medicaid Services (CMS). (2005, December). 2005 annual report: End stage renal disease clinical performance measures project. Department of Health and Human Services, Centers for Medicare & Medicaid Services, Office of Clinical Standards and Quality, Baltimore, MD.

Chavannes, M., Sharma, A.P., Singh, R.N., Reid, R.H., & Filler, G. (2014). Diagnosis by peritoneal scintigraphy of peritoneal dialysis-associated hydrothorax in an infant. *Peritoneal Dialysis International, 34*(1), 140-143.

Cheung, C.K., & Khwaja, A. (2008). Chylous ascites: An unusual complication of peritonealdialysis. A case report and literature review. *Peritoneal Dialysis International, 28*(3), 229-231.

Cho, Y., & Johnson, D.W. (2014). Peritoneal dialysis-related peritonitis: Towards improving evidence, practices, and outcomes. *American Journal of Kidney Disease, 64*(2), 278-289.

Chow, K.M., Szeto, C.C., & Li, P. (2003). Management options for hydrothorax (complicating) complicating peritoneal dialysis. *Seminars in Dialysis, 16*(5), 389-394.

Chuang, Y.W., Shu, K.H., Yu, T.M., Cheng, C.H., & Chen, C.H. (2009). Hypokalemia: An independent risk factor of enterobacteriaceae peritonitis in CAPD patients. *Nephrology Dialysis and Transplantation, 24,* 1603-1608.

Churchill, D.N. (2005). Impact of peritoneal dialysis dose guidelines on clinical outcomes. *Peritoneal Dialysis International, 25*(Suppl. 3), S95-S98.

Covidien. (2011). *Argyle™ peritoneal dialysis catheters.* Retrieved from http://www.covidien.com/imageServer.aspx/doc215777.pdf?contentID=20743&contenttype=application/pdf

Crabtree, J.H. (2006a). Hernia repair without delay in initiating or continuing peritoneal dialysis. *Peritoneal Dialysis International, 26*(2), 178-182.

Crabtree, J.H. (2006b). Rescue and salvage procedures for mechanical and infectious complications of peritoneal dialysis. *International Journal of Artificial Organs, 29*(1), 67-84.

Crabtree, J.H. (2006c). Selected best demonstrated practices in peritoneal dialysis access. *Kidney International, 70,* S27-S37.

Crabtree, J.H. (2010). Who should place peritoneal dialysis catheters. *Peritoneal Dialysis International, 30*(2), 142-150.

Crabtree, J.H., & Burchette, R.J. (2013). Peritoneal dialysis catheter embedment. Surgical considerations, expectations, and complications. *The American Journal of Surgery, 206*(4), 464-471.

Crabtree, J.H., & Fishman, A. (2005). A laparoscopic method for optimal peritoneal dialysis access. *The American Surgeon, 71*(2), 135-143.

Davies, S.J. (2013). Peritoneal dialysis – Current status and future challenges. *Nature Reviews Nephrology, 9*(7), 399-408.

Dell'Aquila, R., Chiaramonte, S., Rodighiero, M.P., Spano, E., Di Loreto, P., & Kohn, C.O. (2007). Rational choice of peritoneal dialysis catheter. *Peritoneal Dialysis International, 27*(Suppl. 2), S119-S125.

De Sousa, E., del Peso-Gilsanz, G., Bajo-Rubio, M.A., Ossorio-Gonzalez, M., & Selgas-Gutierrez, R. (2012). Encapsulating peritoneal sclerosis in peritoneal dialysis. A review and European initiative for approaching a serious and rare disease. *Nefrologia, 32*(6), 707-714.

Diaz-Buxo, J.A. (2005). Clinical use of peritoneal dialysis. In A.R. Nissenson, & R.N. Fine (Eds.), *Clinical dialysis* (4th ed., pp. 421-489). New York: McGraw Hill.

Diaz-Buxo, J.A. (2006). Complications of peritoneal dialysis catheters: Early and late. *The International Journal of Artificial Organs, 29*(1), 50-58.

Diaz-Buxo, J.A. (2007). Peritoneal dialysis solutions low in glucose degradation products: Clinical experience and outcomes. *Advances in Peritoneal Dialysis, 23,* 132-134.

Dombros, N., Dratwa, M., Feriani, M., Gokal, R., Heimbürger, O., Krediet, R., … Verger, C. (2005). European best practice guidelines for peritoneal dialysis. *Nephrology Dialysis Transplantation, 20*(Suppl. 9), ix1-ix37.

Ejaz, A.A. (1998). Peritoneal fluid eosinophilia. *Nephrology Dialysis Transplant, 13,* 2463-2464.

Figueiredo, A., Goh, B.K., Jenkins, S., Johnson D.W., Mactier, R., Ramalakshmi, S., … Wilkie, M. (2010). Clinical practice guidelines for peritoneal access. *Peritoneal Dialysis International, 30*(4), 424-429.

Findlay, A., Serrano, C., Punzalan, S., & Fan, S.L. (2013). Increased peritoneal dialysis exit site infections using topical antiseptic polyhexamethylene biguanide compared to mupirocin: Results of a safety study interim analysis of an open-lable prospective randomized study. *Antimicrobial Agents and Chemotherapy, 57*(5), 2026-2028.

Firanek, C., Sloand, J., & Todd, L. (2013). Training patients for automated peritoneal dialysis: A survey of practices in six successful centers in the United States. *Nephrology Nursing Journal, 40*(6), 481-491.

Foley, R.N., Parfrey, P.S., Harnett, J.D., Kent, G.M., Murray, D.C., & Barre, P.E. (1996). Impact of hypertension on cardiomyopathy, morbidity and mortality in end-stage renal disease. *Kidney International, 49*(5), 1379-1385.

Fourtounas, C., Dousdampanis, P., Hardalias, A., Liatsikos, E., & Vlachojannis, J. (2008). Eosinophilic peritonitis following air entrapment during peritoneoscopic insertion of peritoneal dialysis catheters. *Seminars in Dialysis, 21*(2), 180-182.

Gahl, G.M., & Jorres, A. (2000). Nightly intermittent peritoneal dialysis: Targets and prescriptions (review). *Peritoneal Dialysis International, 20*(Suppl. 2), S89-S92.

Ghaffari, A. (2012). Urgent-start peritoneal dialysis: A quality Improvement Report. *American Journal of Kidney Disease, 59*(3), 400-408.

Gokal, R., Alexander, S., Ash, S., Chen, T.W., Danielson, A., Holmes, C., … Vas, S. (1998). Peritoneal catheters and exit-site practices toward optimum peritoneal access: 1998 update. *Peritoneal Dialysis International, 18*(1), 11-33.

Gokal, R., Khanna, R., Krediet, R.T., & Nolph, K.D. (Eds.). (2000). *Textbook of peritoneal dialysis* (2nd ed.). Dordrecht: Kluwer Academic Publishers.

Gokal, R., Moberly, J., Lindholm, B., & Mujais, S. (2002, October). Metabolic and laboratory effects of icodextrin. *Kidney International,* Suppl. 81, s62-s71.

Healthy People 2010. *Main page.* Retrieved from http://www.healthy people.gov/

Hussain, S.I., Bernardini, J., & Piraino, B., (1998). The risk of hernia with large exchange. Volumes. *Advances in Peritoneal Dialysis, 14,* 105-107.

International Society for Peritoneal Dialysis (ISPD). (2010). *Peritoneal dialysis-related infections recommendations: 2010 update.* Retrieved from http://www.pdiconnect.com/content/30/4/393.full.pdf+html

Jain, S., Crooper, L., & Rutherford, P. (2003). Chylous ascites due to bile duct tumor in a patient receiving automated peritoneal dialysis. *Nephrology Dialysis Transplantation, 18,* 224.

Kaplan, G.G., Manns, B., & McLaughlin, K. (2005). Heparin-induced thrombocytopaenia inintraperitoneal heparin exposure. *Nephrology Dialysis Transplantation, 20,* 2561-2562.

Kathuria, P., Twardowski, Z.J., & Nichols, W.K. (2009). Peritoneal dialysis access and exit-site care including surgical aspects. In R. Khanna & R.T. Krediet (Eds.), *Nolph and Gokal's textbook of peritoneal dialysis* (pp. 371-446). New York: Springer.

Kubey, W., & Straka, P. (2005). Comparison of disinfection efficacy of four PD transfer set change procedures (abstract). *Peritoneal Dialysis International, 25*(Suppl. 1), S9.

Leblanc, M., Ouimet, D., & Pichette, V. (2001). Dialysate leaks in peritoneal dialysis. *Seminars in Dialysis, 14*(1), 50-54.

Lee, P.H., Lin, C.L., Lai P.C., & Yang, C.W. (2005). Octreotide therapy for chylous ascites in a chronic dialysis patient. *Nephrology, 10,* 344-347.

Lew, S.Q. (2007). Hemoperitoneum: Bloody peritoneal dialysate in ESRD patients receiving peritoneal dialysis. *Peritoneal Dialysis International, 27*(3), 226-233.

Lew, S.Q. (2010). Hydrothorax: Plueral effusion associated with peritoneal dialysis. *Peritoneal Dialysis International 30*(1), 13-18.

Li, P., Szeto, C., Piraino, B., Bernardini, J., Figueiredo, A., Gupta, A., … Struijk, D.G. (2010). Peritoneal dialysis-related infections recommendations: 2010 update. *Peritoneal Dialysis International 30*(4), 393-423.

Lo, W.K., Bargman, J.M., Burkart, J., Krediet, R.T., Pollock, C., Kawanishi, H., Blake, P.G., for the ISPD Adequacy of Peritoneal Dialysis Working Group. (2006). Guideline on targets for solute and fluid removal in adult patients on chronic peritoneal dialysis. *Peritoneal Dialysis International, 26*(5), 520-522.

Lo, W.K., Ho, Y.W., Li, C.S., Wong, K.S., Chan, T.M., Yu, A.W., … Cheng, I.K. (2003). Effect of Kt/V on survival and clinical outcome in CAPD patients in a randomized prospective study. *Kidney International, 64*(2), 649-656.

Mahnensmith, R.L. (2014). Urgent-Start peritoneal dialysis: What are the problems and their solutions. *Seminars in Dialysis, 27*(3), 291-294.

Martinez-Mier, G., Garcia-Almazan, E., Reyes-Devesa, H., Garcia-Garcia, V., Cano-Gutierrez, S., Mora y Fermin, R., … Mendez-Machado, G.F. (2008). Abdominal wall hernias in end-stage renal disease patients on peritoneal dialysis. *Peritoneal Dialysis International 28*(4), 391-396.

Maya, I.D. (2008). Ambulatory setting for peritoneal dialysis catheter placement. *Seminars In Dialysis, 21*(5), 457-468.

McCann, L. (1998). *Pocket guide to nutritional assessment of the renal patient* (2nd ed., pp. 3-13). New York: National Kidney Foundation,.

McCormick, B.B., Bargman, J.M., (2007). Noninfectious complications of peritoneal dialysis: Implications for patient and technique survival. *Journal of the American Society of Nephrology, 18,* 3023-3025.

McCormick, B.B., Brown, P.A., Knoll, G., Yelle, J.D., Page, D., Biyani, M., … Lavoie, S. (2006). Use of the embedded peritoneal dialysis catheter: Experience and results from a North American center. *Kidney International, 70,* S38-S43.

McQuillan, R.F., Chiu, E., Nessim, S., Lok, C.E., Roscoe, J.M., Tam, P., & Jassal, S.V. (2012). A randomized controlled trial comparing mupirocin and polysporin triple ointments in peritoneal dialysis patients: The mp3 study. *Clinical Journal of the American Society of Nephrology, 7,* 297-303.

Miller, M., McCormick, B., Lavoie, S., Biyani, M., & Zimmerman, D. (2012) Fluoroscopic manipulation of peritoneal dialysis catheters: Outcomes and factors associated with successful manipulation. *Clinical Journal of the American Society of Nephrology, 7,* 795-800.

Muirhead, N. (2005). Erythropoietic agents in peritoneal dialysis. *Peritoneal Dialysis International, 25*(6), 547-550.

Mujais, S., Nolph, K., Gokal, R., Blake, P., Burkart, J., Coles, G., … Segas, R. (2000). Evaluation and management of ultrafiltration problems in peritoneal dialysis. *Peritoneal Dialysis International, 20*(4), S5-S21.

Nabeel, A., Bernardini, J., Fried, L., Burr, R., & Pirano, B. (2006). Comparison of infectious complications between incident hemodialysis and peritoneal dialysis patients. *Clinical Journal American Society Nephrology, 1,* 1226-1233.

National Kidney Foundation (NKF). (2000). Clinical practice guidelines for nutrition in chronic renal failure. *American Journal of Kidney Diseases, 35*(6, Suppl. 2), S1-S140. Erratum in *American Journal of Kidney Diseases, 38*(4), 917.

National Kidney Foundation (NKF). (2006a). KDOQI clinical practice guidelines and clinical practice recommendations for 2006. Update: Peritoneal dialysis adequacy. *American Journal of Kidney Diseases, 48*(Suppl. 1), S91-175.

National Kidney Foundation. (2006b). KDOQI clinical practice guidelines and clinical practice recommendations for 2006 updates: Hemodialysis adequacy, peritoneal dialysis adequacy, and vascular access. *American Journal of Kidney Diseases, 48*(Suppl. 1), S1-322.

Nissenson, A.R., & Fine, R.N. (Eds.). (2005). *Clinical dialysis* (4th ed.). New York: McGraw Hill.

Paniagua, R., Amato, D., Vonesh, E., Correa-Rotter, R., Ramos, A., Moran, J., & Mujais, S., for the Mexican Nephrology Collaborative Study Group. (2002). Effects of increased peritoneal clearances on mortality rates in peritoneal dialysis: ADEMEX, a prospective, randomized, controlled trial. *Journal American Society of Nephrology, 13*, 1307-1320.

Penner, T., & Crabtree, J.H. (2013). Peritoneal dialysis catheters with back exit sites. *Peritoneal Dialysis International, 33*(1), 93-96.

Peppelenbosch, A., van Kuijk, W., Bouvy, N.D., van der Sande, F.M., & Tordoir, J. (2008). Peritoneal dialysis catheter placement technique and complications. *Nephrology Dialysis Transplantation Plus, 1*(Suppl. 4), iv23-iv28.

Perez-Fontan, M., Garcia-Falcon, T., Rosales, M., Rodriguez-Carmona, A., Adeva, M., Rodriguez-Lozano, I., & Moncalian, J. (1993). Treatment of *Staphylococcus aureus* nasal carriers in continuous ambulatory peritoneal dialysis with mupirocin: Long-term results. *American Journal of Kidney Disease, 22*(5), 708-712.

Piraino, B., Bailie, G.R., Bernardini, J., Boeschoten, E., Gupta, Holmes, C., ... Uttley, L. (ISPD Ad Hoc Advisory Committee).(2005). Peritoneal dialysis-related infections recommendations: 2005 update. *Peritoneal Dialysis International, 25*(2), 107-131.

Piraino, B., Bernardini, J., Brown, E., Figueiredo, A., Johnson, D., Lye, W., ... Szeto, C.C. (2011). ISPD position statement on reducing the risks of peritoneal dialysis-related infections. *Peritoneal Dialysis International, 31*(4), 614-630.

Ponce, D., Balbi, A.L., & Finkelstein, F.O. (2014). Peritoneal dialysis for the treatment of acute kidney injury. In J.T. Daugirdas, P.G. Blake, & T.S. Ing (Eds.), *Handbook of dialysis* (5th ed., pp. 451-463). Philadelphia: Lippincott Williams & Wilkins.

Povlsen, J.V., & Ivarsen, P. (2005). Assisted automated peritoneal dialysis (AAPD) for the functionally dependent and elderly patient. *Peritoneal Dialysis International, 25*(Suppl. 3), S60-S63.

Prischl, F.C., Muhr, T., Seiringer, E.M., Funk, S., Kronabethleitner, G., Wallner, M., ... Kramar, R. (2002). Magnetic resonance imaging of the peritoneal cavity among peritoneal dialysis patients, using the dialysate as "contrast medium." *Journal of the American Society of Nephrology, 13*, 197-203.

Prowant, B.F., Ponferrada, L.P., & Satalowich, R.J. (2008). Peritoneal dialysis access. In C.S. Counts (Ed.), *Core curriculum for nephrology nursing* (5th ed., pp. 765-794). Pitman, NJ: American Nephrology Nurses' Association.

Prowant, B.F., & Twardowski, Z.J. (1996). Recommendations for exit care. *Peritoneal Dialysis International, 16*(Suppl. 3), S94-S99.

Quinlan, C., Cantell, M., & Rees, L. (2010). Eosinophilic peritonitis in children on chronicperitoneal dialysis. *Pediatric Nephrology, 25*, 517-522.

Scanziani, R., Pozzi, M., Pisano, L., Barbone, G.S., Dozio, B., Rovere, G., ... Magri, F. (2006). Imaging work-up for peritoneal access care and peritoneal dialysis complications. *The Journal of Artificial Organs, 29*(1), 142-152.

Shah, H., Chu, M., & Bargman, J.M. (2006). Perioperative management of peritoneal dialysis patients undergoing hernia surgery without the use of interim hemodialysis. *Peritoneal Dialysis International 26*(6), 684-687.

Stylianou, K.G., & Daphnis, K.G. (2014). Selecting the optimal peritoneal dialysis catheter. *Kidney International, 85*, 741-743.

Tapawan, K., Chen, E., Selk, N., Hong, E., Virmani, S., & Balk, R. (2011). A large pleural effusion in a patient receiving peritoneal dialysis. *Seminars in Dialysis, 24*(5), 560-563.

Twardowski, Z.J. (2005). Physiology of peritoneal dialysis. In A.R. Nissenson & R.N. Fine (Eds.), *Clinical dialysis* (4th ed., pp. 357-384). New York: McGraw-Hill.

Twardowski, Z.J., Khanna, R., & Nolph, K.D. (1986). Osmotic agents and ultrafiltration in peritoneal dialysis. *Nephron, 42*(2), 93-101.

Twardowski, Z.J., Nolph, K.D., Khanna, R., Prowant, B.F., Ryan, L.P., Moore, H.L., & Nielsen, M.P. (1987). Peritoneal equilibration test. *Peritoneal Dialysis Bulletin, 7*(3), 138-147.

United States Renal Data System (USRDS). (2011). USRDS 2009 annual data report: Atlas of end-stage renal disease in the United States. Bethesda, MD: National Institutes of Health, National Institute of Diabetes and Digestive and Kidney Disease.

United States Renal Data System (USRDS). (2014). USRDS 2014 annual data report: Atlas of end-stage renal disease in the United States. Bethesda, MD: National Institutes of Health, National Institute of Diabetes and Digestive and Kidney Disease.

Vaux, E.C., Torrie, P.H., Barker, L.C., Naik, R.B., & Gibson, M.R. (2008). Percutaneous fluoroscopically guided placement of peritoneal dialysis catheters – aA 10-year experience. *Seminars in Dialysis, 21*(5), 459-465.

Zanger, R. (2010). Hyponatermia and hypokalemia in patients on peritoneal dialysis. *Seminars in Dialysis, 23*(6), 575-580.

Zorzanell, M.M., Fleming, W.J., & Prowant, B.F. (2004). Use of tissue plasminogen activator in peritoneal dialysis catheters: A literature review and on center's experience. *Nephrology Nursing Journal, 31*(5), 534-537.

CHAPTER **5**
Home Dialysis

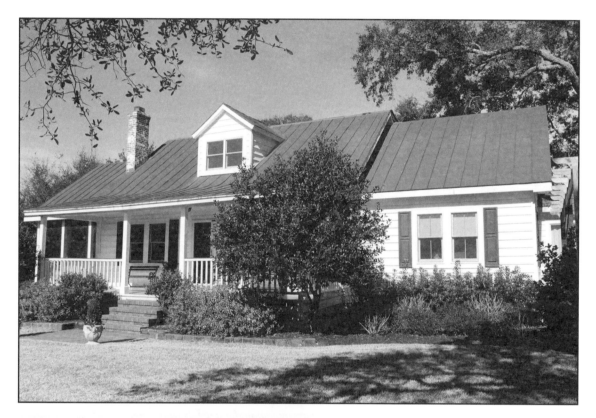

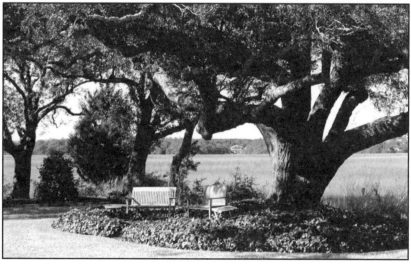

Chapter Editor
Karen E. Schardin, BSN, RN, CNN

Authors
Karen E. Schardin, BSN, RN, CNN
Maria Luongo, MSN, RN
Geraldine F. Morrison, BSHSA, RN
Susan C. Vogel, MHA, RN, CNN

CHAPTER **5**

Home Dialysis

This offering for **1.4 contact hours** is provided by the American Nephrology Nurses' Association (ANNA).

American Nephrology Nurses' Association is accredited as a provider of continuing nursing education by the American Nurses Credentialing Center Commission on Accreditation.

ANNA is a provider approved by the California Board of Registered Nursing, provider number CEP 00910.

This CNE offering meets the continuing nursing education requirements for certification and recertification by the Nephrology Nursing Certification Commission (NNCC).

To be awarded contact hours for this activity, read this chapter in its entirety. Then complete the CNE evaluation found at **www.annanurse.org/corecne** and submit it; or print it, complete it, and mail it in. Contact hours are not awarded until the evaluation for the activity is complete.

Example of reference for Chapter 5 in APA format. Use author of the section being cited. This example is based on Section C – Home Peritoneal Dialysis.

Luongo, M. (2015). Home dialysis: Home peritoneal dialysis. In C.S. Counts (Ed.), *Core curriculum for nephrology nursing: Module 3. Treatment options for patients with chronic kidney failure* (6th ed., pp. 279-310). Pitman, NJ: American Nephrology Nurses' Association.

Interpreted: Section author. (Date). Title of chapter: Title of section. In …

Cover photo by Counts/Morganello.

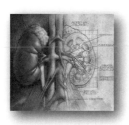

CHAPTER 5

Home Dialysis

Introduction

The patient with chronic kidney disease who will need kidney replacement therapy (KRT) has the option to select home dialysis as the modality of choice. The process of educating the patient and family about dialysis options should ideally occur as part of chronic kidney disease (CKD) management, but may occur later in the patient's healthcare experience. Key to the successful implementation of home dialysis is the patient's motivation to assure self-care responsibility and the support, facilitation, and management of this process by the home training nurse.

Purpose

The purpose of this chapter is to discuss the history, benefits, and requirements of home dialysis, patient selection and training, and the roles of the nurse in managing and monitoring patients. The chapter also provides information that focuses on the concepts and principles related to home hemodialysis (HD) and home peritoneal dialysis (PD), including urgent-start PD.

Objectives

Upon completion of this chapter, the learner will be able to:
1. Describe the principles of home hemodialysis and home peritoneal dialysis.
2. Identify the clinical advantages to patients on home dialysis therapies.
3. Identify the necessary components that are required for a successful home dialysis program.
4. Explain the role of the nursing staff in managing and monitoring patients at home.
5. List three considerations for patient selection related to home dialysis.
6. Identify the training requirements necessary to assure patients are safe and competent to perform home dialysis.
7. Explain two reasons for partner training.

SECTION A
Overview of Home Dialysis
Geraldine F. Morrison

I. Home dialysis – a treatment option (Scribner, 1990).

A. Hemodialysis was the first treatment option available for home dialysis therapy. It took almost 10 more years before peritoneal dialysis caught on as a mainstream home therapy.

B. In 1973, when the Medicare End Stage Renal Disease (ESRD) program became available to ESRD patients, 40% of the 11,000 dialysis patients were on home dialysis. Following Medicare's payments for

treatment, the number of home patients has decreased dramatically with only 0.4% on home hemodialysis and 11% on some form of peritoneal therapy, continuous ambulatory peritoneal dialysis (CAPD), or continuous cycling peritoneal dialysis (CCPD), now recognized as automated peritoneal dialysis (APD). Virtually no patients are at home on intermittent peritoneal dialysis (IPD).

II. Home dialysis – its beginning and its history. See *Significant Dates in the History of Home Hemodialysis* on next page.

During the period of 1960–1970, home hemodialysis accounted for a large proportion of patients treated with dialysis. The first program to perform home hemodialysis remains controversial, as many patients were being simultaneously initiated.

Significant Dates in the History of Home Hemodialysis

1961   First documented case of home hemodialysis by Nose in Japan.

1962   First free-standing outpatient dialysis facility at Seattle Artificial Kidney Center (SAKC).

1963   Sheldon performs first nocturnal treatment.

1964   First documented person to receive home hemodialysis in the United States reported by Curtis and Associates.

1966   Home hemodialysis training program developed at Seattle Artificial Kidney Center.

1969   First study of daily dialysis by DePalma and Associates in Los Angeles.

1972   Bonomini and Associates in Bologna, Italy, first used short daily hemodialysis in the home.

1973   Medicare End Stage Renal Disease Program in effect; 40% of patients on home hemodialysis.

1980   Health Care Financing Administration (HCFA) funded three multicenter studies of home hemodialysis using "paid aides."

1983   Congress introduces "composite rate" reimbursement, excluding payment for home dialysis aides.

1994   Report by Uldall and Associates of slow, overnight (nocturnal) hemodialysis.

1997   Lynchburg Nephrology Dialysis starts a nightly home hemodialysis program in the United States.

2002   Aksys – FDA approved device to be marketed for home hemodialysis.

2005   Aksys – removed from market.

2005   NxStage – FDA approved device to be marketed for home hemodialysis.

2011   K @ Home- FDA approved device to be marketed for home hemodialysis.

2014   NxStage received approval for its Nocturnal Indication from the FDA.

Hemodialysis was not the only form of home therapy. Peritoneal dialysis as a home treatment option emerged in the 1970s and for many patients became the treatment of choice. This was due to the simplicity of performing the treatment and the ability to dialyze at home without an assistant.

A. In 1960, Belding Scribner and colleagues from the University of Washington developed the Teflon arteriovenous shunt, an access that made long-term intermittent hemodialysis possible for the treatment of ESRD (Scribner, 1990). In 1961, equipment such as the Kiil dialyzer was developed and used for ongoing dialysis treatments.

B. As developments with hemodialysis continued during the 1960s, Drs. Fred Boen and Henry Tenchkoff of Seattle were working on methods of providing peritoneal dialysis as therapy for ESRD patients.
   1. A closed peritoneal dialysis fluid supply system was initiated to reduce the risk of peritonitis.
   2. Tenckhoff developed the first indwelling peritoneal catheter which became the industry standard for long-term peritoneal dialysis.

C. The 1960s was a time period during which the medical, social, financial, and ethical problems associated with the treatment of patients with ESRD were discussed.
   1. In 1962, there were no funding sources to cover the cost of dialysis treatments, and the demand for treatment far exceeded the available financial resources.
   2. The financial burden of ESRD treatment led directly to the development of home hemodialysis in the United States.

D. During the 1960s, the University of Washington trained and supported 52 patients, their families, and physicians on home hemodialysis from all over the United States, Chile, Malaysia, the Philippines, and the Sudan.

E. The early beginning of home dialysis.
   1. In 1961, the first patient treated on home hemodialysis was in Japan, dialyzing on a coil dialyzer immersed in an electric washing machine.
   2. A committee in Seattle was mandated to ration the resources of hemodialysis based on selected criteria and denied a 15-year-old girl access to

treatment. That denial began home hemodialysis in the United States.

3. In 1963, home hemodialysis was being performed in India on a wealthy Madras businessman.

4. In 1963 to 1964, John Merrill in Boston was doing home dialysis with a nurse performing the treatments in the patient's home with twin-coil dialyzers.

5. In 1964, Dr. Scribner, in conjunction with Les Babb, built an automated hemodialysis proportioning machine that was used by the first home hemodialysis patient in Seattle (Scribner, 1990).

6. In the same time period, 1964, Stanley Sheldon and colleagues in London were the first to initiate overnight home hemodialysis (10–12 hours) using a setup similar to Seattle's.

7. In 1966, Kolff at the Cleveland Clinic began their home hemodialysis program.

8. It took until 1970 before home IPD (intermittent peritoneal dialysis) became possible for selected patients, although it was not widely used as a therapy.

9. In 1972, Tenckhoff developed a system for in-line peritoneal dialysate using reverse osmosis and an ultraviolet light to sterilize the fluid.

10. In 1972, short daily hemodialysis treatment was introduced as a home therapy by Dr. Bonomini in Bologna, Italy.

11. In 1976, Drs. Popovich and Moncrief in Austin, Texas, developed the technique of CAPD. CAPD was a home peritoneal dialysis method of self-treatment that required no automated equipment.

12. In 1981, Diaz-Buxo initiated CCPD as another form of self-therapy done at home during the night.

13. In 1994, Toronto, Canada, began nocturnal home hemodialysis.

14. In 1997, Lynchberg Nephrology Dialysis in Virginia began a nightly home hemodialysis program patterned after Toronto.

15. Beginning in 2000, innovative changes to home hemodialysis equipment have allowed patients in the United States opportunities to select a variety of therapies for home treatment: standard three treatments per week, short daily, or long nocturnal dialysis.

III. Home dialysis – its decline and resurgence.

As the number of dialysis facilities increases across the country, and care is readily available in a patient's local community, the number of patients selecting home dialysis as a treatment option has declined.

A. Since 1980, home dialysis in the United States has been on a steady decline due to numerous causes.
 1. Increase in the number of dialysis facilities providing in-center treatment.

2. Increase in the ages of patients and the number of comorbidities of patients.

3. Reimbursements to units and physicians better for in-center therapy than for home dialysis.

4. Patients are less independent and have less desire to take responsibility for their own treatment.

5. In-center treatment allows patients to socialize with other patients and therefore not feel isolated.

6. Home dialysis assistants, either family members or others, are not as available due to changes in the work force.

7. Nephrologists have less experience with home dialysis because so few programs in the United States are available and therefore do not promote home as a therapy to their patients.

8. Important dialysis-related medications are not available to home patients.

9. The infrastructure necessary for a successful home program is costly, and many dialysis facilities do not want to incur the additional costs.

B. Since 2000, the focus in the nephrology community has been on the revival of home dialysis. The mandate from CMS to provide regular modality education to all patients with CKD has exposed them to the possibility of other therapies besides in-center.
 1. Because of the mandate to provide modality education, physicians and centers have become more involved in patient education to the home therapies.
 2. New technology will revive home dialysis. Innovative, easy-to-operate equipment offers patients a variety of home dialysis therapies and allows for more frequent and/or longer dialysis sessions.
  a. Short daily treatment (SDHD).
  b. Slow nocturnal dialysis (SNHD).
  c. Daily nocturnal dialysis (DNHD).
  d. Automated peritoneal dialysis (APD).
 3. Patients feel better and promote home to others.
 4. Buttonhole cannulation is easy and less painful for the patient.
 5. There are increased payment incentives since 2005 for physicians to have patients on home dialysis.
 6. Information from the latest USRDS (2014) revealed that:
  a. In 2012, the use of home dialysis among incident patients with CKD stage 5 had increased 35% as compared to figures from 2002.
  b. 49,000 patients received home dialysis in 2012, a number that is 63% higher than a decade ago.
   (1) Home hemodialysis accounted for 16.3%.
   (2) Home peritoneal dialysis (PD) accounted for the other 83.7%.
   (3) There was five times more home HD in 2012 (N = 7,923) than in 2002 (N = 1,563).

IV. Benefits of home dialysis.

The benefits of home dialysis are many and varied. Benefits include clinical advantages, better patient outcomes, and personal benefits for the home dialysis patients. Most advantages are experienced with SDHD, SNHD, DHND, CAPD, or APD home treatments.

A. Clinical advantages and better patient outcomes include:
1. Home hemodialysis has the best survival of any kind of dialysis, about the same as a transplant from a deceased donor. Survival is 2 to 3 times higher in short daily hemodialysis than in three treatments per week in-center patients, with an estimated additional 2.3 to 10.9 years of life (Kjellstrand et al., 2008).
   a. A 2003–2004 Northwest Kidney Center's study of 117 patients on SDHD compared home hemodialysis to USRDS data for three treatments per week patients, which was adjusted for age, sex, and comorbidities.
   b. The study found a 61% better survival rate in home hemodialysis patients (Blagg et al., 2006).
2. More frequent dialysis (5–6 days/week) is efficient at removing waste products by the most physiologic methods.
   a. Predialytic serum urea and creatinine levels are near normal and remain steady during the week.
   b. Conventional 3x/week in-center hemodialysis is not physiologic.
   c. More dialysis = longer life, better health.
3. The relative risk of death was less for home patients.
   a. Cardiac death is 3x more likely after the "weekend" for 3x week patients (Bleyer et al., 2006; Foley et al., 2011).
   b. Risk of death is 30% higher in patients who gain over 3 kg per treatment (Kalantar-Zadeh et al., 2009).
4. A quicker recovery time after treatment (Heidenheim et al., 2003).
5. Improved blood pressure and volume control.
   a. Safer treatment.
   b. Less volume to remove.
   c. Ability to achieve dry weight.
6. Improved acid-base balance.
7. Better phosphate control and decreased need for binders.
8. Increased appetite and improved nutritional state. Diets can remain more normal.
9. Decrease in left ventricular hypertrophy (Culleton et al., 2007).
10. Significantly reduced complications of hypotension, cramps, nausea or vomiting.
11. Reduction in medications.

12. Decreased hospitalizations.
13. Less risk of infection.
14. Better outcomes.

B. Personal benefits.
1. Better quality of life.
2. Ability to sleep better.
3. Increased rehabilitation and ability to work.
4. Increase in sexual functioning.
5. Fewer side effects.
6. No weather or transportation worries.
7. Increased energy, endurance, strength, and feeling of well-being.
8. Improved family and social relationships.
9. Increased independence and travel.
10. Better knowledge about illness and its treatment.
11. Flexible dialysis schedules.

V. Requirements of a home program.

The Medicare Conditions of Coverage (ESRD Program Interpretive Guidelines) provide guidance through regulations on the necessary requirements for an organization to establish and maintain a home dialysis program for either peritoneal or hemodialysis (Centers for Medicare and Medicaid Services, October 3, 2008). A successful home program has many integrated segments that are centered on patient education, support, and follow-up.

A. Conditions of Coverage requirements for a home program.
1. Qualified personnel to provide the self-dialysis training. Training is provided only by an RN with at least 12 months of experience in the provision of nursing care, and at least 3 months' experience in the home modality field in which he/she is training.
2. Services received by home patients must be at least comparable to those provided to patients dialyzing in-center.
3. Home patients and their helpers must be verified as proficient in performance of home dialysis procedures before going home.
4. Surveillance of the patient's home adaptation.
5. Social service and nutrition support.
6. Installation and maintenance of equipment.
7. Oversight of supplies.
8. Monitoring of laboratory, medication, and treatment results.
9. Competency with medication management and administration.
10. Multidisciplinary team for care planning development and review processes.
11. Monitoring of water quality and dialysate sample collection when used with hemodialysis, following

the standards of the Association for the Advancement of Medical Instrumentation (AAMI).
12. Review of daily run logs at least every 2 months to monitor the patient's condition.

B. Additional requirements.
1. Defined policies and procedures specific to each type of home dialysis therapy that clearly define program expectations and patient's responsibilities.
2. On-call nursing, technical support, and medical support 24/7 to respond to emergency and machine problems. A plan is in place for emergency in-center backup as needed.
3. Follow-up clinics.
4. Environment conducive to learning.
5. Variety of teaching methods and materials geared to patient learning.
6. Appropriate and usable dialysis access.
7. Home surveys to assure that storage space and plumbing and electrical supplies are adequate.
8. Home visits as deemed necessary.
9. Home hemodialysis assistants and helpers identified.
10. Documentation of home teaching and training and confirmation of patient helper proficiency.
11. Retain recordkeeping system that guarantees continuity of care and patient privacy.
12. Patient and helper are able to respond appropriately to medical and nonmedical emergencies.
13. Early identification of suitable candidates for home dialysis via early modality education.
14. Trainers skilled in adult education teaching methods.
15. Tools to objectively measure the patient's and helper's skills and competency to perform dialysis treatments.
16. Communication methods to reach patients at home for changes to procedures.
17. Local water and power companies should be informed when there are people on home therapies so they can be placed on a priority for reinstatement of services during water and power failures.

VI. Patient selection.

The main objective in patient selection is to accurately assess a patient's motivation to learn and ability to provide safe and effective dialysis treatments in the home.

A. Considerations.
1. Significant mental health issues.
2. Drug and alcohol abuse.
3. Physical and cognitive abilities.
4. Abusive partner.
5. Reliable support if needed.

B. Factors involved in patient selection (Gomez, 2011).
1. Living circumstances and accommodations. Overview of home environment for:
   a. Space planning for equipment and supply storage.
   b. Absence of pests.
   c. Cleanliness.
   d. Water quality.
   e. Plumbing connections.
   f. Telephone readiness.
2. Learning ability.
   a. Able to learn the necessary skills required to dialyze alone or with a helper.
   b. Has the applicable motor skills to complete self-care at home, or has a helper to do so.
3. Level of patient and/or family anxiety regarding home dialysis.
4. Type and severity of medical condition.
   a. Impact on quality of life.
   b. Rehabilitation potential.
5. Motivation to learn and compliance with treatment regimen.
6. In-center nursing staff, social worker, dietitian, and physician identifying patients to refer to home therapy. Physicians are a key component in patients selecting home dialysis.
7. Availability of an assistant for hemodialysis, or patient is able to dialyze safely alone.
8. Availability to accommodate training schedule.
9. Ability of patient to communicate. English as a second language is not a complete deterrent, but patient or helper must be able to troubleshoot over the phone.

VII. Patient training.

The main objective of any training program for home dialysis is to assure that patients and/or their partners are educated and understand how to perform safe, effective dialysis in the home setting without undue anxiety while achieving maximum independence.

A. Training objectives must be clearly stated and agreed to by the patient and partner.

B. One-on-one training that is tailored to the patient's level of understanding and learning needs seems to be the most effective method of teaching patients and helpers. Patients may be trained in their homes.

C. The amount of time to train patients varies by modality. Both day and evening trainings should be provided to meet patients' needs.
1. Peritoneal training may be up to 5 days.
2. Hemodialysis training may take 3 to 5 weeks or longer.

D. There is a peritoneal dialysis catheter for peritoneal training, or a hemodialysis vascular access for home hemodialysis training, in place and ready to use. An arteriovenous fistula or graft is preferable to a catheter.

E. Programs must provide the necessary dialysis experiences for patients and helpers to become proficient with the procedures.

F. Training manuals should contain procedures that are written at no greater than an eighth grade reading level. It is important to evaluate the patient's and helper's health literacy prior to training.

G. Training should occur both on dialysis and nondialysis days.
   1. On nondialysis days, ancillary training can be done for hemodialysis procedures for water treatment, waste disposal, storage, setups, laboratory work, vital signs, aseptic technique, infection control precautions, machine maintenance, supply ordering, and record keeping.
   2. Review patient/family/helper/primary care nurse roles in education, evaluation, and decision-making processes. Identify and incorporate patient's beliefs, preferences, and cultural impacts on aptitude to learn. Revise education and training materials as needed.

H. Multiple types of teaching methods should be employed to meet individual learning styles.

I. Repetition and feedback is the key to successful patient learning. Teach patient how to establish goals to attain education and training requirements.

J. Having objective ways to assess the patient's knowledge and understanding is critical, whether through tests, checklists, or observational scoring data.

K. If possible, training for self-cannulation should occur while the patient is in-center and before starting formal home training.

L. Training must include several dialysis sessions in the training unit that simulate the patient dialyzing at home, with follow-up in the patient's home.

VIII. Nursing roles and responsibilities.

Nurses have several roles and responsibilities in home dialysis programs. The nurse's prime responsibility is to provide patients with complete, accurate, and understandable information to promote the patient's independence in the home setting.

A. Five major nursing roles and responsibilities include assessment, education, monitoring and oversight, resource and support, and documentation.
   1. Assessments.
      a. Readiness for training.
      b. Adherence to treatment.
      c. Learning style.
      d. Appropriateness of the home environment.
      e. Family dynamics.
   2. Education.
      a. Tailored to individual learning style.
      b. Objective assessments of competency.
      c. Dialysis procedures.
      d. Recordkeeping.
      e. Emergency procedures.
      f. Troubleshooting machine alarms.
      g. Supply ordering.
   3. Monitoring and oversight.
      a. Lab value reviews.
      b. Therapy outcomes compliance with treatment prescription.
      c. Home follow-up visits.
      d. Adaptation to home therapy.
      e. Review of monthly logs.
      f. Communication to physicians.
      g. Problem lists.
      h. Care plans.
   4. Resource and support.
      a. Assistance 24/7.
      b. Coordination of services (technical, supplies, procedural).
      c. Conditions for Coverage.
      d. Regulation compliance.
      e. Communications.
      f. Ongoing patient education.
   5. Complete and thorough ongoing documentation.

B. Safe transition home.
   1. Facilitate safe resettlement of patients who have completed home training, enabling them to perform their own dialysis at home.
   2. For those patients who still feel the need for in-home oversight during the early stages after home training, further home visits and telephone communication should be scheduled as needed.
   3. The home program should continue to provide reasonable levels of support following the early home adjustment.

Section B
Home Hemodialysis
Karen E. Schardin, Susan C. Vogel

I. Background information.

The resurgence of home hemodialysis brings hemodialysis procedures full circle. In the initial days of the ESRD program, it was felt that patients would be able to provide their own treatments in their home to obtain better control over their disease and personal lifestyle. The commercialization of hemodialysis shifted the focus from home hemodialysis to in-center. Now, with improvements in the knowledge of dialysis, coupled with the advances in technology, the renal industry is again interested in home hemodialysis (Blagg, 1997).

II. Why choose home hemodialysis?

A. Conditions for Coverage require that patients are given their treatment options (Centers for Medicare & Medicaid Services [CMS], 2008, April 15).

B. Self-management and patient engagement are beneficial to patients. "Patient engagement is the involvement in their own care by individuals (and others they designate to engage on their behalf), with the goal that they make competent, well-informed decisions about their health and health care and take action to support those decisions" (Sofaer & Schumann, 2013).

C. Patients who choose their own therapy are significantly more likely to live longer and to receive a transplant (Stack & Martin, 2005).

D. Top factors influencing the decision to choose home hemodiaysis (Czajkowski et al., 2013).
1. Having ability to perform dialysis at home.
2. Having control over one's own schedule.

E. Other factors.
1. Potential for better outcomes.
2. Fewer dietary restrictions.
3. Transportation issues.
4. Ability to keep working.

F. Lifestyle motivators for choosing home and/or self-care dialysis (McLaughlin et al., 2008).
1. Ability to take control of one's own care.
2. Greater freedom to travel and freedom from specific time constraints.
3. Greater ability to work and participate in "normal" life activities.
4. Reduced need to travel to and from the dialysis center.

III. Basic concepts of home hemodialysis.

The purpose of this part is to define and describe concepts and principles related to home hemodialysis.

A. Concepts related to solute removal (see Chapter 2 in this module).

B. Concepts related to fluid removal (see Chapter 2 in this module).

C. Types of home hemodialysis.
1. Intermittent hemodialysis (IHD) – conventional/traditional 3-times-a-week therapy.
2. Every-other-day hemodialysis.
   a. Avoids the 2-day interdialytic period, which has been associated with increased sudden death and cardiac death (Bleyer et al., 1999).
   b. Limits complications with more frequent cannulation and increased dialyzer exposure (Diaz-Buxo et al., 2013).
   c. May decrease the burden of therapy associated with more frequent treatments.
3. Hemodialfiltration. Currently there is no FDA approved online hemofiltration fluid equipment available in the United States. It is being used internationally in some areas (Ronco et al., 2006; Vaslaski et al., 2005).
   a. This treatment uses convection as the mechanism for uremic toxin removal.
      (1) Removes the middle molecules more efficiently.
      (2) Generally uses a high-flux membrane.
   b. Uses ultrapure fluid to prevent contamination of fluid delivered to the patient. Ultrapure fluids reduce the risks associated with contaminated dialysate.
      (1) Specifically designed equipment with online generation of ultrapure fluid.
      (2) May also be partially achieved through maximizing internal filtration and back filtration in the dialyzer.
   c. Treatment may be done 3 times per week or daily.
   d. Offers benefits such as correction of anemia, inflammation, oxidative stress, lipid profiles, calcium-phosphate product, as well as improvement in pruritus.
   e. May be associated with increased leakage of albumin and proteins and may compromise nutritional status. New membranes with nano-controlled characteristics may minimize the

loss of important nutrients while maximizing the benefits of middle molecule removal.

4. Daily (quotidian) hemodialysis.
   a. Generally a shortened treatment (2.5 to 3.5 hours) 5 to 7 times per week.
   b. Dialysate flow and blood flow rates may be the same as in-center (depending on equipment used).
   c. Uses a high-efficiency dialyzer, which shows beneficial effects in controlling renal anemia and controlling cost.
   d. Patients generally use an anticoagulation bolus at the beginning of treatment and no infusion during the treatment.
   d. Patients undergoing daily dialysis experience a significant increase in removal of urea, calculated at 20% to 40% when hemodialysis is performed 6 to 7 times per week.
5. Nocturnal (overnight) hemodialysis (Lindsay et al., 2006). NxStage received approval for its Nocturnal Indication from the FDA in December 2014 and is currently the only equipment approved by the FDA for use in nocturnal home hemodialysis in the United States.
   a. Long nightly treatments (6 to 8 hours); may be 3 to 7 nights per week.
   b. Dialysate flow rate (100 mL/min) and blood flow rate (200 to 300 mL/min) run slower than in-center rates.
   c. Home patients may have remote monitoring during therapy.
   d. Requires the use of anticoagulation during the treatment to prevent clotting.
   e. Use of enuresis pads, leak detectors, and safety clips at the needle connections may be beneficial.
   f. Single needles may assist in accidental needle dislodgement
   g. Slow dialysis (6 to 10 hours) may allow for the equilibration of tissue and vascular compartments, which results in better clearance and decreased postdialysis rebound in solutes.
   h. Offers best control of hyperphosphatemia without phosphate binders; may require phosphate replacement in dialysate.
   i. Significant reduction in beta-2 microglobulin levels.

IV. Benefits of home hemodialysis (Young et al., 2012).

A. Potential for greater dialysis delivery.

B. Flexibility of scheduling treatment time.

C. Decreased transportation issues going to center for weekly treatments.

D. Independence and convenience along with a greater sense of control over one's own health and life.

E. Improved survival rates.

F. Decreased hospitalization rates.

G. Improved opportunity for rehabilitation and employment potential.

H. Improved quality of life.

V. Benefits of daily hemodialysis.

A. Less stress on the heart and less risk of cardiac stunning (Ayus et al., 2005; Glick, 2012).

B. Lower risk of death (Blagg et al., 2006; Kjellstrand et al., 2008).
   1. Improvement in left ventricular hypertrophy.
   2. Improvement in inflammatory and related biomarkers; the release of inflammatory cytokines is attenuated with the use of more biocompatible membranes.

C. Improvement in hypertension and decreased need for antihypertensive medications (Chan, 2009; Fagugli et al., 2006; Jaber et al., 2009; Nesrallah et al., 2003).
   1. This is due to improved fluid control and normalization of extracellular volume.
   2. Blood pressure medications may be decreased, which decreases the pill burden and cost of medication.

D. Decreased fluid overload; the effects of intradialytic hypotension may be minimized.

E. Improved anemia control that may decrease medications required.

F. Improved removal of beta-2 microglobulin, which may delay or prevent the progression of amyloidosis (Young et al., 2012).

G. Improved hyperphosphatemia, particularly in nocturnal dialysis (Young et al., 2012).
   1. May contribute to the reduction of morbidities and risk of cardiovascular incidents that are associated with elevated phosphorus and Ca x PO_4 products.
   2. There is a potential decrease in phosphate binders (particularly with nocturnal therapy).

H. Improved patient appetite and measures of nutrition (Galland et al., 2001; Spanner et al., 2003).
   1. Improved albumin/prealbumin, protein intake.
   2. Increase in dry weight and lean body mass.

3. Disappearance of anorexia and improved nutritional status is explained by:
   a. Decreased dietary restrictions.
   b. Improvement in adequacy of dialysis, cardiovascular stability, and interdialytic hydration.

I. Improved quality of life (Young et al., 2012).
   1. Improved energy levels.
   2. Better rehabilitation.
   3. Decreased hospitalizations.
   4. Flexibility of treatment schedule may also improve quality of life.

J. Improved mental and physical scores on SF 36 (Jaber et al., 2010).

K. Decreased depression reported on Beck's Depression Index (Jaber et al., 2010).

L. Improved sleep patterns with a decreased prevalence or improvement in sleep apnea.

M. Decreased intradialytic symptoms resulting from improved homeostasis.
   1. Muscle cramping.
   2. Nausea and/or vomiting.
   3. Headaches.

N. Quicker recovery time after treatment and fewer postdialysis symptoms such as fatigue, cramps, "washed out" feeling, and lightheadedness (Jaber et al., 2010).

O. Reduction in global cost of care due to reductions in costs related to hospitalizations, access complications, medications, and transportation (Young et al., 2012).

P. Improved fertility and fetal outcomes (Tennankore et al., 2012).

VI. Contraindications to home hemodialysis.

A. There are no known contraindications to therapy.
   1. The patient and/or partner must be able to perform the treatments safely.
   2. The patient must be able to have the equipment in the home environment.

B. Concerns.
   1. Poorly functioning access.
   2. Marked arteriosclerosis leading to the possibility of more complications.
   3. Folic acid and vitamin B deficiencies are associated with increased C Reactive Protein levels which may be worsened if not corrected.

4. Blood loss associated with ineffective rinse back volume.
5. Infection associated with increased opportunity for contamination.
6. Need for respite care for patient and/or partner.

VII. Patient selection for home hemodialysis.

A. General considerations.
   1. Home dialysis should be discussed as an option for all patients (CMS, 2008, April 15).
   2. Early referral to nephrologists for patients with chronic kidney disease may allow for early education about modality choices.
   3. Patients with chronic illness can and should take day-to-day management of their illness (Thomas-Hawkins & Zazworsky, 2005).
   4. Healthcare professionals can help patients manage their own care, including home dialysis.
   5. Barriers to home hemodialysis (Young et al., 2012).
      a. Lack of knowledge about the option.
      b. Attitude barriers (e.g., "patients should not dialyze without supervision").
      c. Fear of cannulation.
      d. Fear of failure to perform procedures appropriately.
      e. Fear of social isolation.
      f. Burden of therapy for patients and partners.
      g. Lack of partner.
      h. Mechanical complexity.
      i. Home water treatment.
      j. Physician barriers due to educational gaps regarding home therapy.
   6. Choosing home hemodialysis requires changing knowledge, attitudes, and skills of physicians and nurses as well as patients.
   7. Assessment of the patient's and partner's ability to cope with responsibilities of primary care is important for preventing therapy dropout.

B. Patient assessment.
   1. Interdisciplinary team interview is required to assess the patient's ability to perform or receive home therapy (Gomez, 2011; Leitch et al., 2003).
   2. Motivation for home therapy may be the most important factor to patient success at home.
   3. Vascular access (Shurraw & Zimmerman, 2005).
      a. The access's capability to achieve required blood flow rate for therapy.
      b. The patient's and partner's capabilities to perform cannulation or access catheter.
   4. Literacy.
      a. Assess patient's and partner's abilities to read or memorize skills and abilities to speak or read English.

b. Assess staff's ability to teach patient and partner and provide follow-up care in native language.

5. Vision.
   a. Assess for ability to see various type sizes.
   b. Assess for color blindness.

6. Hearing.
   a. Assess for ability to hear instructions in normal conversation.
   b. Assess for ability to hear alarm sounds.

7. Strength and energy level. Assess motor skills and ability to perform tasks required for therapy (e.g., opening and closing clamps, making connections, hanging solutions, etc.).

8. Comorbid factors. Is the patient medically stable to dialyze at home?

9. Adherence with current treatment plan.
   a. Ability to accommodate therapy into personal schedule.
   b. Recognize and address conflicts that may interfere with therapy.
   c. Identify reasons for nonadherence that may be either intensified by home therapy or may be improved with patient control over schedule and therapy.

10. Home visit to assess the suitability of the environment for home hemodialysis (Gomez, 2011).
    a. Ability to make electrical connections.
    b. Home ownership or rental. If renting, it must be determined whether renovation required is permissible.
    c. Ability to make arrangements required for water testing and connections.
    d. Telephone access.
    e. Space for equipment and supplies.
    f. General cleanliness of home environment.

C. Partner assessment. *Note*: Some facilities do not require a partner for home hemodialysis.
   1. A partner for home hemodialysis is advised to assist with medical emergencies that may arise (Tennankore et al., 2012).
   2. A separate multidisciplinary team assessment can provide insight into a partner's motivation and willingness to provide treatments.
      a. Exploring the relationship and the ability to handle the responsibilities of hemodialysis is important. This should be done as part of the selection process to identify any issues or develop a plan to address concerns so that home therapy can be successful.
      b. The goals are to optimize the use of support and interventional measures to avoid or identify negative effects on the partner's life (Belasco & Sesso, 2002).
      c. Partner burnout can be minimized by encouraging the patient to maintain primary responsibility for care when possible.

d. Early identification and intervention may minimize the partner's burden and improve the quality of life and medical outcome of the patient.

3. It has been reported that partners may experience comorbidities, more psychopathologic states, more physician visits, and have poorer health than counterparts.

4. Types of partners.
   a. Spouse.
      (1) Make up 76% of home dialysis caregivers.
      (2) Women assume most responsibility for health care, including home dialysis.
   b. Family member.
   c. Friend.
   d. Paid aide, with the payment made by the patient or the facility program.
   e. Staff-assisted, with some facilities providing the staff to perform the patient's treatments in the home.
   f. Assess the partner as noted previously for the patient (see B4 to B9).
   g. Assess the partner's availability for the training period and ability to participate in home treatments.
   h. Identify and assist the partner in dealing with stressors associated with home hemodialysis treatments. Most successful patient and partner relationships are found in those with a collaborative approach to home dialysis.
   i. Barriers to rendering care in the home hemodialysis situation.
      (1) Fear of equipment and equipment breakdown.
      (2) Time requirement for treatment and related functions.
      (3) Complexity of home hemodialysis.
      (4) Fear of change in family relationships.
      (5) Fear of stress and demands of responsibility that may include inability to work outside the home due to home hemodialysis requirements.

VIII. Patient and partner training (Harwood & Leitch, 2006).

A. Patient education (see Chapter 3 in Module 2 for general education principles).

B. Prior to training.
   1. Initiate a signed agreement to follow program expectations for home hemodialysis; review program and patient expectations.
      a. The patient and partner should review tasks required for home hemodialysis and agree on the division of tasks.

b. The more the patient can perform, the less burden or stress on the partner.
2. Ensure patient and partner have clear instructions about training program.
    a. Start date and time.
    b. Preparation and participation required.
    c. Length of training days.
    d. Length of training program, etc.
3. Assess the patient's and partner's learning styles and adapt training plan and materials to meet their needs.
4. Training regarding vascular access care and management can be completed prior to home dialysis training.
    a. Minimizes training time.
    b. Allows more flexibility in training multiple patients simultaneously.

C. Training.
1. Use a training plan and review it with patient and partner at each session (Young et al., 2012). Check off as the patient and partner demonstrate their understanding of concepts or ability to perform tasks. Figure 5.1 presents suggested content for home hemodialysis training.
2. Allow patient and partner to gain comfort and confidence with procedures.
3. When teaching motor skills, master one step at a time.
    a. Teach in small sessions, building on the steps.
    b. Allow opportunities for reviewing learned skills.
    c. Use varied learning methods.
4. Training multiple patients can be done.
    a. Train one patient per shift (two patients per day).
    b. Treatment times may be increased as needed during training period.
    c. Stagger patient starts (e.g., start one patient until he or she begins to gain independence, and then start another patient).
    d. Group training.
        (1) Use multiple trainers who have specific roles in the training; work from a clear, well-defined training plan.
        (2) Match the patients' skill levels and compatibility in the group.
5. Assess the patient's and partner's learning through return demonstration, discussion, oral or written exams, and observation.
    a. Document training, assessment of learning, and skill mastery.
    b. It is essential to assure that the patient and the partner retain troubleshooting skills.
6. Allow flexibility in the training plan.
    a. Ongoing evaluation of the patient's and partner's learning is necessary.

Suggested Content for Home Hemodialysis Training

- ❑ Kidney function and kidney failure
- ❑ Kidney complications
- ❑ Infection control
    Hand washing
    Personal protective equipment
- ❑ Aseptic and sterile techniques
- ❑ Access
    Types
    Initiation/discontinuation
    Management and complications
- ❑ Vital signs
    Blood pressure
    Pulse
    Temperature
    Dry weight
- ❑ Hemodialysis fundamentals
    Theory
    Equipment (dialysis and water treatment)
    Operating procedures (setup, monitoring, discontinuing, disinfection)
- ❑ Dialysis prescription (home schedule)
- ❑ Anticoagulation
- ❑ Medication administration
- ❑ Lab analysis
    Drawing labs
    Interpretation
- ❑ Nutrition and dietary considerations
- ❑ Complications
    Management of procedure complications
    Medical complications
- ❑ Treatment documentation
- ❑ Clinic visits
- ❑ Supply inventory and ordering
- ❑ Equipment maintenance
- ❑ Travel
- ❑ Back up requirements/support

Figure 5.1. Checklist for content for home hemodialysis training.

b. Alter the training plan as soon as the need is identified.

7. Optimally, one home training nurse is assigned to train the patient and partner throughout the training process. Using multiple staff for the training is offset by having an organized, well-documented training plan and checklist to assure consistency in training.

8. The training should take place in a quiet atmosphere with minimal distractions and is usually done in a dedicated home training area.

9. The training nurse should assure that the patient and partner can demonstrate all the needed skills to perform home hemodialysis and document completion of training with a certificate of completion.

IX. Clinical management of the home hemodialysis patient.

A. Home visits.
1. Support from the home training nurse at the patient's first home hemodialysis treatment(s) to observe setup and procedure will encourage the patient's and partner's confidence in performing their treatments at home.
   a. The home training nurse can provide insight into organization of the home treatment area to optimize the efficiency of the space.
   b. Many programs use either the nurse or the biomed technician to help the patient determine the best location for equipment and supplies in the home.
2. Annual home visits are necessary to observe the patient in the home environment.

B. Clinic visits are usually performed monthly with the following assessments being made.
1. Fluid status and dry weight: weight, blood pressure, shortness of breath, edema, cramping, etc.
2. Vascular access.
   a. Treatment parameters: blood flow rates, pressure readings during treatment, etc.
   b. Site examination: swelling, redness, drainage, aneurysm, bruising, etc.
3. Laboratory review.
   a. Assure that labs are drawn correctly.
   b. Anemia parameters: hemoglobin, hematocrit, iron stores, erythropoietin stimulating agent dosage, etc.
   c. Bone metabolism and disease: serum Ca, PO_4, and PTH levels; phosphate binders, etc.
   d. Chemistries with emphasis on serum K, CO_2, albumin.
   e. Adequacy of dialysis: pre-and post-BUN, KT/V, creatinine. Compare to previous levels and treatment patient is receiving.

f. Diabetes management if applicable: glucose records, HbA1C, prescribed medicine for diabetes, and other areas of importance (e.g., foot care and visual problems).
   g. Cardiovascular management: lipid profiles and C-reactive protein levels.
4. Medication review.
   a. Verify the medications being taken, whether or not they are being taken as ordered, and if any refills are needed.
   b. If performing daily dialysis, ensure that medications are taken after treatment.
5. Treatment record review and assessment.
   a. Patient flow sheets for treatment settings and treatment completion as ordered.
   b. Symptoms or complications noted but not reported by patient and partner.
   c. Any symptoms not noted by patient and partner.
   d. Alarms noted and appropriate resolution.
   e. Dialyzer appearance at end of treatment which may indicate red cell loss and/or the need to alter heparin dosage.
   f. Overall documentation completeness.
6. Supplies and equipment.
   a. Verify appropriate use and operation.
   b. Discuss any equipment issues and equipment management.
   c. Review supply usage and inventory management.
7. Nutritional assessment.
   a. Usually done by the dietitian.
   b. May include reviews of weight, adequacy, bone metabolism and disease, anemia status, appetite, etc.
8. Psychosocial assessment.
   a. Usually done by the social worker.
   b. Energy level.
   c. Stress levels.
   d. Changes in relationship with partner.
   e. Financial concerns.
   f. Quality of life.
9. Skills review.
   a. The nurse assesses the patient's and partner's competence in performing dialysis procedures and troubleshooting skills.
   b. Semiannual to annual competency observation for patient's and partner's abilities to perform treatments should be conducted in the training department or patient's home setting.

C. Many facilities are using connected health to communicate with patients between clinic visits.
1. Connected health can provide nurses and physicians with treatment data from the equipment, patient vital signs, medications given, and other pertinent data.

2. Having patient data available through connected health allows the healthcare team the ability to review information on a daily basis to analyze trends and detect any issues before clinic visits to help the patient make adjustments in treatment which may avoid complications for the patient.

3. Connected health gives the healthcare team the ability to assure that treatments are completed as prescribed.

4. Some connected health systems have the capability to provide the physicians and nurses with a daily "dashboard" and notification of any values that are outside of limits set by the physician and facility. This gives the healthcare team the opportunity to contact the patient to evaluate what is happening in the home.

5. Connected health can also provide the healthcare team and patient the ability to communicate either live or within minutes.

6. Other applications include the ability to message treatment changes, medication changes, appointment times, or inventory.

D. Patient retention.
   1. Reasons for patients to drop therapy.
      a. Uncontrollable: death, transplant, transfer, health issues, other concerns.
      b. Controllable: burden of therapy for patient or partner, psychological, vascular access.
   2. Home training nurses as well as the interdisciplinary team should be involved in assessing the patient and partner to help them stay on home therapy.
   3. Suggested retention activities should start with the selection process and continue as long as the patient is on therapy. The highest risk for dropping out is in the first 90 days of therapy.
      a. Provide realistic view of home hemodialysis to include accurate expectations.
      b. Use an interdisciplinary team to interview the patient and partner. Consider interviewing the partner separately to accurately gauge his/her commitment.
      c. Focus on the patient motivation for home therapy.
      d. The home training nurse should tailor the training program to the patient's and partner's needs to make them successful. The ability of the nurse to provide customized training is a key to success.
      e. Provide the opportunity to perform independent treatments at the facility before going home to encourage self-confidence.
      f. Home visits for the first treatment help support the patient and partner and help them feel comfortable in performing treatments in the home environment.

      g. Frequent phone calls from the facility home training staff can provide support, answer questions, and resolve concerns in the first several weeks after the patient is at home.
      h. The patient should be coming to the facility for clinic visits, but the home training nurse may have patients come more frequently after they first go home to provide additional support.
      i. The interdisciplinary team can help the patient and partner assess their health and lifestyle benefits from home therapy.
      j. Group support meetings or meetings with peers performing home hemodialysis may be beneficial for both patients and partners.
      k. The patients should continue to be encouraged to perform as much of their treatment as possible.
      l. Providing support 24/7 as needed.
      m. Respite care in the facility or home training area may be helpful for the patient and partner as a means to take a break from the responsibility of treatment.

E. Self-care unit/area.
   1. A self-care unit/area can be used to support the home hemodialysis program.
   2. Allows patient and/or partner to gain confidence prior to going home.
      a. May be used by patient and/or partner to learn or reinforce knowledge and skills regarding care of a new or revised vascular access.
      b. Allows the patient and/or partner to have a routine vacation from the usual responsibilities.
      c. Allows the patient and/or partner respite as needed.
      d. May be used to train new or backup partners.

X. Components of the home hemodialysis system.

A. Equipment requirements are the same as for hemodialysis in a healthcare facility.
   1. The NxStage machine is approved for home hemodialysis by the FDA.
      a. A small, portable system that uses volumetric balancing in a disposable cartridge.
      b. The NxStage system is a volume-based system, much like peritoneal dialysis, where the patient prescription is based on the patient weight or total body water (TBW). Tools such as the Estimated Treatment Time Calculator and Dosing Calculator are available to help the home training team prescribe and adjust patient therapy.
      c. The system has no special electrical requirements and offers an option using sterile bagged dialysate, with no water treatment system.

d. The system may use the PureFlow water purification system, which uses the patient's source (tap) water to make ultrapure water. PureFlow uses a disposable deinonization process to purify the tap water.
   (1) PureFlow SL produces ultra-pure water.
   (2) Mixes the water with the concentrate to make the batch of dialysate.
   (3) Tests the prepared dialysate.
   (4) Warms the dialysate.
   (5) Stores the dialysate.
   (6) Delivers the dialysate to the NxStage System One Cycler when needed for therapy (NxStage, 2012).
e. The NxStage system uses lactate as the buffer for dialysis treatments. Lactate has been used as the buffer for PD successfully for years.

2. The 2008K@home™ is approved for home hemodialysis by the FDA.
   a. It is a smaller version of the conventional Fresenius machine and designed for home patients' use.
   b. The 2008K@home™ is prescribed as a time-based therapy as with conventional hemodialysis treatments.
   c. The system requires electrical and plumbing modifications in the home as per manufacturer guidelines to operate the equipment.
   d. The 2008K@home™ requires a water purification system, generally a reverse osmosis (RO) system as well as carbon tanks to purify the water for dialysis treatments. The RO, depending upon the model used, can be disinfected either with heat or chemical sterilization.
   e. The 2008K@home™ uses bicarbonate as the buffer for the dialysis treatments (Fresenius Medical Care, 2014).

3. Dialysis machines that are not approved specifically for home treatments are currently being used according to a physician's prescription.

B. Dialysate preparation using water purification system dialysate concentrate.
   1. Key component of the water treatment system is a knowledgeable user.
   2. The patient and/or partner must have a clear understanding of the water system, water testing, test results, and alarm conditions to assure safe operation.
   3. Water and dialysate should meet current Association for the Advancement of Medical Instrumentation (AAMI) Standards and be tested per CMS guidelines (see Table 5.1) (Mehrabian et al., 2003).
   4. Refer to Chapter 2 for general information on water treatment in dialysis.

5. Equipment installation in the home must meet electrical and plumbing requirements for the equipment.
6. Maintenance will vary according to design and age of equipment. Follow manufacturer's guidelines for installation, service, and maintenance.
7. Disinfection of equipment must be done at required intervals per manufacturer's guidelines.
   a. NxStage does not require internal equipment disinfection.
   b. 2008K@home™ requires machine disinfection after treatment (see Table 5.2 for a comparison to alternative home purification system for dialysate preparation).

XI. The dialysis procedure (see Chapter 2 in this module).

A. Special considerations for patients on home hemodialysis and their partners.
   1. The patient on home HD and/or partner must learn the same procedures as in-center staff. In some cases, additional procedures may be added to ensure safety and/or individualized care in the home environment.
   2. The treatment documentation recorded by the patient and/or partner should be reviewed at each clinic visit.
   3. Disinfection of the dialysis and water equipment must be done by either the patient and/or partner, or arrangements made with the home training facility to provide this service to comply with the manufacturer's disinfection recommendations.
   4. The patient and/or partner should have a document (using a checklist or other means) indicating that they have been observed in all treatment and equipment procedures and that they are competent to perform these treatments at home.
   5. It is recommended that the partner be present while the patient is undergoing the hemodialysis treatment at home.
   6. Manufacturers may have training tools and plans available for use for home hemodialysis staff and patients.

B. Dialyzer reprocessing in the home (see Chapter 2 in this module).
   1. Reprocessing procedures must meet all of the AAMI's recommended practices for reuse of hemodialyzers.
   2. Arrangements must be made for either the appropriate equipment (AAMI standards) if reprocessing hemodialyzers in the home, or appropriate transportation procedures if dialyzers are transported to the facility for reprocessing.

Table 5.1

PureFlow SL (PFSL) Testing Requirements* per CMS** Guidelines Applicable in the United States Only

(for reference purposes the table also compares the PFSL testing requirements with those for conventional equipment)

Fluid	CMS Interpretive Guideline	Conventional Equipment	PureFlow SL
Product water	Bacterial contamination of water used to prepare dialysate	Quarterly minimum	Not required for the PureFlow SL system
Product water	Maximum level of chemical contaminants in water used to prepare dialysate	Initial and quarterly	**For Source Water from Public Water Supplies:** Initially (first PAK in the patient's home) and annually. **For Source Water from Private Water Supplies:** Initially (first PAK in the patient's home) and at intervals sufficiently spaced in time to capture the possible seasonal variability of the source water quality. **Notes on Product Water Testing** • Testing should be performed at or near the end-of-life of the PAK. • Testing is **NOT** required after installing and priming a new PAK disposable. • Testing is **NOT** required after changing the PureFlow SL Control Unit hardware. • If testing is to be performed on new PAKS (i.e., those that have made three or less 60 liter batches), product water samples should be collected within 4 hours of completing a batch. This will ensure acccurate, interference-free AAMI panel results.
Product water	Total Chlorine/Chloramines	Every treatment	Testing is required prior to the first use of each batch (twice a week on average). **For best results**, it is recommended that the test for Total Chlorine be performed within 2 hours of making a batch or with ultra low total chlorine test strips that are insensitive to interference agents.
Dialysate	Bacterial contamination of dialysate	Quarterly minimum	Minimum of quarterly testing. Even with thorough care and expeditious transfer to labs, false positives can be expected to occur at rates of 2% to 9.1%.*** Follow appropriate retesting and retraining procedures in response to any false positives.

* State and foreign regulations on testing requirements may vary from those of CMS

** US Center for Medicare and Medicaid Services (CMS)

*** Even in best case culture sampling conditions (controlled lab conditions, expert sampling personnel, etc.), false positive rates of 2% to 9.1% have been reported when performing blood cultures in a controlled clinical environment (Norberg, A., Christopher, N.C, Ramundo, M.L., Bower, J.R., Berman, S.A. (2003). Contamination rates of blood cultures obtained by dedicated phlebotomy vs. intravenous catheter, *JAMA*, 289(6), 726-729.

Source: NxStage Medical, Inc. *Dialysate Preparation Primer: Chronic Hemodialysis with the NxStage® PureFlowTM SL* ©2011 NxStage APM231 Rev D, p. 20. Used with permission.

Table 5.2

Comparison to Alternative Home Purification System for Dialysate Preparation

Parameter	Alternative Water Purification System for Dialysis	PureFlow SL
Filtration Technology	Reverse Osmosis (RO) filtration with recirculation capabilities	De-ionization filtration
Product water quality	Product water quality proportionally related to source water quality	Product water quality independent of source water quality. The PureFlow SL consistently produces AAMI and ISO-quality product water from source water that meets the PureFlow SL Source Water Purity Requirements.
Source Water Purity Requirements: Iron	< 0.1 mg/L	< 0.3 mg/L (US EPA SDWA, Secondary Drinking Water Standard)
Manganese	< 0.1 mg/L	< 0.05 mg/L (US EPA SDWA, Secondary Drinking Water Standard)
Free Chlorine	0.0 mg/L	4.0 mg/L
Total Hardness	< 267.7 ppm CaCO3 (or < 15.7 grains per gallon)	No operational limits on Total Hardness and TDS, although there may be contractual limits on TDS
Source Water Temperature	10 to 30° C (50 to 86° F)	5 to 30° (41 ti 90° F)
Source Water Flow Rate	8.33 L/min (132 gallons/hour)	0.2 L/min (3.2 gallons/hour)
Yield (percent of incoming water that is converted to product water)	30% to 70% depending on source water quality, temperature, pH, flow rate, and pressure	100%
Operator Monitoring Requirements	Source water must be monitored, since changes in product water may exceed acceptable limits if source water deteriorates significantly	None required. Continuous monitoring by the PureFlow SL system
Disinfection	Required • Quarterly, minimum • Monthly, if RO water not routinely tested for bio-burden • Whenever the filtration system has been idle for more than 72 hours • Whenever the permanent fluid pathway has been opened and/or changed	None required due to the disposable nature of the Purification Pack (PAK)

Source: NxStage Medical, Inc. *Dialysate Preparation Primer: Chronic Hemodialysis with the NxStage® PureFlowTM SL* ©2011 NxStage APM231 Rev D, p. 17. Used with permission.

3. If reprocessed hemodialyzers are to be used, the patient and/or partner must have documentation of their competency in all procedures that they are required to perform including:
   a. Testing for sterilants.
   b. Testing for absence of sterilants.
   c. Monitoring for complications related to dialyzer reprocessing.
4. Most facilities choose not to reprocess dialyzers for home patients.

C. Vascular access for home hemodialysis patients (see Chapter 3 in this module).
   1. Types of vascular accesses used for home hemodialysis.
      a. Central venous catheter (CVC).
         (1) The CVC must be able to sustain the prescribed blood flow for treatment to assure treatment adequacy.
         (2) CVCs have interlocking connectors for attachment to the patient's bloodlines. Facilities may make recommendations to patients for an additional locking device.
      b. Fistula.
         (1) Fistulas are the preferred dialysis access for home patients.
         (2) Fistulas have the lowest complication rates in home and daily therapies.
         (3) The patient and/or partner may use either the rotating site method or the buttonhole technique. As staff skill in training techniques improves, buttonhole technique may become the preferred method of cannulation for daily treatments (Young et al., 2012).
         (4) Single needles may be used for nocturnal treatments to reduce the number of punctures. It has been considered by some to be safer in case of accidental dislodgement while sleeping.
      c. Graft.
         (1) The patient and/or partner use the rotating site method of cannulation.
         (2) Buttonhole technique is not used for grafts.
   2. Guidelines for vascular access.
      a. The patient or the partner must be taught cannulation technique using proper infection control practices (e.g., hand washing, cleansing of the access, and basic principles of infection prevention as outlined in NKF KDOQI).
      b. The patient and the partner must be taught the signs and symptoms of access infection and the appropriate action to take (e.g., report the problem following the facility protocol and follow through with the treatment prescribed).
      c. Current data does not indicate that daily cannulation is harmful to fistulas or grafts.

   d. Training in cannulation techniques prior to home training may be beneficial to the home training process and in patient selection.
   e. The patient and partner must recognize the symptoms of vascular access complications and be able to report and follow the prescribed treatment plans.

D. Adequacy of dialysis (see Chapter 2 in this module).
   1. The home patient's adequacy testing should meet or exceed the NKF KDOQI Guidelines.
   2. Testing should be done monthly and be evaluated by the attending nephrologist or advanced practice registered nurse (APRN) for necessary changes to the patient's dialysis prescription.
   3. The patient and/or the partner must be taught laboratory drawing procedures and know how the lab samples are transferred to the laboratory.
   4. Post-BUN samples should be drawn according to NKF KDOQI Guidelines using either the low flow or stop flow method.
   5. KT/V is generally the accepted measure of "adequate dialysis." Other factors to be considered are creatinine, potassium, albumin, phosphorus, beta-2 microglobulin, appetite, sleep patterns, energy level, and quality of life.
   6. Standardized KT/V results of 2.0–2.1 are recommended as a minimum standard for adequacy (NKF, 2006)
   7. Minimum single pool KT/V results per treatment (see Figure 5.2).
      a. 1.2 for conventional dialysis.
      b. 0.5 for short daily therapy done 6 times per week.
   8. Physicians may have preferences for higher standards for single pool KT/V results.

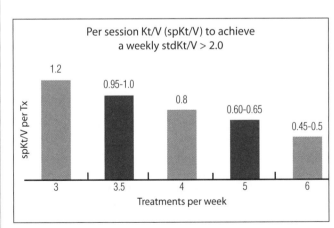

Figure 5.2. Comparison of Standardized Kt/V and spKt/V by treatments per week.

Source: NKF KDOQI™ Clinical Practice Guidelines (2006 updates) and published eKt/V and stdKt/V formulae listed above.
Defined to achieve stdKt/V > 2.0.
The dark blue bars represent extrapolation not in KDOQI guidelines. Graph does not take residual kidney function into account. Used with permission.

9. All patient lab results and general well-being should be considered in assessing adequate treatment.

E. Acute complications (see Chapter 2 in this module).
   1. The home hemodialysis patient and partner must be competent in identification and management of acute complications of hemodialysis and must be able to respond appropriately to medical emergencies.
   2. At a minimum, a partner must be able to recognize signs of a medical emergency, call for emergency assistance if needed, and treat the emergent medical symptoms.
   3. An emergency safety kit is recommended for home patients. Required contents may vary by facility.

F. Infection control (see Module 2, Chapter 6: Infection Control).
   1. The patient and partner must use appropriate infection control practices during all aspects of the home hemodialysis process to help prevent infections.
   2. The patient and partner must be taught to recognize the symptoms of infections, report symptoms, and complete the prescribed treatment.

XII. Role of the home training nurse.

A. The primary role of the nurse is to teach the patient and partner to manage the patient's kidney disease and to safely and effectively perform dialysis procedures in the home. The nurse functions as a presenter, coach, and facilitator in the role.

B. The home hemodialysis training nurse must have:
   1. Documented training in hemodialysis (CMS, 2008, Tuesday, April 15).
   2. Documented training and experience in home hemodialysis training.
   3. An understanding of adult learning principles.
   4. The capability to assess patients for the ability to perform hemodialysis procedures in the home environment.
   5. The ability to develop and execute a training plan, individualized to each patient in home training.
   6. The ability to develop and implement patient selection criteria, patient schedules, and oversight of patients at home.

C. For home hemodialysis programs, minimum staffing is two nurses — one dedicated to home training and another to fill in as backup when required.

D. Having staff available on call for home patients is essential.
   1. Provides optimal home services.
   2. Improves patient outcomes through rapid response.
   3. Prevents waste of resources.
   4. Promotes patient confidence and satisfaction.

XIII. Future of home hemodialysis.

A. Home hemodialysis has shown an increase since 2002. Contributing factors include:
   1. Improved mortality in home hemodialysis patients.
   2. Improved clinical benefits of daily therapy.
   3. New technology in home hemodialysis systems and manufacturer funding for advances in equipment and dialyzer membranes.
   4. Increased interest in convective therapies.
   5. Flexible dialysis prescriptions and scheduling (short daily, nocturnal, every other day, and other combinations) which may allow patients to continue to fit dialysis into their lives and their lifestyles, avoiding dropping out of this form of therapy.
   6. While costs increase, particularly for daily hemodialysis, there are economic benefits for home and daily hemodialysis related to decreased hospitalization rates and lessened needs for medications.
   7. Improved quality of life.
   8. Patient's increased sense of independence and freedom.
   9. Increased physician information and training about benefits of home hemodialysis.
   10. Home hemodialysis allows one nurse to manage more patients than conventional, in-center patients.
   11. Studies indicating that, if educated, more patients would choose and are capable of performing home dialysis.

B. Other considerations.
   1. There is a need for improvement in vascular access outcomes, including the ability to decrease bacterial infection.
   2. There is a need for improved removal of middle molecules, such as beta-2 microglobulin.
   3. Exploring the benefits of ultrapure dialysate may lead to improvements in inflammation, maintenance of kidney function at initiation of dialysis, improvement in nutrition, and improvement in iron utilization and erythropoietin response.
   4. Home dialysis, especially home daily hemodialysis, requires local and national advocacy for appropriate funding models and infrastructure to develop and promote these modalities. The federal government must have a role in understanding the

benefits and costs of home and daily dialysis through the development of a tiered payment system to reflect hemodialysis dose and in funding of a randomized, controlled study of the effects of short daily and nocturnal dialysis.

SECTION C
Home Peritoneal Dialysis
Maria Luongo

I. Definition of terms.

A. Continuous ambulatory peritoneal dialysis (CAPD). The patient performs 4 to 5 manual exchanges of dialysis solution daily through a surgically implanted catheter in the home setting.

B. Continuous cycled peritoneal dialysis (CCPD) or automated peritoneal dialysis (APD).
   1. Dialysis is performed by a machine during the night in the home.
   2. The nighttime exchanges are called cycles.
   3. The cycler does a final fill in the morning before the patient is disconnected from the machine.
   4. Some patients may need to do additional manual exchanges during the day depending on the individual patient's clinical issues (Luongo & Prowant, 2009).

II. Interviewing the potential patient for peritoneal dialysis.

A. Potential candidates for peritoneal dialysis (Blake, 2012; Campbell, 2001; Diaz-Buxo, 1996; Luongo & Prowant, 2009; Singh & Kari, 2014).
   1. Patients ready to discuss dialysis options.
   2. Patients who self-select peritoneal dialysis.
   3. Patients who have uremic symptoms and must make a timely decision regarding dialysis.
   4. Hospitalized patients who must select a dialysis option before discharge. These patients may be newly diagnosed and may not have had the benefit of CKD education and disease management.
   5. Patients currently on hemodialysis and experiencing vascular access issues.
   6. Patients on hemodialysis and wishing to switch to PD.
   7. Patients with a failed transplant who must choose a dialysis modality.
   8. Patients unable to assume responsibility for self-dialysis and are cared for by a spouse, family member, or caretaker.
   9. Infants and very young children.
   10. Patients with severe cardiac disease.
   11. Patients who desire to travel frequently.

B. The interview process (Babcock & Miller, 1994; Luongo & Kennedy, 2004; Luongo & Prowant, 2009; Redman, 2004) (see Figure 5.3).
   1. The goals of the interview.
      a. Provide the patient and family with information about peritoneal dialysis.
      b. Assess the patient's readiness to assume self-care responsibility.
      c. Provide a supportive environment.
      d. Identify the unique needs of each patient.
      e. Identify the individual patient needs with other members of the healthcare team.
   2. Prerequisites for the PD nurse interviewer.
      a. Knowledge of physical assessment.
      b. Knowledge of nursing diagnosis.
      c. Knowledge of adult education principles.
      d. Documentation skills.
      e. Appreciation of cultural diversity.
      f. Ability to individualize information.
      g. Understanding of the process of chronic disease.
      h. Understanding of CKD disease management.
      i. Knowledge of principles of peritoneal dialysis.
      j. Ability to communicate effectively.
      k. Ability to coordinate participation of other members of renal healthcare team.
      l. Ability to involve family members and/or significant others as indicated.
   3. Obtaining patient medical history.
      a. Document prior medical history.
      b. Obtain physical assessment information from primary care provider.
      c. Obtain physical assessment information from nephrologists.
      d. List current medications.
      e. List other healthcare providers (e.g., surgeons, specialists, consultants, etc.).
      f. List family members and significant others.
      g. Include adherence history.
      h. Include patient's current understanding of health needs.
   4. Identify patient's cultural beliefs and needs.
      a. The individual cultural needs of the patient.
      b. The patient's ethnicity.
      c. Specific cultural issues identified by the patient.
      d. The religious beliefs of the patient and family.
      e. The primary language of the patient.
      f. Arrange for interpreter if necessary.
   5. Preparation of the interview environment.
      a. Well-ventilated room.
      b. Comfortable seating.
      c. Seating for family and significant others.
      d. Appropriate lighting.

Patient Information Sheet

Name: _____   Date: _____

Address: _____   Home Phone Number: _____

_____   Work Phone Number: _____

_____   Email Address: _____

Nephrologist: _____

Primary Care Physician: _____

Specialty Physicians: _____

_____

_____

_____

Medical/Surgical History: _____

_____

_____

_____

_____

_____

_____

Medication List:

_____

_____

_____

_____

_____

_____

_____

_____

Allergies (medications, food, others):

_____

_____

_____

Insurance Information:

Primary:

Secondary:

Medication Coverage: ____Yes   ____No

Employment: ____Full time ____Part time ____Unemployed ____Retired

Transportation: Do you drive?   ____Yes   ____No

Family/friend drives?   ____Yes   ____No

Do you use public transportation?   ____Yes   ____No

Do you use taxis?   ____Yes   ____No

Do you use assisted transportation?   ____Yes   ____No

Figure 5.3. Patient information sheet.

Source: Luongo, M., & Kennedy, S. (2004). Interviewing prospective patients for peritoneal dialysis: A five-step approach. *Nephrology Nursing Journal, 31*(5), 513-520. Used with permission.

6. The interviewing process.
   a. Introduce yourself and identify your role.
   b. Explain why the interview is necessary.
   c. Include family members but establish patient as primary focus.
   d. Monitor the response of the patient and others present.
   e. Identify sensory needs (e.g., hearing loss, visual problems, language barrier).
   f. Monitor the patient for fatigue or confusion.
   g. Ask one question at a time.
   h. Do not interrupt the patient.
   i. Restate question if patient seems confused.
   j. Use language the patient can understand.
   k. Validate the patient's fears and anxieties.
   l. Stop if the patient is overwhelmed.
   m. Use humor if appropriate.
   n. Be a good listener.
7. The nurse must be aware of warning signs or situations that may be predictive of future problems. The use of clinical judgment, previous experience, and professional expertise is extremely important.
   a. Does the patient state that he or she cannot take self-responsibility for care?
   b. Does the patient live alone without the benefit of family and friend interaction and support?
   c. Does the patient have a documented history of nonadherence to medications and/or the plan of care?
   d. Does the patient have multiple physical and tactile impairments?
   e. Does the patient need a partner to successfully do home PD?
   f. Is there an available partner who is willing to assume responsibility?
   g. Does the patient have transportation to the dialysis unit?
   h. Does the patient express unusual concern about disruption of body image?
   i. Does the patient demonstrate an unusual level of anxiety?
   j. Do you need to stop the interview?
   k. Do you need to enlist the help of the social worker, the nephrologist, or APRN (advanced practice registered nurse)?
   l. Do you need to provide additional interview time?
8. Interviewing the geriatric patient.
   a. Identify age-related changes in hearing, vision, and cognition.
   b. Schedule appointment early in day to diminish fatigue.
   c. May need an additional interview appointment.
   d. Provide quiet, uninterrupted environment.

e. Sit directly in front of patient to facilitate hearing.
f. Ask one question at a time. Repeat if necessary.
g. Refocus the patient when necessary.
h. Involve family in the process.
i. Be patient.
9. The patient with language barriers.
   a. Use a professional interpreter to ensure accurate communications.
   b. Instruct interpreter to translate information and response exactly as stated.
   c. The use of a family member may be uncomfortable for patient in regard to confidentiality and cultural beliefs.
   d. Family members may interject their own biases.
   e. Use of interpreter will lengthen the time of the interview.
10. The patient with a hearing impairment.
    a. Sit directly in front of patient so the patient has a clear view of your lips and facial expressions.
    b. Speak slowly.
    c. Frequently repeat information and questions.
    d. Provide written information.
11. The patient with a visual impairment.
    a. Patient may be light sensitive.
    b. Adjust lighting to avoid glare; dim lights; close shades.
    c. Written information must be in large print on nonglossy paper.
12. The unusually anxious patient.
    a. Stop the interview if necessary.
    b. Open the door to the interview room.
    c. Offer the patient some refreshments.
    d. Reschedule if necessary.
    e. Discuss anxiety with the patient's nephrologist or APRN.
    f. Enlist the help of family members if necessary.
    g. Enlist the help of a home PD patient to provide a patient-to-patient experience if appropriate.
13. Documentation of the interview.
    a. Share results with other members of healthcare team.
    b. Develop specific interview forms if appropriate.
    c. Document specifics of interview and recommendation.
    d. Place documentation in patient's medical record.

III. Individualized patient training for the PD program.

A. Training for the PD patient should be planned to meet the patient's individual needs.
   1. Family members and/or significant others may be included to provide support for the patient (Bernardini, Price, & Figueiredo, 2006; Hall et al., 2004; Luongo & Prowant, 2009).
   2. The length of the training session should be based on the patient's ability to concentrate without feeling overwhelmed and anxious.
   3. The PD nurse not only provides the training experience, but also evaluates the patient's progress and readiness to assume responsibility for home dialysis performance (Luongo & Prowant, 2009; Prowant, 2001).

B. Review adult learner principles. (See Module 2, Chapter 3.)

C. Possible locations for training.
   1. Peritoneal dialysis unit training room.
   2. Hospital setting for hospitalized patient.
   3. Patient's home.

D. Length of training session.
   1. Determined by the patient's attention span, current uremic symptoms, and ability to process information.
   2. Influenced by transportation issues and family participation.
   3. The need for an interpreter will usually increase the time needed for training (Bernardini, Price, & Figueiredo, 2006).

E. Number of training sessions.
   1. Depends on the patient's ability to learn and feel comfortable with home PD procedures.
   2. Limited by reimbursement. The PD nurse must be aware of the possible restrictions and guidelines.

F. Content of training sessions. The content must be individualized for each patient. The PD nurse must be very careful in presenting information that the patient can assimilate without being overwhelmed by technical terminology and/or the amount of the information. Topics include (Bernardini, Price, & Figueiredo, 2006; Luongo & Prowant, 2009):
   1. Basic explanation of kidney function.
   2. Theory of how PD works as a kidney replacement therapy.
   3. Aseptic technique.
   4. Weight and blood pressure measurement.
   5. Setup of the home environment for an exchange.
   6. Performing a CAPD exchange. This involves multiple demonstrations by the PD nurse and return demonstrations by the patient and/or family.
   7. Addition of medications to the dialysis solution bags.
   8. Techniques for warming the dialysis solution bags using dry heat.
      a. Moist heat must be avoided due to the danger of waterborne organisms.
      b. Use of the microwave to warm the solution

bags must be avoided due to the danger of:
(1) Thermal burns.
(2) Leaching of plastics into solution creating possible chemical irritation to the peritoneal membrane.
9. Proper hand-washing techniques.
a. The proper use of antibacterial soap.
b. The use of waterless hand cleaners if antibacterial soap and water are not available.
10. Proper use of a face mask.
a. During exchange procedure.
b. When adding medications to the dialysis solution bags.
c. When performing exit-site care.
11. Problem solving in the home, including:
a. Obstruction to flow of dialysis solution.
b. Recognition of change in color of effluent.
c. Presence of fibrin in effluent and appropriate use of heparin.
d. Accidental disconnections.
(1) How to clamp the catheter.
(2) Report the event to PD nurse immediately.
e. Recognition of a tear or hole in catheter.
(1) How to clamp the catheter.
(2) Report the event to PD nurse immediately.
f. How to report a fall or tugging of catheter that may or may not result in tissue trauma (Khanna & Krediet, 2009).
12. Recognition of the signs and symptoms of peritonitis and seeking appropriate treatment, including (Khanna & Krediet, 2009):
a. Cloudy effluent.
b. Abdominal pain.
c. Fever, chills.
d. Nausea, vomiting, diarrhea.
13. Fluid balance.
a. Recognition of the signs and symptoms of hypovolemia and hypervolemia.
b. Specific instructions and guidelines for fluid balance management.
14. The importance of monitoring and recording:
a. Daily weight.
b. Frequency of exchanges, dextrose percentage, and amount of fluid infused and drained.
c. Daily blood pressure if able.
15. Guidelines concerning weight, blood pressure, and the appropriate use of the different dextrose concentrations.
16. Formulation of an acceptable daily dialysis routine by the PD nurse and the patient. This routine plan is based on the individual dialysis needs and lifestyle of the patient. Consideration is given to:
a. Social and family support systems.
b. Family members who live with the patient and their involvement in daily care.
c. Plan for routine, low impact exercise if able.

d. Employment status.
e. Student status.
17. A daily hygiene plan that includes:
a. Reminders about frequent hand washing and use of face mask.
b. Daily showers if able to stand or sit in shower stall.
c. Use of antibacterial soap.
d. Cleansing of exit site per facility protocol, inspecting the catheter, and appropriately securing the catheter to prevent trauma to the exit site.
e. Applying antibacterial cream to exit site as ordered.
18. Recognition of the signs and symptoms of an exit-site infection.
a. How to seek appropriate intervention.
b. Potential signs and symptoms include fever, erythema, pain, and tenderness at the exit site or along the catheter tunnel.
19. Reproductive and sexual concerns.
20. Individualized plan to prevent constipation.
21. Medication review to include medication's name, purpose, schedule, route of administration, precautions, and potential side effects.
22. Storage of supplies, maintenance of the home inventory, and ordering additional supplies.
23. How to contact nephrologist, APRN, or PD nurse by telephone and/or email.
24. Identification of emergency situations and how to seek emergency help.
25. Consultation with the social worker.
26. Consultation with the dietitian.
27. Copy of the unit's specific training manual for home reference.
28. Copies of forms for medical records at home.
29. Routine assessment of adequate dialysis that includes:
a. Determination of membrane characteristics.
b. Periodic dialysate collection for Kt/V assessment.

G. Home dialysis is initiated when the patient and the PD nurse mutually agree that the patient is ready for the responsibility.

IV. Initiation of peritoneal dialysis in the home.

A. Prerequisites for home dialysis initiation (Farina, 2001; Luongo & Prowant, 2009; Prowant, 2001). See Table 5.3 for advantages and limitations of home visits.
1. Patient has completed home training program.
2. Patient agrees to home visit.
3. Supplies are ordered and in place in the home.
4. Appropriate orders written by the nephrologist or APRN.

Table 5.3

Advantages and Limitations of Home Visits

Advantages	Limitations
• Assessment of home environment	• Time-consuming process
• Observation and correction of potential or real hazards	• Staffing issues
• Assessment of supplies, equipment, and medicines	• Costly
• Evaluation of procedures demonstrated during PD training	• Some environments cannot be changed
• Reinforcing the patient as an active partner as a healthcare team member	• Potentially dangerous environment for the visitor
• Enables patient and family to discuss concerns and issues specific to the home setting	
• Observation of family adaptation skills and burnout	
• Reinforce patient's confidence in the dialysis unit by providing support and encouragement of self-care behaviors	
• Assessment for the need to provide services to accommodate the home for a patient with a disability	
• Assessment of motivation and adaptation skills	
• Assessment of compliance	
• Initiation and reinforcement of patient education	

Source: Farina, J. (2001). Peritoneal dialysis: A case for home visits. *Nephrology Nursing Journal, 28*(4), 423-428. Used with permission.

5. PD nurse arranges home visit.
6. Family members and significant others involved as appropriate.

B. Components of the home visit (Farina, 2001; Luongo & Prowant, 2009) (see Figure 5.4 for interview guide).
   1. A home visit may be done prior to training program.
   2. A home visit may be done on the first day of home dialysis or other designated alternative day.
   3. Consideration is given to where the patient lives (e.g., an apartment, a home that is owned, a home that is rented, a foster home, a skilled nursing facility, a shelter, or the patient may be homeless).
   4. Who else lives in the home?
   5. Is there running water and electricity?
   6. Infection control issues are considered.
      a. Are there adequate facilities for hand washing? Review hand-washing technique.
      b. Where will patient do exchanges? Is there a clean surface area? Is the area away from open windows, blowing fans, air conditioners, or heating vents?
      c. Are there pets in the home? If so, is the pet removed from the site of the dialysis exchange?
      d. Dialysis solution bags warmed by dry heat mechanism.
   7. Safety issues are considered (e.g., storage of syringes and medications safely out of the reach of small children).
   8. Consideration is given to supplies.

   a. Initial supplies are unpacked by patient and/or PD nurse.
   b. Initial supplies are inventoried and appropriately organized.
   c. Is there adequate storage space?
   d. Are supplies safely stored in a dry, clean, climate-controlled area?
   e. How frequently will the patient need delivery of supplies; e.g., every 2 weeks, every 4 weeks?
   f. Who will contact the vendor for supplies – the staff of the PD unit or the patient?
   9. The first exchange is prepared by and performed by patient under the supervision of the PD nurse.
   10. Family member or significant other may be present and participating.
   11. Documentation of exchanges by patient is reviewed and reinforced.
   12. The PD nurse and patient review:
      a. Patient's individualized daily dialysis routine.
      b. The written training manual with particular attention given to problem solving and troubleshooting in the home.
      c. Emergency contact numbers (include the family members or significant others).
      d. Home environment including the possible need for changes to ensure a safe dialysis environment.
      e. Medications supply and schedule with the patient if necessary.
      f. Administration, storage, and documentation of erythropoiesis-stimulating agents (ESAs) in the

Interview Worksheet Guidelines (Page 1 of 2)

Social History

Patient age:

Marital Status: ☐ Single   ☐ Married   ☐ Divorced   ☐ Widow/Widowed

Is the patient employed?   ☐ No   ☐ Yes If yes, ☐ Full time ☐ Part time

　　Occupation:

Is the patient retired?   ☐ Yes   ☐ No

Is the patient disabled?   ☐ Yes   ☐ No

Does the patient live: ☐ Alone   ☐ With spouse ☐ With significant other

　　With significant others: If yes, with whom? _____

Does the patient have children?   ☐ No ☐ Yes If yes, how many?_____

Does the patient have extended family?   ☐ No ☐ Yes If yes, who? _____

Are family members/friends involved in the patient's life?   ☐ No ☐ Yes If yes, who?_____

What are the patient's usual daily activities? _____

What are the patient's special interests or hobbies? _____

Does the patient travel nationally or internationally?   ☐ No ☐ Yes If yes, where? _____

Home Environment

Where does the patient live?   ☐ Apartment   ☐ Home-rented   ☐ Home-owned

　　　　　　　　　　　　　☐ Foster home   ☐ Skilled nursing facility   ☐ Homeless

Where will the patient do exchanges? _____ Is there sufficient privacy? ☐ Yes   ☐ No

How many individuals live in the household? _____

Is there running water?   ☐ Yes   ☐ No   Electricity? ☐ Yes ☐ No

Where will supplies be stored? _____

Are there pets in the household?   ☐ Yes   ☐ No

Language/Education

What is the patient's primary language? _____

What is the patient's secondary language? _____

Highest grade of school completed: _____

Can the patient read English?   ☐ Yes ☐ No   Write English?   ☐ Yes ☐ No

Read another language?   ☐ Yes ☐ No   Write another language? ☐ Yes ☐ No

Physical Limitations

Visual:　　Does the patient wear glasses?   ☐ No   ☐ Yes

　　　　　Have Cataracts?   ☐ No   ☐ Yes, Left Eye ☐ Yes, Right Eye

　　　　　Have Glaucoma?   ☐ No   ☐ Yes, Left Eye ☐ Yes, Right Eye

　　　　　Is the patient legally blind?   ☐ No   ☐ Yes

Hearing:　Hard of hearing?   ☐ No   ☐ Yes

　　　　　Uses a hearing aid?   ☐ No   ☐ Yes, Left Ear ☐Yes, Right Ear

Tactile: Is the patient's sense of touch impaired?   ☐ No   ☐ Yes If yes, specifics_____

Extremities: Arm/leg impairments?   ☐ No   ☐ Yes If yes, specifics_____

　　　　　Amputations?   ☐ No   ☐ Yes If yes, specifics_____

　　　　　Paralyzed limbs?   ☐ No   ☐ Yes If yes, specifics_____

　　　　　Hand strength problems?   ☐ No   ☐ Yes If yes, specifics_____

Daily activities: ☐ Independent ☐ Needs assistance ☐ Dependent

Does the patient have a history of CVA?   ☐ No   ☐ Yes If yes, specifics_____

General Questions

　　Previous experience with CKD dialysis? _____

　　Does the patient have a family member/friend with CKD? _____

　　Is the family member/friend on hemodialysis? _____PD?_____Transplant recipient?_____

　　How does the patient handle stress? _____

　　What is the most stressful situation the patient has experienced? _____

　　How does the patient make decisions? ☐ Self directed ☐ Relies on family/spouse/other. If yes, who? _____

Financial Issues

Does the patient have: ☐ Insurance   ☐ Medicare   ☐ State assistance   ☐ Self pay

How does the patient pay for medications?   ☐ Insurance   ☐ Self pay

Chronic Kidney Disease Education

Has the patient had previous CKD education?   ☐ No   ☐ Yes If yes, by whom? _____

What does the patient recall? _____

Figure 5.4. Interview worksheet guidelines, page 1 of 2.

Interview Worksheet Guidelines (Page 2 of 2)

Kidney Replacement Therapy Education and Information
 Brief review of normal kidney function
 Brief review of diseased kidney function
 Describe symptoms of kidney failure

Hemodialysis:
 In-center hemodialysis
 Home hemodialysis
 Access placement:
  Fistula
  Graft
 Catheter
 Describe hemodialysis session
 Role of nurse and technician
 Short-term/Long-term management
 Responsibilities and participation of patient

Transplantation:
 Living-related donor
 Living, nonrelated donor
 Nonliving donor
 Medical evaluation
 Surgical evaluation
 Waiting for transplant
 Preoperative routine
 Postoperative routine
 Role of immunosuppression
 Role of medications
 Follow-up
 Usual transplant clinic routine
 Possible complications

Peritoneal Dialysis:
 Review how PD works
 Surgical evaluation
 Catheter insertion routine
 Postoperative catheter routine
 Changes in body image
 PD solution exchange demonstration
 Allow patient to handle the PD tubing/equipment
 Daily routine of PD
 Clinic visit routine including frequency
 Roles of the PD nurse, social worker, dietitian
 Prevention of infection
 Possible complications
 Outline of the events of the first month on PD, 6 months on PD, long term
 What is included in training sessions
 Emergency interventions

Self-Care Issues:
 Adherence to medications
 Communication with health care team
 Consistent follow-up care
 Attendance at appointments
 What is the patient's previous experience with self-care?

Figure 5.4. Interview worksheet guidelines, page 2 of 2.

Adapted from Bates, 1991; DeHaan, 2003; Prowant, 2001. Reprinted in Luongo, M., & Kennedy, S. (2004). Interviewing prospective patients for peritoneal dialysis: A five-step approach. *Nephrology Nursing Journal, 31*(5), 513-520. Used with permission.

home environment. (This is a requirement in some states.)

    g. Completion of home record form(s).

    h. Disposal plan for dialysate effluent and used dialysis equipment.

    i. Patient's or family member or significant other's questions and concerns.

    j. The plan for the next PD clinic visit and the frequency of phone call reporting.

    k. The plan for obtaining supplies from the vendor.

    l. Initial inventory of supplies.

    m. All questions and concerns.

13. The PD nurse and patient may complete additional exchanges together if deemed necessary.

14. The PD nurse observes the interactions of patient with family members and/or significant others and documents appropriately.

15. The PD nurse documents the activities of the home visit in the patient's medical record.

16. The PD nurse shares the patient's progress with the other members of the healthcare team.

C. Additional home visits may be needed to evaluate unexplained clinical changes, repetitive infections, and/or changes in family unit. State regulations may differ in regard to frequency of required home visits.

D. Some patients may receive home peritoneal dialysis in the nursing home or extended care facility. Careful administrative and educational planning must be implemented to provide a safe clinical environment for the patient (Farina, 2001).

1. Establish administrative liaison and contract with nursing home or extended care facility.

2. Organize dialysis supply delivery and monthly ordering.

3. Identify training objectives and curriculum with nursing home staff.

4. Provide training for nursing home staff.

5. Provide competency list for nursing home staff.

6. Organize periodic retraining of nursing home staff to ensure safe clinical skills.

7. Inspect facility prior to patient admission to sure safe patient care.

8. Provide home visits on a routine basis per referring PD Unit and state regulations.

9. Establish documentation requirements for both referring PD unit and nursing home facility.

10. Establish plan for weekly or more frequent patient follow-up.

11. Identify emergency situations with nursing home staff and appropriate communication pathway with referring PD unit.

12. Arrange for routine clinic visits for patients on PD in a nursing home.

V. Management of home peritoneal dialysis patient (Luongo & Prowant, 2009).

A. Home management.
1. PD procedures.
2. PD access.
3. PD disease management.
4. PD complications.
5. PD adequacy.

B. Provision of dialysis care follow-up.
1. The PD patient should be seen monthly or more frequently in the PD unit.
2. Specific forms for the monthly visit should be developed and include:
    a. Vital signs, weight, and blood pressure.
    b. Review of current dialysis prescription.
    c. Review and list of current medications.
    d. Assessment and review of systems.
    e. Review of home record forms.
    f. Inspection and documentation of condition of PD catheter.
    g. Review of home supply inventory.
    h. Documentation of serum blood studies.
    i. Collection and documentation of PD adequacy parameters.
    j. Documentation of current plan of care.
    k. Arrangements for next follow-up appointment with nephrologists or APRN and the PD unit.
3. Other forms.
    a. Quarterly or semiannual care plans.
    b. Transplant preparation care plans.
    c. Consent forms.
    d. Problem list.
    e. Dialysis order sheets.
    f. Assessments by social worker, dietitian, and other healthcare workers.
    g. Documentation of insurance information.
    h. Confidentiality release forms.
    i. Unit specific forms.
    j. Assessments required by CMS and individual state regulatory agencies.

VI. The roles of the home peritoneal dialysis nurse.

The role of the home PD nurse is multifaceted and may vary in different clinical settings. Included are the specific actions and competencies that the home PD nurse must use when initiating peritoneal dialysis in the home setting. These actions and competencies are not all inclusive but focus on the early education and initiation of home peritoneal dialysis (Luongo & Prowant, 2009; Marquis & Huston, 2003).

A. As a facilitator of care, the PD nurse will:
   1. Organize the interview with the patient and family.
   2. Plan home training program.
   3. Clarify plan with healthcare team.
   4. Order appropriate supplies.
   5. Plan for routine follow-up after initiation of home dialysis.
   6. Collaborate with social worker and dietitian for specific interventions.

B. As an educator, the PD nurse will (Bernardini, Price, & Figueiredo et al., 2006, Prowant, 2006, 2008):
   1. Develop the content for dialysis options and interview process.
   2. Develop the content of training sessions.
   3. Coordinate educational content with the healthcare team.
   4. Share the individualized training plan with patient and significant others.
   5. Identify patient and family learning styles.
   6. Provide safe environment for training.
   7. Assess patient's motor skills.
   8. Assist patient with step-by-step procedures and appropriate repetition.
   9. Offer feedback each session to support learning.
   10. Identify problem-solving methods with the patient.
   11. Provide written educational materials.
   12. Evaluate patient's comprehension of educational materials.
   13. Adjust plan to accommodate special needs and/or language barrier.
   14. Document patient's training accomplishments and individualized needs.
   15. Plan frequent retraining sessions as repetitive educational reinforcement.
   16. Document short-term and long-term patient outcomes.

C. As a clinician, the PD nurse will (Bernardini, Price, & Figueiredo, 2006; Bernardini, Price, Figueiredo, Riemann, & Leung, 2006; Prowant, 2006):
   1. Collaborate with the nephrologist or APRN to develop an appropriate home dialysis prescription for the patient.
   2. Evaluate the effectiveness of the prescription in regard to fluid balance, blood pressure, and dialysis adequacy.
   3. Identify risks of infection.
   4. Ensure infections are treated and establish follow-up interventions.
   5. Review medication program with patient.
   6. Evaluate patient's adherence with the dialysis regimen and medications.
   7. Delineate short-term and long-term disease management goals with patient and healthcare team.
   8. Document plan of care, patient health assessment, daily progress, and ESRD required forms.
   9. Facilitate disease management strategies.
   10. Identify peritoneal dialysis complications and intervene appropriately.
   11. Develop a relationship with the patient on PD that focuses on trust and support (Blake, 2006).
   12. Collect PD unit specific data and evaluates outcomes.

VII. Urgent-start peritoneal dialysis.

A. Introduction.
   1. The option of urgent-start peritoneal dialysis may be used for the patient with CKD stage 5 who is not a candidate for the more traditional elective transition to home peritoneal dialysis. Potential reasons for urgent-start include:
      a. Late referral for dialysis.
      b. Poor vascular access.
      c. Delay in traditional peritoneal dialysis access placement.
      d. Avoidance of central venous catheter placement for emergent HD; possible complications of infection, septicemia, and vascular injury can be prevented.
   2. Providing urgent-start peritoneal dialysis depends on the appropriate clinical environment, patient clinical assessment and management, availability of nursing support, supplies, and established procedures.
   3. The peritoneal dialysis nurse will function as the facilitator of care, clinician, and educator as expected for all patients on peritoneal dialysis. This PD nurse has the additional responsibility of providing direct dialysis care in a clinical setting several days per week.
   4. Transition to home peritoneal dialysis care will be individualized based on the patient's clinical improvement, ability to be safely trained, and acceptance of responsibility for home peritoneal dialysis (Chaudhary et al., 2011; Groenhoff et al., 2014).

B. Program components for urgent-start peritoneal dialysis (Chaudhary et al., 2011; Groenhoff et al., 2014).
   1. Education and initiation at peritoneal dialysis clinic.
      a. Emergent or immediate education for patient and family.
      b. Education may be provided in clinic or hospital setting.
      c. Reinforcement of previous education.
      d. Urgent-start plan of care developed with patient and family.
      e. Initial patient assessment completed.

2. Access placement.
   a. Laparoscopy.
   b. Interventional radiology.
   c. Surgical.
3. Clinical setting.
   a. Safe, clean environment.
   b. Reclining chair.
   c. Climate controlled.
   d. Appropriate lighting.
   e. Call button for nursing assistance.
4. Nursing staff.
   a. Must be determined by each unit.
   b. Will require additional nursing hours.
5. Urgent-start dialysis modality is determined by each unit, i.e., cycled dialysis or low volume manual exchanges.
6. Clinical management is focused on:
   a. Fluid balance and blood pressure management.
   b. Assessment including:
      (1) PD catheter exit-site healing and integrity.
      (2) Early catheter complications (leaking at site or subcutaneous, migration).
      (3) Uremic symptoms that may require intervention.
   c. Patient psychosocial adjustment to peritoneal dialysis.
7. Training/transition to home PD.
   a. Observational training by patient and family during urgent-start sessions.
   b. Initiation of home peritoneal dialysis training is determined by the patient's clinical improvement, healing of the exit site, and the patient's readiness to learn.
8. Supplies.
   a. Adequate dialysis and ancillary supplies to support patient's daily dialysis for 1 to 2 weeks of urgent peritoneal dialysis care.
   b. Appropriate storage area for supplies to support this option.
9. Policies and procedures.
   a. Separate policies and procedures are established for urgent-start peritoneal dialysis care.
   b. Documentation guidelines are created to reflect clinical, training progress, and transition to home self-care.
10. Outcome and data collection.
    a. Data collection; for example: patient's clinical improvement, catheter complications, and ease of transition to home care.
    b. Quality improvement program with interdisciplinary involvement.

C. The development and implementation of an urgent-start program is the decision that must be made by the individual peritoneal dialysis unit. Providing nurse-assisted daily dialysis for patients who are late referrals for dialysis care is dependent on appropriate staffing, safe environment, assessment, and management of clinical parameters and adequate supplies. The role of the PD nurse is crucial in providing clinically safe care for the patient in this particular pathway.

References

Ayus, J.C., Mizani, M.R., Achinger, S.G., Thadhani, R., Go, A.S., & Lee, S. (2005). Effects of short daily versus conventional hemodialysis on left ventricular hypertrophy and inflammatory markers: A prospective, controlled study. *Journal of the American Society of Nephrology, 16*, 2778-2788.

Babcock, D., & Miller, M. (1994). *Client education*. St. Louis: Mosby.

Bates, B. (1991). *A guide to physical examination*. Philadelphia: Lippincott.

Belasco, A.G., & Sesso, R., (2002). Burden and quality of life of caregivers for hemodialysis patients. *American Journal of Kidney Diseases, 39*(4), 805-812.

Bernardini, J., Price, V., & Figueiredo, A. (2006.) Peritoneal dialysis patient training. *Peritoneal Dialysis International, 26*(6), 625-632.

Bernardini, J., Price, V., Figueiredo, A., Riemann, A., & Leung, D. (2006). International survey of peritoneal dialysis training programs. *Peritoneal Dialysis International, 26*(6), 658-663.

Blagg, C.R. (1997). The history of home dialysis: A view from Seattle. *Home Hemodialysis International, 1*(1), 1-7.

Blagg, C.R., Kjellstrand, M., Ting, G., & Young, B.A. (2006). Comparison of survival between short-daily hemodialysis and conventional hemodialysis using the standardized mortality ratio. *Hemodialysis International, 10*(4), 371–374.

Blake, P. (2006). The importance of the peritoneal dialysis murse. *Peritoneal Dialysis International, 26*(6), 623-624.

Blake, P. (2012). Peritoneal dialysis and the process of modality selection. *Peritoneal Dialysis International, 33*(3), 233-241.

Bleyer, A.J., Hartman, J., Brannon, P.C., Reeves-Daniel, A., Satkol, S.G., & Russell, G. (2006). Characteristics of sudden death in hemodialysis patients. *Kidney International, 69*, 2268–2273.

Bleyer, A.J., Russell, G.B., & Satko, S.G. (1999). Sudden and cardiac death rates in hemodialysis patients. *Kidney International, 55*, 1553-1559.

Campbell, D. (2001). Client education in the nephrology setting. *Dialysis and Transplantation, 30*(9), 571-574.

Centers for Medicare and Medicaid Services (CMS). (2008, October 3). *ESRD program interpretive guidelines*, Version 1.1. Retrieved from https://www.cms.gov/Medicare/Provider-Enrollment-and-Certification/SurveyCertificationGenInfo/downloads/SCletter09-01.pdf

Centers for Medicare & Medicaid Services (CMS). (2008, April 15). Final rule. Conditions of coverage for end stage renal disease facilities. Medicare and Medicaid Programs, *Federal Register, 73*, 20370-20484. Retrieved from http://www.cms.gov/Regulations-and-Guidance/Legislation/CFCsAndCoPs/downloads/esrdfinalrule0415.pdf

Chan, C.T. (2009). Cardiovascular effects of home intensive hemodialysis. *Advanced Chronic Kidney Disease, 16*(3), 173-178.

Chaudhary, K., Sangha, H., & Khanna, R. (2011). Peritoneal dialysis first: Rationale. *Clinical Journal of the American Society of Nephrology, 6*(2), 447-456. doi: 10.2215/CJN.07920910

Czajkowski, T., Piekos, S., & Doss-McQuitty, S. (2013). First exposure to home therapy options – Where, when and how. *Nephrology Nursing Journal, 40*(1), 29-34.

Diaz-Buxo, J. (1996). Patient selection and the success of peritoneal dialysis. *Nephrology News and Issues, 3*, 7-19.

Diaz-Buxo, J.A., White, S., & Himmele, R., (2013). Frequent hemodialysis: A critical review. *Seminars in Dialysis*, 1-12.

Fagugli, R.M., Pasini, P., Pasticci, G., Cicconi, B., & Buonocristiani, U. (2006). Effects of short daily hemodialysis and extended standard hemodialysis on blood pressure and cardiac hypertrophy: A comparative study. *Journal of Nephrology, 19*(1), 77-83.

Farina, J. (2001). Peritoneal dialysis: A case for home visits. *Nephrology Nursing Journal, 28*(4), 423-428.

Foley, R.N., Gilbertson, B., Murray, T., & Collins, A. (2011). Long interdialytic interval and mortality among patients receiving hemodialysis. *New England Journal of Medicine, 365*, 1099-1107.

Fresenius Medical Care. (2014). *2008K@home user's guide, Rev D, March 14 10.* Retrieved from http://www.fmcna.com/fmcna/OperatorsManuals/operators-manuals.html

Galland, R., Traeger, J., Arkouche, W., Delawari, E., & Fouque, D., (2001). Short daily hemodialysis and nutritional status. *American Journal of Kidney Diseases, 37*(1)(Suppl. 2), s95-s98.

Glick, J.D. (2012, April 27). Stunning consequences of thrice-weekly in-center dialysis. *Medscape.* Retrieved from http://www.medscape.com/viewarticle/762480

Gomez, N. (Ed.). (2011). *Nephrology nursing scope and standards of practice* (7th ed., 159-160). Pitman, NJ: American Nephrology Nurses' Association.

Groenhoff, Delgado, E., McClernon, M., Davis, A., Malone, L., Majirsky, J., & Guest, S., (2014). Urgent-start peritoneal dialysis: Nursing aspects. *Nephrology Nursing Journal, 41*(4), 347-352.

Hall, G., Bogan, A., Dreus, S., Duffy, A., Greene, S., & Kelley, K. (2004). New directions in peritoneal dialysis training. *Nephrology Nursing Journal, 31*(2), 149-154,159-163.

Harwood, L., & Leitch R. (2006). Home dialysis therapies. In A. Molzahn & E. Butera (Eds.), *Contemporary nephrology nursing: Principles and practice* (2nd ed., pp. 605-626). Pitman, NJ: American Nephrology Nurses' Assocation.

Heidenheim, A.P., Muirhead, M., Moist, L., & Lindsay, R.M. (2003). Patient quality of life on quotidian hemodialysis. *American Journal of Kidney Diseases, 42*(Suppl. 1), 36-41.

Jaber, B.L., Collins, A.J., Finkelstein, F.O., Glickman, J.D., Hull, A.R., Kraus, M.A. … Sprys, L.A. (2009, October 29). *Daily hemodialysis (DHD) reduces the need for antihypertensive medications.* Abstract presented at American Society of Nephrology Conference.

Jaber, B.L., Lee, Y., Collins, A.J., Hull, A.R., Kraus, M.A., McCarthy, J. … Finklestein, F. (2010). Effect of daily hemodialysis on depressive symptoms and postdialysis recovery time: Interim report from the FREEDOM Study (Following rehabilitation, economics and everyday-dialysis outcome measurements). *American Journal of Kidney Diseases, 56*(3), 531-539.

Kalantar-Zadeh, K., Regidor, D.L., Kovesdy, C.P., Van Wyck, D., Bunnapradist, S., Horwich, T.B., & Fonarow, G.C. (2009). Fluid retention is associated with cardiovascular mortality in patients undergoing long-term hemodialysis. *Circulation, 119*, 671-679.

Khanna, R., & Krediet, R. (2009). *Nolph and Gokal's textbook of peritoneal dialysis* (3rd ed.). New York: Springer.

Kjellstrand, C.M., Buoncristiani, U., Ting, G., Traeger, J., Piccoli, G.B., Sibai-Galland, R., Young, B.A., & Blagg, C.R. (2008). Short daily haemodialysis: Survival in 415 patients treated for 1006 patient-years. *Nephrology Dialysis Transplantation, 23*(10), 3283-3289.

Leitch, R., Ouwendyk, M., Ferguson, E., Clement, L., Peters, K., Heidenheim, A.P., & Lindsay, R.M. (2003). Nursing issues related to patient selection, vascular access, and education in quotidian hemodialysis, *American Journal of Kidney Diseases, 42*(Suppl. 1), 5-60.

Lindsay, R.M., Heidenbaum, P.A., Nesrallah, G., Garg, A.X., & Suri, R. (and on behalf of the Daily Hemodialysis Study Group London Health Sciences Centre). (2006). Minutes to recovery after a hemodialysis session: A simple health related quality of life question that is reliable, valid and sensitive to change. *Clinical Journal of the American Society of Nephrology, 5*, 952-959.

Luongo, M., & Prowant, B.F. (2009). Peritoneal dialysis program management and organization. In R. Khanna & R. Krediet (Eds.), *Nolph and Gokal's textbook of peritoneal dialysis* (3rd ed., 335-370). New York: Springer.

Luongo, M., & Kennedy, S. (2004). Interviewing prospective patients for peritoneal dialysis: A five step approach. *Nephrology Nursing Journal, 31*(5), 513- 520.

Marquis, B., & Huston, C. (2003). *Leadership roles and management: Functions in nursing* (4th ed.). Philadelphia: Lippincott Williams & Wilkins.

McLaughlin, K., Jones, H., VanderStraeten, C., Mills, C., Visser, M., Taub, K., & Manns, B. (2008). Why do patients choose self-care dialysis? Oxford Journals. *Nephrology Dialysis Transplantation, 23*(12), 3972-3976.

Mehrabian, S., Morgan, D., Schlaeper, C., Kortas, C., & Lindsay, R.M., (2003). Equipment and water treatment considerations for the provision of quotidian home hemodialysis, *American Journal of Kidney Diseases, 42* (Suppl. 1), 66-70.

National Kidney Foundation (NKF). (2006). NKF-K/DOQI clinical practice guideline for hemodialysis adequacy: Update 2006. *American Journal of Kidney Diseases, 48*(1), S2-S90. doi: http://dx.doi.org/10.1053/j.ajkd.2006.03.051

Nesrallah, G., Suri, R., Moist, L., Kortas, C., & Lindsay, R.M. (2003). Volume control and blood pressure management in patients undergoing quotidian hemodialysis. *American Journal of Kidney Diseases, 42*(1)(Suppl. 1), S13-S17.

NxStage Medical, Inc. (2014). *Dialysate preparation primer: Chronic hemodialysis with the NxStage® PureFlow™ SL* ©2011 NxStage APM231 Rev D.

Prowant, B. (2008). Peritoneal dialysis. In C.S. Counts (Ed.), *Core curriculum for nephrology nursing* (5th ed., pp.768-851). Pitman, NJ: American Nephrology Nurses' Association.

Prowant, B.F. (2006). Determining if characteristics of peritoneal dialysis home training programs affect clinical outcomes: Not an easy task (Editorial). *Peritoneal Dialysis International, 26*(6), 643-644.

Redman, B.K. (2004). *Advances in patient education* (Chapter 3. Patient education and ethical standards, pp. 39-51). New York: Springer.

Ronco, C., Bowry, S., & Tetta, C. (2006). Dialysis patients and cardiovascular problems: Can technology help solve the complex equation? *Blood Purification, 24*, 39-45.

Scribner, B.H. (1990). A personalized history of hemodialysis. *American Journal of Kidney Disease, 15*, 215.

Sofaer, S., & Schumann, M.J. (2013, March 15). White paper, fostering successful patient and family engagement: Nursing's critical role. *Nursing Alliance for Quality Care.* Retrieved from http://www.naqc.org/WhitePaper-PatientEngagement

Shurraw, S., & Zimmerman, D. (2005). Vascular access complications in daily dialysis: A systematic review of the literature, *Minerva Urological E Nephrologia, 57*, 151-63.

Singh, A., & Kari, J. (2014). Management of CKD stages 4 and 5: Preparation for transplantation, dialysis, or conservative care. In J. Daugirdas, P. Blake, & T. Ing (Eds.), *Handbook of dialysis* (5th ed.). Philadelphia: Lippincott Williams & Wilkins.

Spanner, E., Suri, R., Heidenheim, A.P., & Lindsay, R.M. (2003). The impact of quotidian hemodialysis on nutrition. *American Journal of Kidney Diseases, 42*(1)(Suppl. 1), S30-S35.

Stack, A.G., & Martin, D.R. (2005). Association of patient autonomy with increased transplantation and survival among new dialysis patients to the US. *American Journal of Kidney Diseases, 45*(4), 730-742.

Tennankore, K., Chan, C., & Curran, S.P. (2012). Intensive home hemodialysis: Benefits and barriers, *Nature Reviews Nephrology, 8*(9). doi:10:10.1038/nrnneph 2012.145

Thomas-Hawkins, C., & Zazworsky, D. (2005). Self-management of chronic kidney disease. *American Journal of Nursing, 105*(10), 40-48.

United States Renal Data System (USRDS). (2014). *Annual data report: Atlas of end-stage renal disease in the United States.* Bethesda, MD: National Institutes of Health, National Institute of Diabetes and Digestive and Kidney Diseases.

Vaslaki, L., Major, L., Berta, K., Karatson, A., Misz, M., Pethoe, F. ... Passlick-Deetjen, J. (2005). On line hemofiltration versus haemodialysis: Stable haematocrit with less erthropoetin and improvement of other relevant blood parameters. *Blood Purification, 24*(2), 163-73.

Young, B., Chan, C., Blagg, C., Lockridge, R., Golper, T., Finkelstein, F., & Shaffer, R. (2012). How to overcome barriers and establish a successful home HD program, *Clinical Journal of the American Society of Nephrology, 7*(12), 2023-2032.

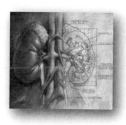

SELF-ASSESSMENT QUESTIONS FOR MODULE 3

These questions apply to all chapters in Module 3 and can be used for self-testing. They are not considered part of the official CNE process.

Chapter 1

1. Mortality rates are higher during what phase of the kidney transplant process?
   a. During preoperative desensitization.
   b. During transplant surgery.
   c. Immediately following transplantation.
   d. Peritransplantation period.

2. Immediate postoperative management of the kidney transplant recipient includes monitoring fluid and electrolyte balance by
   a. reviewing daily electrolyte levels.
   b. observing for hypotension.
   c. administering diuretics as prescribed.
   d. all of the above.

3. Discharge planning after kidney transplantation includes all of the following except
   a. the patient should resume low intensity activities as before transplant such as gardening.
   b. the patient should monitor daily weight, blood pressure, intake and output.
   c. the patient should call the transplant center for fever or decreased urine output.
   d. the patient should be able to describe name, dose, action, frequency, and side effects of medications.

4. Acute rejection may be treated with
   a. glucocorticoids and antithymocyte globulin.
   b. cyclosporine and cyclophosphamide.
   c. tacrolimus.
   d. mycophenolate mofetil.

5. Chronic causes of kidney allograft dysfunction include
   a. toxic levels of mycophenolate mofetil.
   b. T and B lymphocyte mediated rejection.
   c. calcineurin inhibitor toxicity, nephrosclerosis, and chronic obstruction.
   d. both b and c.

6. The most common form of cancer following kidney transplantation is
   a. lung cancer.
   b. colon cancer.
   c. breast cancer.
   d. squamous cell skin cancer.

7. Medication management in kidney transplant recipients with HIV is challenging because
   a. patients must take both immunosuppressive and antiretroviral medications.
   b. patients with HIV are not able to take immunosuppressive medications.
   c. patients with HIV must stop the antiretroviral medications prior to transplant.
   d. both b and c.

8. Kidney transplant recipients that are infected with hepatitis C virus create management challenges due to all of the following except
   a. difficulty in detecting acute kidney allograft rejection.
   b. difficulty in detecting progression of liver fibrosis.
   c. higher mortality risk.
   d. .higher incidence of glomerulonephritis.

Chapter 2

9. The main principle for hemodialysis solute removal is based on
   a. osmosis.
   b. diffusion.
   c. hemofiltration.
   d. convection.

10. Which hemodialysis dialyzer properties contribute the most to membrane solute clearance?
    a. Method used to obtain dialyzer sterility.
    b. Method used to prime the dialyzer.
    c. Membrane fiber thickness and pore size.
    d. Membrane fiber alignment and organization .

11. Equilibration of urea and most electrolytes occurs within
    a. 3 to 6 hours postdialysis.
    b. 30 to 60 minutes postdialysis.
    c. 24 hours postdialysis.
    d. 10 minutes postdialysis.

12. The most important component of any dialysate preparation system is
    a. the operator.
    b. the carbon tanks.
    c. the reverse osmosis membrane.
    d. the length of the distribution loop.

13. Total chlorine is removed by
    a. the reverse osmosis membrane.
    b. the carbon tanks.
    c. the deionization tanks.
    d. the distribution loop

14. In preparing acid or bicarbonate concentrates from powders, it is important that the mixing ratios "match." A mixing ratio refers to
    a. the ratio between amount of calcium and potassium.
    b. the ratio between the amount of bicarbonate and acid used to make dialysate.
    c. the ratio between the amount of water and acid used to make dialysate.
    d. the ratio between the amount of water, acid, and bicarbonate used to make dialysate.

15. Determining target weight loss prior to initiation of hemodialysis needs to include a
    a. comparison of the predialysis weight with their last postdialysis weight.
    b. comparison of their clothing attire from their last dialysis treatment.
    c. dietary recount over the past 48 hours.
    d. fluid intake over the past 48 hours.

16. The ultrafiltration rate that is thought to provide the safest upper threshold for fluid removal during hemodialysis is
    a. 15 mL/kg/hour.
    b. 17 mL/kg/hour.
    c. 10 mL/kg/hour.
    d. 6 mL/kg/hour.

17. A delayed hemolytic transfusion reaction might be detected by
    a. seizures.
    b. chills and fever
    c. a higher than expected increase in hemoglobin posttransfusion.
    d. a fall in hemoglobin below the pretransfusion level 1 to 2 weeks later.

18. The most common complications that occur during hemodialysis include all of the following except
    a. hypotension
    b. confusion .
    c. cramps.
    d. nausea and vomiting.

19. Which of the following strategies could be used to help prevent development of intradialytic hypotension?
    a. In selected patients, lower the dialysate temperature to 35°C.
    b. Give food or glucose orally about the middle of the treatment.

    c. Use only acetate containing dialysate.
    d. Instruct patient to take alpha-adrenergic agent prior to dialysis.

20. Which one is not a desired quality outcome?
    a. Achieving a serum albumin level of 3.0 g/dL by the BCP method.
    b. Achieving an intact parathyroid hormone level of 8 times upper limit of normal.
    c. Achieving a serum phosphorus level between 5 and 6 mg/dL.
    d. Achieving a normalized hemoglobin level.

21. Muscle cramps during hemodialysis may be caused by
    a. excessive or rapid fluid removal.
    b. using a higher sodium dialysate.
    c. low ultrafiltration rate.
    d. IV iron administration.

22. Methemoglobinemia may be a result of elevated copper, nitrate, and/or chloramine levels in R/O water. Signs and symptoms include
    a. bright red (cherry) colored bloodlines.
    b. back pain.
    c. seizures
    d. cyanosis.

23. Life-threatening alkalosis as a complication of hemodialysis can be prevented by
    a. reducing a patient's dietary intake of fatty and salty foods.
    b. reducing a patient's dietary intake of high biological value protein.
    c. calculating the total buffer received from the machine bicarbonate display and the acetate contained within the acid concentrate.
    d. calculating the total buffer received from the machine bicarbonate display and the concentration of glucose within the acid concentrate.

24 A potential risk to a patient who participates in a dialyzer reuse program is
    a. inadequate dialysis.
    b. air embolus.
    c. severe hypertension.
    d. hypercalcemia.

25. Hypokalemia tends to occur immediately following hemodialysis, it is most appropriate when detected to
    a. treat immediately with a potassium oral suspension.
    b. not treat unless there are extenuating circumstances.
    c. obtain a 12-lead EKG even if the patient is asymptomatic.
    d. obtain a cardiac troponin I (cTn) to determine risk for arrhythmias.

26. Pruritus that occurs in a patient receiving chronic hemodialysis is most concerning when it
    a. occurs with certain clothing.
    b. occurs during the winter months.
    c. occurs during episodes of diaphoresis .
    d. occurs only during dialysis.

Chapter 3

27. Referral for vascular access surgery should begin early, and most recommend referral when the eGFR reaches
    a. 60 mL/min/1.72 m².
    b. 90 mL/min/1.72 m².
    c. 14 mL/min/1.72 m².
    d. 30 mL/min/1.72 m².

28. If a tunneled hemodialysis catheter is unavoidable, then best practice would include which action?
    a. Use the noncuffed catheter to avoid venous and soft tissue injury.
    b. Use the smallest French diameter catheter to avoid venous injury.
    c. Limit catheter length to avoid venous injury.
    d. Limit catheter days to a minimum.

29. What time frame is usually required to obtain adequate maturity of a native vessel arteriovenous fistula?
    a. 3 to 6 months.
    b. 2 to 3 weeks.
    c. 1 month.
    d. 2 months.

30. The mean primary patency period for an AV fistula is
    a. 4 years.
    b. 9 months.
    c. 7 years.
    d. 3 years.

31. The leading pathologic cause of access infections is
    a. *Staphylococcus aureus.*
    b. *Pseudomonas.*
    c. *Enterococcus.*
    d. *Candida.*

32. Signs and symptoms of central vein stenosis include
    a. swelling of the access arm.
    b. development of collateral veins in the upper arm and chest.
    c. pain in the arm during dialysis.
    d. all of the above.

33. Which of the following suggests an anatomic problem with an arteriovenous access?
    a. Prolonged INR without anticoagulation.
    b. Prolonged bleeding after dialysis.

c. KT/V trending up.
    d. No pain with cannulation.

34. What is the difference between an aneurysm and a pseudoaneurysm?
    a. Aneurysms are always larger.
    b. A pseudoaneurysm is not contained by the vessel wall.
    c. Pseudoaneurysms pose no threat to the patient.
    d. Aneurysms are a natural progression in the maturation process.

35. The rate and degree of native vessel arteriovenous fistula maturation is enhanced by what physiologic variable?
    a. Good venous in flow and wall shear stress.
    b. Good cardiac output and wall shear stress.
    c. A low left ventricular ejection fraction.
    d. Presence of a juxta-anastamosis stenosis.

36. The AV graft is used
    a. as a first-line choice for arteriovenous access.
    b. when no autologous option exists for a native vessel fistula.
    c. as a last-resort access.
    d. as a primary site for pediatrics.

Chapter 4

37. An absolute contradiction to someone's candidacy for doing peritoneal dialysis would include which of the following?
    a. Poor visual acuity.
    b. Overweight.
    c. Reduced dexterity.
    d. Hypercatabolism.

38. All of the following events affect solute transport during peritoneal dialysis except which one?
    a. Infection of the peritoneum.
    b. Increased dietary protein.
    c. Temperature of the dialysis solution.
    d. Electrical charge.

39. Current KDOQI Clinical Practice Guidelines recommendations for adequate peritoneal dialysis (PD) include that an absolute minimum Kt/V urea over 1.7 be achieved by
    a. All patients on PD therapy regardless of the type of PD used.
    b. Patients receiving continuous ambulatory peritoneal dialysis.
    c. Patients using cycler peritoneal dialysis only in daytime.
    d. Patients using cycler peritoneal dialysis only at night.

40, Preservation of the peritoneal membrane is an important aspect of care in patients receiving peritoneal dialysis. Efforts to promote this would include (select all that apply)
   a. prevention of catheter-related infections.
   b. avoiding a KT/V that exceeds 1.7.
   c. using low-glucose degradation products (GDP).
   d. avoiding the use of the abdomen for injection of ESAs.

41. Peritoneal dialysis outflow failure is most likely caused by
   a. frequent use of lower concentration dianeal.
   b. frequent use of higher concentration dianeal.
   c. increased fibrin or constipation.
   d. increased total body water and salt.

42. Noninfectious causes of peritoneal dialysis complications with a symptom of cloudy dialysate include all of the following except which?
   a. Hemoperitoneum.
   b. Chyloperitoneum.
   c. Eosinophillia.
   d. Heparin-induced thrombocytopenia.

Chapter 5

43. What aspects of care or conditions are considered to be the most important in determining the success of an integrated home dialysis program?
   a. Patient education, support, follow-up.
   b. Assessment, patient selection, home size.
   c. Conditions of Coverage, patient selection, education.
   d. Equipment, supplies, laboratory monitoring.

44. One of the most important components to consider in developing a home dialysis educational program is
   a. Program objectives clearly stated.
   b. Training occurs on dialysis and nondialysis days.
   c. Cannulation is taught before training actually begins.
   d. Employing multiple types of teaching methods.

45. What are the major roles and responsibilities of the nurse functioning in a home dialysis program?
   a. Provide frequent assessment, education, monitoring, support, and documentation.
   b. Provide complete, accurate, and complete details of the program during the first day of training.
   c. Review laboratory data, complete care plans, and assess the patient's adaptation to the home within the first week after training.
   d. Review laboratory data, complete care plans, and assess the patient's adaptation to the home within 48 hours after training.

46. Benefits of daily home hemodialysis are
   a. no transportation required for in-center treatments.
   b. patient independence and sense of control over health and treatment.
   c. improved quality of life.
   d. improved level of comfort.
   e. all of the above.

47. A key factor in maintaining water systems for hemodialysis in the home is:
   a. Follow the manufacturer's specifications as well as state and CMS regulations for use of the water treatment system.
   b. Follow the ESRD Network's specifications as well as the city water's guidelines for water treatment.
   c. Conserve water within the home by reducing showers, baths, and washing.
   d. Conserve water within the home by reducing watering of the yard.

48. If the patient and care partner are showing signs of treatment burnout, it is important to provide
   a. respite care for both within a skilled nursing facility that provides dialysis.
   b. referral to another home training program that allows more flexibility .
   d. a time to discuss what issues are concerning the patient and care partner.
   e. all of the above.

49. When interviewing and evaluating the prospective peritoneal dialysis patient, all of the following should be considered except
   a. capacity and motivation to learn
   b. distance of home from the training facility.
   c. nutritional status and any chronic gastrointestinal issues.
   d. prior abdominal surgeries and presence of hernias.

50. Problem-solving techniques that are taught to the home peritoneal patient dialysis include
   a. what to do to correct obstruction of dialysate flow.
   b. recognizing the color and clarity of the effluent.
   c. what to do when the transfer set or catheter adapter is disconnected.
   d. all of the above.

51. When initiating home peritoneal dialysis and providing home care management, the peritoneal dialysis nurse must be able to
   a. provide appropriate education for the patient and family.
   b. coordinate the members of the health care team.
   c. establish a professional relationship with the patient and family.
   d. all of the above.7

Answer Key

Chapter 1
1. d
2. d
3. a
4. a
5. d
6. d
7. a
8. a

Chapter 2
9. b
10. c
11. b
12. a
13. b
14. d
15. a
16. c
17. d
18. b
19. a
20. d
21. a
22. d
23. c
23. c
24. a
25. b
26. d

Chapter 3
27. d
28. d
29. a
30. d
31. a.
32. d
33. b
34. b
35. b
36. b

Chapter 4
37. d
38. b
39. a
40. a & c
41. c
42. d

Chapter 5
43. a
44. d
45. a
46. e
47. a
48. d
49. b
50. d
51. d

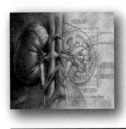

INDEX FOR MODULE 3

Page numbers followed by **f** indicate figures.
Page numbers followed by **t** indicate tables

Peritoneal sclerosis
    encapsulating
        peritoneal dialysis and, 272
Peritoneum
    blood supply to, 241
Peritonitis
    peritoneal dialysis and, 273–274
PET. *See* Peritoneal equilibration test (PET)
Phobia(s)
    needle, 189, 189t
Phoenix system, 82, 83f
Plasma refill rate
    in hemodialysis, 127–129, 127f, 128f
Pneumocystis jiroveci pneumonia
    prevention of
        after kidney transplantation in HIV-positive patient, 56
Pneumocystosis
    kidney transplantation–related, 21
Pneumonia
    Pneumocystis jiroveci
        after kidney transplantation in HIV-positive patient, 56
Pneumoperitoneum
    peritoneal dialysis and, 268
Polyclonal antibody preparation
    in kidney transplantation, 30
Potassium
    in hemodialysis concentrate, 89–90
Pregnancy
    after kidney transplantation, 21
Pseudoaneurysm
    in hemodialysis
        AVF-related, 185, 185t, 186f
        AVG-related, 202, 202f
Psychosocial issues
    kidney transplantation–related, 19
Pulmonary system
    in kidney transplant recipients
        preoperative assessment of, 12
PureFlow SL (PFSL) testing requirements
    in United States, 295t
Pyogenic reaction
    hemodialysis and, 145–146

Q

QAPI. *See* Quality Assessment Performance Improvement (QAPI)
Quality Assessment Performance Improvement (QAPI)
    activities for water and dialysate
        in hemodialysis, 113

R

Red blood cell transfusion
    adverse effects of, 120–122
    in hemodialysis, 120–122
Rejection
    kidney transplantation–related. *See* Kidney transplantation, rejection in
Renal artery thrombosis
    kidney transplantation–related, 18
Renal vein thrombosis
    kidney transplantation–related, 18
Residual kidney function (RKF)

in peritoneal dialysis adequacy, 255–258, 258t
Rituximab
    for antibody-mediated acute rejection, 31
RKF. *See* Residual kidney function (RKF)

S

Seizure(s)
    hemodialysis and, 154–155
Self-care abilities
    in chronic peritoneal dialysis assessment, 261
Sepsis
    pancreas transplantation and, 37
Simultaneous pancreas–kidney (SPK) transplantation, 31–43
    candidates for
        evaluation of, 33–34
    described, 35
    goal of, 33
    indications for, 33
    patient education after, 42t
    patient outcomes of, 41t
    rejection of
        signs and symptoms of, 38, 38t
Sodium
    in hemodialysis concentrate, 88–89
Solute removal
    in hemodialysis, 74, 74f, 76–79, 76f–79f, 78t, 79t
SPA. *See* Standard Peritoneal Permeability Analysis (SPA)
SPK transplantation. *See* Simultaneous pancreas–kidney (SPK) transplantation
Standard Peritoneal Permeability Analysis (SPA), 246
Starling's curve
    in hemodialysis, 129, 130f, 130t
Steal syndrome
    in hemodialysis
        AVF-related, 187
        AVG-related, 202–203
Stenosis
    in hemodialysis
        AVG-related, 199–201, 200f
Surveillance
    defined, 217
Swan-neck Missouri presternal peritoneal dialysis catheter, 232, 233f

T

T lymphocytes, 22
Tacrolimus
    in kidney transplantation, 28–29, 28t
Thrombocytopenia
    heparin-induced
        peritoneal dialysis and, 272
Thrombosis(es)
    in hemodialysis
        AVF-related, 183–185
        AVG-related, 201–202
    renal artery
        kidney transplantation–related, 18
    renal vein
        kidney transplantation–related, 18

Tidal dialysis, 255
Toxoplasmosis
    after kidney transplantation in HIV-positive patient
        prevention of, 56
Transfusion(s)
    adverse effects of, 120–122
    red blood cell
        in hemodialysis, 120–122
Transplantation, 1–68. *See also specific types*
    in chronic peritoneal dialysis patients, 266
    heart
        chronic kidney disease after, 47–51. *See also* Chronic kidney disease, after heart transplantation
    islet cell, 42–43
    kidney, 2–31. *See also* Kidney transplantation
    lung
        chronic kidney disease in, 51–52
    pancreas, 31–42. *See also* Pancreas transplantation
    SPK, 31–43. *See also* Simultaneous pancreas–kidney (SPK) transplantation
Tubular necrosis
    acute
        kidney transplantation–related, 18–19
Tunnel infection
    CVCs-related, 210, 211f
Tunnel infections
    peritoneal dialysis and, 239–240

U

Ultrafiltration
    in fluid removal in hemodialysis, 80–82, 81f, 81t, 82f
    reverse
        in dialyzer reprocessing, 159
Ultrafiltration profile
    in hemodialysis, 85–86, 86f
United Network for Organ Sharing (UNOS)
    in kidney transplantation, 7–8
UNOS. *See* United Network for Organ Sharing (UNOS)
Urea kinetic modeling
    in hemodialysis, 94–100, 95f, 98f, 100f
        application of, 95–97
        background of, 94–95, 95f
        indications for, 97–99, 98f
        integrative component of, 99–100, 100f
        Kt/V in, 97–99, 99f
        limitations of, 100
        rationale for, 94–95, 95f
        treatment parameters related to, 97
        URR calculation in, 100
Urea reduction rate (URR)
    in hemodialysis, 100
Urgent-start peritoneal dialysis
    in home, 307–308
Urinary tract
    in kidney transplant recipients
        preoperative assessment of, 10–11
Urinary tract infection (UTI)